Immunoglobulins

Comprehensive Immunology

Series Editors: ROBERT A. GOOD and STACEY B. DAY

Sloan-Kettering Institute for Cancer Research
New York, New York

1 Immunology and Aging
Edited by TAKASHI MAKINODAN and EDMOND YUNIS

2 Biological Amplification Systems in Immunology
Edited by NOORBIBI K. DAY and ROBERT A. GOOD

3 Immunopharmacology
Edited by JOHN W. HADDEN, RONALD G. COFFEY, and FEDERICO SPREAFICO

4 The Immunopathology of Lymphoreticular Neoplasms
Edited by J. J. TWOMEY and ROBERT A. GOOD

5 Immunoglobulins
Edited by GARY W. LITMAN and ROBERT A. GOOD

Immunoglobulins

Edited by

GARY W. LITMAN, Ph.D.

Sloan-Kettering Institute for Cancer Research
Rye, New York

and

ROBERT A. GOOD, Ph.D., M.D.

Sloan-Kettering Institute for Cancer Research
New York, New York

PLENUM MEDICAL BOOK COMPANY
New York and London

Library of Congress Cataloging in Publication Data

Main entry under title:

Immunoglobulins.

(Comprehensive immunology; v. 5)
Includes bibliographies and index.
1. Immunoglobulins. I. Litman, Gary W. II. Good, Robert A., 1922-   III. Series.
[DNLM: 1. Immunoglobulins. W1 CO4523 v. 5/QW601 I33]
QR186.7.I45   599'.02'9   78-1439
ISBN-13: 978-1-4684-0807-2   e-ISBN-13: 978-1-4684-0805-8
DOI: 10.1007/978-1-4684-0805-8

Contributors

Silvio Barandun   Institute for Clinical and Experimental Cancer Research, University of Berne, Tiefenau-Hospital, Berne, Switzerland

J. Donald Capra   Department of Microbiology, University of Texas Health Science Center at Dallas, Southwestern Medical School, Dallas, Texas 75235

Renata E. Cathou   Department of Biochemistry and Pharmacology, Tufts University School of Medicine, Boston, Massachusetts 02111

Yong Sung Choi of Memorial Sloan-Kettering Cancer Center, New York, New York 10021

Charlotte Cunningham-Rundles   Memorial Sloan-Kettering Cancer Center, New York, New York 10021

Ø. Førre   Institute of Immunology and Rheumatology, Rikshospitalet University Hospital, Oslo, Norway

Blas Frangione   Department of Pathology, Irvington House Institute, New York University Medical Center, New York, New York 10016

Fred Karush   Department of Microbiology, University of Pennsylvania School of Medicine, Philadelphia, Pennsylvania 19104

J. Michael Kehoe   Department of Microbiology/Immunology, The Northeastern Ohio Universities College of Medicine, Rootstown, Ohio 44272

William H. Konigsberg   Department of Molecular Biophysics and Biochemistry and of Human Genetics, Yale University, New Haven, Connecticut 06510

Gary W. Litman   Memorial Sloan-Kettering Cancer Center, New York, New York 10021

T. E. Michaelsen   Institute of Immunology and Rheumatology, Rikshospitalet University Hospital, Oslo, Norway

Andreas Morell   Institute for Clinical and Experimental Cancer Research, University of Berne, Tiefenau-Hospital, Berne, Switzerland

J. B. Natvig   Institute of Immunology and Rheumatology, Rikshospitalet University Hospital, Oslo, Norway

Susumu Ohno   Department of Biology, City of Hope National Medical Center, Duarte, California 91010

Benvenuto Pernis   Departments of Microbiology and Medicine, College of Physicians and Surgeons of Columbia University, New York, New York 10032

Roberto J. Poljak   Department of Biophysics, Johns Hopkins University School of Medicine, Baltimore, Maryland 21205

Frank F. Richards   Department of Medicine, Yale University School of Medicine, New Haven, Connecticut 06510

Robert W. Rosenstein   Department of Medicine, Yale University School of Medicine, New Haven, Connecticut 06510

Janos M. Varga   Department of Dermatology, Yale University School of Medicine, New Haven, Connecticut 06510

An-Chuan Wang   Department of Basic and Clinical Immunology and Microbiology, Medical University of South Carolina, Charleston, South Carolina 29401

Horace H. Zinneman   Department of Medicine, Veterans Administration Hospital and University of Minnesota Medical School, Minneapolis, Minnesota 55417

Foreword

Since the discovery more than thirty years ago that antibody activity could be localized to discrete plasma protein fractions, the study of immunoglobulin structure and function has dominated the field of immunochemistry. During this time, sources of homogeneous immunoglobulin molecules have been discovered, the subunit nature of the proteins has been defined, and the three-dimensional structures of the antigen-recognition portion of several antibody molecules have been elucidated. Insights into the complicated genetic control of these proteins are being gained rapidly through analysis of amino acid sequences of naturally occurring and induced homogeneous immunoglobulins. Immunoglobulins have been analyzed by protein chemists as models of complex multimeric systems, examined by geneticists studying serum protein polymorphisms, and employed by molecular biologists as highly selective probes capable of distinguishing minor features of molecular topography. Clinical applications have ranged from the now routine quantitation of immunoglobulin levels to the use of antibodies to detect trace levels of a variety of natural products and drug metabolites. All these applications have depended ultimately on a thorough understanding of the immunoglobulin and its antigen-combining site.

To cover the entire field of immunoglobulin structure and function would require many volumes this size; therefore, subjects presented in this volume represent those which we felt contribute most to our current understanding of this protein family. The first chapters deal with the structure and function of the immunoglobulin molecule. The next group of chapters deals with various aspects of the genetic control of immunoglobulin synthesis, including the evolutionary origins of the immunoglobulins. Additional chapters deal with abnormalities in immunoglobulin structure, the synthesis and secretion of immunoglobulin, and the nature of cell-surface immunoglobulin. Other, related topics will be developed in subsequent volumes of this series devoted to molecular immunology. As can be expected for a multiauthored work, the content of the individual chapters reflects the viewpoint and concern of the authors. While the contributions vary in length and scope, authors, where indicated, have provided references to recent comprehensive reviews to correct apparent deficiencies.

It is our sincere hope that this volume will provide both a background and a source of direction for investigators concerned with the structure, function, and genetic control of immunoglobulins and the role of antibody in host defense.

Gary W. Litman
Robert A. Good

Contents

Chapter 1

Studies on the Three-Dimensional Structure of Immunoglobulins 1

    Roberto J. Poljak

  1. Introduction   1
  2. X-Ray Crystallographic Techniques   5
  3. Immunoglobulins and Fc Fragments   9
  4. Three-Dimensional Structure of Light Chains   10
  5. Fab Fragments   12
  6. Antibody Combining Sites   21
  7. Structure of Fab–Hapten Complexes   23
  8. Structure and Genetic Control of V_L and V_H Regions   26
  9. Conclusions   29
 10. Note Added in Proof   30
     References   31

Chapter 2

Solution Conformation and Segmental Flexibility of Immunoglobulins 37

    Renata E. Cathou

  1. Introduction   37
  2. Immunoglobulin G   39
  3. Immunoglobulin M   56
  4. Immunoglobulin A   67
  5. Immunoglobulin D   70
  6. Immunoglobulin E   72
  7. Concluding Remarks   76
     References   76

Chapter 3

The Affinity of Antibody: Range, Variability, and the Role of Multivalence   85

> *Fred Karush*

1. Introduction   85
2. Affinity for Monovalent Ligands   88
3. Role of Multivalence   104
4. Structural Analysis of Combining Sites   112
5. Closing Statement   113
   References   113

Chapter 4

Antibody Combining Regions   117

> *Frank F. Richards, Robert W. Rosenstein, Janos M. Varga, and William H. Konigsberg*

1. Background   117
2. Structural Properties of Antibody Combining Regions   122
3. Structural and Functional Correlates of Antigen-Binding   135
4. Biological Significance of Antigen-Binding   142
5. Summary   147
   References   148

Chapter 5

The Secretory Component and the J Chain   155

> *Charlotte Cunningham-Rundles*

1. Introduction   155
2. The Secretory Component   155
3. The J Chain   162
   References   169

Chapter 6

The Structural Basis for the Biological Properties of Immunoglobulins   173

> *J. Michael Kehoe*

1. Introduction   173
2. Nature of Immunoglobulin Biological Properties   173
3. Submolecular Localization of Immunoglobulin Biological Properties   186
4. Summary and Conclusions   192
   References   192

Chapter 7

The Significance of Gene Duplication in Immunoglobulin Evolution (Epimethean Natural Selection and Promethean Evolution) 197

Susumu Ohno

1. Introduction   197
2. Epimethean Nature of Evolution by Natural Selection   199
3. Why the Promethean Evolution of the Immune System?   200
4. Strategy of Promethean Evolution   201
5. Conclusions   203
   References   204

Chapter 8

The Phylogenetic Origins of Immunoglobulin Structure   205

Gary W. Litman and J. Michael Kehoe

1. Introduction   205
2. Invertebrate Humoral Immunity—Agglutinins   206
3. Immunoglobulins of Ostracoderm-Derived Vertebrates   208
4. Immunoglobulins of Placoderm-Derived Vertebrates   209
5. Conformation and Active Sites   214
6. Proteolytic Cleavage Products of Immunoglobulins from Lower Species   217
7. Primary Structure   217
8. Cell-Surface Immunoglobulin and Immunoglobulin-Related Structure(s)   219
9. Summary and Conclusions   223
   References   224

Chapter 9

Evidence for and the Significance of 'Two Genes, One Polypeptide Chain'   229

An-Chuan Wang

1. Basic Immunoglobulin Units   229
2. History   229
3. Allotypes of Rabbit Heavy-Chain Variable Regions   230
4. Sharing of a Single Constant Region by Variable Regions   231
5. Sharing of a Single Variable Region by Constant Regions   232
6. Reciprocal Sharing of Variable and Constant Regions in Heavy Chains   233
7. DNA–RNA Hybridization   234
8. Fusion of the Variable and Constant Regions   235
9. Three Linkage Groups   241

10. More Than Two Genes for One Polypeptide Chain?   242
11. Specific Gene Activation and Differential Gene Expression   243
12. Genetic Switch   245
13. Summary   246
    References   247

Chapter 10

Structure of Atypical Immunoglobulins—Relationship to Genetic Control Mechanisms   257

Blas Frangione

1. Introduction   257
2. Heavy-Chain Variants: Heavy-Chain-Disease Proteins   258
3. Myelomas with Altered Heavy Chains   263
4. Myelomas with Altered Light Chains   265
5. Hybrid Molecules   266
6. Nonsecretors   267
7. Discussion   267
   References   269

Chapter 11

Patterns of Sequence Variability in Immunoglobulin Variable Regions: Functional, Evolutionary, and Genetic Implications   273

J. Michael Kehoe and J. Donald Capra

1. Introduction   273
2. Variable Regions Defined: Molecular Limits and Phylogenetic Occurrence   274
3. Variable Region–Constant Region Transition   276
4. Subgroups Defined and Their Distribution in Phylogeny   277
5. Phylogenetically Associated Residues   280
6. Nature of Idiotypy and Its Relationship to Hypervariable Regions and the Antibody Combining Site   281
7. Genetic Origin of Variable-Region Sequence Diversity   284
8. Conclusions   291
   References   291

Chapter 12

Genetic Control of Immunoglobulin Synthesis in Man   297

Andreas Morell and Silvio Barandun

1. Introduction   297
2. Evidence for Genetic Control of Antibody Synthesis in Experimental Animals   298

3. Evidence for Genetic Control of Immunoglobulin Synthesis in Man   300
   References   308

Chapter 13

Heavy-Chain Variable (V_H) Subgroups among Myeloma Proteins, Antibodies, and Membrane Immunoglobulins of Lymphocytes   311

J. B. Natvig, Ø. Førre, and T. E. Michaelsen

1. Introduction   311
2. Anti-V_H-Subgroup Antisera   312
3. Comparison of V_H Subgroups of the Same Proteins Determined Serologically and by Amino Acid Sequence Analysis   313
4. Serologically Determined V_H Subgroups in Myeloma Proteins with Previously Unknown V_H Subgroups   314
5. Relative Amounts of the V_H Subgroups in Different Human Sera   316
6. Restriction of Immune and Natural Human Antibodies for V_H Subgroups   316
7. V_H Subgroups of Membrane Immunoglobulin of Normal Human Lymphocytes   317
8. V_H Subgroups of Membrane Immunoglobulin of Chronic Lymphocytic Leukemia Cells   317
9. Comments   319
   References   320

Chapter 14

Cryoglobulins and Pyroglobulins   323

Horace H. Zinneman

1. Cryoglobulins   323
2. Pyroglobulins   335
   References   338

Chapter 15

Biosynthesis and Secretion of Immunoglobulins   345

Yong Sung Choi

1. Introduction   345
2. Methods   345
3. Synthesis of Light and Heavy Polypeptide Chains   346
4. Assembly of Immunoglobulin Molecules   347
5. Secretion of Immunoglobulins   348
6. Differentiation of B Lymphocytes   351
   References   353

Chapter 16

Lymphocyte Membrane Immunoglobulins: An Overview   357
Benvenuto Pernis

1. Introduction   357
2. Basic Data on Membrane Immunoglobulins   358
3. Cells That Carry Actively Synthesized Membrane Immunoglobulins   360
4. Membrane Immunoglobulin Idiotypes, Allotypes, and Isotypes   361
5. Effects of the Interaction between Membrane Immunoglobulins and
   Antiimmunoglobulin Antibodies   365
   References   369

Immunoglobulins

1

Studies on the Three-Dimensional Structure of Immunoglobulins

ROBERTO J. POLJAK

1. Introduction

One of the central problems in immunochemistry is that of defining the structural basis for the activity, specificity, and physiological function of antibody molecules. Although several experimental approaches such as amino acid sequence determination and affinity labeling have provided important clues to the solution of this problem, it is generally accepted that X-ray crystallographic analysis is the only technique currently available to reveal the complete three-dimensional structure of proteins. In recent years, several laboratories have succeeded in obtaining atomic-resolution models of immunoglobulins (Ig's) by X-ray diffraction methods. A review of the major conclusions achieved in these studies is the aim of this chapter.

A brief introduction to the polypeptide chain structure of Ig's will be presented first. The reader is referred to other chapters in this volume for a detailed discussion of this topic.

The study of Ig's is greatly facilitated by the occurrence of homogeneous pathological Ig's produced by monoclonal neoplastic lymphocytic cells in mice and in humans. These myeloma proteins, associated with the spontaneous occurrence of multiple myelomatosis and other pathological lymphoproliferative disorders in man and with experimentally induced tumors in mice, have been shown to be closely related to normal Ig's and antibodies by a number of structural and functional properties. Myeloma proteins can be obtained in large quantities and can be readily purified to homogeneous molecular species, thus providing suitable material for detailed structural studies. In general, these myeloma proteins can be isolated as complete molecules, but sometimes only a portion of the molecule is

ROBERTO J. POLJAK • Department of Biophysics, Johns Hopkins University School of Medicine, Baltimore, Maryland 21205.

present, most frequently the "light (L) chain" of the polypeptide structure (see below). Bence Jones proteins are L chains (isolated from urine) that display a peculiar thermal behavior: they precipitate at 40–60°C, redissolve at 95–100°C, and reprecipitate on cooling.* Ig's can be divided into major classes or isotypes called IgM (macroglobulins, mol. wt. approximately 900,000), IgA (mol. wt. approximately 170,000–500,000), IgG (mol. wt. approximately 150,000), and IgD and IgE (mol. wt. approximately 180,000). In the serum of normal individuals, IgM, IgA, and IgG are found to constitute approximately 5–10, 10–20, and 70–80%, respectively, of the total circulating Ig. These three classes contain carbohydrates that range from 2–3% of the total weight for IgG to about 10–12% for IgA and IgM. The covalently attached carbohydrates are largely hexose and hexosamine with smaller amounts of sialic acid and fucose. IgD and IgE are quantitatively minor components.

The IgG class of Ig's has been the most intensively studied. A diagrammatic structure of a human IgG molecule is shown in Figure 1. The molecule consists of two identical L polypeptide chains (mol. wt. 20,000–25,000) and two identical "heavy" (H) polypeptide chains (mol. wt. 50,000–55,000), which are linked by interchain disulfide bonds to form a covalent arrangement of four chains. Noncovalent interactions between the H and the L chains require the use of drastic conditions (e.g., acid pH, urea) for the separation of this structure into individual polypeptide chain components after reduction of the interchain disulfide bonds. The L chains of human IgG can be antigenically classified into two classes called κ and λ, each characterized by unique sequences in their C-terminal regions. Human IgM, IgA, IgD, and IgE also include the same type of L chain (κ or λ), but their H chains are different and are specific to each class.

A major finding in the determination of the multichain structure of IgG was made by Porter (1959), who found that controlled enzymatic digestion of rabbit IgG produces two kinds of fragments, Fab (antigen-binding) and Fc (constant). The Fab fragment (Figure 1, mol. wt. 50,000) retains the antibody activity of the parent molecule, except that it can behave only as a monovalent antibody. No complement-fixation activity can be observed in the immune Fab–antigen complex, indicating that the Fc region is required for complement fixation. Controlled digestion of a human or rabbit IgG protein by pepsin produces a major fragment called F(ab')$_2$ (Nisonoff *et al.*, 1960). By reduction and alkylation of the inter-H-chain disulfide bond(s), the Fab' fragment (Figure 1) is readily obtained. Fab and Fab' consist of a complete L chain and a piece (called Fd or Fd', respectively) that is the N-terminal half of the H chain. Human Fd' is about ten amino acid residues longer than Fd. Similar Fab fragments have been obtained by the use of other proteolytic enzymes such as trypsin. All these proteolytic enzymes split peptide bonds in a region that appears openly accessible and that has been called the "hinge" region ("flexibly") connecting Fab and Fc.

Amino acid sequence studies of the L- and H-chain components of Ig's have shown that these chains possess unique structural features. When the first human myeloma L chains were sequenced, it became clear that L chains of the same class (κ or λ) consist of a C-terminal half of constant amino acid sequence and an N-terminal half of variable sequence. Because of the possible genetic implications, the

*See Humphrey and Owens (1972) for a detailed review of plasma cell dyscrasias and pathological Ig's.

patterns of variability of L-chain sequences have been extensively analyzed. Thus, it has been observed that within a given class of L chains, there are sequences that are very similar and can be included in one "subgroup." Three subgroups have been recognized in human κ chains and at least four in human λ chains. All chains within a subgroup are very similar in sequence except at certain positions where a pattern of extreme variability is observed (Wu and Kabat, 1970). It is believed that these hypervariable sequences constitute the regions of the L-chain structure that come in contact with antigen, so that the presence of different sequences is correlated with the occurrence of different antibody specificities. Studies on H chains have shown that the region of constant sequence extends to about three quarters of the length of the chain beginning at the C-terminus. As in the case of the L chains, the region of variable sequence occurs toward the N-terminus of the molecule and spans a length of about 110 amino acid residues. The first H-chain sequences that were determined, in the Fc region of rabbit IgG (Hill *et al.*, 1966), showed another important feature of structure: the existence of sequence homology regions. Two sequences are homologous when they contain chemically related amino acids in the same positions in the polypeptide chain (e.g., serine in the first sequence and threonine at the same position in the second sequence). Another criterion for homology between two sequences is to examine amino acid differences in terms of the minimum mutational events that are necessary to change the

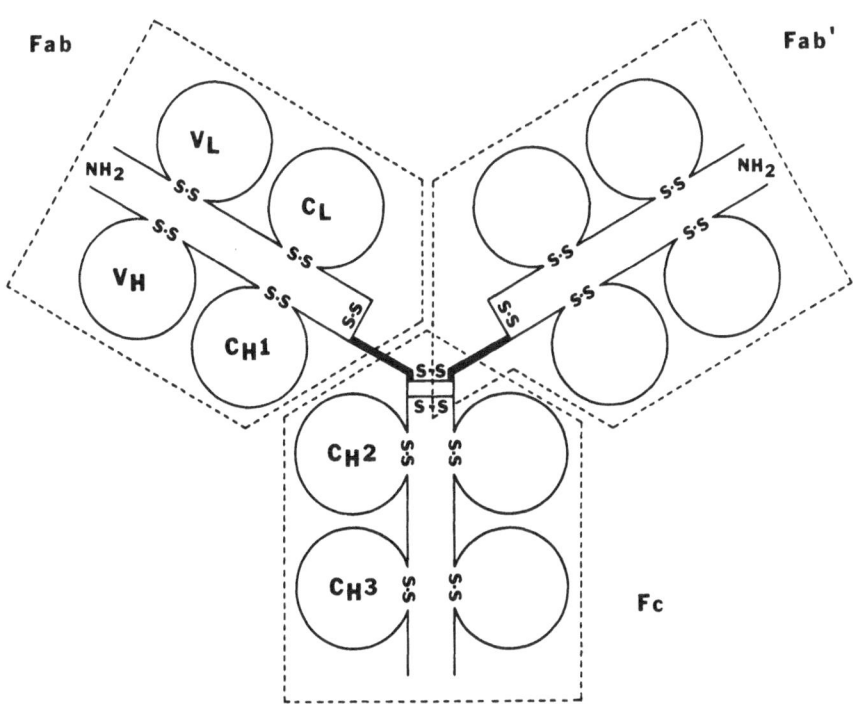

Figure 1. Diagrammatic structure of a human IgG1 molecule. The L chains are divided into two homology regions, V_L (variable) and C_L (constant). The thicker lines in the H chains correspond to the "hinge" region. The four homology regions (V_H, C_H1, C_H2, and C_H3) of the H chains, the interchain and intrachain disulfide bonds, the N-terminal regions of both chains, and the major fragments (Fab, Fab', and Fc) are indicated. Reproduced from Poljak (1973) with permission.

nucleotide sequence specifying the first chain to that specifying the second polypeptide chain. If the number of mutations is smaller than can be expected from random chance, then the sequences are said to be homologous. By either of the two criteria mentioned above, one can define four constant "homology regions": C_H1, C_H2, and C_H3 in the H chains and C_L in the L chains (Figure 1). The N-terminal, variable regions V_L and V_H (Figure 1) are homologous with each other and have a weaker homology with C_L, C_H1, C_H2, and C_H3. It is interesting to observe that the pattern of a single intrachain disulfide loop of similar length is present in each one of these regions (Figure 1). In addition to their genetic implications, these findings also suggest that the overall three-dimensional folding of IgG molecules is determined by the existence of the homology regions. Inspired by these and other observations, several proposals were made about the folding of the H and L polypeptide chains (Singer *et al.*, 1967; Putnam *et al.*, 1967; Edelman *et al.*, 1969; Welscher, 1969; and others) that can be summarized by describing the tertiary structure of Ig's as consisting of globular "domains," each corresponding to a homology region.

Electron-microscopic (EM) studies have provided the first direct pictures of the general shape and structure of Ig's. The elegant experiments of Valentine and Green (1967), in which a divalent hapten [bis-N-dinitrophenyl-(DNP)-octamethyl-enediamine] was used as a link between several anti-DNP antibodies, provided a picture of the general shape of an IgG molecule and of the arrangement of the Fab and Fc regions (Figure 2). When combined with antigen, the shape is that of the letter Y, with variable separations for the two arms (Fab) of the Y depending on the number of IgG molecules connected by the bis-DNP hapten. The flexibility required to obtain a variable separation is thought to reside in the "hinge" region connecting Fab to Fc. Electron micrographs of an IgA protein produced by the (laboratory-induced) mouse plasma cell tumor MOPC 315 (Green *et al.*, 1971) indicated that the IgA structure consists of globular units or domains. In this study on IgA, a divalent bis-DNP hapten was also used, taking advantage of the fact that the MOPC 315 myeloma protein has the specificity of an anti-DNP antibody. No such globular subunits or domains had been consistently observed in electron micrographs of IgG.

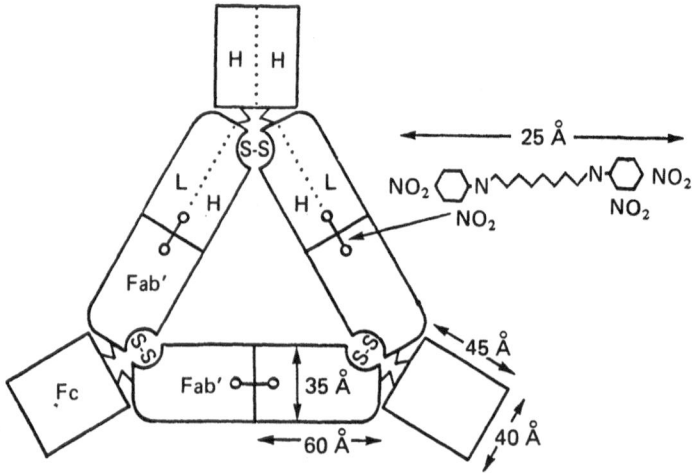

Figure 2. Diagram illustrating a hapten-linked trimer of anti-DNP rabbit IgG antibody molecules. Reproduced from Valentine and Green (1967) with the permission of Academic Press, New York.

Affinity-labeling experiments have contributed to the knowledge of the location and topography of antigen binding sites. In these experiments, a haptenic group is specifically (reversibly) bound and covalently attached to an amino acid side chain on the antibody molecule by means of a chemically reactive group on the hapten. In principle, amino acid side chains that are part of the combining site of antibody molecules or are close to it can be specifically labeled and identified. Using a number of different reactive haptens and antibodies (and also some myeloma proteins that behave like antibodies), a picture had emerged in which the antigen-binding site was defined by the V_L and the V_H regions. Amino acid side chains in, or close to, the regions of hypervariable sequence in L and H chains have been labeled (Singer *et al.*, 1967; Haimovich *et al.*, 1970; Cebra *et al.*, 1971), thus supporting the hypothesis that these regions contribute to (or determine) the antigen-binding site of antibodies. Synthetic antigens have been used as an experimental tool in analyzing the specificity of antibodies, the role of immunodeterminant groups in the antigen–antibody reaction, and the dimensions of the combining sites. With different antigens, the most exposed end of an immunodeterminant group has consistently been found to make the larger contribution to the energy of the binding reaction (Kabat, 1966; Sela, 1969; Schechter, 1971). The dimensions of the binding site have been estimated to be of the order of $35 \times 10\text{--}15 \times 6\text{--}10$ Å by using antigenic polysaccharides (Kabat, 1966) and polypeptides (Maurer, 1964; Sage *et al.*, 1964; Haber *et al.*, 1967).

2. X-Ray Crystallographic Techniques

Extensive, up-to-date reviews on this subject are available (e.g., Holmes and Blow, 1965; Dickerson, 1964; *Cold Spring Harbor Symposium,* 1971; Matthews, 1976), and the reader is referred to them for a more extensive account of principles and methods. This outline will be a brief, qualitative description of principles and techniques intended for immunologists and immunochemists.

X-ray diffraction has the potential for providing a high-resolution picture of matter in the solid or crystalline state. The basis for this potential is that X rays with wavelengths of the order of magnitude of interatomic distances can be used to obtain diffraction patterns of crystals. There is, however, one major difficulty in producing the desired image of the atomic arrangement: the relative phase of the X-ray waves cannot be measured directly from an X-ray diffraction experiment. Since no X-ray lenses are available, reconstitution of the image from the diffraction spectra must be obtained by the use of a "mathematical lens" function (a Fourier series transformation) in which both the amplitudes and the phases of the diffracted rays are required. The missing phase information can be obtained by a variety of techniques, including "direct methods" in which relationships among the intensities of the diffracted waves are analyzed mathematically to obtain the required phases. For large, complex molecules such as proteins, the only successful and widely used method of determining phases is that of isomorphous heavy-atom substitution. When the phase of each diffracted wave has been determined, amplitudes and phases can be used to calculate a map of the distribution of electron-dense X-ray scatterers (atoms or groups of atoms) that displays their relative densities and positions. In the following sections, some major points of the theory and practice of X-ray diffraction will be considered in more detail.

2.1. Crystallization of Proteins

In most cases, crystals have been obtained at an advanced stage in the isolation and purification of proteins. Since the ideal crystal is formed by a three-dimensional repetition of identical molecules, purifications to a single homogeneous molecular species should, in general, help in obtaining crystals. Conditions that render a protein insoluble (e.g., pH, type of ions, ionic strength, temperature, protein concentration) are favorable for the nucleation and growth of crystals. A classic example is the crystallization by "salting out" of protein molecules in solution. Frequently, the same protein can be obtained in several different crystal forms by changing the conditions of crystallization. In the few cases in which these different crystalline forms of the same (or related) proteins were analyzed by X-ray diffraction, the same three-dimensional structure was found to be present in all, although the contact points between the molecules and the volume taken by the solvent vary from one crystal form to another. Most of the indirect evidence obtained suggests that the structure of a protein in the crystalline state is very similar to the structure of the protein in solution, since many reactions (e.g., enzymatic activity) that take place in solution can also be shown to take place in the crystalline state. Detailed analysis of all the available evidence could be briefly summarized by saying that the structure in the crystalline form is at least one of several possible "ground states" of the molecule. Since X-ray diffraction measurements of proteins take place over extended periods of time (hours), only stable conformations can be studied by this method.

2.2. Diffraction Techniques

Protein crystals are mounted in sealed thin glass or quartz capillaries surrounded by their "mother liquor" (buffer or solution from which they were crystallized), any drying being carefully avoided during the crystal-mounting operation. The ideal dimensions for such crystals are about $0.5 \times 0.5 \times 0.5$ mm (i.e., they are visible to the eye). Crystals should measure at least 0.05 mm on each side before they can be used for single-crystal X-ray diffraction experiments. Smaller crystals (which are frequently obtained with many proteins) do not usually diffract strongly enough to permit observation of their single-crystal diffraction patterns.

X rays are produced by water-cooled stationary- or rotating-anode tubes (both commercially available). A copper anode from which CuK_α X rays of wavelength $\lambda = 1.542$ Å are obtained is most frequently used in protein work. Photographic techniques are always used for preliminary studies such as the investigation of the crystallinity of the material, its unit cell dimensions, and its symmetry. Precession photographs provide a picture of the "reciprocal lattice" (i.e., the diffraction pattern) of a crystal and make the determination of its unit cell dimensions and symmetry a relatively simple operation. The unit cell dimensions, symmetry (the way in which molecules are packed in the crystal), and crystal density can be used to calculate the molecular weight contained in the "asymmetrical unit" of the crystal. By measuring the amount of solvent, the molecular weight of an individual molecule (or molecules) contained in the volume of an asymmetric unit can be determined.

As the size of the asymmetrical unit of a crystal increases, with increasing molecular weight, so do the number of X-ray reflections that must be measured to determine the molecular structure. Furthermore, as the size of the asymmetrical unit increases, the reflections become closer and generally weaker and their measurement more time-consuming and inaccurate. Thus, the difficulty in obtaining diffraction data from larger macromolecules (such as Ig's and crystalline viruses) necessitates special techniques for intensity measurements. Computer-controlled X-ray diffractometers have been most widely used for the automatic measurement of X-ray intensities from protein crystals. In these instruments, the crystal and an X-ray counter (scintillation or proportional) are set to the appropriate angular values to measure a given reflection. The angular values are calculated by a computer that is connected "on-line" to the diffractometer. Since reflections must be measured in a temporal sequence that extends over periods of several hours, a highly stabilized X-ray source is required. Photographic techniques, which were used in the early days of X-ray diffraction experiments, are regaining an important role in protein crystallography because their use allows the recording of many reflections simultaneously. In this way, the speed of data collection is increased, providing an invaluable help when the crystalline material is damaged by radiation. The diffraction films may then be measured by film scanners that provide the output information in a form suitable for further computer processing (e.g., on magnetic tape).

2.3. The Phase Problem

As stated above, the intensities of the X rays diffracted by a crystal can be measured by films or by radiation counters, but the relative phases of these reflections cannot be measured directly. Several methods, ranging from purely mathematical to combined analytical and experimental, have been used to solve this problem. In the case of protein crystals, the only method that has provided positive results when the three-dimensional structure of the molecule under study is totally unknown is the method of isomorphous heavy-atom substitution. This method consists of introducing one or a few atoms of high electron density (i.e., "heavy" atoms) into specific sites in the asymmetrical unit of the crystal without altering the conformation of the protein molecule under study or the relative positions of the molecules in the crystal. If this condition is achieved, the native protein crystals and those in which solvent or other atoms have been replaced by the heavy atoms are said to be *isomorphous*. Intensity changes, which can be seen by comparing the diffraction pattern of the native protein crystals with that of isomorphous crystals containing heavy atoms, are an indication of a possible heavy-atom substitution. The Fourier transform of the measured intensity changes (in the form of a two- or three-dimensional autocorrelation map called the *Patterson function*) can be analyzed to determine the location of the heavy atoms. If this analysis has been successfully completed for two or more different heavy-atom substituents, the contribution of the heavy-atom derivatives can be calculated, and the phases thus obtained can be used to determine the native protein phases. An example of a heavy-atom substitution is the titration of a (Cys-) SH group of a protein by a mercurial such as p-chloromercuribenzoic acid. In such a case, the substitution can be performed before or after crystallization. In most cases, heavy atoms are introduced by diffusion into already grown crystals by "soaking" the crystals in a solution containing heavy atoms. Coordination of the substituent in a favorable environment of protein side chains accounts for their binding at the few specific sites that are required.

A few rules can be mentioned here to summarize the preceding statements about heavy-atom isomorphous substitution:

1. It is important that the isomorphism be as perfect as possible so that distortions of the protein configuration will not interfere with the determination of its structure. This criterion becomes more exacting as the resolution of the analysis is increased.
2. The substitution should take place at a few sites in one molecule and in all or most molecules in the crystal, leading to a few sites with high occupancy. A high occupancy is particularly desirable for a large protein so that the heavy-atom scattering can be measured accurately over that of the large number of (lighter) atoms of the protein.
3. A minimum of two heavy atoms (at different sites) is necessary to solve the protein phases. A number in excess of two is desirable to increase and improve the phase information. If the number of reflections to be measured for the native protein crystals is N, the minimum number of reflections to be measured for all the derivatives will be $N(n + 1)$, where n is the number of heavy-atom derivatives that are used in the process of phase determination.
4. Heavy-atom attachment to crystalline proteins is, in most cases, a trial and error process. Fortunately, results can be analyzed by X-ray diffraction methods; visual inspection of photographs is enough to detect the intensity changes that occur if substitution has taken place.

Because it is unpredictable, isomorphous heavy-atom substitution remains one of the most difficult and elusive steps in the study of protein structures by X-ray crystallographic methods.

2.4. Interpretation of Fourier Maps

Heavy-atom parameters such as positional coordinates, relative occupancies, and a measure of their thermal vibrations in space can be refined by least-squares techniques from the intensities of the diffraction pattern. Refinement of these parameters leads to more precise phase information. An index called the *figure of merit* is frequently used to express the average error in the phase angles for all the reflections that were calculated. The average figure of merit m is a measure of the cosine of the average angular error in the calculated phase angles. The range of m is, evidently, 0–1. A value above 0.7 is considered satisfactory; i.e., the average error in phase angle is less than 45°. The value of m tends to decrease as the resolution increases, due to factors such as poorer experimental data and lack of strict isomorphism.

The problem of resolution in protein crystallography will be considered next. Although in theory resolution depends on the wavelength of the radiation used, in practice, the intensity of the X-ray diffraction pattern of proteins decreases rapidly with increasing diffraction angle, so that it is difficult to measure reflections beyond 2 Å, which would be needed for atomic resolution. [A 2-Å reflection can be visualized as obtained from an imaginary set of parallel planes spaced 2 Å apart following the condition known as Bragg's law, $\lambda = 2d \sin \Theta$, where λ is the wavelength of X-rays, d is the (2-Å) spacing of the set of planes, and Θ is the angle made by both the incident and the diffracted beams and the planes.] Because of crystalline disorder, it is frequently observed that the diffraction pattern of proteins fades at much lower resolutions. In these cases, only a gross structure of the molecule can be determined. Features of secondary structure such as polypeptide chains in α-helical configuration can be detected at a resolution of 6 Å, as has been demonstrated by the X-ray analyses of myoglobin and hemoglobin. When the helical content of a protein is small, it is mostly features of tertiary and quaternary structure that can be determined at a low resolution such as 6 Å.

The number of reflections to be measured increases sharply with increasing resolution. If the number of reflections to be measured for a resolution of 6 Å is N, the number of reflections will be (approximately) $2N$ for a resolution of 4 Å, $5N$ for a resolution of 3.3 Å, and $25N$ for a resolution of 2 Å. If one considers that N is of the order of 10^3 for a native protein crystal (and for each heavy-atom derivative), the increasing amount of work with increasing resolution becomes clear. It is also clear that if 2–3 Å is the resolution limit that can be attained with a given protein crystal, it will be necessary to have access to the amino acid sequence for a complete interpretation of the Fourier map of the electron density even if good phase information is available.

Fourier maps of the electron density describe the structure under study. In low-resolution maps (e.g., 6 Å), it is possible to define the shape of a molecule. In regions of the map in which one molecule comes into contact with another, however, this task may be difficult and may require noncrystallographic information (such as a knowledge of the approximate molecular shape by light scattering or EM) or an arbitrary decision. An electron-dense "marker" such as the heme group in hemoglobin can be easily located and used as a reference point in the interpretation of low- and high-resolution maps. Despite their higher electron density, disulfide bonds cannot be easily located in low-resolution maps. In high-resolution maps (3-Å or smaller spacings), runs of continuous polypeptide chains can be seen, and if sequence information is available, amino acid side chains can be matched with the electron-density map. Some side chains or the ends of a polypeptide chain may be freely rotating, and thus they are difficult to locate in a map. Solid models are usually built of a material such as balsa wood from low-resolution maps. They represent features of electron density above the background due to the intermolecular solution of crystallization. Skeletal wire models of amino acids are used to interpret high-resolution maps in terms of polypeptide chains. A good fit of the amino acid sequence to the electron-density map constitutes the ultimate test of the determination of a protein structure.

3. Immunoglobulins and Fc Fragments

A crystallographic analysis of a whole IgG molecule was reported by Sarma *et al.* (1971). These studies were carried out on IgG Dob, a human cryoglobulin that crystallizes spontaneously on cooling. One L chain and one H chain are contained in the asymmetrical unit of the crystal and are related to the other H and L chains by a two-fold axis of symmetry that runs through the inter-H-chain disulfide bonds. The X-ray diffraction pattern of IgG Dob does not extend to high resolution because of structural disorder, making it difficult to measure intensities with Bragg spacings smaller than 6 Å. Also, the crystals are damaged by irradiation after relatively short exposures, thus making the collection of intensity data a difficult problem even at low resolution. Under these experimental conditions, an X-ray diffraction study becomes a very difficult problem. A Fourier map of the electron density at a nominal resolution of 6 Å was interpreted as indicating two globular regions (Sarma *et al.*, 1971). Since one of these regions is located around a two-fold axis of symmetry, it was assigned to the Fc part of the molecule, where two identical C_H2 and two identical C_H3 moieties (see Figure 5) are related by an exact two-fold axis of symmetry (Goldstein *et al.*, 1968). The other globular region should correspond to the Fab part of the molecule. Four possible ways of assembling a complete IgG Dob molecule were found in this study, and of these, one was chosen as a tentative structure. In this model, the IgG molecule is T-shaped; however, an EM study of the same crystalline material (Labaw and Davies, 1971) showed a Y-shaped molecule similar in this respect to those observed by Valentine and Green (1967) in rabbit anti-DNP antibody preparations. Given the experimental difficulties mentioned above, the tentative nature of the model should be emphasized; furthermore, it should be considered that Dob may not be a typical IgG molecule, since it has a deletion in its hinge region (Lopes and Steiner, 1973), a factor that could influence the shape of the molecule. Also, lattice forces may induce a T shape in this particular crystal form, a shape that may be changed in solution or after glutaraldehyde fixation prior to EM.

Small-angle X-ray scattering studies were conducted on a human myeloma Ig by Pilz *et al.* (1970) and on rabbit antibodies by Pilz *et al.* (1975). The slopes of the X-ray scattering curves obtained in these experiments are a measure of the shape of the molecule. From these studies, it was concluded (Pilz *et al.*, 1970) that IgG molecules are T-shaped in solution. In considering this conclusion, it is hard to decide whether there are other possible approximations to the shape of the molecule that could fit the data equally well, since molecular shape could be a rather complex function even at low resolution. The importance of this problem should be considered in the light of antibody properties, such as complement fixation or binding to target cells, that may depend on a conformational change of the molecule after antigen-binding. In another small-angle X-ray scattering study, Pilz *et al.* (1975) found a volume contraction of about 10%, and a decrease in radius of gyration of about 8%, when 90% of the antigen-binding sites or rabbit anti-poly-D-alanyl antibodies where titrated with a tetra-D-alanine hapten. This finding is in agreement with a potential for conformational change that resides in the "segmental flexibility" of the molecule around its hinge regions (Yguerabide *et al.*, 1970).

Fc fragments from human and rabbit IgGs have been the subject of X-ray diffraction studies in several laboratories. However, difficulties in obtaining isomorphous heavy-atom derivatives, pronounced damage after X-ray irradiation, and other technical problems have slowed down the expected progress in the structural analysis of Fc. In view of these difficulties, it is not surprising that a structural model of Fc has not yet been obtained.

4. Three-Dimensional Structure of Light Chains

Detailed crystallographic analyses have been reported for human λ chains (Schiffer *et al.*, 1973; Edmundson *et al.*, 1974) and human κ chains (Epp *et al.*, 1974). In addition to these studies on crystalline L chains, work on Fab fragments (see Section 5) has also produced atomic resolution models of the structure of human and murine L chains.

A 3.5-Å-resolution Fourier map allowed Edmundson and his colleagues (Schiffer *et al.*, 1973) to trace the polypeptide-chain backbone of the two λ chains present in the asymmetrical unit of the Mcg Bence Jones dimer (Figure 3). Although an atomic model was not built at this stage of the work, many side chains could be located. The most prominent features of the electron-density map were identified as the four intrachain disulfide bonds. The density of the interchain disulfide bond was much lower, a feature that was attributed in part to the fact that this bond is at a surface region of the molecule with more freedom of motion. The V and C domains as well as the "switch" region connecting both were traced in this map. The switch regions are made of exposed, easily accessible, extended polypeptide chains (see Figure 3), a finding that explains the ease with which L chains can be cleaved into two globular domains, V and C (Solomon and McLaughlin, 1969; Karlsson *et al.*, 1972). Although the two L chains are identical in amino acid sequence, they differ in their three-dimensional structure: in one of the chains, the major axes of the V and C regions make an angle of 110°; in the other, the angle is 70°, an observation reminiscent of the L- and H-chain structure of Fab (see Section 5). The V and C domains closely resemble each other in shape and in polypeptide-chain folding. Residues 48–60, which include the second hypervariable region, have no equivalent in the C domain. At one end of the V regions, there is a cavity in the shape of a truncated cone about 15 Å wide and 10 Å deep. This cavity is lined by the hypervariable segments of both chains and constitutes the equivalent of the antigen-binding site of the Fab region of antibody molecules.

The structure of a crystalline dimer of the variable region V_κ of Bence Jones protein Rei has been determined to a resolution of 2.8 Å. About 50% of all amino acid residues are located in one of the two β-sheets present in a V_κ monomer. The

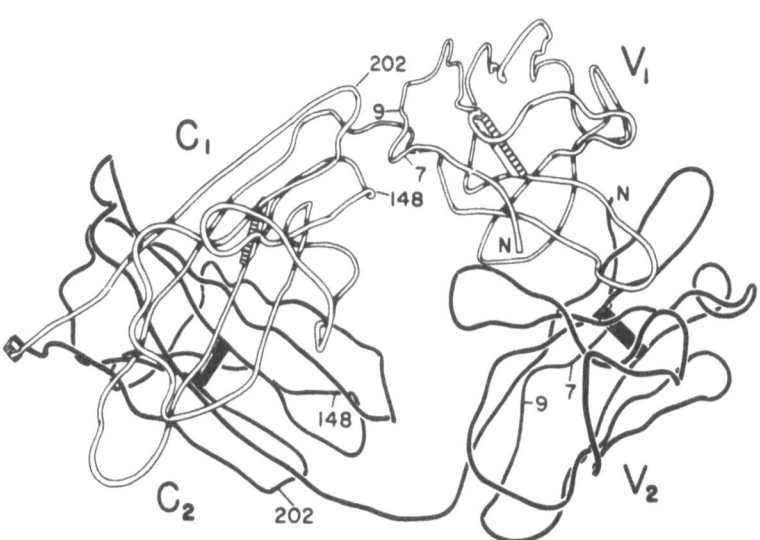

Figure 3. Tracing of the polypeptide chain of the Mcg λ-chain Bence Jones dimer, obtained from a 3.5-Å-resolution Fourier map. The C_L (C_1, C_2) and V_L (V_1, V_2) homology regions are indicated. Disulfide bonds are indicated by bars. *N*-termini are labeled N; *C*-termini are joined by the interchain disulfide bond. In the two monomers, the V and C regions differ in their relative orientation as shown by the distances between points labeled 7, 9 (V), and 148, 202 (C). Reproduced from Schiffer *et al.* (1973) with permission.

two β-sheets cover a hydrophobic interior formed by invariant or semiinvariant residues. Only one turn of a distorted α (or π) helix could be determined in the model, in agreement with circular dichroism experiments on Ig's and L chains. As in the case of the λ chains discussed above, a large cavity around a local two-fold axis of symmetry is lined up by amino acid residues belonging to the hypervariable regions. The V_κ monomers form a dimer that closely resembles the V_λ domains of the λ-chain dimer discussed above. This can be taken as an indication that the V regions can associate independently of the interchain contacts that occur in the C regions. Other features of this thorough structural anaylsis of the V_κ dimer will be discussed in the next section in connection with the Fab' structure.

5. Fab Fragments

Fragments Fab and Fab' from human myeloma proteins were crystallized by Rossi and Nisonoff (1968) and by Rossi et al. (1969). X-ray diffraction patterns of the crystalline Fab and Fab' fragments (Avey et al., 1968; Humphrey et al., 1969) from IgG1 (λ) New and IgG1 (λ) Hil gave identical intensity patterns, indicating that they have the same structure. It would normally be expected that since Fab' is about ten amino acid residues longer than Fab (in its Fd' chain), the X-ray intensity patterns should reflect this difference. Subsequent high-resolution studies of Fab' New indicated that the C-termini of the Fd' and Fd chains do not make any significant contribution to diffracted X-ray intensities, probably due to random motion of the ends of the polypeptide chains. It follows that Fab' New and Fab New are equivalent for crystallographic studies; thus, Fab' and Fab can be used as equivalent terms for the purpose of this review.

5.1. Low-Resolution Studies

The 6-Å-resolution study of Fab' New (Poljak et al., 1972) showed that the Fab' fragment consists of two discrete globular domains, V and C, containing the V_L and V_H and the C_L and $C_H 1$ homology regions, respectively. Despite the limitations of a low-resolution study, the two polypeptide chains, L and Fd', were found to be two, continuous, independent stretches of electron density, which originate in one of the globular subunits and, after a region of globular folding in that subunit, extend to the other subunit through a narrow outer bridge of polypeptide chain (Figure 4). The overall scheme is that of a tetrahedral arrangement of four globular subunits, two of which (V_L and C_L) are formed by the L chain and the other two (V_H and $C_H 1$) by the Fd' chain. This type of arrangement is roughly similar to that observed in hemoglobin (Perutz et al., 1960), in which four globular subunits are arranged in tetrahedral configuration, although in hemoglobin there are four independent (two α, two β) polypeptide chains.

The 6 Å Fab New structure provides a three-dimensional model to explain some of the physicochemical properties of Ig molecules. For example, fragments of L chains that appear to be of catabolic origin were reported in human urine samples (Solomon and McLaughlin, 1969; Baglioni et al., 1966). In vitro cleavage of human myeloma L chains by controlled enzymatic digestion was shown (Solomon and McLaughlin, 1969; Karlsson et al., 1972) to generate fragments having a more compact shape, as judged by the radius of gyration and frictional coefficient, than the parent L chain. Studies of allotypic and idiotypic markers (Solomon and

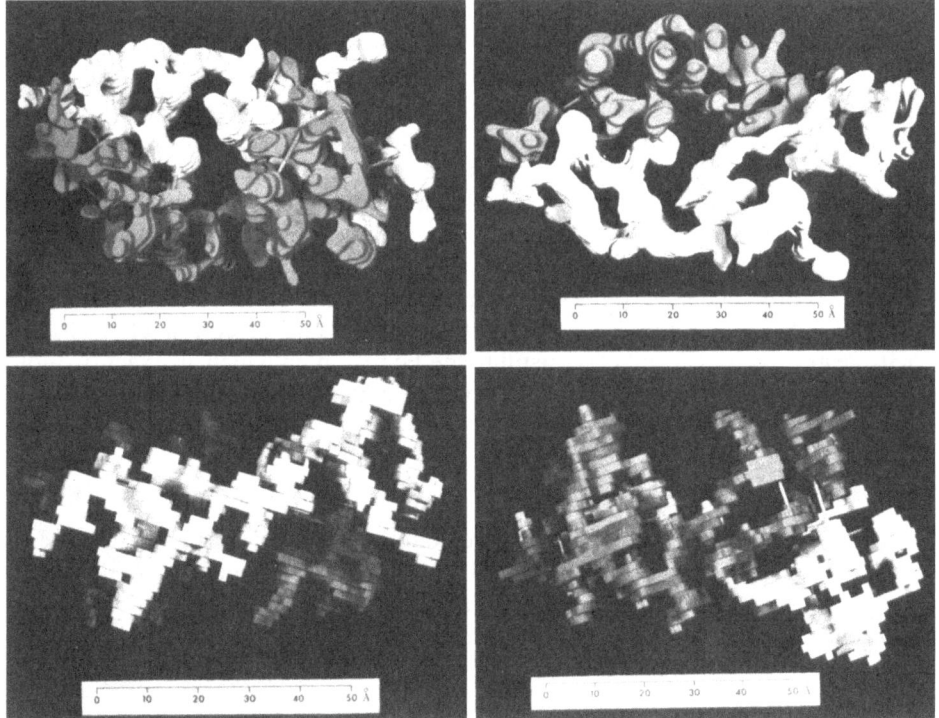

Figure 4. "Top" (upper left), "bottom" (upper right), and "side" views of the 6-Å-resolution model of Fab' New. The two continuous chains of electron density described in the text are shown in white (L chain) and gray (Fd' chain). The two globular domains V (left) and C (right) are separated by an internal cleft and joined by two easily accessible connections. The two side views show the tetrahedral arrangement of the V_L, V_H, C_L and C_H1 homology subunits. Reproduced from Poljak *et al.* (1972) with the permission of *Nature*.

McLaughlin, 1969), peptide mapping, and partial amino acid sequence data (Karlsson *et al.*, 1972) indicate that the fragments obtained by enzymatic action on L chains correspond to the V_L and C_L homology regions. Cleavage of the parent polypeptide chain occurs at the "switch" connecting the V_L and C_L homology regions, which is probably easily accessible to proteolytic attack by enzymes. In the Fab model, both L and Fd chains do indeed show easily accessible linear regions around the middle of their total length that connect the globular V and C subunits described above. Cleavage at the middle point of the L chain would generate two L-chain fragments of globular shape with a radius of about 15–20 Å, which compares well with the value of 16 Å obtained for the radius of gyration of several C_L and V_L fragments (Karlsson *et al.*, 1972). The model of Fab New suggests that it should be possible to cleave Fab itself into two fragments of molecular weight 25,000 each, one of which should correspond to the V subunit and could presumably retain antigen-binding activity. In fact, Givol and co-workers (Inbar *et al.*, 1972) demonstrated that cleavage of an Fab' fragment by pepsin can generate a fragment (called F_V), consisting of the V_L and the V_H regions. It is interesting to note that a similar type of cleavage can be obtained in the Fc region (Turner and Bennich, 1968), leading to the appearance of an Fc' fragment of molecular weight approximately 25,000.

The X-ray crystallographic model of Fab New also shows a definite correlation between the internal homologies in amino acid sequence and the tertiary structures of Ig's. In fact, it verifies that the homology regions fold into compact structures or domains linked by linear connecting regions. The striking structural feature of Fab is the presence of two globular subunits, V and C, each comprised of two distinct polypeptide chains. This finding suggests that gene duplication (Hill *et al.*, 1966) determined a structural duplication resulting in increasingly larger precursors of Ig molecules by the addition of globular subunits. The structure obtained for Fab New can then be extended to the whole IgG molecule to provide the scheme shown in Figure 5. In this schematic representation, the V subunit consists of the homology regions V_L and V_H, C1 consists of C_L and C_H1, and C2 and C3 consist of $(C_H2)_2$ and $(C_H3)_2$, respectively. C2 and C3 constitute the Fc region, in which an exact two-fold axis of symmetry relates two C_H2 and two C_H3 domains (Goldstein *et al.*, 1968).

5.2 High-Resolution Studies

The conclusions outlined above were confirmed by high-resolution studies on the crystalline Fab' New (Poljak *et al.*, 1973, 1974). In these studies, atomic models were built using amino acid sequence data and Fourier maps at 2.8- and 2.0-Å resolution. An Fab fragment from the murine myeloma protein McPC 603 was also analyzed to a resolution of 3.1 Å by Segal *et al.*, 1974). Some of the results obtained from these studies will be discussed below.

The overall dimensions of the Fab molecule are $80 \times 50 \times 40$ Å. A centrally located cleft divides the molecule into two structural domains, V and C (see Figure 6). Four "homology subunits" that correspond to the homology regions V_L, V_H, C_L, and C_H1 can be clearly differentiated. The C_L and C_H1 subunits interact very closely and appear more tightly packed than the V_L–V_H subunits. The C_L, C_H1, V_L, and V_H subunits are strikingly similar in their three-dimensional folding, as would be expected from the homology in their amino acid sequences. However, although V_L and V_H share the basic "immunoglobulin-fold" of C_L and C_H, they include an additional length of polypeptide chain in the form of a loop not present in C_L and C_H1 (see Figure 7). In the L (λ) chain of IgG New, a deletion of seven amino acids in V_L (Figure 8, positions 54–60) results in a shortening of this additional loop of the polypeptide chain, making the V_L structure of IgG New more similar to that of the C_L and C_H1 subunits than to V_H. The deleted amino acid residues can be readily placed in the model of V_L by comparison with the folding of the V_H subunit.

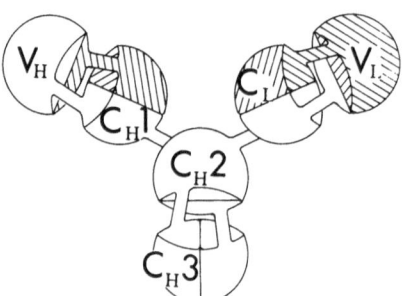

Figure 5. Schematic model of the structure of an IgG molecule incorporating the structural features determined for the Fab fragment and extrapolating these structural features to the Fc region. Reproduced from Poljak *et al.* (1972) with the permission of *Nature*.

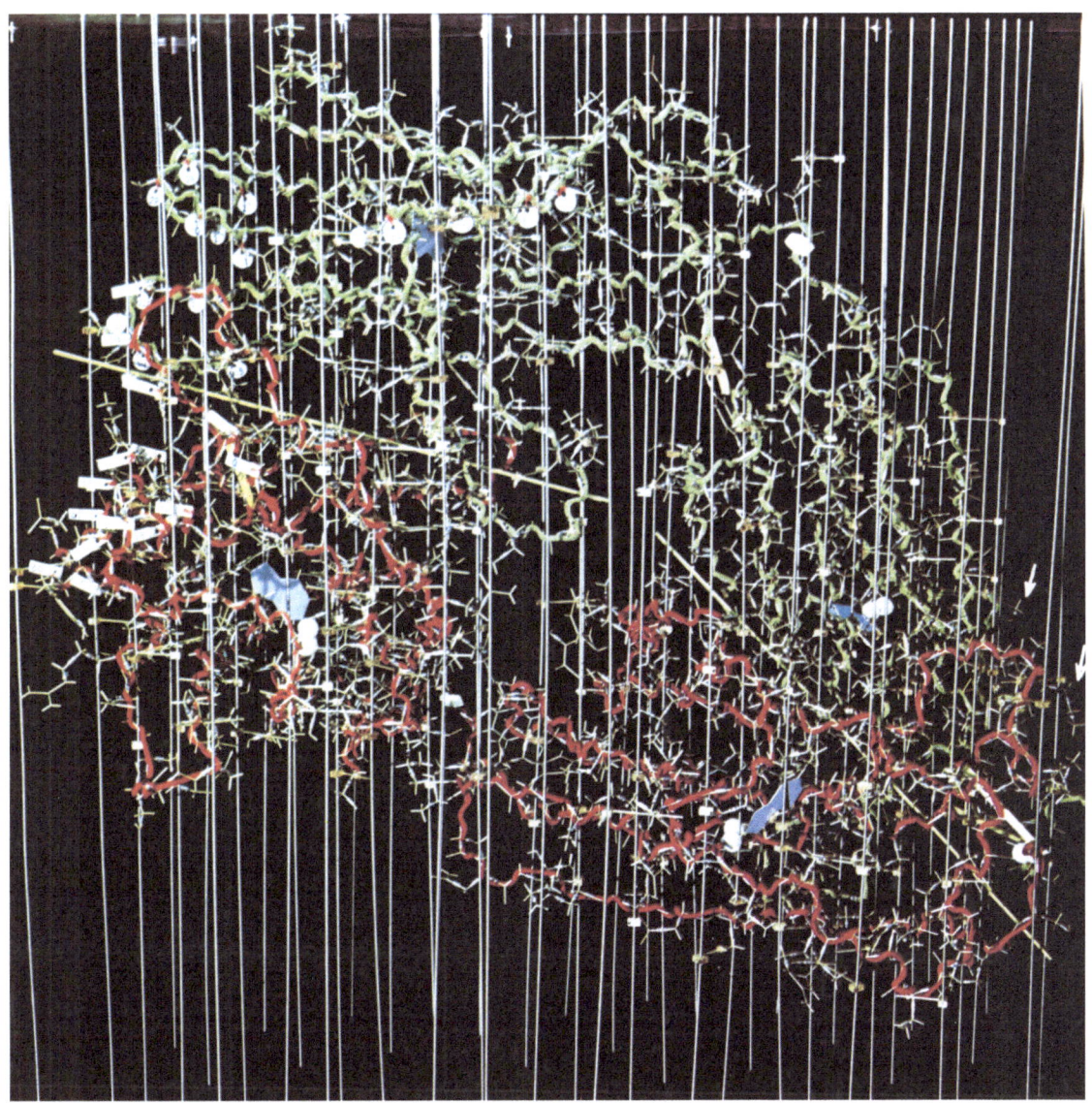

Figure 6. Model of Fab′ New at 2.8-Å resolution. The orientation of this model is close to that in the upper left section of Figure 4. The L and H (Fd′) chains are shown in green and red, respectively. A central cleft divides the structure into V (left) and C (right) domains connected by the "switch regions." White spheres mark the four intrachain and the interchain disulfide bonds; constant Trp residues located near the intrachain disulfides in each homology subunit are indicated with blue tags. α-Carbon positions of residues that form disulfide bonds in other Ig's are connected by yellow tapes. Arrows point to Ser 154 and Lys 191, which correlate with the Kern and Oz serological markers of λ chains, respectively. The "hypervariable regions" of the L and H chains are numbered with circular (L-chain) and rectangular (H-chain) tags; they occur at the left end of the molecule in close spatial proximity, except for the second hypervariable region of the L chain, which precedes a special deletion (see Figure 8).

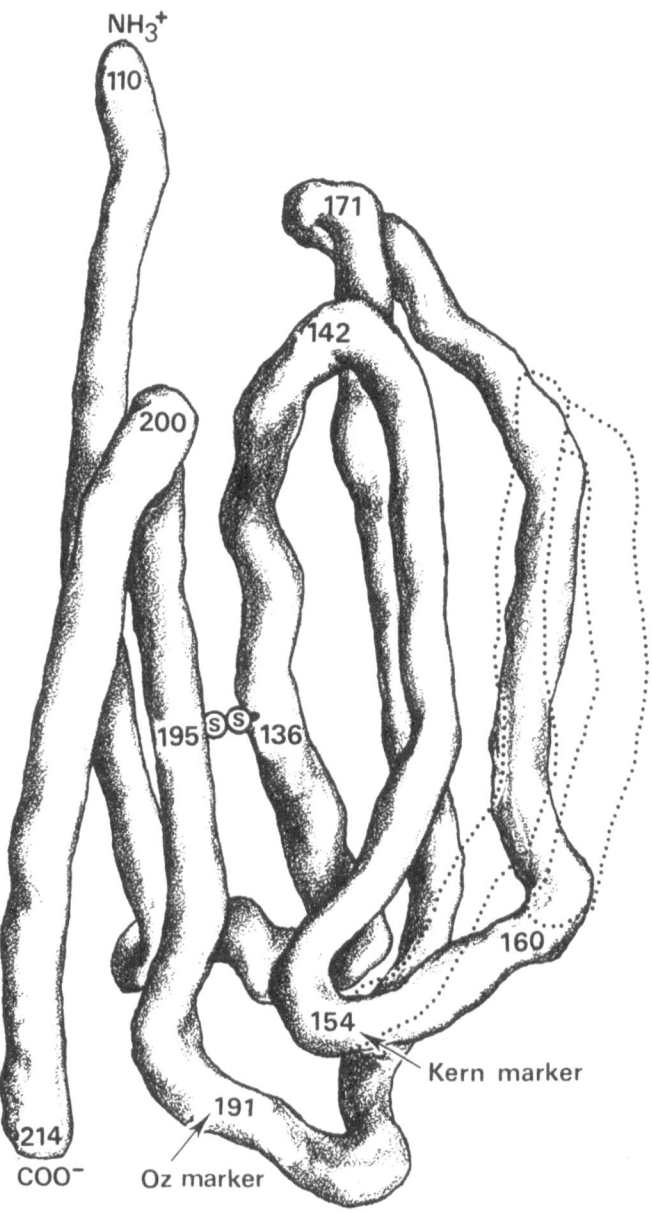

Figure 7. Diagram of the polypeptide-chain folding of a homology region of an Ig: "immunoglobulin-fold." The solid trace shows the folding of the polypeptide chain in the constant subunits; the numbers designate human C_λ residues, beginning at "NH_3^+," which corresponds to residue 110. The dotted lines indicate the additional loop of polypeptide chain characteristic of the V_L and V_H homology subunits. Reproduced from Poljak *et al.* (1973).

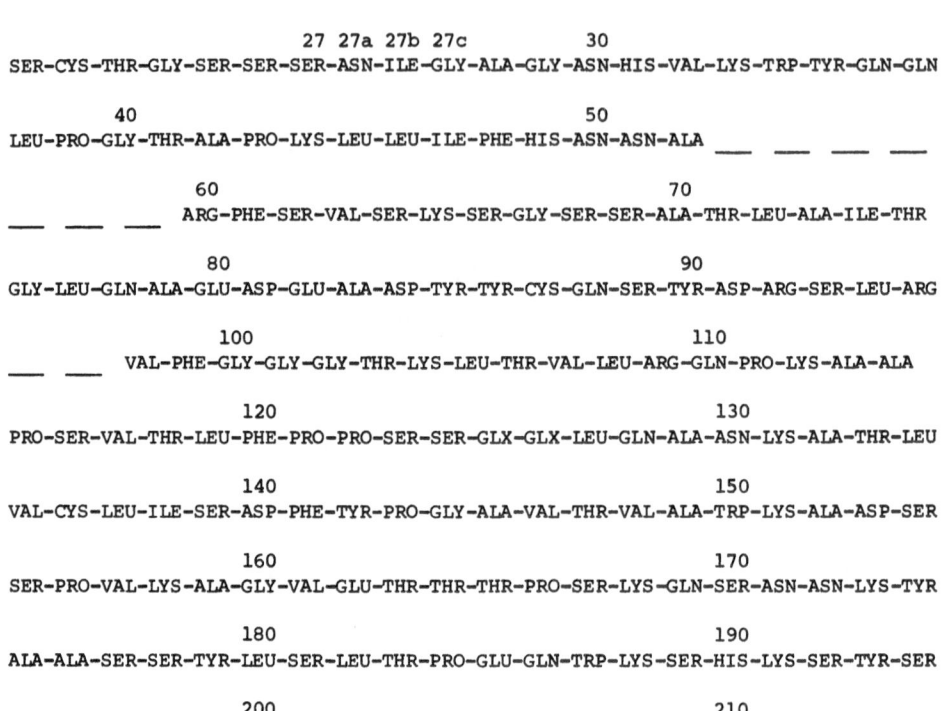

Figure 8. Amino acid sequence of the L chain from IgG new. Numbers 27a–c and gaps (53–59 and 96–97) are introduced to maximize homology with other λ chains. The gap extending from residues 53 to 59 appears unique to this λ chain. Data from Chen and Poljak (1974).

The structure of the homology subunits can be described as consisting of two β-pleated sheets formed by several strands (seven in C_L and C_H1) of antiparallel polypeptide chain. The C_L homology subunit, for example, consists of a β-pleated sheet made up by four hydrogen-bonded antiparallel chains (residues 116–120, 132–140, 160–169, and 173–182) and another β-pleated sheet containing three antiparallel chains (residues 147–151, 193–199, and 202–208) (see Figure 9). These two twisted and roughly parallel sheets surround a tightly packed interior of hydrophobic side chains including the intrachain disulfide bond that links the two sheets in a direction approximately perpendicular to their planes. About 60% of the C_L residues are included in these two β-pleated sheets. The homologous subunits C_H1, V_L, and V_H (Figure 9) can be described in similar terms. In addition to the features of secondary structure just discussed, in Fab′ New, V_L residues 26–27c appear in a helical conformation close to that of a π-helix. Also, V_L residues 78–82, and the homologous V_H residues 87–91, fold with the conformation of a distorted π- or α-helix. In general, the precise conformation of amino acid residues that do not belong to the regions of secondary structure discussed above is more difficult to define, especially when they correspond to regions of lower electron density on the surface of the molecule.

Amino acid sequence comparisons have been extensively used in several laboratories to align the primary structures of different Ig molecules and their homology regions. The alignment of V_L and V_H sequences with those of the C_L and C_H homology regions is less straightforward than alignments between V_L and V_H or between C_L and C_H regions. This problem has been approached by matching their similar three-dimensional structures and aligning residues that occupy an identical or similar position in the constant pattern of the tertiary structure of the homology subunits. Alignments obtained by this procedure, which is independent of amino acid sequence homologies, are shown in Figure 10.

Some of the variable and constant features of V_L sequences can be discussed in terms of the three-dimensional structure of V_λ New. Hairpin bends in the polypeptide chain of V_λ New occur around positions 14–15, 27–30, 39–40, 67–68, and 92–93, and an approximate 90° bend around residues 75–76. Except for the bend at positions 92–93 (a hypervariable region), all others involve a Gly residue that is constant in human λ-chain sequences. Most of these bends also involve a constant

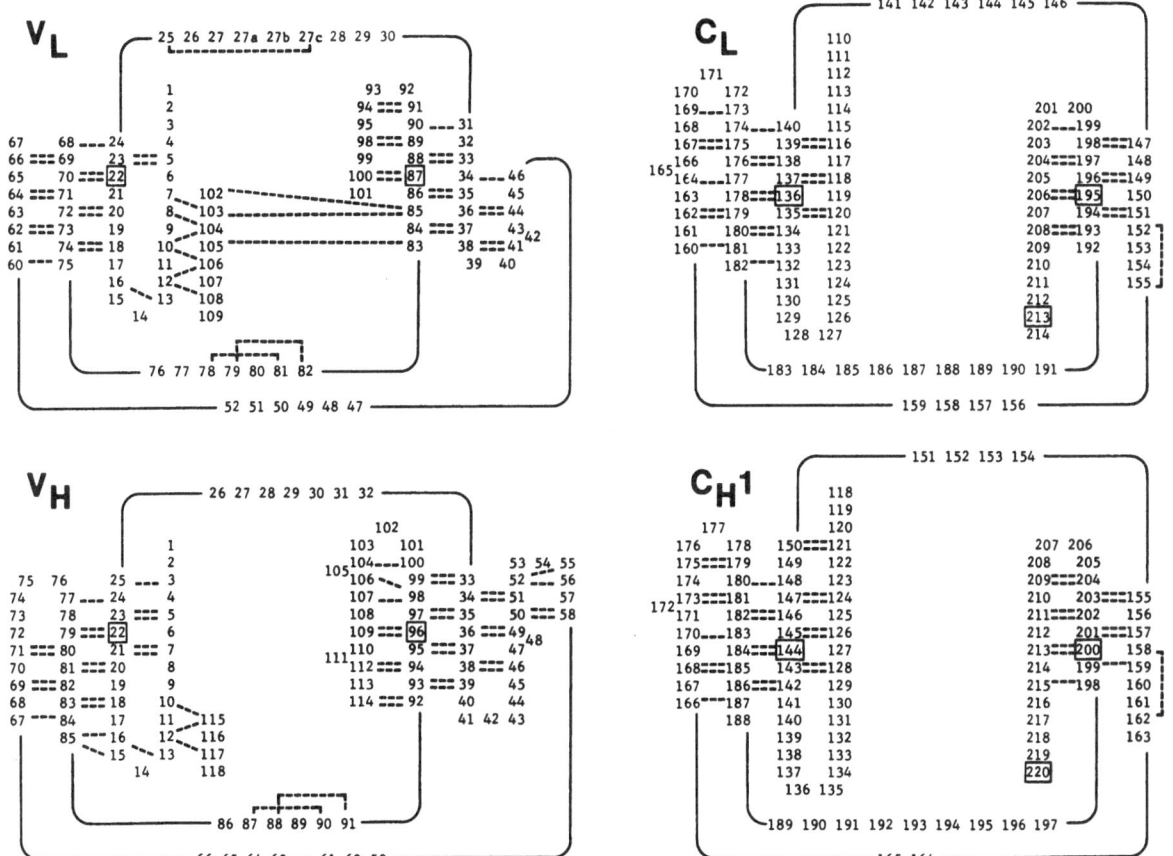

Figure 9. Diagram of the hydrogen bonds (----) between main chain atoms for V_L, V_H, C_L, and C_H1. The two hydrogen-bonded clusters correspond to the two β-pleated sheets of each homology subunit (see the text). Cysteine residues that participate in the intrachain disulfide bonds linking the two β-sheets are enclosed in rectangles; C_L residue 213 and C_H1 residue 220 form the interchain disulfide bond and are also enclosed in squares. The numbers refer to the amino acid sequence as given in Figure 8. Reproduced from Poljak *et al.* (1974).

ROBERTO J. POLJAK

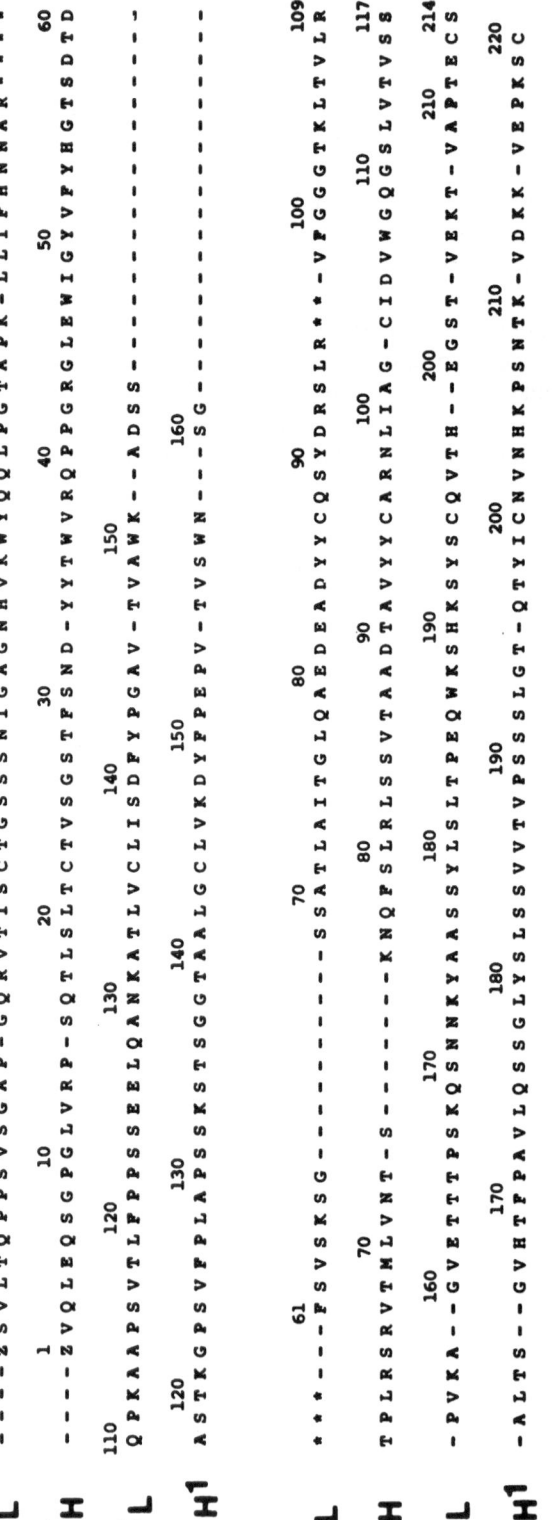

Figure 10. Alignment of the amino acid sequences of the V_L, V_H, C_L, and C_H1 homology regions of Fab' New obtained by comparison of their three-dimensional structures. The V_H sequence is as given by Poljak et al. (1977); the C_H1 sequence is as given by Edelman et al. (1969). The one-letter code for amino acids is as given by Dayhoff (1972).

or nearly constant Pro-Gly or (Ser,Thr)-Gly sequence. A similar conclusion was obtained from the study of a crystalline V_κ fragment (Epp *et al.*, 1974). Glycine residues also contribute to a constant sequence (Phe-Gly-Gly-Gly, positions 99–102) that is not part of a bend. The constant character of this sequence in all λ chains can be explained by the following observations: (1) Phe 99 is located in an internal, interchain hydrophobic pocket that includes the homologous constant Trp 108 in V_H, related to Phe 99 by a local pseudo two-fold axis of symmetry; it can be assumed that Phe 99 (and Trp 108) make an interchain contact that is important for V_L–V_H assembly; (2) Gly 100 in V_λ (or Gly 109 in V_H) is tightly packed between the intrachain disulfide bond and Leu 4 (a constant residue in V_L and V_H); (3) Gly 101 is relatively close to the constant Gln 6, although here there is room for a side chain as observed in V_κ (Gln 101) or in V_H (position 110); (4) Gly 102 (111 in V_H) is very close to a constant aromatic residue (Tyr/Phe, 86 in V_λ or 95 in V_H), so that the limited space available requires the presence of a Gly residue at this position. Some other residues that are constant in V_λ or that show only a limited degree of variability, such as Tyr 35, Gln 37, Ala 42, Pro 43, and Asp 84 are involved in close contacts with the V_H subunit. Other constant residues such as Gln 37 and Tyr 85, Glu 83 and Tyr 142 (C_L) make internal hydrogen bonds. In addition to the residues just discussed, most of the nonpolar, hydrophobic amino acids that occur in the interior of the structure between the two β-sheets are invariant or are replaced by other hydrophobic residues. They are Leu 4, Gln 6, Val 10, Val 18, Ile 20, Cys 22, Val 32, Trp 34, Leu 46, Phe 61, Val 63, Ala 70, Leu 72, Ile 74, Leu 77, Ala 83, Tyr 85, Cys 87, Ser 89, Val 98, Thr 103, Leu 105, and Val 107. Thus, residues that appear at bends or contribute to intra- and intersubunit bonds and that seem to have an important structural role are invariant or semiinvariant.

In the C_L subunit, Ser 154 and Lys 191, which correlate with the serological nonallelic human λ-chain markers Kern⁻ and Ox⁺, respectively, appear at the outside of the molecule in close spatial proximity, about 8 Å from each other. The *Inv* allotypic markers of human κ chains were shown (Milstein *et al.*, 1974b) to involve Ala/Val and Val/Leu substitutions at positions 153 and 191, respectively, which correspond closely to the positions of the Kern and Oz markers in human λ chains. Replacements at positions 153 and 191 in κ chains will also affect antigenic determinants of the molecule that are recognized by antiallotypic antisera. Since the distance between the α-carbon atoms of the homologous residues is about 8–10 Å, replacements involving both positions can be simultaneously recognized by an antiallotypic antibody molecule.

The similarity of the folding pattern of the homology regions of Fab' and the fact that the allotypic markers of human κ chains can be correlated with structural features of a human λ chain suggest that the structural model of Fab' is valid for other Ig's of different isotype or even different animal species. Supporting evidence for this postulate was obtained by an analysis of the interchain and intrachain disulfide bonds (Poljak *et al.*, 1973), which will be reviewed below.

The L and H chains of Ig's are covalently linked by a disulfide bond [with the exception of some IgA molecules in which two L chains are linked to each other by a disulfide bond (Grey *et al.*, 1968)]. The L-chain cysteine residue that contributes to this bond is at the *C*-terminus of the chain (as in human κ chains) or adjacent to it (as in human λ chains) (see Figure 11). In different isotypes of H chain, and in different animal species, the cysteine residue that completes the S–S bond is either at position 214 or at about position 131 (Figure 11). The bonding scheme illustrated

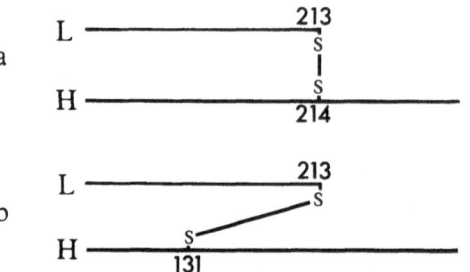

Figure 11. Diagram of two different patterns of disulfide bonds connecting the H and L chains of different isotypes of Ig's (see the text).

in Figure 11a applies to human IgG1 (Steiner and Porter, 1967) Ig's such as IgG New. The interchain disulfide bond illustrated in Figure 11b, in which the H-chain cysteinyl residue occurs at position 131, is found in human IgG2, IgG3, and IgG4 (De Preval *et al.*, 1970), in human IgM (Putman *et al.*, 1971), in rabbit IgG (O'Donnell *et al.*, 1970), in guinea pig IgG2a (Birshtein *et al.*, 1971), and in mouse IgG2a and IgG2b (De Preval *et al.*, 1970). In the three-dimensional model of Fab' New, the H-chain Cys 214 is at a distance of about 6 Å from L-chain Cys 213, to which it is linked by a disulfide bond. Position 131 in C_H1 also occurs at a distance of 6 Å from L-chain Cys 213, however, so that its replacement by a cysteinyl residue could lead to an alternative interchain disulfide bond as is found in the Ig molecules listed above.

Unusual intrachain disulfide bonds that have been observed in several Ig's can be explained on the basis of the model of Fab New (Poljak *et al.*, 1973). One of these bonds is the intra-H-chain disulfide observed in rabbit IgG, linking the polypeptide chain at positions 131–221 (O'Donnell *et al.*, 1970). An unusual disulfide bond observed in the V_H region of a human γ1 chain from IgG Daw (Press and Hogg, 1970) can also be explained by the close spatial proximity (about 6 Å) of the homologous residues in Fab New. Perhaps the most interesting interchain disulfide bond that has been reported is the one that links V_L position 80 to C_L position 171 in rabbit antibodies of restricted heterogeneity (Poulsen *et al.*, 1972; Appella *et al.*, 1973). A comparison of the sequences of these rabbit κ chains and the human λ chain from IgG New indicates that Cys 80 and Cys 171 in rabbit κ chains correspond to Ala 79 and Asn 172, respectively, in IgG New. The side chains of V_L Ala 79 and C_L Asn 172 face each other, and the distance between their α-carbon atoms is about 5.5 Å, compatible with the presence of a disulfide bond linking the two homology subunits as observed in rabbit κ chains. Thus, the Fab' model provides an adequate structural framework for the various patterns of interchain and intrachain disulfide bonds that have been established by sequence analyses and gives further support to the postulate that κ and λ L chains have the same overall three-dimensional structure and that the V_H and C_H regions of different classes of H chains (e.g., α, γ, μ) also have the same overall pattern of polypeptide chain folding. Further support for this postulate was given by the results of the crystallographic analysis of the $V_κ$ Rei dimer and the murine McPC 603 IgA-Fab (Segal *et al.*, 1974), in which the overall three-dimensional folding of the polypeptide chains is the same as that observed in the human Fab fragment. At the present stage of the structural analysis of Ig's, the postulate that they all have a common pattern of three-dimensional structure (see Figure 7) can be accepted with reasonable confidence. The hinge region that connects Fab to Fc and determines the segmental flexibility observed in some Ig's is not included in this pattern. Also, the region that determines the conformation and specificity of an antibody-combining site allows for variability in structure and function.

6. Antibody Combining Sites

As outlined above, "hypervariable" sequences have been recognized by a statistical analysis of L chains (Wu and Kabat, 1970; Kabat and Wu, 1971), around positions 30, 50, and 95. A similar conclusion was obtained by comparison of H chains, although since fewer H-chain sequences have been studied, the location of hypervariable regions was less definitive (Kabat and Wu, 1971). In addition, comparison of the sequences of human subgroup III H-chains (Kehoe and Capra, 1971) indicated the presence of a hypervariable region around residues 86–91 that had not been detected before. Amino acid sequence determination and affinity-labeling studies led to the recognition of three hypervariable regions in guinea pig H chains (Cebra *et al.*, 1974) that occur around positions 25–30, 55–65, and 100–110. The hypervariable regions of Ig's were postulated to specify the conformation of the antigen-binding sites. Support for this postulate was obtained by affinity-labeling studies (Singer *et al.*, 1971; Goetzl and Metzger, 1970; Franek, 1971; Ray and Cebra, 1972; Givol *et al.*, 1971; Fleet *et al.*, 1972), which, in general, labeled residues of V_L and V_H sequences coincident with, or adjacent to, hypervariable positions. Cross-linking of H and L chains by affinity labels (Givol *et al.*, 1971) clearly indicated that H and L chains occur in close spatial proximity at the antigen-binding site, or near it.

Independently of the results outlined above, the study of human myeloma proteins (Slater *et al.*, 1955) and of induced antibodies (Kunkel *et al.*, 1963; Oudin and Michel, 1963; Oudin, 1966) revealed the existence of "idiotypic" antigenic determinants that are unique and characteristic of every molecule studied. Quantitative investigations of the reaction between rabbit anti-*p*-azobenzoate antibodies and their antiidiotypic antisera showed that the reaction could be inhibited by the specific benzoate hapten and some of its derivatives (Brient and Nisonoff, 1970). A main conclusion derived from this finding was that the location of the hapten-binding site partially or totally overlapped with that of the idiotypic determinants. Furthermore, the work of Potter and colleagues (Barstad *et al.*, 1974) showed that mice myeloma proteins that share idiotypic (and hapten-binding) specificities also share a common amino acid sequence through the first hypervariable region of both the L and H chains. In a study of mice myeloma proteins with antidextran activity, Carson and Weigert (1973) showed that idiotypic specificity resides in both L and H chains. Reconstituted Ig molecules in which the L chain differed from the original L chain by substitution of three amino acid residues (at positions 25, 52, and 97) had a recognizably altered idiotypic constitution.

In the model of Fab' New, the regions of hypervariable sequences of both H and L chains are fully exposed to the solvent, at one end of the molecule. These regions occur at adjacent, exposed bends of tightly packed polypeptide chains that are part of the β-pleated sheets of V_H and V_L. The hypervariable positions in the L chain are related to the hypervariable positions of the H chain by an approximate two-fold rotation symmetry, with the exception of H-chain residues 86–91, which are unrelated to the other hypervariable positions (see Figure 12). A similar

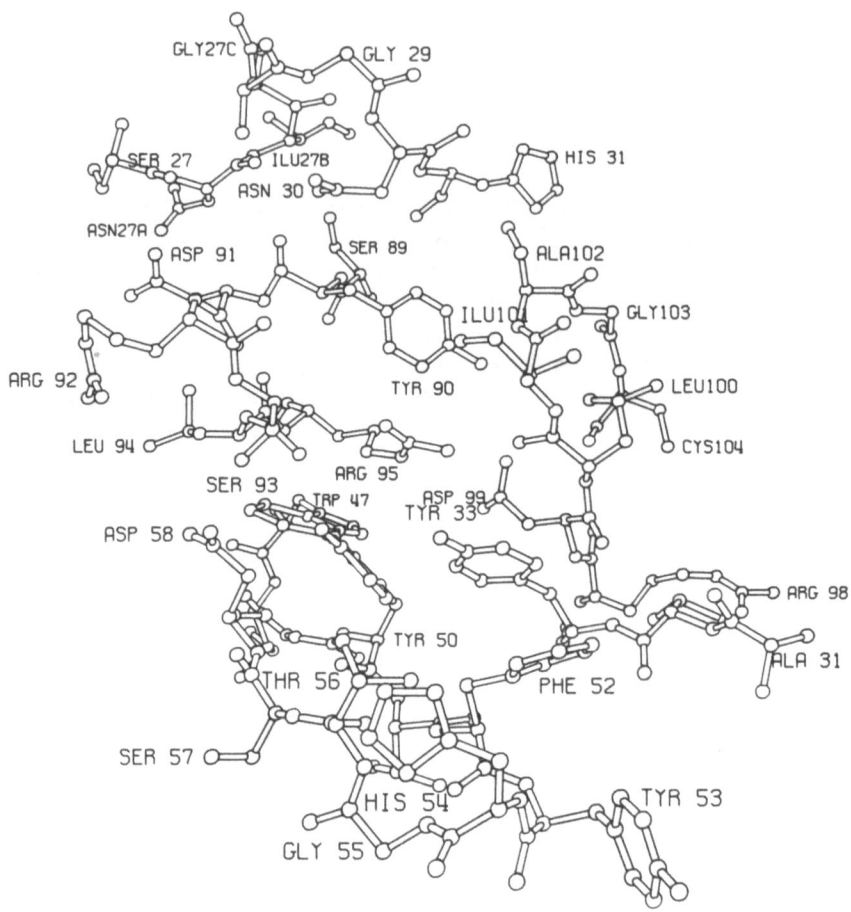

Figure 12. View of some of the amino acid residues at the active site of IgG New. The numbers refer to the amino acid sequence as given in Figures 8 and 9. Reproduced from Poljak *et al.* (1974).

observation was made in the structure of Fab from the McPC 603 IgA (Segal *et al.*, 1974) and in the L-chain dimers Mcg (Schiffer *et al.*, 1973) and Rei (Epp *et al.*, 1974). Thus, different Ig's will present unique structures at this end of the molecule, a fact that correlates with their unique idiotypic specificities.

In IgG New, the region of the combining site is relatively flat with a central channel or pocket 15 Å long, about 6–7 Å wide at its center, and about 6 Å deep. L-chain residues 27–30 delineate the "upper" limit and H-chain residues 55–65 and 30–33 the "lower" limit of this channel. Its sides are made of L-chain residues 90–95 to the left and H-chain residues 102–107 to the right. The combining center of McPC 603 IgA is deeper (about 12 Å) than that observed in IgG New. This increased depth can be attributed in part to the fact that the first hypervariable region of the κ (L) chain of McPC 603 is longer by an "insertion" of six amino acid residues (as in human $V_{\kappa III}$ sequences) than other murine and human κ and λ chains. This inserted sequence protrudes to form a "deeper" combining site and "eclipses" the second L-chain hypervariable region, which does not contribute directly to the combining site. In different H chains, the V_H hypervariable sequences around positions 100–110 have been found to consist of a variable number of amino acid residues, ranging from 13 to 20 when counted from Cys 96 to Trp 108. This hypervariable loop of V_H does not conform to the approximate local two-fold axis of symmetry relating V_L to V_H, since it bends toward the L chain, thus narrowing the central channel at the combining site. It can be concluded that the pattern of insertions or deletions, or both, characteristic of the hypervariable regions (in particular around residue 105 in human H chains) will be a major determinant of the dimensions of the active site. Variations in sequence or amino acid replacements that are also a characteristic of those regions will determine the chemical environment of the site. Thus, different antibodies may display unique antigen complementarity sites, although they share a common three-dimensional structure. A vast number of recognition specificities can be incorporated in this design while maintaining a constant, compact immunoglobulin-fold. In addition, it must be considered that since both H and L chains contribute to the combining site, random pairing could give rise to a large number of different combining sites (n^2) with a much smaller number (n) of H and L chains, further extending the economy of structural design. This aspect will be analyzed in Section 8.2. Also, as outlined above, in the L-chain dimers Mcg (Schiffer *et al.*, 1973) and Rei (Epp *et al.*, 1974), there is a cavity surrounded by the hypervariable regions of both chains that resembles the combining sites of the Fab fragments, although it is wider and symmetrical around a central two-fold rotation axis.

With the model of Fab' New as a basic structural framework, a correlation between the structure and function of the well-studied MOPC 315 anti-DNP mouse myeloma protein was made by Poljak *et al.* (1974). The L (λ) chains of IgG New and MOPC 315 (Francis *et al.*, 1974) are highly homologous and contain an equal number of residues in the third hypervariable region between the constant amino acid residues Cys 89 and Phe 99. Also, a comparison of the tentative sequence of V_H New (see Figure 10) and that of V_H MOPC 315 indicates that the third hypervariable regions of V_H in both chains between the constant Cys 96 and Trp 108 include the same number of amino acid residues. It is therefore feasible to fit the MOPC 315 sequence to the basic V_L and V_H structures obtained in the 2.0-Å Fourier map of Fab' New. The model of the MOPC 315 binding site that emerges from this comparison includes a crevice similar to that shown in Figure 12, in which L-chain Tyr 34 forms the "upper" limit; H-chain Trp 47 and Phe 50 form the "lower" limit; L-chain Phe 99, H-chain Tyr 104 and Phe 34 contribute to the "sides"; and L-chain Trp 98 and Phe 103 and H-chain Phe 105 form the 6- to 10-Å deep "floor." The high density of adjacent aromatic side chains that line this crevice, at the center of the active region, is striking and correlates with the observed specificity of MOPC IgA for DNP and other haptens that include benzene and naphthalene aromatic rings. The relatively shallow depth of the active center is in agreement with the EM study of a complex between MOPC 315 IgA and the bifunctional hapten bis(DNP-β-alanyl)-diaminosuccinate (Green *et al.*, 1971) in which the DNP groups that join the Fab arms of different IgA molecules end to end are only 15 Å apart.

7. Structure of Fab-Hapten Complexes

Human and murine myeloma Ig's are capable of reacting with a variety of haptens or antigens in a way that resembles closely the behavior of induced antibodies (see the reviews by Metzger, 1969; Krause, 1970; Potter, 1973; Seligmann and Brouet, 1973; Warner, 1975). Views that myeloma Ig's are abnormal and lack antibody activity have had to be abandoned because of mounting evidence of the antigen-binding specificities that they display. For example, human myeloma Ig's frequently possess anti-Fc and antibacterial specificities (Seligmann and Brouet, 1973). The general concept that has emerged from these and other studies is that myeloma Ig's share structural and functional properties with induced antibodies, although the definition of their specificities may require extensive screening. Key points in defining the specificity of a myeloma protein are: (1) that the affinity constant for the myeloma Ig–hapten complex should be comparable to that of induced antibodies, usually higher than 10^4–10^5 liters/mol; (2) that the number of bound ligands should be two for an IgG protein, giving rise to a linear Scatchard plot; (3) that the ligand be specifically bound by the Fab in a competitive reaction with antiidiotypic antibodies.

Myeloma proteins of murine origin have been found to bind a number of haptens such as nitrophenol, 1–6 galactans, α, 1–3 dextrans, and phosphorylcholine. These carbohydrate haptens are widely present in bacteria that inhabit the gut of the BALB/c mice in which tumors are experimentally induced. A number of phosphorylcholine-binding proteins have been obtained, and, as referred to above, one of them, McPC 603 IgA, was the object of detailed crystallographic analysis (Segal *et al.*, 1974). By diffusion of phosphorylcholine into crystals of Fab from McPC 603 IgA, a crystalline hapten–Fab complex was obtained and studied crystallographically. Phosphorylcholine binds at one end of the Fab in the cavity that is formed by hypervariable residues of the L and H chains. The binding is with amino acid residues of the H chain. Interactions with Arg (52), Lys (54), and Glu (35) are in agreement with the presence of negative and positive charges on phosphorylcholine at neutral pH. Since this hapten occupies only a small part of the binding site, a true antigenic determinant should be larger to involve all the amino acid residues at the combining site.

IgG New was submitted to a screening assay (Varga *et al.*, 1974) that led to the identification of several compounds such as uridine, orceine, menadione, and others that bind with a low-affinity constant ($K \approx 1 \times 10^3$ liters/mol) and a γ-hydroxy derivative of vitamin K_1, namely, vitamin K_1OH (Figure 13) that binds with a higher-affinity constant ($K = 1.7 \times 10^5$ liters/mol) Crystallographic analysis of the vitamin K_1OH–Fab' New complex to 3.5-Å resolution (Amzel *et al.*, 1974) indicated that vitamin K_1OH is bound to the active site region of Fab' New. The menadione moiety of vitamin K_1OH is bound to the upper part of the pocket at the center of the combining site and surrounded by hypervariable residues of both the L and H chains (Figure 13). It makes close contacts with the side groups of Tyr 90 and the peptide chain of Gly 29 and Asn 30 in V_L and with residues 100–102, 47 (a constant Trp residue in human V_H sequences), 50, and 58 in V_H. Crystallographic studies of the Fab' New complexes with the low-affinity ligands menadione, orceine, and uridine indicated that these ligands bind to the same part of the active site to which the methyl naphthoquinone rings of vitamin K_1OH are bound. Since the affinity constants of these compounds are substantially lower than that observed with the Fab' New–vitamin K_1OH complex, it was concluded that the total binding energy of the Fab'New–vitamin K_1OH complex is derived from the contacts made by the quinone rings and by the phytyl chain with the Fab' fragment.

No major conformational change was observed after binding of vitamin K_1OH

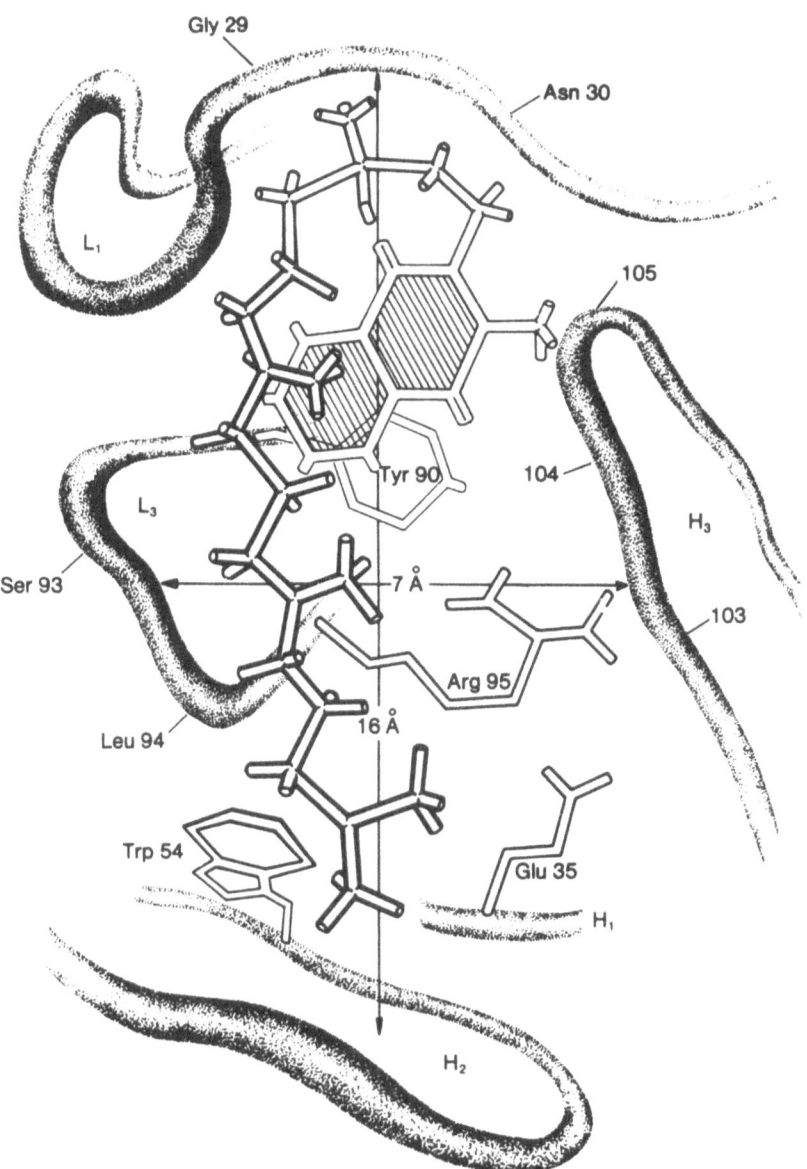

Figure 13. Drawing of vitamin K_1OH bound to the combining site of Fab New, based on a model built from a 3.5-Å-resolution difference Fourier map. (H_1, H_2, and H_3) Hypervariable segments of the H chain sequence; (L_1, L_3) first and third hypervariable regions of the L chain, respectively. L-chain Tyr 90 and Arg 95 are at the bottom of the active site, between the L and H chains. Compare this drawing with Figure 12 and see the text for a more complete description of this complex. Reproduced from Amzel *et al.* (1974).

to Fab' New. These results are similar to those obtained by Padlan *et al.* (1973), who examined the phosphorylcholine–Fab McPC 603 complex to 4.5-Å resolution and concluded that there was no major conformational change after hapten binding.

Crystallographic studies of the hapten–Fab complexes provide a structural model for the interactions between antigens and antibodies. The interactions with haptens of variable size, as seen in Fab New, are formally consistent with the notion of a combining site consisting of subsites (Schechter, 1971; Givol, 1973). The size of the combining site is in general agreement with that estimated by the experiments of Maurer (1964), Sage *et al.* (1964), Kabat (1966), Haber *et al.* (1967), and Weigert *et al.* (1974).

Binding studies and crystallographic characterization of the complexes have also been published for the λ-Mcg Bence Jones dimer (Edmundson *et al.*, 1974). A number of DNP ligands such as ε-dansyl-lysine, colchicine, 1,10-phenanthroline, menadione, and others are bound in the crystalline state. The ligands occupy the cavity that corresponds to the combining site of the Fab fragments. Although no affinity constants or other physicochemical data are given in this work, it is suggested that the Mcg Bence Jones dimer can be considered as a model for a primitive antibody.

8. Structure and Genetic Control of V_L and V_H Regions

8.1. Variable and Constant Sequences

Variable and constant features of V_L and V_H sequences can be discussed in terms of the three-dimensional structure of Ig's. Most of the bends in the polypeptide chain (hairpin bends) involve a constant Gly residue, in a sequence Pro-Gly or Ser(Thr)-Gly. In λ (L) chains, Gly residues form part of a nearly constant Phe-Gly-Gly-Gly sequence (positions 99–102); in κ chains and in H chains, the homologous sequences Phe-Gly-Gln-Gly and Trp-Gly-Gln-Gly, respectively, are frequently observed. The invariant or semiinvariant character of this sequence has been explained above by the fact that Phe 99 (or Trp 108 in V_H) make an interchain contact that is important for V_L–V_H assembly. Gly 100 in V_λ, V_κ, or Gly 109 in V_H is tightly packed between the intrachain disulfide bond and Leu 4 (constant in V_L and V_H). Gly 102 (111 in V_H) is very close to a constant aromatic residue (Tyr or Phe, 86 in V_λ, 95 in V_H); the limited space available prevents substitution by other residues at this position. V_λ residues Tyr 35, Gly 37, Ala 42, Pro 43, Tyr 86, and Phe 99 provide for close interaction with V_H and are invariant or semiinvariant. Other constant residues such as Gln 37 and Tyr 85, Glu 82, and Tyr 142 (C_L) make internal hydrogen bonds. In addition to the residues just discussed, most of the nonpolar, hydrophobic amino acids that occur in the interior of the structure between the two β-sheets are invariant or are replaced by other hydrophobic residues. In V_L, they are Leu 4, Gln 6, Val 10, Val 18, Ile 20, Cys 22, Val 32, Trp 34, Leu 46, Phe 61, Val 63, Ala 70, Leu 72, Ile 74, Leu 77, Ala 83, Tyr 85, Cys 87, Ser 89, Val 98, Thr 103, Leu 105, and Val 107. All the constant or nearly constant residues that appear at bends or contribute to intra- and intersubunit bonds seem to be important for the preservation of structure. Mutations that alter any of these residues, which constitute more than 50% of the total number of residues of the V_λ sequence, cannot be considered to be neutral or modulating. Different combinations of these invariant and semiinvariant residues that are compatible with the requirements of the constant three-dimensional structure of the homology subunits can be better explained by a process of evolutionary germ-line gene divergence than by random somatic mutations. By contrast, the nature of the residues that occur in the regions of hypervariable sequence, at one end of the molecule and fully exposed to the solvent, is not limited by any visible structural constraints.

Insertions or deletions, or both, frequently observed in Ig sequences can also be closely correlated with the three-dimensional structure. A striking example of this correlation is that of positions 27a, 27b, and 27c in human λ chains. These residues form part of a single-turn helical loop that can be deleted without creating a gap or other major alteration in the path of the polypeptide chain (Poljak *et al.*, 1973). Deletions also occur in segments of the polypeptide chains of Ig's outside the hypervariable regions. Two examples with a clear structural correlation can be given here. The first is that of the deletion of residues numbered 54–60 in the amino acid sequence of the L chain of IgG New (Poljak *et al.*, 1973). These residues very nearly constitute the loop of polypeptide chain that is characteristic of the variable regions (V_L, V_H) of Ig's and that does not occur in the constant regions C_L and C_H1 in Figure 7. An integral deletion of this loop can be easily visualized in a three-dimensional model of V_L (Figure 7) and evidently results in a stable tertiary structure similar to that of C_L. The second example to be considered here is that of the deletion of an entire homology region, which occurs in H chains synthesized by human tumor cells in the "heavy-chain disease" (Cooper *et al.*, 1972; Wolfenstein-Todel *et al.*, 1974) and in murine myeloma H chains (Milstein *et al.*, 1974a; Preud'homme *et al.*, 1975), beginning at the start of the C_H1 region (position 119) or before, and ending at position 215, close to the beginning of the C_H2 region. In the three-dimensional structure the sequence . . . Val-Ser-Ser shared by γ and μ chains (Florent *et al.*, 1974) clearly constitutes the end of V_H, and after a sharp bend, position 119 marks the beginning of the C_H1 homology subunit. Complete deletion of C_H1 should not affect the molecular interactions of C_H2 and C_H3, leading to a compact, stable Fc-line molecule with an *N*-terminal appendix of variable length.

8.2. Association of Heavy and Light Chains

As discussed in Section 6, the conformation of the active site of antibodies is determined by regions of hypervariable amino acid sequences occurring at exposed, adjacent bends of the homologous H and L polypeptide chains. A large number of recognition specificities can be incorporated by this design while maintaining the constant overall three-dimensional Ig structure. If H and L chains could recombine to form new Ig molecules, their permutation would give rise to a large number (N^2) of specificities with a minimum number (N) of H and L chains, further extending the economy of structural design. A germ-line gene hypothesis postulating that every V region of the L and H chains (V_L, V_H) is encoded by an inherited gene would thus become an attractive explanation of antibody diversity. Experimental evidence of *in vitro* recombination of H and L chains has been obtained in several laboratories. Although the possibility that *in vitro* recombination is restricted to mutually compatible subgroups of H and L chains has been submitted to experimental test (Stevenson and Mole, 1974; Capra and Kehoe, 1975), these tests do not cover all possible recombinations. Study of the three-dimensional model of a human

Fab' (Poljak *et al.*, 1975a) indicates that the close interactions between V_L and V_H involve the side chains of residues at positions 35, 37, 42, 43, 86, and 99 (L-chain sequence) and at positions 37, 39, 43, 45, 47, 95, and 108 (V_H sequence). These positions are occupied by constant residues or by fairly conservative replacements in human V_L and V_H sequences as well as in V_L and V_H sequences that have been studied from other animal species. It is striking that human λ and κ chains are very similar in their amino acid sequences at these positions: almost all human L chains have Tyr (35), Gln (37), Ala (42), Pro (43), Tyr (86), and Phe (99). L-chain positions 88 and 90 occur at the active site and also appear to provide for V_L–V_H interactions, but the importance of these interactions is more difficult to evaluate because they could be affected to some degree by the conformation of the last hypervariable region of V_H; even so, there are preferred residues at these positions: Gln (88) and Trp/Tyr (90). Undoubtedly, associations could occur *in vivo* under mechanisms of genetic control, but the interactions between V_H and V_L, which should provide the stereochemical basis for the unique association of H, L chain pairs, appear to be independent of H- and L-chain "subgroups" or even L-chain class.

8.3. Subgroups and Combining Sites

Although the notion of subgroups does not seem to be useful in predicting associations of H and L chains, and in this way the conformation of combining sites, a clear structural and functional meaning can be assigned to the notion of "subgroup" in human λ and κ chains. Since such "subgroups" are defined mainly by the presence of insertions or deletions or both in the hypervariable regions (in particular the first hypervariable region), they define different conformations of the active site. For example, human κ chains of subgroup III ($V_{κIII}$) with insertions of up to six amino acid residues in their first hypervariable region will delineate a "deeper" active site such as that observed in the murine myeloma protein McPC 603 than will a κ chain of subgroup I or a human λ chain. It is interesting to observe that murine λ chains appear to lack the pattern of deletions or insertions, or both, at the hypervariable regions characteristic of murine κ chains and human κ and λ chains. Murine λ chains would thus make a smaller contribution to the diversity of antibody specificity so that the number of genes encoding λ chains, or their expression in mice, would be limited relative to κ chains as reflected in the κ/λ serum ratio (Weigert *et al.*, 1970).

8.4. Multispecificity of Combining Sites

The capacity of individual Ig's to bind different ligands has been taken as support for the postulate that an antibody molecule can be multispecific (Eisen *et al.*, 1967; Richards *et al.*, 1975; Poljak *et al.*, 1975b). X-ray crystallographic studies (Amzel *et al.*, 1974) showed that IgG New can bind at the same locus in the active site a number of ligands with different chemical properties. A comparison has been made between IgG New and the MOPC 315 IgA, which has high affinity for DNP and also competitively binds other ligands, such as menadione, with high affinity. As pointed out in Section 6, the amino acid sequences of IgG New and those of IgA MOPC 315 are highly homologous and contain a similar number of amino acid residues in their hypervariable regions. Consequently, a tentative model of the binding site of IgA MOPC 315 can be built based on that determined for IgG New. Both Ig's have nearly equal avidities for vitamin K_1, and each binds additional ligands that are not bound by the other. These results can be taken as an indication that antibodies are multispecific and can bind different haptens at the same general site in the active region. The mode of binding, e.g., by formation of charge-transfer complexes involving aromatic side chains of the antibody, could be operative for a given chemical class of ligands such as DNP, menadione, and flavin mononucleotide (Michaelides and Eisen, 1974) for which one would expect different affinity constants reflecting different degrees of chemical interaction. In addition, small conformational changes at the active site could play a significant role in promoting the binding of different haptens to the same antibody molecule.

Independent of the role of somatic-mutation mechanisms of diversification, a gene pool encoding multispecific antibodies would be smaller than one encoding monospecific antibodies and would naturally be subject to repeated induction and expression. The advantages of carrying such a genetic pool would ensure its maintenance against genetic drift and deleterious mutations.

9. Conclusions

Some of the conclusions obtained from the X-ray crystallographic studies of the three-dimensional structure of Ig's, reviewed in the preceding sections, can be briefly summarized as follows:

1. Fab consists of four tetrahedrally arranged, globular units of three-dimensional structure containing the amino acid sequence of a homology region. V_L and V_H form a globular domain (V), C_L and C_H1 another globular domain (C). This arrangement can be tentatively extended to the Fc region as indicated in Figure 5.

2. The C_L and C_H1 "homology subunits" consist of a β-sheet made up by four antiparallel strands of polypeptide chain and another β-sheet containing three antiparallel strands. The V_L and V_H subunits can be described in similar terms. Over 50% of the amino acid residues are folded in β-pleated sheets; there is almost no helical conformation in the structure. The two irregular, roughly parallel β-sheets of each homology subunit surround a tightly packed core of hydrophobic side chains that are invariant or semiinvariant in the V_L and V_H subunits and that include the intrachain disulfide bonds that join the two sheets.

3. C_L, C_H1, V_L, and V_H share an overall pattern of polypeptide-chain folding. An additional length of polypeptide chain is characteristic of V_L and V_H (see Figure 7). The common pattern of three-dimensional structure of V_L, V_H, C_L, and C_H1 supports the proposal of gene duplication as the mechanism that gave rise to Ig genes (Hill *et al.*, 1966).

4. Although the V and C subunits share an overall pattern of three-dimensional structure, the interactions between V_L and V_H and those between C_L and C_H1 occur through different, nonhomologous regions of the polypeptide chains. Thus, when the sequences of the homology regions are compared, the hydrophobic residues that provide the interchain contacts and those that face out and interact with solvent (mostly hydrophilic) are at different positions along the primary structure. This feature, and the additional length of polypeptide chain characteristic of the V subunits, makes sequence alignments between V and C regions more

difficult than those between different V regions or between different C regions. By matching residues that occupy similar positions in the tertiary structure of the homologous subunits, an alignment can be obtained, as shown in Figure 10. Since β_2-microglobulin is highly homologous with C_H1 and C_L (Peterson *et al.*, 1972), it can be concluded that β_2-microglobulin shares the same pattern of tertiary structure.

5. Different L chains that have been studied (human and murine κ and λ chains) and different V_H and C_H1 regions of γ and α-H chains show the same overall pattern of three-dimensional structure. Various patterns of interchain disulfide bonds that have been observed in other isotypes (such as IgM) can be explained with the same model of tertiary structure. It can be concluded that the structures of the Fab fragments and the "immunoglobulin-fold" (Figure 7) occur in all Ig classes of different animal species.

6. The regions of "complementarity-determining" residues occur at one end of the molecule and include hypervariable sequences of the H and L chains, in close spatial proximity. They determine the conformation of the antigen (hapten)-combining site of antibodies. Amino acid replacements, insertions, or deletions that occur in these hypervariable regions confer unique antigen-binding and idiotypic antigenic specificities on monoclonal Ig molecules.

7. Crystallographic studies of hapten–Fab complexes show that the haptenic groups interact with a number of amino acid residues of the H and L chains at the combining site. No major conformational changes occur in the crystalline Fab structures after hapten binding.

8. At least in the case of the L chains, the notion of subgroup can be clearly correlated with the conformation of the combining site of Ig's, since different subgroups define deletions or insertions or both at the hypervariable regions.

9. The amino acid residues that constitute the contacts between V_H and V_L are invariable or semiinvariable even when different classes of chains (such as κ and λ-L chains) are compared. Thus, it appears that different L and H chains have the potential to recombine to form Ig molecules of new specificity, in agreement with experimental evidence obtained in several laboratories.

10. Amino acid replacements and deletions frequently observed in Ig sequences can be correlated with the three-dimensional structure. Integral deletions of a homology region do not affect the contacts between the remaining homology regions, which can still interact to form a stable, viable molecule. Many invariant and semiinvariant residues occupy positions that can be shown to be important for the maintenance of three-dimensional structure. The regions of hypervariable sequences are not under visible structural constraints.

10. Note Added in Proof

Since this manuscript was completed several important developments have taken place in the study of the three-dimensional structure of immunoglobulins. Some of these developments will be briefly mentioned below.

The three-dimensional structure of the human Fc fragment has been solved to a resolution of 3.5 Å (Deisenhofer *et al.*, 1976). The tertiary structures of C_H2 and C_H3 conform to the immunoglobulin fold; C_H2 and C_H3 are connected by a loosely folded segment of polypeptide chain (Ser 337 to Gln 342) which is exposed to solvent and to proteolytic attack by enzymes. The C_H3 domains interact very closely in a pattern which is similar to the C_H1–C_L interactions described in a preceding section for Fab. The C_H2 domains show no close interaction with each other, in fact carbohydrate chains lie in between the C_H2 domains. The site of attachment of the carbohydrate chain (Asn 297) is at an accessible turn of the polypeptide chain in agreement with the notion of a posttranslational insertion of carbohydrate molecules by specific transferases.

A human myeloma IgG1 protein (Kol) has been studied by X-ray diffraction (Colman *et al.*, 1976). Two interesting features were revealed by this study: (1) the Fc region could not be traced out in the crystal, a fact compatible with movement around the hinge region; (2) the Fab arms of the molecule are more extended than in the crystalline Fab fragments discussed above. These observations led Huber *et al.* (1976) to propose a structural model by which a conformational change could be transmitted from the antigen combining site to $C_\gamma2$ and $C_\gamma3$, the putative binding sites of effector functions. In this model, extended Fab arms (as observed in IgG Kol) are characteristic of the "relaxed" or "unliganded" structure in which segmental flexibility is structurally allowed by an extended hinge region. A more rigid or "minimum disorder" model, with Fab arms in the contracted conformation observed in Fab crystals and with a retracted hinge region is proposed as the liganded antibody molecule. Antigen binding would induce this conformation via longitudinal amino acid side-chain contacts from V_L to C_L, V_H to C_H1, C_H1 to C_H2, etc., decreasing segmental flexibility and bringing about the structural conformation necessary for binding of complement and for other effector functions. Although this structural model has several attractive features, it fails to explain some of the facts related to complement fixation. Moreover, a recent determination of the structure of the Fab fragment from IgG Kol carried out in Huber's laboratory shows that in the isolated Fab parts the same "relaxed" conformation present in whole IgG Kol is actually observed (P. M. Colman and J. Deisenhofer, personal communication). This observation is in disagreement with the proposed model.

Comprehensive reviews of these and related topics of immunoglobulin structure and function have recently been made by Beale and Feinstein (1976), Davies *et al.* (1975), and Poljak *et al.* (1976).

ACKNOWLEDGMENTS

The author is grateful to his colleagues who helped to obtain some of the results outlined in this chapter through several years of work in his laboratory. During the course of this work, substantial support was derived from National Institutes of Health and American Cancer Society research grants and from an N.I.H. Research Career Development Award.

References

Amzel, L. M., Poljak, R. J., Saul, F., Varga, J. M., and Richards, F. F., 1974, The three-dimensional structure of a combining region–ligand complex of IgG New at 3.5-Å resolution, *Proc. Natl. Acad. Sci.* **71**:1427–1430.

Appella, E., Roholt, O. A., Chersi, A., Radziminski, G., and Pressman, D., 1973, Amino acid sequence of the light chain derived from a rabbit anti-*p*-azobenzoate antibody of restricted heterogeneity, *Biochem. Biophys. Res. Commun.* **53**:1122–1129.

Avey, H. P., Poljak, R. J., Rossi, G., and Nisonoff, A., 1968, Crystallographic data for the Fab fragment of a human myeloma immunoglobulin, *Nature (London)* **220**:1248–1249.

Baglioni, C., Alescio-Zonta, L., Cioli, D., and Carbonara, A., 1966, Allelic antigenic factor Inv(a) of the light chains of human immunoglobulins: Chemical basis, *Science* **152**:1517–1519.

Barstad, P., Rudikoff, S., Potter, M., Cohn, M., Konigsberg, W., and Hood, L., 1974, Immunoglobulin structure: Amino terminal sequences of mouse myeloma proteins that bind phosphorylcholine, *Science* **183**:962–964.

Beale, D., and Feinstein, A., 1976, Structure and function of the constant regions of immunoglobulins, *Quart. Rev. Biophys.* **9**: 135–161.

Birshtein, B. K., Hussain, Q. Z., and Cebra, J. J., 1971, Structure of heavy chain from strain 13 guinea pig immunoglobulin-G(2). III. Amino acid sequence of the region around the half cystine joining heavy and light chains, *Biochemistry* **10**:18–25.

Brient, B. W., and Nisonoff, A., 1970, Quantitative investigations of idiotypic antibodies, *J. Exp. Med.* **132**:951–962.

Capra, J. D., and Kehoe, J. M., 1975, Distribution and association of heavy and light chain variable region subgroups among human IgA immunoglobulins, *J. Immunol.* **114**:678–681.

Carson, D., and Weigert, M., 1973, Immunochemical analysis of the cross-reacting idiotypes of mouse myeloma proteins with anti-dextran activity and normal anti-dextran antibody, *Proc. Natl. Acad. Sci. U.S.A.* **70**:235–239.

Cebra, J. J., Ray, A., Benjamin, D., and Birshtein, B. K., 1971, Localization of affinity label within the primary structure of γ2 chain from guinea pig IgG(2), in: *Progress in Immunology* (B. Amos, ed.), pp. 269–284, Academic Press, New York.

Cebra, J. J., Koo, P. H., and Ray, A., 1974, Specificity of antibodies: Primary structural basis of hapten binding, *Science* **186**:263–265.

Chen, B. L., and Poljak, R. J., 1974, Amino acid sequence of the (λ) light chain of a human myeloma immunoglobulin (IgG New), *Biochemistry* **13**:1295–1302.

Cold Spring Harbor Symposium, 1971, Structure and function of proteins at the three-dimensional level, *Cold Spring Harbor Symp. Quant. Biol.* **36**.

Colman, P. M. Deisenhofer, J., Huber, R., and Palm, W., 1976, Structure of the human antibody molecule Kol (IgG1): An electron density map at 5 Å resolution, *J. Mol. Biol.* **100**:257–272.

Cooper, S. M., Franklin, E. C., and Frangione, B., 1972, Molecular defect in a gamma-2 heavy chain, *Science* **176**:187–189.

Davies, D. R., Padlan, E. A., and Segal, D. M., 1975, Three-dimensional structure of immunoglobulins, *Annu. Rev. Biochem.* **44**:639–667.

Dayhoff, M. O., 1972, *Atlas of Protein Sequence and Structure,* Vol. 5, p. D-2, National Biomedical Research Foundation, Silver Spring, Maryland.

Deisenhofer, J., Colman, P. M., Epp, O., and Huber, R., 1976, Crystallographic structural studies of a human Fc fragment. II. A complete model based on a Fourier map at 3.5 Å resolution, *Hoppe-Seyler's Z. Physiol. Chem.* **357**:1421–1433.

De Preval, C., Pink, J. R. L., and Milstein, C., 1970, Variability of interchain binding of immunoglobulins, *Nature (London)* **228**:930–932.

Dickerson, R. E., 1964, X-ray analysis and protein structure, in: *The Proteins* (H. Neurath, ed.), pp. 603–778, Academic Press, New York.

Edelman, G. M., Cunningham, B. A., Gall, W. E., Gottlieb, P. D., Rutishauser, U., and Waxdal, M. J., 1969, The covalent structure of an entire γG immunoglobulin molecule, *Proc. Natl. Acad. Sci. U.S.A.* **63**:78–85.

Edmundson, A. B., Ely, K. R., Girling, R. L., Abola, E. E., Schiffer, M., Westholm, F. A., Fausch, M. D., and Deutsch, H. F., 1974, Binding of 2,4-dinitrophenyl compounds and other small molecules to a crystalline λ-type Bence–Jones dimer, *Biochemistry* **13**:3816–3827.

Eisen, H. N., Little, J. R., Osterland, C. K., and Simms, E. S., 1967, A myeloma protein with antibody activity, *Cold Spring Harbor Symp. Quant. Biol.* **32**:75–81.

Epp, O., Colman, P., Fehlhammer, H., Bode, W., Schiffer, M., and Huber, R., 1974, Crystal and molecular structure of a dimer composed of the variable protions of the Bence–Jones protein Rei, *Eur. J. Biochem.* **45**:513–524.

Fleet, G. W. J., Knowles, J. R., and Porter, R. R., 1972, The antibody binding site: Labeling of a specific antibody against the photo-precursor of an aryl nitrene, *Biochem. J.* **128**:499–508.

Florent, G., Lehman, D., and Putnam, F. W., 1974, The switch point in μ heavy chains of human IgM immunoglobulins, *Biochemistry* **13**:2482–2498.

Francis, S. H., Leslie, R. G. Q., Hood, L., and Eisen, H. N., 1974, Amino acid sequence of the variable region of the heavy (α) chain of a mouse myeloma protein with anti-hapten activity, *Proc. Natl. Acad. Sci. U.S.A.* **71**:1123–1127.

Franek, F., 1971, Affinity labeling by *N*-nitrobenzenediazonium fluoroborate of porcine anti-dinitrophenyl antibodies, *Eur. J. Biochem.* **19**:176–183.

Givol, D., 1973, Structural analysis of the antibody combining site, in: *Contemporary Topics in Molecular Immunology,* Vol. 2 (R. A. Reisfeld and W. J. Mandy, eds.), pp. 27–50, Plenum Press, New York.

Givol, D., Strausbauch, P. H., Hurwitz, E., Wilchek, M., Haimovich, J., and Eisen, H. N., 1971, Affinity labeling and cross-linking of the heavy and light chains of a myeloma protein with anti-2,4-dinitrophenyl activity, *Biochemistry* **10**:3461–3466.

Goetzl, E. J., and Metzger, H., 1970, Affinity labeling of a mouse myeloma protein which binds nitrophenyl ligands: Sequence and position of a labeled tryptic peptide. *Biochemistry* **9**:3862–3871.

Goldstein, D. J., Humphrey, R. L., and Poljak, R. J., 1968, Human Fc fragment: Crystallographic evidence for two equivalent subunits, *J. Mol. Biol.* **35**:247–251.

Green, N. M., Dourmashkin, R. R., and Parkhouse, R. M. E., 1971, Electron microscopy of human and mouse myeloma serum IgA, *J. Mol. Biol.* **56**:203–208.

Grey, H. M., Abel, C. A., Yount, W. J., and Kunkel, H. G., 1968, A subclass of human γA-globulins (γA2) which lacks the disulfide bonds linking heavy and light chains, *J. Exp. Med.* **128**:1223–1236.

Haber, E., Richards, F. F., Spragg, J., Austen, K. F., Vallotton, M., and Page, L. B., 1967, Modifications in the heterogeneity of the antibody response, *Cold Spring Harbor Symp. Quant. Biol.* **32**:299–310.

Haimovich, J., Givol, D., and Eisen, H. N., 1970, Affinity labeling of the H and L chains of a myeloma protein with anti-2,4-dinitrophenyl activity, *Proc. Natl. Acad. Sci. U.S.A.* **67**:1656–1661.

Hill, R. L., Delaney, R., Fellow, R. E., Jr., and Lebowitz, H.E., 1966, The evolutionary origins of the immunoglobulins, *Proc. Natl. Acad. Sci. U.S.A.* **56**:1762–1767.

Holmes, K. C., and Blow, D. M., 1965, The use of X-ray diffraction in the study of protein and nucleic acid structure, *Methods Biochem. Anal.* **13**:113–239.

Huber, R., Deisenhofer, J., Colman, P. M., Matsushima, M., and Palm, W., 1976, Crystallographic structure studies of an IgG molecule and an Fc fragment, *Nature (London)* **264**:415–420.

Humphrey, R. L., and Owens, A. H., Jr., 1972, Immunoglobulins and the plasma cell dyscrasias, in: *The Principles and Practice of Medicine* (A. H. Harvey, R. J. Johns, A. H. Owens, Jr., and R. S. Ross, eds.), pp. 1206–1240, Appleton-Century-Crofts, New York.

Humphrey, R. L., Avey, H. P., Becka, L. N., Poljak, R. J., Rossi, G., Choi, T. K., and Nisonoff, A., 1969, X-ray crystallographic study of the Fab fragments from two human myeloma proteins, *J. Mol. Biol.* **43**:223–226.

Inbar, D., Hochman, Y., and Givol, D., 1972, Localization of antibody-combining sites within the variable portions of heavy and light chains, *Proc. Natl. Acad. Sci. U.S.A.* **69**:2659–2662.

Kabat, E. A., 1966, The nature of an antigenic determinant, *J. Immunol.* **97**:1–11.

Kabat, E. A., and Wu, T. T., 1971, Attempts to locate complementarity-determining residues in the variable positions of light and heavy chains, *Ann. N. Y. Acad. Sci.* **190**:382–391.

Karlsson, F. A., Peterson, P. A., and Berggord, I., 1972, A structural feature of human immunoglobulin light chains, *J. Biol. Chem.* **247**:1065–1073.

Kehoe, M. J., and Capra, J. D., 1971, Localization of two additional hypervariable regions in immunoglobulin heavy chains, *Proc. Natl. Acad. Sci. U.S.A.* **68**:2019–2021.

Krause, R. M., 1970, The search for antibodies with molecular uniformity, in: *Advances in Immunology,* Vol. 12 (F. J. Dixon, Jr., and H. G. Kunkel, eds.), pp. 1–56, Academic Press, New York.

Kunkel, H. G., Mannick, M., and Williams, R. C., Jr., 1963, Individual antigenic specificity of isolated antibodies, *Science* **140**:1218–1219.

Labaw, L. W., and Davies, D. R., 1971, An electron microscopic study of human γG1 immunoglobulin crystals, *J. Biol. Chem.* **246**:3760–3762.

Lopes, A. D., and Steiner, L. A., 1973, A structural defect in a crystallizable myeloma protein, *Fed. Proc. Fed. Am. Soc. Exp. Biol.* **32**:1003.

Matthews, B. W., 1976, X-ray crystallographic studies of proteins, *Ann. Rev. Phys. Chem.* **27**:493.

Maurer, P. H., 1964, Use of synthetic polymers of amino acids to study the basis of antigenicity, *Prog. Allergy* **8**:1–40.

Metzger, H., 1969, Myeloma proteins and antibodies, *Am. J. Med.* **47**:837–844.

Michaelides, M. C., and Eisen, H. N., 1974, The strange cross-reaction of menadione (vitamin K₃) and 2,4-dinitrophenyl ligands with a myeloma protein and some conventional antibodies, *J. Exp. Med.* **140**:687–702.

Milstein, C. P., Adetugbo, K., Cowan, N. J., and Secher, D. S., 1974a, Clonal variants of myeloma cells, in: *Progress in Immunology II*, Vol. 1 (L. Brent and E. J. Holborow, eds.), pp. 157–168, North-Holland, Amsterdam.

Milstein, C. P., Steinberg, A. G., McLaughlin, C. L., and Solomon, A., 1974b, Amino acid sequence change associated with genetic marker Inv (2) of human immunoglobulin, *Nature (London)* **248**:160–161.

Nisonoff, A., Wissler, F. C., Lippman, L. N., and Woer, D. L., 1960, Separation of univalent fragments from the bivalent rabbit antibody molecule by reduction of disulfide bonds, *Arch. Biochem. Biophys.* **89**:230–244.

O'Donnell, I. J., Frangione, B., and Porter, R. R., 1970, The disulfide bonds of the heavy chain of rabbit immunoglobulin G, *Biochem. J.* **116**:261–268.

Oudin, J., 1966, Genetic regulation of immunoglobulin synthesis, *J. Cell. Physiol.* **67**(Suppl. 1):77–108.

Oudin, J., and Michel, M., 1963, Une nouvelle forme de'allotypie des globulines γ du serum de lapin, apparemment liee a la fonction et a la specificite anticorps, *C. R. Acad. Sci.* **257**:805–808.

Padlan, E. A., Segal, D. M., Spande, T. F., Davies, D. R., Rudikoff, S., and Potter, M., 1973, Structure at 4.5 Å resolution of a phosphorylcholine-binding Fab, *Nature (London) New Biol.* **245**:165–167.

Perutz, M. F., Rossman, M. G., Cullis, A. F., Muirhead, H., Will, G., and North, A. C. T., 1960, Structure of hemoglobin: A three-dimensional Fourier synthesis at 5.5 Å resolution obtained by X-ray analysis, *Nature (London)* **185**:416–422.

Peterson, P. A., Cunningham, B. A., Berggard, I., and Edelman, G. M., 1972, β₂-Microglobulin—A free immunoglobulin domain, *Proc. Natl. Acad. Sci. U.S.A.* **69**:1697–1701.

Pilz, I., Puchwein, G., Kratky, O., Herbst, M., Naager, O., Gall, W. E., and Edelman, G. M., 1970, Small angle X-ray scattering of a homogeneous γG1 immunoglobulin, *Biochemistry* **9**:211–219.

Pilz, I., Kratky, O., Licht, A., and Sela, M., 1975, Shape and volume of fragments Fab' and (Fab')₂ of anti-poly (D-alanyl) antibodies in the presence and absence of tetra-D-alanine as determined by small-angle X-ray scattering, *Biochemistry* **14**:1326–1333.

Poljak, R. J., 1973, X-ray crystallographic studies of immunoglobulins, in: *Contemporary Topics in Molecular Immunology* (R. A. Reisfeld and W. J. Mandy, eds.), Vol. 2, pp. 1–26, Plenum Press, New York.

Poljak, R. J., Amzel, L. M., Avey, H. P., Becka, L. N., and Nisonoff, A., 1972, Structure of Fab' New at 6 Å resolution, *Nature (London) New Biol.* **235**:137–140.

Poljak, R. J., Amzel, L. M., Avey, H. P., Chen, B. L., Phizackerley, R. P., and Saul, F., 1973, Three-dimensional structure of the Fab' fragment of a human immunoglobulin at 2.8-Å resolution *Proc. Natl. Acad. Sci. U.S.A.* **70**:3305–3310.

Poljak, R. J., Amzel, L. M., Chen, B. L., Phizackerley, R. P., and Saul, F., 1974, The three-dimensional structure of the Fab' fragment of a human myeloma immunoglobulin at 2.0-Å resolution, *Proc. Natl. Acad. Sci. U.S.A.* **71**:3440–3444.

Poljak, R. J., Amzel, L. M., Chen, B. L., Phizackerley, R. P., and Saul, F., 1975a, Structural basis for the association of heavy and light chains and the relation of subgroups to the conformation of the active site of immunoglobulins, *Immunogenetics* **2**:393–394.

Poljak, R. J., Amzel, L. M., Chen, B. L., Phizackerley, R. P., and Saul, F., 1975b, Structure and specificity of antibody molecules, *Philos. Trans. R. Soc. London B* **272**:43–51.

Poljak, R. J., Amzel, L. M., and Phizackerley, R. P., 1976, Studies on the three-dimensional structure of immunoglobulins, *Prog. Biophys. Molec. Biol.* **31**:67–93.

Poljak, R. J., Nakashima, Y., Chen, B. L., and Konigsberg, W., 1977, Amino acid sequence of the V_H region of a human myeloma immunoglobulin (IgG New), *Biochemistry* **16**:3412–3420.

Porter, R. R., 1959, The hydrolysis of rabbit γ-globulin and antibodies with crystalline papain, *Biochem. J.* **73**:119–127.

Potter, M., 1973, The developmental history of the neoplastic plasma cell in mice: A brief review of recent developments, *Semin. Hematol.* **10**:19–32.

Poulsen, K., Fraser, K. J., and Haber, E., 1972, An active derivative of rabbit antibody light chain composed of the constant and the variable domains held together only by a native disulfide bond, *Proc. Natl. Acad. Sci. U.S.A.* **69**:2495–2499.

Press, E. M., and Hogg, N. M., 1970, The amino acid sequences of the Fd fragments of two human γ1 heavy chains, *Biochem. J.* **117**:641–660.

Preud'homme, J. L., Birshtein, B. K., and Scharff, M. D., 1975, Variants of a mouse myeloma cell line that synthesize immunoglobulin heavy chains having an altered serotype, *Proc. Natl. Acad. Sci. U.S.A.* **72**:1427–1430.

Putnam, F. W., Titani, K., Wikler, M. and Shinoda, T., 1967, Structure and evolution of kappa and lambda light chains, *Cold Spring Harbor Symp. Quant. Biol.* **32**:9–30.

Putnam, F. W., Shimizu, A., Paul, C., Shinoda, T., and Kohler, H., 1971, The amino acid sequence of human macroglobulins, *Ann. N. Y. Acad. Sci.* **190**:83–102.

Ray, A., and Cebra, J. J., 1972, Localization of affinity-labeled residues in the primary structure of anti-dinitrophenyl antibody raised in strain 13 guinea pigs, *Biochemistry* **11**:3647–3657.

Richards, F. F., Konigsberg, W. H., Rosenstein, R. W., and Varga, J. M., 1975, On the specificity of antibodies, *Science* **187**:130–137.

Rossi, G., and Nisonoff, A., 1968, Crystallization of fragment Fab of human IgG myeloma proteins, *Biochem. Biophys. Res. Commun.* **31**:914–918.

Rossi, G., Choi, T. K. and Nisonoff, A., 1969, Crystals of fragment Fab': Preparation from pepsin digests of human IgG myeloma proteins, *Nature (London)* **223**:837–838.

Sage, H. J., Deutsch, H. F., Fasman, G., and Levine, L., 1964, The serological specificity of the poly-alanine immune system, *Immunochemistry* **1**:133–144.

Sarma, V. R., Silverton, E. W., Davies, D. R., and Terry, W. D., 1971, The three-dimensional structure at 6 Å resolution of a human γG1 immunoglobulin molecule, *J. Biol. Chem.* **246**:3753–3759.

Schechter, I., 1971, Mapping the combining sites of antibodies specific to polyalanine chains, *Ann. N. Y. Acad. Sci.* **190**:394–418.

Schiffer, M., Girling, R. L., Ely, K. R., and Edmundson, A. B., 1973, Structure of a lambda-type Bence–Jones protein at 3.5-Å resolution, *Biochemistry* **12**:4620–4631.

Segal, D. M., Padlan, E. A., Cohen, G. H., Rudikoff, S., Potter, M., and Davies, D. R., 1974, The three-dimensional structure of a phosphorylcholine-binding mouse immunoglobulin Fab and the nature of the antigen binding site, *Proc. Natl. Acad. Sci. U.S.A.* **71**:4298–4302.

Sela, M., 1969, Antigenicity: Some molecular aspects, *Science* **166**:1365–1374.

Seligmann, M., and Brouet, J. C., 1973, Antibody activity of human myeloma globulins, *Semin. Hematol.* **10**:163–177.

Singer, S. J., Solbin, L. I., Thorpe, N. O., and Fenton, J. W., 1967, On the structure of antibody active sites, *Cold Spring Harbor Symp. Quant. Biol.* **32**:99–109.

Singer, S. J., Martin, N., and Thorpe, N. O., 1971, Affinity labeling of the active sites of antibodies and myeloma proteins, *Ann. N. Y. Acad. Sci.* **190**:342–351.

Slater, R. J., Ward, S. M., and Kunkel, H. G., 1955, Immunological relationships among the myeloma proteins, *J. Exp. Med.* **101**:85–108.

Solomon, A., and McLaughlin, C. L., 1969, Bence–Jones proteins and light chains of immunoglobulins, *J. Biol. Chem.* **244**:3395–3404.

Steiner, L. A., and Porter, R. R., 1967, The interchain disulfide bonds of a human pathological immunoglobulin, *Biochemistry* **6**:3957–3970.

Stevenson, G. T., and Mole, L. E., 1974, The specificity of chain interactions among immunoglobulins: Combination of γ chains with kappa chains of the same subgroup as in the parent immunoglobulin G, *Biochem. J.* **139**:369–374.

Turner, M. W., and Bennich, H., 1968, Subfragments from the Fc fragment of human immunoglobulin G: Isolation and physicochemical characterization, *Biochem. J.* **107**:171–178.

Valentine, R. C., and Green, N. M., 1967, Electron microscopy of an antibody–hapten complex, *J. Mol. Bio.* **27**:615–617.

Varga, J. M., Lande, S., and Richards, F. F., 1974, Immunoglobulins with multiple binding functions, *J. Immunol.* **112**:1565–1570.

Warner, N. L., 1975, Autoimmunity and the pathogenesis of plasma cell tumor induction in NZB inbred and hybrid mice, *Immunogenetics* **2**:1–20.

Weigert, M. G., Cesari, I. M., Yonkovice, S. J., and Cohn, M., 1970, Variability in the lambda light chain sequences of mouse antibody, *Nature (London)* **228**:1045–1047.

Weigert, M. G., Raschke, W. C., Carson, D., and Cohn, M., 1974, Immunochemical analysis of the

36

ROBERTO J. POLJAK

idiotypes of mouse myeloma proteins with specificity for levan or dextran, *J. Exp. Med.* **139**:137–147.

Welscher, H. D., 1969, Correlations between amino acid sequence and conformation of immunoglobulin light chains, *Int. J. Protein Res.* **1**:253–265.

Wolfenstein-Todel, C., Mihaesco, E., and Frangione, B., 1974, "Alpha chain disease" protein Def: Internal deletion of a human immunoglobulin A_1 heavy chain, *Proc. Natl. Acad. Sci. U.S.A.* **71**:974–978.

Wu, T. T., and Kabat, E. A., 1970, An analysis of the sequences of the variable regions of Bence–Jones proteins and myeloma light chains and their implications for antibody complementarity, *J. Exp. Med.* **132**:211–250.

Yguerabide, J., Epstein, H. F., and Stryer, L., 1970, Segmental flexibility in an antibody molecule, *J. Mol. Biol.* **51**:573–590.

2

Solution Conformation and Segmental Flexibility of Immunoglobulins

RENATA E. CATHOU

1. Introduction

The immune response is highly complex and is regulated by an interwoven network of feedback mechanisms in which antibody molecules play a central role. One of the major functions of antibody is to initiate biological effector functions after binding to specific antigens. These effector functions are varied and include: (1) recognition of incoming antigen by specific memory cells, leading to differentiation of the small B lymphocyte to an antibody-producing plasma cell; (2) complement activation, which has several end results, e.g., cell lysis, as well as elaboration of chemotactic and inflammatory factors; (3) immediate hypersensitivity, which involves release of histamine from mast cells and basophils; (4) T-cell helper and suppressor functions, which control the immune response; (5) cell-mediated immunity. All these processes share in common the specific combination of antibody and antigen (the recognition step), which then triggers more general biochemical events (the biological effector steps). In the case of T-cell function, the role of immunoglobulin (Ig) has not been firmly established, but there is recent evidence for an Ig-like molecule on the surface of T cells that can bind antigen (reviewed by Marchalonis, 1975).

Antibody thus acts as a transducer that transmits a signal from the antigen-combining sites, which are located at one end of the molecule, to distally located effector-molecule-binding sites. The transmission of such information typically occurs over distances of greater than 80 Å and across several conformational domains.

To fulfill these functions, antibody molecules have evolved into a set of structures with highly unusual conformations and with appropriate dynamic proper-

---

RENATA E. CATHOU • Department of Biochemistry and Pharmacology, Tufts University School of Medicine, Boston, Massachusetts 02111.

ties. All Ig's are multisubunit proteins with similarities in their basic architecture. The IgG molecule, which can be considered to be a prototype for other classes, consists of four polypeptide chains—two heavy (H) and two light (L)—held together by strong noncovalent forces as well as by disulfide bonds. Perhaps the most intriguing feature of the structure is the folding of the chains into reasonably separate and compact regions that have been designated *domains* (Edelman *et al.*, 1969). Since the various functions of Ig's can be localized to different domains (see Figure 1), it is clear that the molecular mechanism of information transfer will depend inherently on the arrangement of the domains in both time and space.

In this chapter, we will be concerned primarily with the conformation as defined to be the spatial relationship of structural entities the size of domains, or larger. The arrangement of the constituent polypeptide chains and amino acid residues within domains is more appropriately considered as the secondary and tertiary structure, which is discussed in Chapter 1. We will, however, discuss conformation at all levels in the context of conformational changes that occur on antibody–antigen binding. The dynamic change in spatial arrangement of domains, specifically those changes observed to occur on a nanosecond time scale, will also be considered. Finally, this chapter does not attempt to be comprehensive; rather, it presents a selection of reports that is intended to give the reader an overall view of the current state of thinking on the subject. For a more detailed discussion, the reader is referred to the recent reviews by Dorrington and Tanford (1970) and Cathou and Dorrington (1975).

The problem of determining the complete conformation in solution at atomic

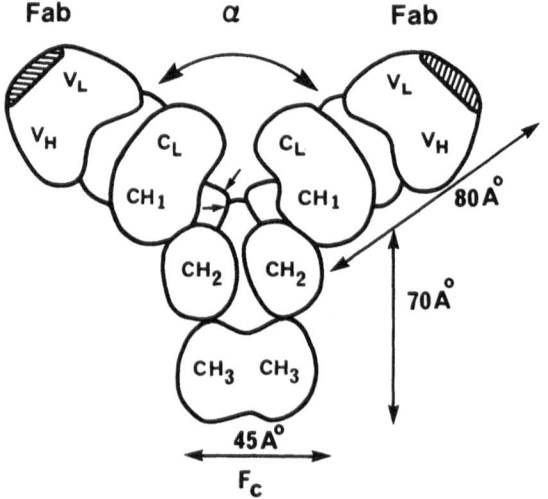

Figure 1. Schematic structure of IgG. The Fab and Fc fragments are each composed of several homology regions or domains. Fab contains the variable (V) regions of the L (V_L) and H (V_H) chains as well as the constant (C) region of the L chain (C_L) and the first C region of the H chain (C_H1); the shapes of domains in the diagram approximate those found by X-ray diffraction studies (Poljak *et al.*, 1973; Segal *et al.*, 1974). Fc consists of the second (C_H2) and third (C_H3) C regions of the H chains; recent evidence suggests that the C_H2 domains are farther apart than indicated and have a combined width of about 70 Å (Deisenhofer *et al.*, 1976). The two antigen-combining sites are located at the outer tips of the Fab and are shown as shaded areas. Binding of the first component of the classic complement cascade occurs in C_H2. Cell fixation is localized in C_H3. Cleavage in the hinge region by papain occurs *N*-terminal to the inter-H-chain disulfide(s), one of which is shown, as in rabbit IgG (Cys 226), to yield Fab and Fc fragments. Cleavage on the other side of the disulfide produces (Fab')$_2$. Cleavage points are shown by small arrows. Cys 226 has been estimated to be 7.5 Å (Colman *et al.*, 1976) to 16 Å (Bunting and Cathou, 1974) distant from the L–H disulfide, which is at the lower end of the Fab fragment. In isolated Fc fragments, the hinge peptide may lie between the C_H2 domains (Deisenhofer *et al.*, 1976). The angle α between Fab fragments is larger than 80–100°, and in the crystallized human IgG1 protein Ko1 was found to 125° (Colman *et al.*, 1976).

resolution of a molecule as large as an Ig is awesome. Only one technique, X-ray diffraction of single crystals, has sufficient potential information content to define the entire three-dimensional structure. This approach has been successfully applied to elucidation of the structures of Fab (antigen-binding) and Fc (constant) fragments, Bence–Jones proteins, and V-region domains of L chains (Poljak *et al.*, 1973; Segal *et al.*, 1974; Schiffer *et al.*, 1973; Epp *et al.*, 1974; Deisenhofer *et al.*, 1976). Application of this technique to whole Ig's, however, has been possible only at lower resolution so far (Sarma *et al.*, 1971; Colman *et al.*, 1976). Furthermore, by its very nature, crystallography provides a static picture of a molecule that is in a single conformation.

Fortunately, other biophysical methods exist that, if resourcefully applied, can yield information on the size, shape, and dynamic properties of Ig's, and although no one technique can provide all the desired information, parallel studies from a variety of approaches have led to considerable detail.

2. Immunoglobulin G

2.1. Conformation

The four polypeptide chains of IgG are folded to give three large substructures, two of which, denoted Fab, are identical and each of which contains an antigen-combining site, and an Fc (see Figure 1). Proteolytic digestion by a number of enzymes (i.e., papain, pepsin, trypsin) results in cleavage of the molecule in the same general area to give these Fab and Fc fragments, although with pepsin, Fc is not recovered (Porter, 1958; Nisonoff *et al.*, 1960; Givol and DeLorenzo, 1968). The Fab fragment contains all the L chain and the amino-terminal half of the H chain (Fd), whereas Fc includes the carboxy-terminal halves of the two H chains. The chains are further folded into "domains" (see Chapter 1 for more details). Examination of the gross conformation of Fab and Fc by a variety of crystallographic and hydrodynamic techniques has shown that they can be reasonably approximated as ellipsoids with an axial ratio of about 2, even though each fragment is composed of four domains and there is a relatively empty space in the middle of each fragment (Noelken *et al.*, 1965; Yguerabide *et al.*, 1970; Pilz *et al.*, 1970; Brochon and Wahl, 1972; Poljak *et al.*, 1973; Deisenhofer *et al.*, 1976). In the native molecule, these three structures, two Fab and one Fc, are joined via short sections of H chain, susceptible to enzymatic cleavage, designated as the *hinge regions* (see Figure 1).

From a comparison of the hydrodynamic properties of IgG and of the proteolytic fragments, Noelken *et al.* (1965) first proposed that the native molecule consisted of three globular regions linked together by a more exposed, flexible, and hydrated stretch of each H chain that corresponded to the hinge region (see Figure 2). Later models proposed by other laboratories have essentially confirmed the correctness of the model of Noelken and co-workers, although the descriptions of the hinge region differ somewhat and have included more information on the spatial relationship of the fragments.

The antigen-combining site is located in the V region at or very near the tip of the Fab arm, as shown by electron-microscopic (EM) (Valentine and Green, 1967), energy-transfer (Werner *et al.*, 1972), and X-ray diffraction (Segal *et al.*, 1974; Amzel *et al.*, 1974) studies.

RENATA E. CATHOU

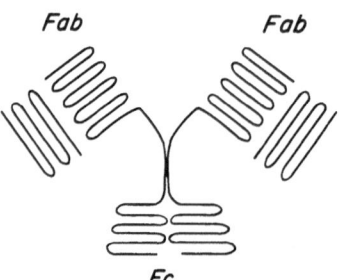

Fab   *Fab*

Fc

Figure 2. Schematic structure of IgG proposed by Noelken *et al.* (1965). The basic features of this model are: (1) compact Fab and Fc regions and (2) a loose, hydrated hinge region. Adapted from Noelken *et al.* (1965).

Early attempts to visualize antibody molecules by EM led to variable results, and most micrographs of free antibody molecules showed a disappointing lack of characteristic structure (reviewed by Green, 1969). Micrographs of antigen-bound antibody taken by a number of workers suggested rodlike molecules, however, and under the right conditions, single antibody molecules could be observed to be bent in the middle or into a loop linking neighboring antigenic determinants when these determinants were on the same virion. Feinstein and Rowe (1965) were able to tentatively identify Fab and Fc regions of antiferritin antibodies and stressed that the angle between the arms of the molecule was variable.

Valentine and Green (1967), employing the brilliant expedient of a small bivalent hapten combined with antibody, obtained soluble polymers from which the shape of the constituent antibody molecules could be deduced. From these micrographs, it could be seen that the structure of an antibody molecule was in the shape of the letter Y, with the Fab fragments forming the arms and Fc forming the tail (see Figure 3). A wide range of angles was observed between Fab arms in any given molecule in the different polymers, however, and there was no suggestion of a preferred angle. Furthermore, the Fc was not always symmetrically disposed between the Fab arms and was not confined to the plane defined by them. Although these observations suggested the presence of a flexible hinge region, the latter was not extended as suggested by Noelken *et al.* (1965), but appeared instead to be compact with no evidence of strain penetration. More recently, electron micrographs of antibodies specific to ribosomal proteins complexed to ribosomal subunits have been obtained (Tischendorf *et al.,* 1975; Wittman, 1976). In these micrographs, antibody molecules, singly or doubly linked to ribosomes, could be seen to generally have a very open Y, but not quite T, shape.

Although EM clearly revealed the subunit nature of IgG molecules and the arrangement of Fab and Fc moieties into a basic Y shape, it left unanswered a number of questions: (1) What is the average disposition of the Fab's and Fc in solution and before attachment to antigen (the "resting" state)? (2) What is the degree of inherent flexibility? Further, it was not clear whether an antibody molecule opened or closed on combination with antigen. To try to answer these questions, other approaches had to be employed.

Determination of the conformation of a large and complex molecule such as an Ig is an inherently difficult task. The methods that have been employed, i.e., small-angle X-ray scattering, transient electric birefringence, resonance-energy transfer, and attempts to intramolecularly cross-link the two antigen-binding sites on antibody molecules with long bivalent haptens, must, by their nature, be directed to elucidating specific and limited aspects of molecular conformation. Further, the

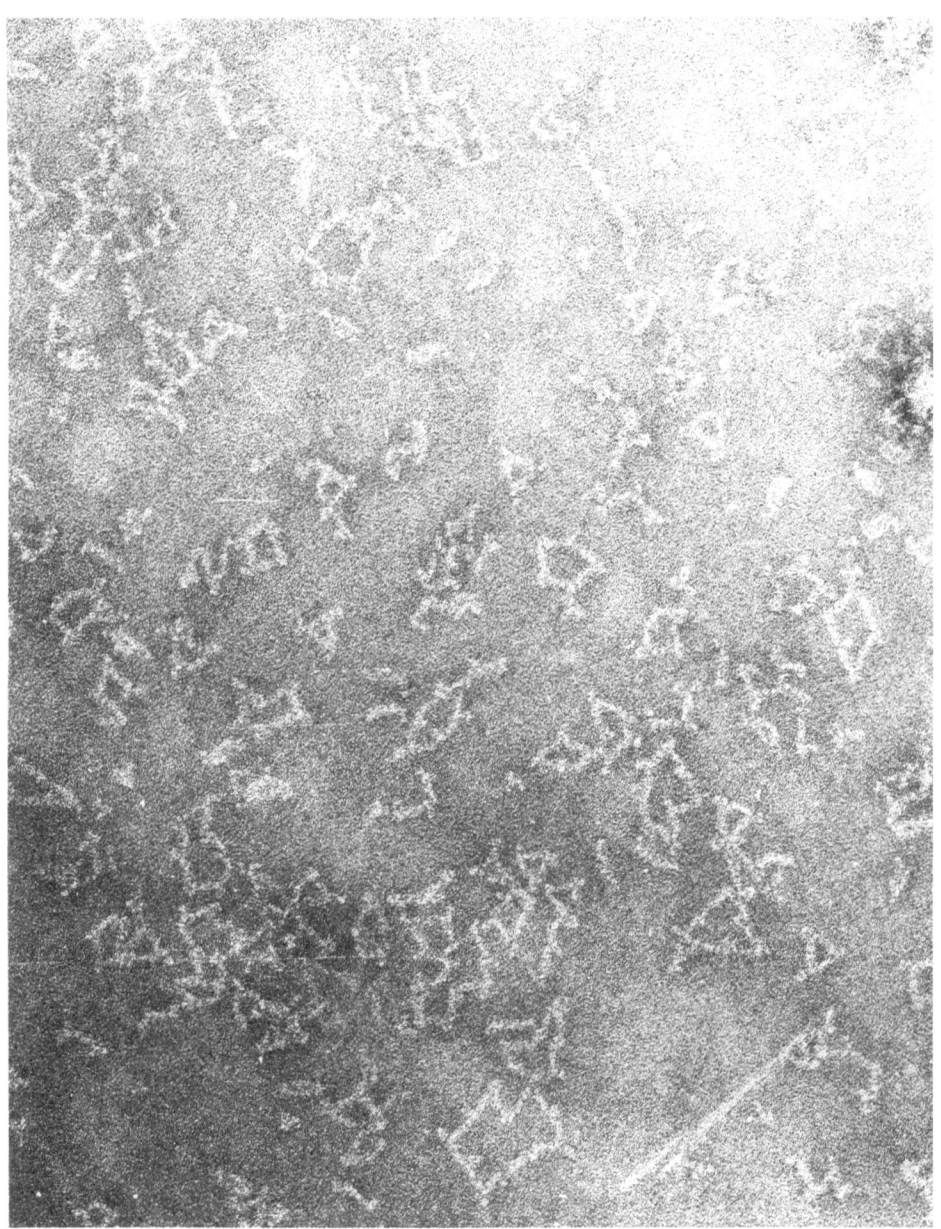

Figure 3. Electron micrograph of polymers produced by reaction of rabbit anti-dinitrophenyl (DNP) IgG with an equivalent amount of the divalent hapten bis-DNP-octamethylene-diamine. The antibody molecules are centered at the corners of the polygonal shapes. The Fc fragments are the knobs at the corners, and the Fab fragments form the edges of the polygons. The hapten is too small to be seen, but links adjacent Fab fragments. Adapted from Green (1969).

experimental data must usually be rationalized in terms of a simplified model. Each method will thus have certain limitations. To overcome these limitations, a number of laboratories have used widely differing techniques with respectively different basic assumptions that should thus, it is to be hoped, yield independent estimates of conformation.

Small-angle X-ray scattering results of a human IgG1 myeloma protein and of two rabbit IgG antibodies were interpreted in terms of a T-shaped model (Pilz *et al.*, 1970, 1973). In this method, it is necessary to assume simplified models that approximate the expected shapes and to compare calculated scattering curves expected from such models with the experimentally observed data. The best agreement was obtained with a model in which the Fab arms are at an angle of 180° with respect to each other and at 90° with respect to Fc and no space is allowed for extended flexible chains between the fragments. At the same time, the best agreement necessitated inclusion of holes between the V and C domains of the Fab as was observed by high-resolution X-ray crystallography (Poljak *et al.*, 1973).

Similarly, transient electric birefringence studies of rabbit anti-DNP antibody complexed with dipeptide α-DNP-Glu-Asp were interpreted in terms of a very open Y-shaped model in which the average angle between Fab arms is about 150° if the center of rotation of the molecule and the intersection of the Fab arms are assumed to coincide (Cathou and O'Konski, 1970). This method, when applied, as in this experiment, to ionized hapten bound to antibody molecules, measures primarily the permanent dipole moment provided by the ionic charge on the hapten over the distance from the combining sites to the center of rotation of the molecule. A basic assumption in the interpretation of these data was that α-DNP-Glu-Asp was fully ionized when bound in the active site. Since the center of rotation and the hinge region need not coincide, the proposed model may not in fact be very different from a T shape.

As an independent estimate of shape, Werner *et al.* (1972) attempted to measure the distance between the two combining sites in a rabbit antibody by the technique of resonance-energy transfer, a method that has been shown to be applicable to measurements of distances of the order of molecular dimensions (Wu and Stryer, 1972). The authors prepared a hybrid antibody molecule in which one combining site specifically bound the energy donor, DNS-Lys, while the other specifically bound the energy acceptor, fluorescein. The fluorescence lifetime of the bound DNS-Lys groups will decrease if there is energy transfer between them and the bound fluorescein molecule. The extent of transfer is determined by the distance and relative orientation between the transition dipole moments of the chromophore pair, by their spectral properties, and by the refractive index of the medium through which transfer occurs. The spectral properties can be measured and a reasonable value for the refractive index assigned. The only major uncertainty is the orientation factor. In favorable cases, this factor can be estimated (Dale and Eisinger, 1975). Usually, however, random orientation is assumed or the experiment is set up in such a way as to favor random orientation (Bunting and Cathou, 1973). In the case of the hybrid antibody, the orientations of the bound DNS-Lys and fluorescein were unknown. The antibody preparations, hwever, were known to be at least somewhat heterogeneous, which would result in some randomization of orientation in the ensemble of molecules, and second, antibody molecules were known to exhibit some segmental flexibility (see Section 2.2) during the lifetime of the excited state of the energy donor, which would result in further randomization. The spectroscopic properties of this donor–acceptor pair were such that energy transfer should be observed up to distances of about 90 Å. In fact, no transfer was observed, setting a lower limit of 90 Å to the distance between combining sites. The actual distance is probably even greater, since the Fab fragments oscillate at a point in the hinge region; thus, if the average position of Fab arms were at this minimum distance, R = 90 Å, some energy transfer would be observed, since there would be a high probability that the donor–acceptor pair would spend some time at a shorter distance. A more reasonable minimum distance, based on measurements of segmental flexibility (see Section 2.2), is 100–120 Å. This in turn sets minimum values of the angle between Fab arms to 80–100°.

It should be kept in mind, however, that one of the basic assumptions employed in this interpretation of the results is that the energy donor and acceptor transition dipole moments are not at 90° to each other when the chromophores are bound in their respective combining sites. Although this possibility appears to be unlikely, especially since the Fab segments are free to move during the fluorescence lifetime of the donor (see below), no direct evidence on this point is available. Second, these experiments were performed on a hybrid antibody in which the inter-H-chain disulfide was reduced and alkylated. IgG shows somewhat more flexibility under these conditions and the average conformation may be somewhat different from that in a molecule in which the interchain disulfide is intact (see Section 2.2.2).

The open conformation was recently confirmed by an entirely different method, namely, an attempt to intramolecularly cross-link combining sites via long bivalent haptens (Gopalkrishnan and Karush, 1974). These authors synthesized several haptens, the longest of which in an extended conformation has a length of 86 Å. It was expected that if intramolecular cross-linking occurred, the binding constant would be enhanced (Hornick and Karush, 1972). In fact, utilizing equine antilactosyl antibody and lactosyl bivalent haptens, no enhancement was observed. The authors ruled out the possibilities of antibody dimer formation and of a compact hapten structure. The most likely conclusion is thus that the binding sites are more than 86 Å apart, although the possibility that the haptens were not fully extended could not be excluded.

Taken together, all the evidence strongly suggests that antibody molecules in solution do, in general, have a very open Y-, possibly T-, shaped structure. Thus, in those antibody–antigen complexes in which the angle between Fab arms is observed to be less than about 90°, a conformational change has most likely occurred.

The discussion up to this point has implicitly assumed that the quaternary structure of the domains in the Fab moiety is similar for all Ig's. This situation does in fact exist in the human IgG1 protein New (Poljak *et al.*, 1973) and the murine IgA protein McPC 603 (Segal *et al.*, 1974), as well as in a human L-chain dimer of protein McG (Schiffer *et al.*, 1973). A common feature of these proteins is that the angle subtended by the local axes of symmetry in the V and C parts of the structure (the "Fab angle") is around 120°. In contrast, Colman *et al.* (1976) found that the Fab angle in in another human IgG1, protein Kol, is 170°. The difference in quaternary structure caused by this difference in Fab angle is shown in Figure 4. In all cases, the L–Fd dimerization pattern within V and C domains is similar, so that the Fab angle is due to the spatial relationship of V and C domains as determined by

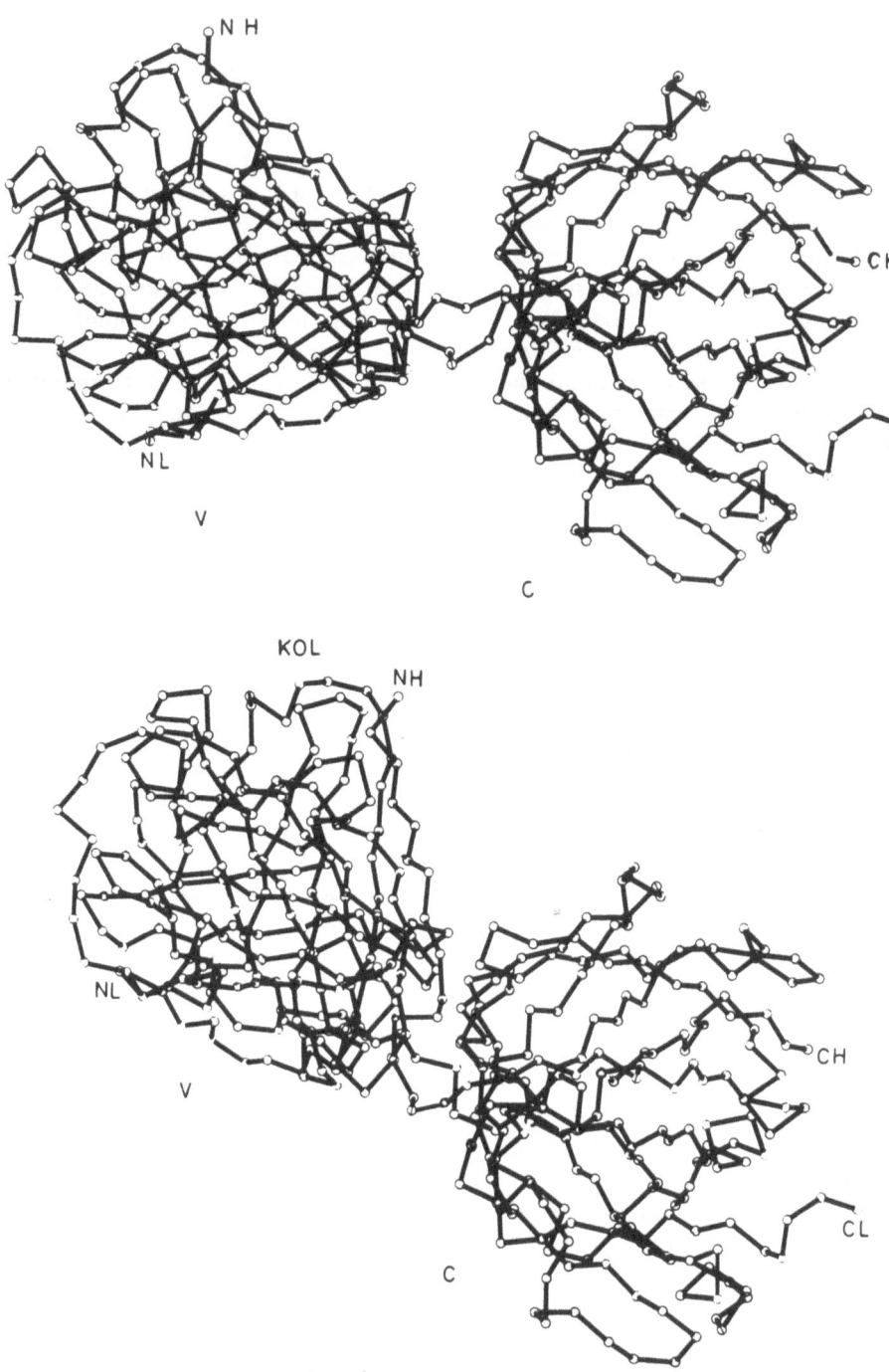

Figure 4. Comparison of the structures of Fab from the human IgG1 myeloma protein Kol (Colman *et al.*, 1976) (*top*) and from the murine IgA myeloma protein McPC 603 (Segal *et al.*, 1974) (*bottom*). V domains are to the left, with L chain at the bottom. Amino- and carboxy-terminal residues are indicated. Orientation of the C regions is similar. Note the difference in orientation of the V regions with respect to the C regions. Adapted from Colman *et al.* (1976).

the switch peptides. We must therefore seriously entertain the possibility that at least two Fab conformations are possible, and that a given protein will crystallize in one or the other conformation. Further, a transition between conformations might be caused by antigen-binding at the combining site. These possibilities will be considered in more detail in Sections 2.2 and 2.3.

The electron-density map of protein Kol (an intact and undeleted IgG1) at 5-Å resolution clearly showed the disposition of the Fab moieties to be at an angle of 125° (Colman *et al.*, 1976). Extrapolation of the structure of the Fab fragment of McPC 603 to an intact Ig leads to an angle between Fabs of about 145°. Both these angles are compatible with the results of the solution studies.

Curiously, although protein Kol contains an intact Fc, little electron density could be associated with this region of the molecule. The most reasonable interpretation of this observation is that Fc is not cylindrical about a two-fold symmetry element, and the disymmetry in the intact molecule might be caused by different three-dimensional structures of the two hinge peptides that link C_H1 and C_H2 (Colman *et al.*, 1976; Deisenhofer *et al.*, 1976). The observations made by Valentine and Green (1967) that the Fc was not always symmetrically disposed would be consistent with the X-ray crystallographic results.

The basic features of the IgG molecule considered so far can be summarized as follows: (1) The overall arrangement of Fab and Fc moieties is in the shape of an open Y, as shown in Figure 1; the average angle between Fab fragments is large, certainly at least 90°, but not always as large as 180°. (2) The antigen-combining sites are located at the outer tips of the Fab moieties: the complement- and cell-binding sites are in, respectively, the C_H2 and C_H3 domains in Fc, although their precise locations cannot yet be assigned to amino acid residues within these domains. (3) The Fc is probably not symmetrically disposed between the Fabs or confined to the plane defined by them. (4) The molecule exhibits restricted flexibility. (5) The hinge region, where the Fab and Fc moieties meet, is reasonable compact, so that the Fabs and Fc appear to abut each other. This last conclusion has profound implications for the transfer of information from the tip of the Fab to the domains in the Fc because it allows for long-range changes in conformation or flexibility, and will be considered in more detail in Section. 2.3.

2.2. Flexibility

The presence of a region in the H chains that is particularly susceptible to proteolytic cleavage might be expected to impart some flexibility to the IgG molecule. Such flexibility is inherent in the model proposed by Noelken *et al.* (1965) (see Figure 2).

2.2.1. Evidence for Flexibility

Electron micrographs of rabbit anti-DNP antibodies in combination with short bivalent haptens showed polymeric figures (see Figure 3) (Valentine and Green, 1967). In these polymers, the Fab arms of antibody molecules subtended apparent angles of anywhere from 0 to 180° with respect to each other. Since the Fab regions appeared to be rigid and compact, these different possible angles must result from some flexibility in the hinge. Since the molecules were connected by hapten, however, distortion may have occurred in the cross-linking process, and it is not possible to obtain a quantitative measure of the degree of inherent flexibility from these studies.

Flexibility is most directly studied by the technique of fluorescence depolarization. In this method, a fluorophore on the protein (usually extrinsic) is excited by plane-polarized light; subsequent depolarization of the emitted light, which is initially plane-polarized, yields information on the rotational modes of the protein (Weber, 1953). There are two types of fluorescence measurements that can be employed: steady-state (Weber, 1953) and time-resolved (Stryer, 1968; Yguerabide, 1972). The latter technique provides more information, but because of the more complex instrumentation involved, has been employed only recently. Historically, the steady-state approach was initially utilized on Ig's; however, apparently conflicting results were obtained (Weltman and Edelman, 1967; Knopp and Weber, 1969; Zagyansky *et al.*, 1969; Tumerman *et al.*, 1972). In retrospect, this is not surprising, considering the inherent limitations of this method and the variety of experimental conditions employed (for a discussion of these factors, see Cathou *et al.*, 1974). Most of these studies did, however, strongly suggest the presence of some flexibility, although determination of the sites was not possible. For example, Zagyansky *et al.* (1969) showed that the average rotational correlation time that was experimentally observed for rabbit and human IgG, $\bar{\phi} = 20$ nsec, was much smaller than the calculated value expected for a rigid ellipsoidal molecule, $\bar{\phi} = 73$ nsec.

Yguerabide *et al.* (1970) employed time-resolved measurements in their studies on rabbit IgG anti-dimethylnaphthalenesulfonyl (DNS) antibodies. These antibodies, with the fluorescent DNS-Lys chromophore rigidly held in the combining sites, showed depolarization curves that could be fit by two major rotational correlation times, one of $\phi_S = 33$ nsec and the other of $\phi_L = 168$ nsec (see Figure 5). The shorter of these times was that found for the Fab fragment alone, and thus may represent segmental flexibility of the Fab, while the longer one is probably due to tumbling motion of the whole molecule. The 33-nsec value is compatible with the mean correlation time of a hydrated rigid ellipsoid with a molecular weight of 50,000 and an axial ratio of 2 (Poljak *et al.*, 1973). Thus, even though V and C domains in Fab are separated by a cleft and do not show extensive regions of contact, the Fab behaves hydrodynamically as a rigid unit in the nanosecond time range. On the other hand, the time-dependent anisotropy curves of whole antibody and of the (Fab')$_2$ fragment were curved, indicating the presence of more than one rotational correlation time. The curvature in both cases was too great to be accounted for by the motions of any equivalent ellipsoid. Hence, such curvature is most easily interpreted as resulting from flexibility of the Fab arms with respect to each other and to Fc. Further, the presence of flexibility in the (Fab')$_2$ fragment, but not in Fab, established the site of flexibility as the hinge region. Some possible modes of flexibility are illustrated in Figure 6. This is, of course, a *minimal* model.

We recently confirmed the results of Yguerabide *et al.* (1970) on rabbit anti-DNS antibody (Chan and Cathou, 1977). The values of correlation times that we obtained, however, were $\phi_S = 26$ nsec and $\phi_L = 110$ nsec; the latter value is smaller than that obtained by Yguerabide *et al.* (1970). To explore the possible effects of choice of fluorophore and antibody specificity on measured rotational correlation times, we elicited antibodies to pyrene-butyric acid (Lovejoy *et al.*, 1975, 1977). When pyrene-butyric acid was bound in the antibody-combining sites, it exhibited a

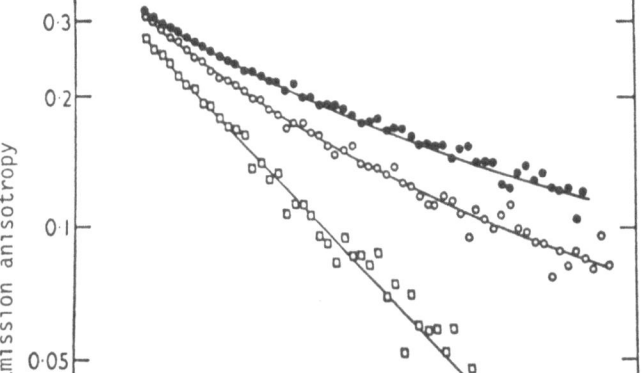

Figure 5. Time dependence of the fluorescence emission anisotropy of DNS-Lys in the combining sites of rabbit IgG anti-DNS (●), (Fab')$_2$ fragment (○), and Fab fragment (□). For Fab, ϕ (rotational correlation time) = 33 nsec. For IgG, the data were fit with the equation $A(t) = A_0[f_s \exp(-t/\phi_s) + f_L \exp(-t/\phi_L)]$ where $f_s = 0.44$, $\phi_s = 33$ nsec, $f_L = 0.56$, $\phi_L = 168$ nsec, and $A_0 = 0.32$. Adapted from Yguerabide *et al.* (1970).

fluorescence lifetime of 118 nsec in air-saturated solutions, a value much longer than that exhibited by DNS-Lys bound to anti-DNS, i.e., 23.6 nsec, and allowed statistically significant depolarization data to be obtained up to 300 nsec. A lifetime of this magnitude should not be required to study the depolarization behavior of IgG conjugates, but does allow one to detect the presence of any longer rotational correlation times that may be present or to determine more accurately the value of

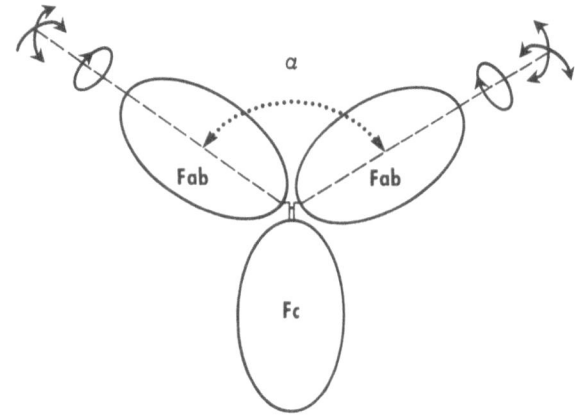

Figure 6. Possible modes of segmental flexibility in IgG. Fab motion can occur in the directions indicated by the solid arrows. Flexibility occurs around an average conformation in which the angle α is probably larger than 80–100°.

ϕ_L. Again, two correlation times of ϕ_S = 24–33 nsec and ϕ_L = 131–140 nsec were obtained (Lovejoy *et al.*, 1977). Thus, the choice of fluorophore had no significant effect on the values of the correlation times, and neither did the specificity of the antibody.

Attachment of the DNS fluorophore to Cys 226, which normally participates in the single H–H interchain disulfide bond, resulted in primarily a single rotational correlation time with a value of 130 nsec (Chan and Cathou, unpublished). Cys 226 is in the hinge region, and is thus at or near the center of rotation of the IgG molecule (O'Donnell *et al.*, 1970); the only modes of rotation that a fluorophore at this location could detect would be flexibility of the hinge region itself and tumbling of the whole molecule. The value of 130 nsec thus clearly represents tumbling motion and gives us an independent estimate for it. A very short correlation time was also observed; whether this is due to some free rotation of the probe itself, or to some flexibility of the hinge peptide, is unclear. Even in this reduced and alkylated preparation, however, the hinge peptide could not be completely flexible, since a long value of ϕ was still observed.

That a value of ϕ_L = 110 nsec is obtained when the fluorophore is bound in the combining site, which is located at the outer end of the Fab fragment, whereas ϕ_L = 130 nsec when the fluorophore is located at or near the center of rotation, suggests that an additional mode of flexibility, besides the segmental flexibility of individual Fab fragments, is present. This possibility is considered further in Section 2.2.5.

The measurement of the same value of the shorter correlation time, ϕ_S = 26 nsec, with both anti-DNS and antipyrene antibodies strongly suggests that the identity of the bound hapten does not affect segmental flexibility. These experiments do not answer, however, the question whether or not the *presence* of bound hapten affects flexibility. This question is unfortunately more difficult to answer, and no satisfactory experiments have been performed. To do so requires a comparison of the rotational modes of an antibody preparation in the presence and absence of hapten and extrinsically labeled with a fluorophore at locations different from the active site (so as not to interfere with hapten binding). Second, the fluorophore should be so situated as to detect motion of the Fab arms, i.e., away from the center of rotation. Finally, the fluorophore should have little or no independent rotation of its own, since the short correlation time for rotation of a covalently linked fluorophore could easily mask the intermediate value for segmental flexibility. Two laboratories have obtained results pertinent to the question of effects of hapten on flexibility, but opposite interpretations were made. Tumerman *et al.* (1972) compared the steady-state polarization of DNS-Lys bound to anti-DNS and of DNS-conjugated IgG. Values of the average rotational correlation time of 37 and 20 nsec, respectively, were obtained. These results were interpreted to mean that the presence of bound hapten made the antibody molecule more rigid. On the other hand, Brochon and Wahl (1972), employing DNS-conjugated IgG, performed time-resolved depolarization experiments and obtained rotational correlation times of ϕ_1 = 2.4 nsec and ϕ_2 = 95–115 nsec; these results were interpreted to mean that IgG (in the absence of hapten) was rigid. Both sets of experiments can be understood when one takes into account that covalently bound DNS in some environments is exposed to the aqueous solution; this results in: (1) independent or only partially hindered rotation of the fluorophore and an accompanying short value of ϕ (i.e., ϕ = 2–4 nsec: Brochon and Wahl, 1972) and (2) shorter fluorescence lifetimes, a situation that leads to noisier data at longer times, at least in the case of time-resolved experiments. Thus, Tumerman *et al.* (1972) had to contend with at least four values of ϕ in the DNS-conjugated IgG and three values of ϕ in the DNS-Lys–anti-DNS complex. Clearly, the average values of ϕ_1 in these two experimental situations would be different. In the case of the measurements of Brochon and Wahl (1972), at least four values of ϕ_1 were also probably present, and these were not resolved to yield intermediate values.

The number of interchain disulfide bonds in the hinge region might also affect segmental flexibility. Rabbit IgG has one interchain disulfide (O'Donnell *et al.*, 1970). Human IgG, on the other hand, has two to five, depending on the subclass. No complete study of the effect of hinge structure on flexibility has been reported. Nezlin *et al.* (1973) showed, however, that the average rotational correlation time for IgG1 is 21 nsec, whereas the value for IgG2 is 30 nsec. IgG1 has two interchain disulfides (Edelman *et al.*, 1969), while IgG2 has four (Frangione *et al.*, 1969). Thus, IgG2 appears to be slightly more rigid.

2.2.2. Flexibility of Reduced and Alkylated IgG

A number of years ago, Schur and Christian (1964) noted that on reduction and alkylation of the single inter-H-chain disulfide bond at Cys 226 of rabbit IgG antibodies, the ability to fix complement was lost. More recently, Schlessinger *et al.* (1975) reported that a univalent ligand-induced conformational change occurs in Fc, but that on reduction and alkylation of the inter-H-chain disulfide, the change is abolished. Studies on isolated C_H2 fragments of human IgG1 suggest that the disulfide bond itself is not part of the complement-fixation site (Isenman *et al.*, 1975). One possible explanation for these observations is that in the absence of antigen, the close proximity of Fab to Fc may cover the C1q binding site of C_H2; on interaction with antigen, a conformational change is transmitted to Fc that results in uncovering of the site (Isenman *et al.*, 1975). Reduction and alkylation of the interchain disulfide bond might then alter the interaction between Fab and Fc. If this is the case, then the conformation and flexibility of the reduced and alkylated IgG should also be changed. To test this hypothesis, we recently compared the time-resolved fluorescence depolarization of DNS-Lys bound to intact rabbit anti-DNS antibody and to mildly reduced and alkylated anti-DNS in which only the inter-H-chain disulfide was reduced (Chan and Cathou, 1977). The time-dependent aniso-tropy curves are shown in Figure 7; the values of rotational parameters are given in Table 1. Although the value of ϕ_s changes slightly under reduction, the values of f_s and f_L change considerably. As will be discussed below, f_L can be correlated with the angular range of flexibility. Thus, the Fab fragments in reduced and alkylated antibody appear to have greater freedom of motion. The average conformation of the reduced IgG is one in which the active sites are more than 100–120 Å apart and the corresponding minimal angle between Fabs is 80–100° (Werner *et al.*, 1972). In human IgG1, the two polypeptide chains that comprise the C_H2 domains do not have a strong tendency to associate (Dorrington and Painter, 1974), and according to a recent 4-Å resolution X-ray crystallography model of the Fc fragment, adjacent C_H2 domains show little or no interactions with each other (Deisenhofer *et al.*, 1976). By analogy, the same lack of association is expected to occur in rabbit IgG. Once the inter-H-chain disulfide bond is broken, the Fab fragments may have less

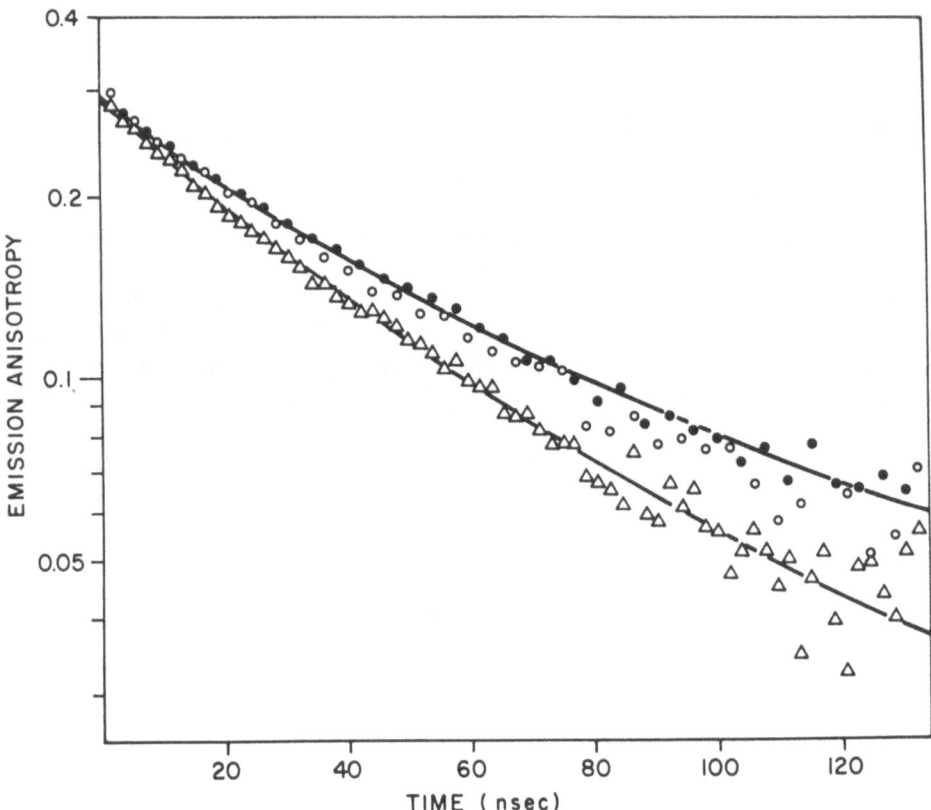

Figure 7. Time-dependent emission anisotropy of rabbit IgG anti-DNS antibody (●), antibody in which the inter-H-chain disulfide bond was reduced and alkylated (△), and reoxidized antibody (○). The points are experimental data. The solid lines were calculated according to the following equations:
upper curve:

$$A(t) = 0.294 \left[0.34 \exp\left(-t/26.3\right) + 0.66 \exp\left(-t/110.5\right)\right]$$

lower curve:

$$A(t) = 0.286\left[0.76 \exp\left(-t/41.2\right) + 0.24 \exp\left(-t/153\right)\right]$$

(Adapted from Chan and Cathou, 1977.)

TABLE 1. Rotational Correlation Times of Intact and Reduced and Alkylated Rabbit Anti-DNS Antibody[a]

Antibody	f_s	ϕ_s (nsec)	f_L	ϕ_L (nsec)
Intact anti-DNS	0.34	26	0.66	110
Reduced and alkylated anti-DNS[b]	0.76	41	0.24	153

[a]From Chan and Cathou (1977). Time-dependent anisotropy curves were analyzed by means of a weighted least-squares fit to the function: $A(t) = A_0[f_s \exp\left(-t/\phi_s\right) + f_L \exp\left(-t/\phi_L\right)]$ where $A_0 = 0.294$ for intact anti-DNS and 0.286 for reduced and alkylated anti-DNS.
[b]Reducing agent: 0.01 M 2-mercaptoethanol.

steric hindrance, and flexibility might also occur between the C_H2 and C_H3 domains. In this conformation, the Fab arms may permanently cover up the C1q binding sites or sufficient torsion may not be generated on combination with antigen to cause a required conformational change for exposure of the C1q sites. Reduction and alkylation, however, does not significantly alter the optical properties of human (Dorrington and Smith, 1972) or rabbit (Bjork and Tanford, 1971) IgG, so that any changes in conformation that occur in this process do not alter the environment of aromatic side chain residues or secondary structure. The changes are thus most likely in the quaternary structure.

2.2.3. Range of Flexibility

From the value of the weighting factor, f_L (see Table 1), it is possible to obtain an estimate of the angular range of segmental flexibility of the Fab arms. Weber (1952) showed that if an "attached" molecule (in this case the Fab segments) executes rapid rotation restricted to a few degrees and if the absorption and emission oscillators are coincident, the angular range of motion, Θ, can be described by $\cos^2 \Theta = (2f_L + 1)/3$, where f_L is the weighting factor for the longer correlation time, ϕ_L. The calculated value for Θ is 44° when one employs the values of f_L and ϕ_L given in Table 1. These values are probably still small enough to fulfill the requirement given above. These values cannot be directly translated into a description of the motion of Fab segments because the direction of such motion is unknown; in fact, several types of motion are possible (see Figure 6). It can be seen, however, that the flexibility in both intact and reduced and alkylated antibody is restricted, although less so in the latter case.

2.2.4. Primary Site of Segmental Flexibility

Time-resolved fluorescence depolarization measurements on intact antibody and (Fab')₂ and Fab fragments (Yguerabide *et al.*, 1970) and electron micrographs (Valentine and Green, 1967) clearly localized the primary site of flexibility to the hinge region. Knowledge of the amino acid sequence and the tertiary structure in this area of the molecule allows us to pinpoint the site even more closely. The pertinent stretch of the hinge region sequence of rabbit IgG is (Smyth and Utsumi, 1967; Givol and DeLorenzo, 1968)

$$
\begin{array}{c}
\text{(CHO)} \\
221 \qquad\qquad | \qquad 226 \\
\text{-Cys-Ser-Lys-Pro-Thr-Cys-Pro-Pro-Pro-Glu} \\
| \\
\text{-Cys-}
\end{array}
$$

Cys 221 is part of an intrachain disulfide bond that is adjacent to the L–H interchain disulfide bond (O'Donnell *et al.*, 1970). Both these disulfide bonds are located, in terms of the three-dimensional structure, near the end of the Fab fragment (Poljak *et al.*, 1973; Bunting and Cathou, 1974). Since Fab is rigid and since the (Fab')₂ fragment displays segmental flexibility, the site of flexibility must be in the stretch from Cys 221 to Cys 226.

In the *dl2* rabbit allotype, position 225 is Thr (Prahl *et al.*, 1970) and carries carbohydrate with an average composition of one galactosamine, one galactose, and one or two sialic acid residues (Fanger and Smyth, 1972). The presence of this oligosaccharide effectively blocks papain attack between Thr 225 and Cys 226, so that in the *d12* allotype, cleavage occurs instead between Cys 221 and Ser 222 and between Ser 222 and Lys 223 (Smyth and Utsumi, 1967). In the *d11* allotype, however, Thr 225 is replaced by Met, which cannot carry any carbohydrate. The effect of the oligosaccharide on flexibility is unknown at present. It would be most interesting to compare the flexibilities of antibodies prepared from homozygous *d11* and *d12* allotypic rabbits.

2.2.5. Additional Sites of Flexibility

Flexibility Within Fab. Through the use of spin labels covalently attached to various Ig's and their fragments, Käiväräinen *et al.* (1973) proposed that the Fab moieties exist primarily in two conformations that are in slow equilibrium with each other.

These conformations are thought to be structures in which the V and C domains of both H and L chains are at different distances from each other. Conformation B, the looser one, is postulated to predominate in free antibody. The mean lifetime of each conformer must be greater than 100 nsec; otherwise, only an average conformation would be detected by electron spin resonance (ESR) measurements. These two conformations were observed in Fab and (Fab')$_2$ fragments as well as in dimers of normal rat and human L chains (Käiväräinen *et al.*, 1973; Käiväräinen and Nezlin, 1976). When the L-chain dimers were split into V and C halves (Bjork *et al.*, 1971), the ESR spectrum showed the presence of only one conformation, which resembled conformer B (Käiväriänen and Nezlin, 1976). When the Ig was rabbit antihemoglobin or anti-IgG, on binding of the appropriate antigen, conformer A was preferentially stabilized.

These two conformers, A and B, could be similar to ones in which the Fab angle is 120 or 170° as shown by X-ray crystallography (see Section 2.1). Nezlin *et al.* (1973) estimated the mean rotational correlation times of human IgG in these two conformations to be 35 nsec for A and 23 nsec for B. These values should represent the average correlation time of motions in the macromolecule itself, since the average correlation time of the spinlabel has been extracted. That the values are still average values is clearly shown by a comparison with rotational correlation times of Fab, (Fab')$_2$, and IgG antibodies in which the spin label was bound in the combining site: for Fab, $\bar{\phi} = 18$ nsec; for (Fab')$_2$, $\bar{\phi} = 30$ nsec, and for IgG, $\bar{\phi} = 32$ nsec (Käiväräinen *et al.*, 1974).

The detection of two conformers implies flexibility at or near the switch peptides that connect V_L with C_L or V_H with C_H1, or both. In the case of rabbit IgG, the presence of a disulfide that bridges V_L and C_L probably limits flexibility to the H chain (Poulsen *et al.*, 1972; Appella *et al.*, 1973). Since the mean lifetime of each conformer is longer than 100 nsec, such flexibility is much slower than that observed by fluorescence spectroscopy. The rotational correlation times corresponding to each conformer should be sampled, however, by time-resolved fluorescence techniques over the time of the experiment, which typically is in hours. Thus, even if the two correlation times are present and cannot be resolved, some average value should be observed, and, based on the sizes of the domains, this value should be considerably shorter than 35 nsec. In fact, values of 26–33 nsec were observed

(Yguerabide *et al.*, 1970; Lovejoy *et al.*, 1975). One way of explaining this discrepancy would be to conclude that all the anti-DNS and antipyrene antibodies were in the more rigid conformation A. If this were the case, then the anti-spin-label antibodies with spin label bound in the combining site should also be in conformation A; however, a value for Fab or ϕ = 18 nsec, rather than 26–33 nsec, was obtained (Käiväräinen *et al.*, 1974). Although there is considerable evidence at present to suggest that a conformational change of some sort does occur on binding of antigen to antibody (see p. 54), the relationship of such a change of flexibility and the minimum size of hapten necessary to effect such a change remain unclear. More data are obviously necessary.

Flexibility Below the Hinge.   Colman *et al.*, (1976) suggested that lack of electron density corresponding to the Fc moiety in X-ray crystallographic studies of protein Kol may be due in part to flexibility in the H chains *C*-terminal to the inter-H-chain disulfide bonds. If such flexibility is present on a nanosecond time scale, a corresponding rotational correlation time between 33 and 100 nsec should be observed in time-resolved fluorescence depolarization measurements. Limitations of precision of data acquisition at present do not justify analysis of depolarization curves in terms of more than two rotational correlation times. However, that a value of ϕ_L = 110 nsec is obtained, whereas independent experiments show that the value of ϕ associated with tumbling of the whole molecule is at least 130 nsec, strongly suggests that 110 nsec represents the average of at least two correlation times; one of these times could represent motion of the $(\text{Fab}')_2$ fragment as a unit, while the other could be global rotation of the IgG.

Conformational Changes on Antigen-Binding.   Because the binding of antibody and antigen can be correlated with the initiation of a number of physiological processes, including antibody synthesis, the complement cascade, tolerance, and histamine release from skin mast cells, it has long been assumed that a conformational change in the antibody molecule must play a central role. Attempts to document such conformational changes have occupied many investigators, and until recently, this area of research has been a particularly frustrating one. In some cases, evidence for a conformational change was presented, although there was always an ambiguity in the interpretation. For example, Grossberg *et al.* (1965) reported the inhibition of release of radioactive chymotryptic peptides from iodinated anti-benzene-arsonate and anti-trimethylammonium antibodies by the presence of hapten. They concluded that a conformational change had occurred in the antibody. This could very well be the case; unfortunately, in experiments such as these, it is different to determine whether such inhibition is related to a shielding of critical peptide bonds in or near the combining site unless the sequences of the released peptides are also determined. Such an experiment could fruitfully be repeated on a homogeneous antibody preparation with the more advanced sequencing techniques that are now available. In other cases, no change was observed in the secondary or tertiary structure. For example, the optical rotary dispersion (ORD) and circular dichroism (CD) spectra of anti-DNP antibodies and of their Fab fragments in which more than 90% of the combining sites were saturated with ϵ-DNP-Lys showed no differences when compared with the spectra of antibody or Fab alone (Steiner and Lowey, 1966; Cathou *et al.*, 1968). Also, with the myeloma proteins New and McPC 603, which were studied by high-resolution X-ray diffraction, no changes were observed on binding with vitamin K_1 and phosphorylcholine, respectively (Amzel *et al.*, 1974; Segal *et al.*, 1974).

It is now becoming clear that an allosteric conformational change of some sort probably does occur on binding of hapten or antigen to antibody. The change, however, appears to be small, and is manifested primarily as a change in the quaternary structure or in the tertiary structure, or in both, rather than in the secondary structure. Furthermore, there may be a minimum size of hapten or antigen necessary, so that all haptens do not necessarily cause a detectable conformational change, although as increasingly more sensitive techniques are utilized, previously undetectable changes may become apparent. Table 2 lists examples of

TABLE 2. Allosteric Conformational Changes in Antibody–Hapten Complexes

Antibody	Antigen or hapten	Method[a]	References
A. No change detected			
McPC 603 (IgA)	Phosphorylcholine	X ray	Segal et al. (1974)
Human myeloma New	Vitamin K_1	X ray	Amzel et al. (1974)
Rabbit anti-DNP	ϵ-DNP-Lys	CD, DS	Cathou et al. (1974), Warner and Schumaker (1970)
Human macroglobulin Wag (IgM)	p-Nitrophenyl-ϵ-aminocaproate	CD	Ashman et al. (1971)
Rabbit anti-phenyl-β-lactoside (IgM)	p-Aminophenyl-β-lactoside	CF	Brown and Koshland (1975)
B. Change detected			
Rabbit anti-Type III pneumococcus	Hexasaccharide	CD	Holowka et al. (1972), Jaton et al. (1975a)
Rabbit anti-Type III pneumococcus	Tetra- to octasaccharide, 16-residue oligomer, polysaccharide	CPL	Jaton et al. (1975b)
Rabbit antiphenyl-β-lactoside	Lactose, Lac dye; p-azophenyl-β-lactoside derivative	DS, SA X ray	Warner et al. (1970), Pilz et al. (1974)
Rabbit antiphenyl-β-lactoside (IgM)	Mono-Lac-RNase	CF	Brown and Koshland (1975)
Rabbit anti-RNase	RNase	CPL	Schlessinger et al. (1975)
Rabbit antilysozyme "loop"	Lysozyme "loop"	CPL	Schlessinger et al. (1975)
Rabbit anti-poly (D-Ala)	Poly-(DL-Ala)-poly-(L-Lys)	CPL	Schlessinger et al. (1975)
Rabbit anti-poly (D-Ala)	(D-Ala)$_4$	SA X ray	Pilz et al. (1973)
TEPC 15 (IgA)	Phosphorylcholine	CD	D. H. Morris et al. (1974)
Rabbit anti-hemoglobin	Hemoglobin	ESR	Käiväräinen and Nezlin (1976)
F_v of MOPC 315 (IgA)	N-(1-oxyl-2,2,6,6-tetramethyl-4-piperidinyl)-2,4-dinitrobenzene; N-(1-oxyl-2,2,5,5-tetramethyl-3-methylaminopyrolidinyl)-2,4-dinitrobenzene	ESR, F	Dwek et al. (1976)

[a](CD) Circular dichroism; (CF) complement fixation; (CPL) circularly polarized luminescence; (DS) differential sedimentation; (ESR) electron spin resonance; (F) fluorescence; (SA X ray) small-angle X-ray scattering.

some antibody–hapten systems that do cause a detectable change and some that do not. (This list is by no means complete.)

Some tentative conclusions can be drawn, based on the available data. First, the size or type of hapten is important. For example, ε-DNP-Lys does not trigger any detectable changes in anti-DNP antibodies (Cathou *et al.*, 1968; Warner and Schumaker, 1970). Phosphorylcholine, another small hapten, causes a change in the case of TEPC 15 but not of McPC 603 (Morris, D. H., *et al.*, 1974; Segal *et al.*, 1974). Lactoside haptens do not enhance complement fixation in IgM (Brown and Koshland, 1975), but do cause other detectable changes (Warner *et al.*, 1970; Pilz *et al.*, 1974); for complement fixation to occur, a monovalent lactoside-conjugated protein carrier is necessary (Brown and Koshland, 1975). A minimum area of interaction between hapten and combining site thus appears to be necessary for the detection of a conformational change. Perhaps sufficient contact must be made with both L and H chains. Second, the conformational changes that are observed are seen as a volume contraction of the antibody, but not as a change in basic shape (Warner *et al.*, 1970; Pilz *et al.*, 1973, 1974), and as rather small changes in the environment of one or more tyrosine and tryptophan residues (Holowka *et al.*, 1972; Jaton *et al.*, 1975a,b; Schlessinger *et al.*, 1975). ESR measurements also suggest increased "rigidity" of the antibody (Käiväräinen and Nexlin, 1976). In some cases, the changes in Fab and Fc (Schlessinger *et al.*, 1975; Jaton *et al.*, 1975b) can be separated. Dwek *et al.* (1976) also observed small, apparently localized, changes in the Fv fragment of MOPC 315 on binding of lanthanide metals and DNP spin-label haptens that form a ternary complex. These changes were manifested primarily in decreased binding constant of metal on binding of hapten, and vice versa, and, at least in the case of metal binding, involved only a few residues. The results were interpreted in terms of two different conformers of Fv that were in equilibrium with each other, one of which is present in the absence of hapten and metal and binds hapten more strongly, while the other binds metal more strongly. Whether these conformational changes are really localized, or are also manifested as changes in quaternary structure, is still unknown. To observe changes ascribed to the Fc region, however, the interchain disulfide bond at the hinge must be intact (Schlessinger *et al.*, 1975). Finally, the volume changes seen by small-angle X-ray scattering also require the presence of intact Fc; no changes were seen in isolated Fab or (Fab')$_2$ fragments (Pilz *et al.*, 1975).

Several molecular mechanisms can be envisioned to account for these diverse results; perhaps the simplest that is consistent with all the data obtained so far is that ligand binding causes a small change in the spatial orientation between V_L and V_H that is then translated into a change in the spatial orientation between the V_L–V_H and C_L–C_H1 domains. Transmission could occur via the switch peptides (Colman *et al.*, 1976) or the limited contact areas between V_L and C_L and between V_H and C_H1. Contact certainly exists between V_L and C_L, and in the case of rabbit κ chains (the predominant class), these two regions are linked by a disulfide bond (Poulsen *et al.*, 1972; Appella *et al.*, 1973). The change(s) in spatial orientation would then lead to: (1) a change in the quaternary structure of Fab (perhaps a change in the Fab angle) (Colman *et al.*, 1976), and (2) small changes in the environment of one or more tyrosine residues in C_L (Holowka *et al.*, 1972) and one or more tryptophan residues the locations of which within Fab are unknown (Holowka *et al.*, 1972; Jaton *et al.*, 1975a,b; Schlessinger *et al.*, 1975).

Most of the changes in environment of aromatic side chains were observed in the isolated Fab fragments (Jaton *et al.*, 1975a,b; Schlessinger *et al.*, 1975), so that the associated conformational change is stable (although the possibility that these particular changes occur directly within the combining site has not been ruled out) (Holowka *et al.*, 1972). On the other hand, change in quaternary structure has been documented only with intact antibodies, and in fact has *not* been found in isolated Fab or (Fab′)₂ fragments (Pilz *et al.*, 1975), although ESR evidence is suggestive (Kävaräinen and Nezlin, 1976). In this connection, it would be of great value to compare the ESR spectra of extrinsically spin-labeled Fab and (Fab′)₂ fragments of antibodies in the presence and absence of antigen. The presence of Fc may be necessary to stabilize the altered quaternary structure and may do so by providing rigidity. Since the H chain in the hinge region is partially flexible (see Section 2.2), rigidity could be best supplied by contact between Fab and Fc. Such contact could then transmit a conformational change to the C_H2 domain, where complement fixation occurs. Although its location has not been ascertained, a change in the environment of one or more tryptophans in Fc was seen by Schlessinger *et al.* (1975).

In addition to the allosteric mechanism, a conformational change at or below the hinge region could also occur by a suitable change in the spatial orientation of the Fab moieties with respect to each other and to Fc. Such changes in IgG were inferred from electron micrographs of antibody–multivalent-hapten complexes (Valentine and Green, 1967) and from hydrogen-exchange measurements that indicated that complex formation between sheep antibodies to poly-$(Glu^{60} Ala^{30} Tyr^{10})_n$ and the antigen results in release of hydrogen ions, presumably at the hinge (Liberti *et al.*, 1972).

Finally, the allosteric conformational changes that have been observed in IgG antibodies are not sufficient, in themselves, to trigger complement fixation (Jaton *et al.*, 1976). Antibody–antigen complexes containing more than three antibody molecules are necessary.

3. Immunoglobulin M

3.1. Conformation

3.1.1. Covalent Structure

Since the initial observations of Heidelberger and Pedersen (1937) of a macroglobulin antibody against pneumococcus polysaccharide in the horse, immunoglobulin M (IgM) has been recognized as a major class of antibodies in humans and other mammals, as well as in vertebrates as phylogenetically distant as the elasmobranchs (Sharks). In serum, it is generally found as a pentamer of five disulfide-linked subunits, each composed of two L and two H (μ) chains that are held together by disulfide bridges and noncovalent interactions (reviewed in Metzger, 1970). A third unrelated chain, known as the joining (J) *chain,* is also present in IgM and is probably involved in its assembly from the subunits (Koshland, 1975). The overall molecular weight of the pentamer is about 900,000 (Dorrington and Tanford, 1970). Functionally, the IgM pentamer has ten potential antigen-binding sites, one on each Fabμ (Kim and Karush, 1973; Riesin *et al.*, 1975), and is capable of binding C1q in the Fc region to initiate the classic complement pathway (Sledge and Bing, 1973;

Müller-Eberhard, 1974). The 7 S subunit is thought to act as one of the major cell-surface receptors for antigens on small B lymphocytes (Vitetta and Uhr, 1975).

The arrangement of chains in IgM is shown schematically in Figure 8. It can be seen that the μ chain contains five homology domains (V_H and $C\mu 1$ through $C\mu 4$); the molecular weight is also higher than that of the γ chain: 56,000–60,000 as compared with 50,000 after subtraction of the contribution by oligosaccharides (Dorrington and Mihaesco, 1970; Dorrington and Tanford, 1970; Putnam *et al.*, 1973; Watanabe *et al.*, 1973). The disulfide bridges that link the IgMs subunits in the native pentamer have been reported to be at Cys 414 (Beale and Feinstein, 1969;

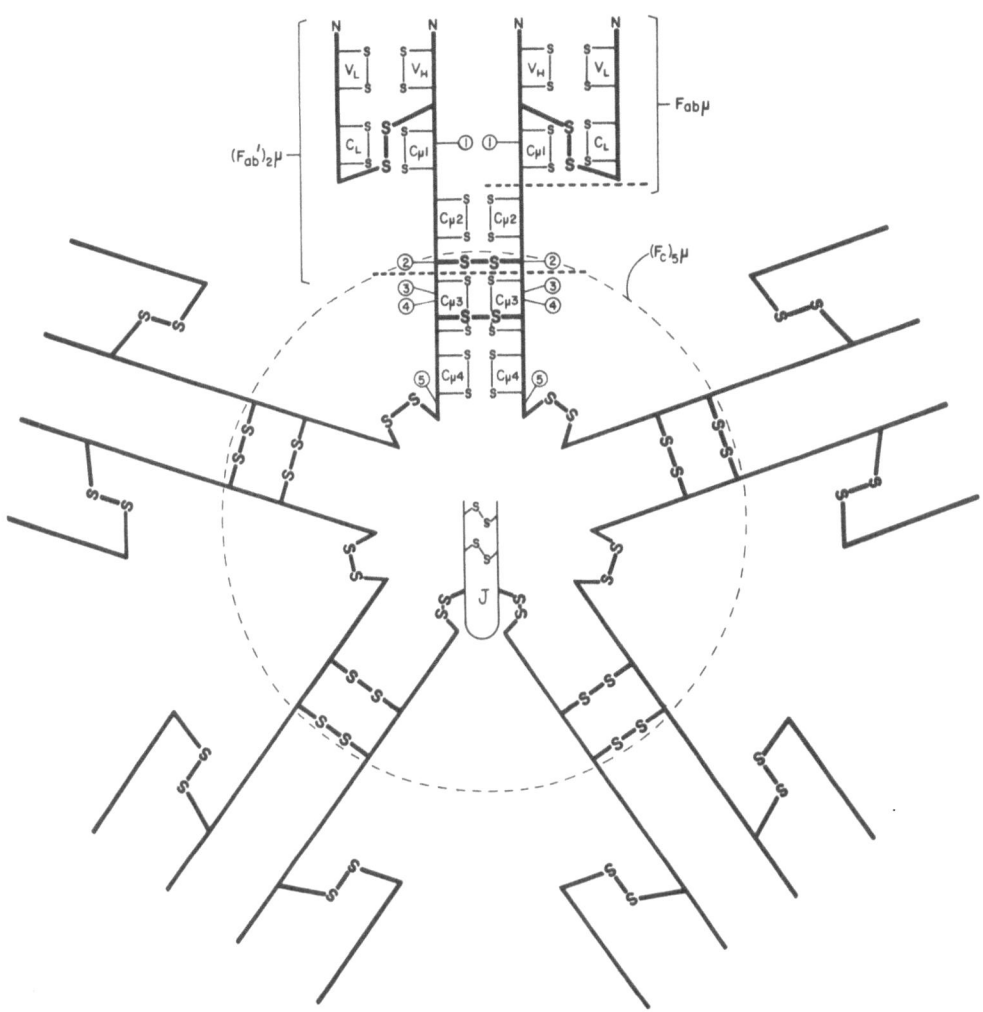

Figure 8. Schematic structure of mamalian IgM. The circular arrangement of the IgMs subunits is shown, as are the homology domains of the L chains (V_L and C_L) and the H chains (V_H and $C\mu 1$). The interchain disulfides are shown at Cys 575 as proposed by Chapuis and Koshland (1974), but substantial evidence also suggests that Cys 414 residues are involved in linking IgMs subunits (Morris, J. E., and Inman, 1968; Beale and Feinstein, 1969; Frangione *et al.*, 1971). The positions of the five oligosaccharides (1–5) are from sequence studies (Putnam *et al.*, 1973; Watanabe *et al.*, 1973). Also indicated are the enzymatic fragments of interest and the probable location of the J chain (Mestecky and Schrohenloher, 1974).

Frangione *et al.*, 1971), although this view was recently challenged (Chapuis and Koshland, 1974), since J chain is located at Cys 575 (Mestecky and Schrohenloher, 1974). J Chain most likely links two adjacent IgMs (Chapuis and Koshland, 1974), so that the remaining intersubunit disulfides must be between μ chains. The controversy over the location of the intersubunit bridges is due to the finding that on selective reduction and alkylation with radioactive iodoacetate under conditions that produce primarily intact IgMs, label is found exclusively at Cys 414 (Beale and Feinstein, 1969), whereas symmetry arguments require that if J chain is located at Cys 575, the remaining Cys 575 residues must also link subunits. On the other hand, Milstein *et al.* (1975) recently found that the most likely arrangement of interchain disulfides in mouse IgM (MOPC 104E) is one in which Cys 575 residues link the IgMs subunits, and that there is no apparent counterpart to the Cys 414 bridges. In any case, there seems to be substantial agreement that in both human and murine IgM, Cys 337 links two adjacent μ chains within IgMs subunits (Beale and Feinstein, 1969; Frangione *et al.*, 1971; Milstein *et al.*, 1975). The J chain is added, and polymerization of five IgMs to IgM occurs just prior to or during secretion from the antibody-synthesizing cell (for a review, see Koshland, 1975). The molecular weight of J chain is small, i.e., 15,000, and its presence does not appear to contribute significantly to the conformation of IgM.

The additional homology domain in the μ chain appears to be Cμ2, which is located between Fab and the hinge-region inter-μ-chain disulfides; we will return to the properties of Cμ2 later. The Fc region is comprised of the Cμ3 and Cμ4 domains. Interestingly, complement fixation has been reported to occur in the Cμ4 domain, rather than in Cμ3 (Hurst *et al.*, 1974).

3.1.2. Subunit Arrangement

When viewed in the electron microscope, IgM appears as a pentameric stellar structure in which each IgMs, or monomer, looks strikingly similar to the open Y structure seen for IgG (see Figure 9). The arms of the Y correspond to Fab; the Cμ2 domains may correspond to the base of the Y, which can occasionally be seen between the Fab arms and the central (Fcμ)$_5$ disk. Electron micrographs of murine, human, rabbit, sheep, chicken, and dogfish IgM all show similar structures (Shelton and McIntire, 1970; Parkhouse *et al.*, 1970; Feinstein *et al.*, 1971).

Early sedimentation and optical studies on human IgMs suggested that no significant noncovalent interactions occurred among subunits. Miller and Metzger (1965) reported that the subunits obtained by reduction with 0.05 M cysteine did not associate. Comparison of the ORD spectra of similarly prepared subunits and the parent IgM showed that between 220 and 300 nm, these spectra were identical within experimental error (Dorrington and Tanford, 1968). On the other hand, Tomasi (1973) found that reduction of IgM with 20 mM mercaptoethanolamine and alkylation led to a mixture of "IgM" (60%) and IgMs (40%). The "IgM" dissociated into IgMs in 4 M guanidine HCl or 1 M propionic acid. Similar noncovalent interactions were observed in murine IgM reduced with 0.5 mM dithioerythritol; the presence of oligomers (dimers or larger) was, however, necessary (Parkhouse, 1974). On sufficient reduction to convert all the IgM into monomers, noncovalent interactions were no longer present. Noncovalent association in IgMs from porcine IgM was also reported (Beale, 1974).

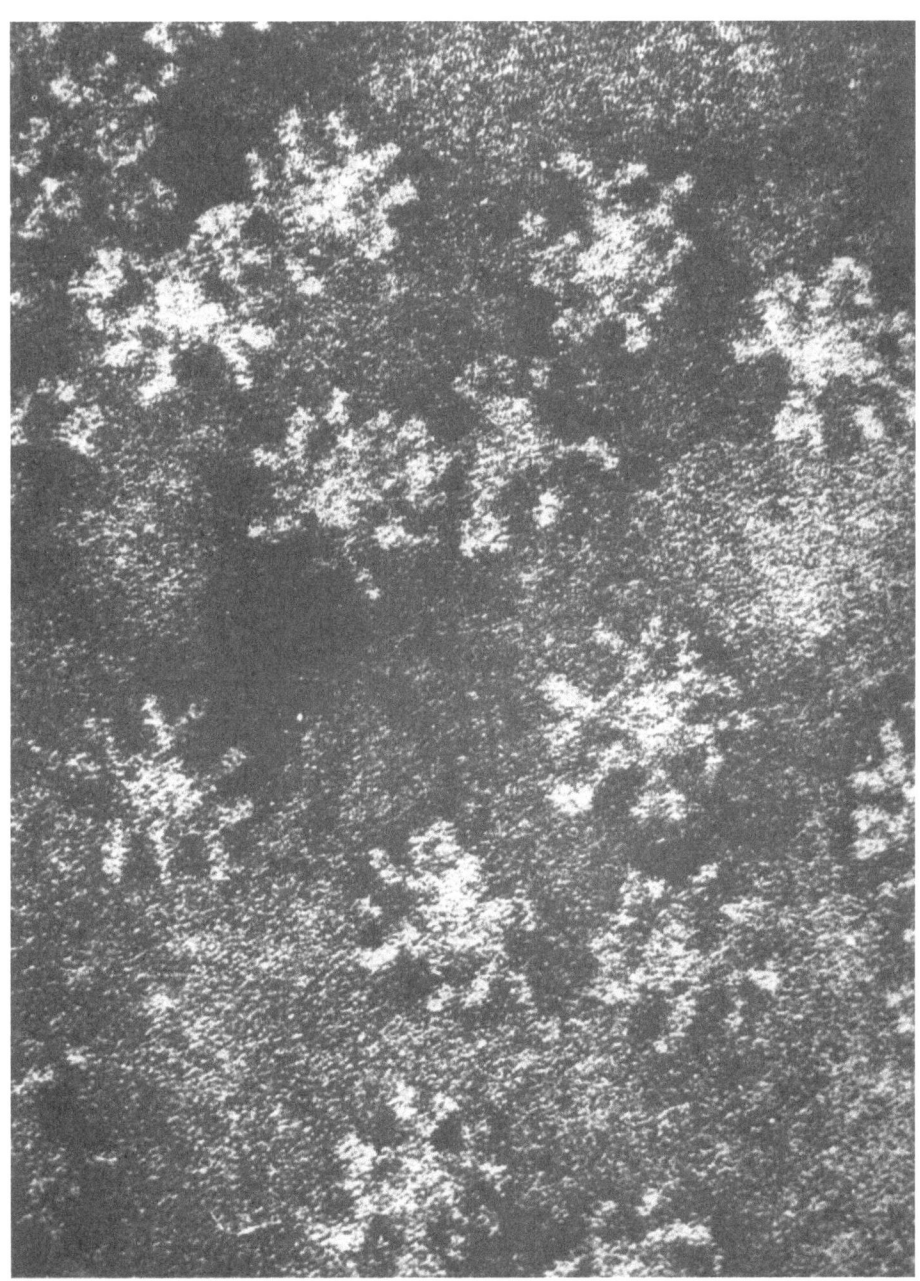

Figure 9. Electron micrograph of the IgM produced by the murine myeloma cell line MOPC 104E. ×
660,000. Courtesy of R. Dourmashkin.

Since all these studies on noncovalent interactions were carried out on reduced and alkylated IgM, one can ask whether or not the reduction process caused a conformational change that then resulted in a change in such interactions. Some disulfide rearrangement may occur on reduction, since the intersubunit bridge is thought to be at Cys 575, whereas alkylation is found at Cys 414. This question has not yet been satisfactorily resolved (see, for example, Percy and Percy, 1975). The CD spectra of $(Fc\mu)_5$ and $Fc\mu$ show an identical negative band at 218 nm that is usually ascribed to β-pleated sheet of the polypeptide backbone, and similar, although not identical, bands in the aromatic side chain region of 260–300 nm (Ghose, 1971). Thus, any conformational changes could not be very extensive. The possibility of subtle conformational changes resulting in substantial changes in noncovalent interactions cannot, however, be ruled out.

3.1.3. Proteolytic Fragments

Because of the presence of the additional domain, $C\mu 2$, in the μ chain, proteolytic digestion occurs in several stages, with destruction of the $C\mu 2$, rather than limited cleavage, in many cases. Temperature, enzyme, and species from which the IgM was obtained all affect that type of fragments produced. For example, trypsin digestion at 60°C of human and equine IgM results in $Fab\mu$ and $(Fc\mu)_5$ fragments; $C\mu 2$ is completely destroyed (Zikán and Bennett, 1973; Putnam *et al.*, 1973; Holowka and Cathou, 1976a). At 37°C, however, trypsin digestion for 18 hr of human IgM results in the destruction of Fc and a mixture of $Fab\mu$ and $(Fab\mu')_2$ (Miller and Metzger, 1966). Limited digestion (16 min at 37°C) of $(Fc\mu)_5$ yields fragments of molecular weight 21,000, 13,800, and 6800; the smallest fragment is derived from the $C\mu 4$ region and fixes complement (Hester *et al.*, 1975; Hurst *et al.*, 1974). Porcine IgM is unaffected by trypsin at either temperature unless IgMs subunits are first produced (Beale, 1974). Papain at 37°C results in $Fab\mu$ and $(Fc\mu)_5$ from human and equine IgM (Onoue *et al.*, 1968; Holowka and Cathou, 1976a). Finally, pepsin digestion of human and equine IgM produces a mixture of $Fab\mu$ and $(Fab'\mu)_2$ (Kishimoto *et al.*, 1968; Holowka and Cathou, 1976a) and $Fab\mu$ and $(Fc\mu)_5$ from porcine IgM (Beale, 1974). These differences in enzymatic proteolysis probably reflect differences in the folding, interaction, and stability, or in any or all, of the $C\mu 2$ domains and Fc region.

The $Fab\mu$ fragments of equine IgM produced by either papain or pepsin exhibited rotational correlation times similar to the value found for $Fab\gamma$ (Holowka and Cathou, 1976b; Yguerabide *et al.*, 1970); no evidence was found for flexibility at the switch peptides in the nanosecond time scale.

There appear to be only limited noncovalent interactions between adjacent μ chains in the Fc region of human IgM; $Fc\mu$ produced by reduction of $(Fc\mu)_5$ by either 0.05 M cysteine or 5 mM DTT exhibited a molecular weight of 31,500–33,500, indicating that it consisted of single chains (Dorrington and Mihaesco, 1970; Hester *et al.*, 1975).

3.1.4. Conformation of IgM in Solution

The solution conformation of IgM has been studied in far less detail than that of IgG. This is not surprising, considering the higher complexity of IgM and its usually transient appearance in the immune response. Most studies have been done on human Waldenström macroglobulins.

Some information on the secondary and tertiary structure of several human IgM has been obtained from CD and ORD measurements. A negative band at 217 nm, indicative of β-pleated sheet, is present (Ashman *et al.*, 1971; Ghose, 1971); comparison of the CD spectra of $(Fc\mu)_5$ and $F\gamma$ suggests that the $(Fc\mu)_5$ contains more β structure (Ghose, 1971). On the other hand, in the aromatic amino acid absorbing region of the spectrum, $Fc\gamma$ shows a larger contribution from tyrosines and tryptophans in asymmetrical environments (Ghose, 1971). This observation is consistent with the number of aromatic residues present: seven tyrosines and four tryptophans in the Fc region of μ chain (Putnam *et al.*, 1973) and nine tyrosines and three tryptophans of a $\gamma 1$ chain (Edelman *et al.*, 1969).

Miller and Metzger (1965) utilized sedimentation and diffusion coefficients to calculate a frictional ratio (f/f_{min}) that is related to the hydrodynamic asymmetry of IgM; they obtained a value of 1.92, which is consistent with either a rigid, highly asymmetrical or a more hydrated, and flexible, structure. In view of fluorescence depolarization measurements (discussed in Section 3.2), the latter interpretation is more plausible.

When viewed in the electron microscope, not all the Fab regions of intact IgM are always seen, an observation that led Feinstein and Munn (1969) to suggest that the plane of the $(Fab')_2\mu$ may be perpendicular to the plane of the Fc ring. The distance between the tips of the Fab fragments in a given IgMs subunit has been estimated from electron micrographs to be in the range of 115–150 Å, which is similar to that indicated for IgG (Metzger, 1970).

On binding to particulate antigen, the stellar configuration of IgM is dramatically changed to a staple conformation in which the $(Fab')_2\mu$ regions are bent out of the plane of the central $(Fc)_5\mu$ disc (Feinstein *et al.*, 1971). Such a conformational change is necessary for optimal utilization of the multiple combining sites, at least in the case of a large antigen with repetitive determinants, and may be correlated with enhancement of complement fixation.

3.2. Flexibility

3.2.1. Segmental Flexibility

Several steady-state fluorescence depolarization studies of IgM clearly showed that some internal flexibility was present. Metzger *et al.* (1966), using a DNS-conjugated human Waldenström macroglobulin, found low values for the mean rotational correlation time, i.e., $\bar{\phi} = 27$ nsec. Zagyansky *et al.* (1972), using three DNS-conjugated Waldenström macroglobulins, also obtained low values of $\bar{\phi}$ i.e., 27–47 nsec. Knopp and Weber (1969), employing pyrenebutyryl conjugate of a human IgM, obtained a value of $\bar{\phi} = 330$ nsec, which they interpreted as rotation of the entire macromolecule, although they pointed out the presence of additional degrees of freedom with much shorter correlation times. Holowka and Cathou (1974) measured a value of $\bar{\phi} = 82$ nsec with DNS-Lys bound in the combining sites of equine anti-DNS IgM. In a phylogenetic comparison, Zagyansky and Ivannikova (1974) studied the IgM from a number of species. They obtained values of $\bar{\phi} = 147$ nsec for shark, 128 nsec for carp, 135 nsec for frog, and 103 nsec for tortoise, and thus concluded that the degree of overall flexibility decreases with the level of phylogeny.

It could not be ascertained, however, at what point in the molecule such flexibility occurred. Because of the presence of the additional domain, $C\mu 2$, flexibility might, in fact, occur in several regions. To try to answer this question, Holowka and Cathou (1976a,b) elicited anti-DNS IgM antibodies so that the fluorophore would be rigidly bound in the combining sites and measured fluorescence depolarization by time-resolved spectroscopy.

Figure 10 shows the nanosecond decay of emission anisotropy, $A(t)$, of DNS-Lys bound in the combining sites of IgM from three species: horse, pig, and nurse shark. In each case, curvature is observed that indicates that several rotational correlation times must be present. For comparison, in Figure 10a, the dotted line depicts the decay expected for the rotation of IgM as a rigid hydrated sphere with $\phi_0 = 380$ nsec. This line represents the fastest decay that could be expected if IgM behaved hydrodynamically as an inflexible macromolecule. This is clearly not the case, since at least one rotational correlation component, as estimated by the slope of a tangent to the curve at any point, is considerably less than 380 nsec in all three cases. Further, it can be seen that such a correlation time must be smaller than 0.95 ϕ_0, so that we are not observing the motion of a rigid and highly asymmetrical molecule (Tao, 1969).

The nurse shark curve (Figure 10c) consists of at least two components with correlation times shorter than 380 nsec and an additional very long component. On analysis, the very fast initial decay had a value of ϕ that ranged from 3 to 13 nsec and is too short to be attributed to the rotation of a rigid $Fab\mu$-like fragment, which would be expected to have a ϕ value of at least 20 nsec. It may be due to some partially hindered rotation of DNS-Lys withing the combining site rather than macromolecular rotation, and we will not consider it further.

Analysis of the anisotropy decay curves in Figure 10 in terms of two correlation times gave the values of ϕ_i listed in Table 3. In the case of nurse shark IgM, the analysis was applied to the curve after the decay of the initial fast component. These results clearly show that internal flexibility is present in the IgM from all three species.

On exposure of the equine IgM to 1 M acetic acid, the anisotropy decay curve changed dramatically (Figure 11). Analysis gave values of $f_s = 0.69$, $\phi_s = 40$ nsec, $f_L = 0.31$, and $\phi_L = 355$ nsec. Thus, one of the effects of acid is to decrease ϕ_s from 61 to 40 nsec. Analysis of the decay curve of the $(Fab')_2\mu$ fragment prepared from acid-exposed IgM gave a similar value for ϕ_s, 38 nsec. For comparison, $\phi = 32$ nsec for free $Fab\mu$ and $\phi = 41.5$ nsec for free $Fab'\mu$ [prepared by reduction and alkylation of $(Fab')_2\mu$]. Thus, the most likely candidate for the rotational subunit in the acid-treated IgM is the $Fab'\mu$, which must have some freedom of rotation within the molecule. For this rotation to occur, interactions between the $C\mu 2$ domains on adjacent H chains must be weak. Lack of significant interaction is supported by the observation that on reduction and alkylation of the acid-exposed $(Fab')_2\mu$, the resulting $Fab'\mu$ fragments do not remain associated.

In the case of native IgM, the value of ϕ_s is longer than that observed for isolated $Fab\mu$ or $Fab'\mu$ fragments. This strongly suggests that the $C\mu 2$ domains in the native molecule are associated with each other to a sufficient degree to hinder the rotational freedom of $Fab'\mu$.

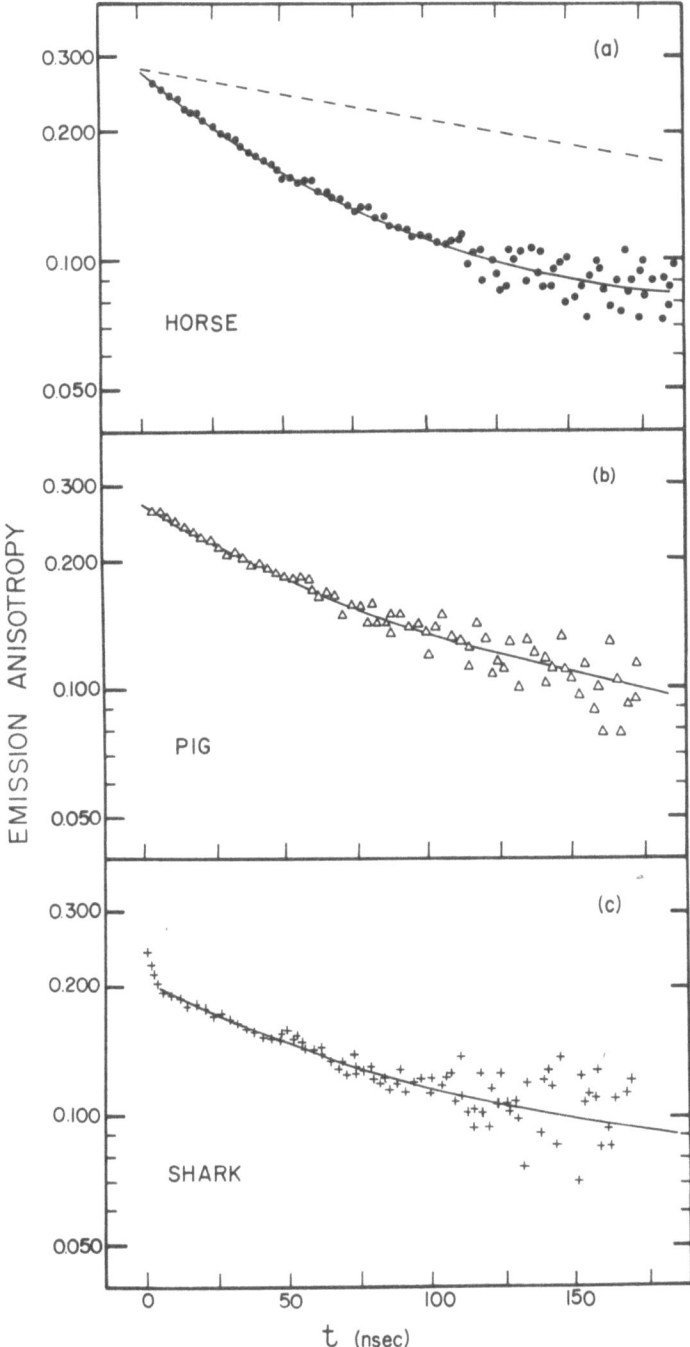

Figure 10. Time dependence of the emission anisotropy of ε-DNS-Lys in the combining sites of IgM. (•, Δ, +) Representative data points; (———) nonlinear least-squares best fit of the observed data to a sum of two exponential decays. The dashed line in 10a represents the calculated decay for a rigid, hydrated sphere of the same volume as IgM. Adapted from Holowka and Cathou (1976b).

TABLE 3.   Rotational Correlation Times of IgM[a]

Species	f_s	ϕ_s (nsec)	f_L	ϕ_L (nsec)
Equine	0.71	61	0.29	> 1000
Porcine	0.57	69	0.43	568
Nurse shark	0.63	93	0.37	> 1000

[a]From Holowka and Cathou (1976b).

It is more difficult to interpret the actual physical significance of the short rotational correlation times obtained for native equine and porcine IgM. The values of ϕ_s are of similar magnitude (60–69 nsec), and suggest a more hindered Fabμ or Fab'μ rotation than is present in the acid-eluted equine IgM. A more precise description of the nature of such motion does not appear warranted at present. Perhaps a more reasonable, albeit more complex, interpretation is that the values of ϕ_s seen in the native equine and porcine IgM really represent an average of several values of ϕ_i, and hence several modes of motion, such as the rotation of Fabμ *and* of the entire (Fab')$_2\mu$. The latter type of motion would be expected to exhibit a rotational correlation time in the range of 80–135 nsec when the Cμ2 domains are associated. If one assumes average values of ϕ_i of 35 and 105 nsec for the rotations of Fabμ (or Fab'μ) and (Fab')$_2\mu$, respectively, a harmonic average in which the latter component contributes twice as much as the former would yield a mean rotational correlation time of roughly the same magnitude as ϕ_s obtained for native equine and porcine IgM. These two basic modes of motion are illustrated in Figure 12. Note that the bending of (Fab')$_2\mu$ may take place on either side of the μ–μ

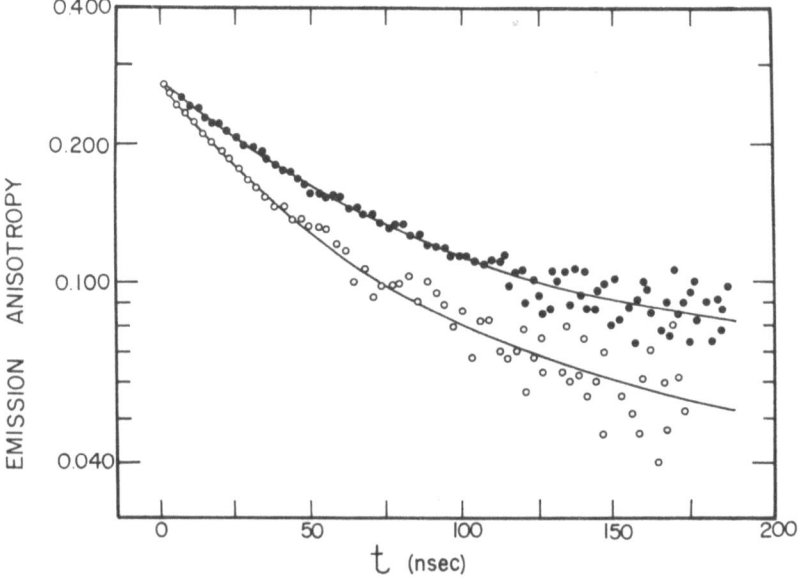

Figure 11. Comparison of the time dependence of emission anisotropy of native (●) and acid-treated (○) equine anti-DNS IgM. (———) Non-linear least-squares best fit of the observed data points (●, ○) to a sum of two exponential decays.

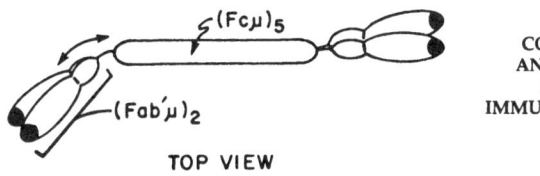

TOP VIEW

Figure 12. Modes of segmental flexibility of IgM. Two possible types of motion are shown. Only two of the five $(Fab')_2$ moieties are depicted in the side view. Adapted from Holowka and Cathou (1976b).

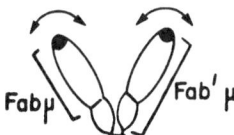

interchain disulfide bond, a feature that was recently suggested for the hinge region of IgG by the X-ray crystallographic studies of Colman *et al.* (1976). These two basic modes of motion, along with the rotation of the entire IgM, are sufficient to account for all of nanosecond depolarization data. They are also compatible with the electron micrographs of IgM that show stellate structures with varying orientations of the Fab segments, and "staple" configurations when IgM is antigen-bound.

The nurse shark anti-DNS IgM depolarization is even more complex than that of the horse and pig IgM. The very fast initial depolarization component is too short to be attributed to the rotation of an Fab-like fragment. With the exception of this very short component, there does not seem to be any component of less than 80 nsec that can be attributed to macromolecular rotation. With anti-DNS IgM from two different nurse sharks, the value of ϕ_s ranged from 88 to 117 nsec. This result shows that there is no contribution from an Fab-like rotation, since these values of ϕ_s are closer to the value expected for rotation of a fragment the size of $(Fab')_2\mu$. The $C\mu2$ domains in shark IgM may be more strongly associated (and possibly more compact) than the analogous domains in IgM of mammalian origin. Papain or trypsin digestion of shark IgMs yields only $(Fab')_2$ and no Fab; after reduction of the IgM$_s$, however, the susceptible bond or bonds become exposed and Fab can be obtained (Klapper *et al.*, 1971). Our results are in agreement with the conclusions of Zagyansky and Ivannikova (1974), who employed steady-state fluorescence polarization to examine DNS-conjugated shark IgM, and concluded that this Ig was less flexibile than those of the higher vertebrates. The steady-state results, however, did not give any indication as to the nature of the flexible segments. In this regard, it is also of interest that our steady-state polarization studies did not detect the difference between hapten and acid-eluted equine IgM, and the higher value of ϕ obtained for porcine IgM, $\phi = 93$ nsec, was not considered to be outside the experimental error of the measurements (Holowka, 1975; Cathou *et al.*, 1974).

For native equine IgM, the component with a long rotational correlation time is probably due to the rotation of the whole molecule. This correlation time could probably be measured more accurately with a longer-lifetime fluorophore such as pyrenebutyrate in an antipyrene combining site. For the porcine IgM, the value of ϕ_L is shorter, i.e., about 570 nsec. This difference may be due to the use of somewhat different purification procedures for the two antibodies. The horse anti-DNS was eluted from immunoadsorbent with hapten, whereas the porcine anti-DNS was eluted with 0.2 M acetic acid and immediately neutralized.

3.2.2. Conformational Lability of the Cμ2 Domains

Weak interactions between the Cμ2 domains may be particularly sensitive to external perturbing agents that lead to irreversible conformational changes. In addition to the effects of acetic acid on flexibility discussed above, the effects of other agents have also been noted. The differential effects of heat (Plaut and Tomasi, 1970) and urea (Shimizu *et al.*, 1974) on the trypsin digestion of human IgM can be accounted for by an irreversible exposure of trypsin-sensitive sites in the Cμ2 domain following these treatments. Equine IgM antipneumococcal antibodies were shown to be especially sensitive to heat treatment with regards to their complement-fixing ability (Deutsch and Amiraian, 1968), and similar correlations of heat and urea treatment with the destruction of complement fixation by rabbit IgM were reported (Cunniff *et al.*, 1968). Recently, it was found that exposure of rabbit IgM to acid pH (pH < 4) also destroyed complement fixation, even though antigen-binding was not affected (Stollar *et al.*, 1976). Thus, it is tempting to speculate that Cμ2–Cμ2 domain interaction may be involved in the activation of binding of the first component of complement (C1q) by antigen. The proper interaction of these domains, governed by a particular spacing of the antigenic determinants in the antigen–IgM complex, may be the trigger that exposes the C1q-binding sites on the $(Fc)_5\mu$ region. Acid treatment of IgM, which prevents the proper antigen-induced conformation necessary for tight C1q binding, would do so by destroying the Cμ2–Cμ2 noncovalent interaction. It should be noted, however, that acid treatment also appears to make the $(Fc)_5\mu$ more susceptible to enzymatic digestion (Holowka and Cathou, 1976a), so that complement-fixation-sensitive alterations may be occurring in that region as well. Recent evidence that monovalent antigen is sufficient to trigger complement activation in rabbit IgM (Brown and Koshland, 1975) is difficult to explain without invoking an allosteric mechanism, but in this case, the integrity of the Cμ2 conformation may be necessary to transmit a signal from the Fab to the $(Fc)_5\mu$ region. The precise role of conformational changes still remains to be assessed.

3.2.3. Role of Flexibility in Function

The finding that IgM from both mammalian species studied, as well as from the immunologically primitive nurse shark, clearly exhibits some segmental motion implicates such motion as a fundamental requirement for the function of this Ig class. It is likely that such flexibility would have advantages in the formation of antigen–antibody complexes. Although the entropy factor is minimized during the formation of multisite antigen–antibody complexes when the antibody-combining sites are as close together as possible (Crothers and Metzger, 1972), flexibility should not decrease such holding power as long as these minimal site-to-site distances are attainable. On the other hand, the capturing power of a multivalent antibody such as IgM should be enhanced by flexibility with respect to the angular orientation factor and also the minimum antigenic site density that is required (Crothers and Metzger, 1972). It is not immediately obvious, however, why the *rate* of segmental rotation should be as rapid as it is. Since the dissociation rate for a monovalent antigen–antibody interaction is maximally about 10^3–10^4 sec^{-1} (Froese and Sehon, 1965; Haselkorn *et al.*, 1974), one would anticipate that segmental rotation in the microsecond rather than nanosecond time range would be sufficient to enhance the multivalent avidity effect.

Thus, it is more likely that the requirement for segmental flexibility extends beyond the binding-enhancement effect. The correlation between the ability of IgM to fix complement and the need to maintain some control over the degree of flexibility that the effects of acid exposure suggest may be the key to the understanding of the conformationally subtle transfer of information from the combining site to a physically distant effector site in the IgM antibody molecule.

4. Immunoglobulin A

4.1. Conformation

4.1.1. Ultrastructure

IgA occurs in several polymeric forms. In serum, it is found primarily as monomer, but dimer or higher oligomers also occur. The polymeric forms contain 1-mole J chain per polymer (Koshland, 1975). When secreted by mucosal surfaces, it is designated *secretory IgA* and contains 1 mole each of J chain and secretory component.

Electron micrographs of dimeric serum IgA of human and murine myeloma origin show that the molecule consists of two Y-shaped 7 S subunits linked at the base of each Fc (Munn *et al.*, 1971; Dourmashkin *et al.*, 1971) (see Figure 13). The joint between adjacent Fc regions appears to be rigid, whereas considerable flexibility is present at the hinge region between Fab and Fc, judging from the variable disposition of individual Fab moieties. The J chain, which is attached at the joint between the two Fc regions (Mestecky *et al.*, 1974; Halpern and Koshland, 1973; Chapuis and Koshland, 1974), cannot be seen.

Secretory IgA, on the othe hand, which also contains two IgA monomers, appears to have a different conformation. The two monomers are superimposed on each other in sandwich fashion (Svehag and Bloth, 1970).

Evidence of the domain structure of IgA was first seen in electron micrographs (Green *et al.*, 1971) and later confirmed by high-resolution X-ray diffraction studies on the Fab fragment of McPC 603 (Segal *et al.*, 1974). In the meantime, Inbar *et al.* (1972) demonstrated that peptic cleavage of MOPC 315 yielded a small fragment that was composed of the variable halves of the L chain and Fd, linked noncovalently, which they designated Fv fragment. This fragment retained the binding activity for DNP haptens. Furthermore, the two chains could be dissociated in 8 M urea and then reassociated to give an active fragment (Hochman *et al.*, 1973). Subsequently, an Fv fragment was also prepared from another murine IgA, XRPC-25 (Sharon and Givol, 1976).

Apart from the EM studies, little information is available on the gross conformation of IgA in solution. The three-dimensional structure of the Fab fragments is very similar to that of IgG Fab (Segal *et al.*, 1974). CD spectra of human serum IgA (monomers and dimers) and secretory IgA are similar to those exhibited by IgG (Underdown and Dorrington, 1974). The structure of Fc remains to be elucidated.

4.1.2. Conformational Changes on Antigen-Binding

On binding of MOPC 315 IgA to bivalent haptens, unusual structures were observed in electron micrographs (Munn *et al.*, 1971; Green *et al.*, 1971). These structures consisted for the most part of a double central bar with eight subunits,

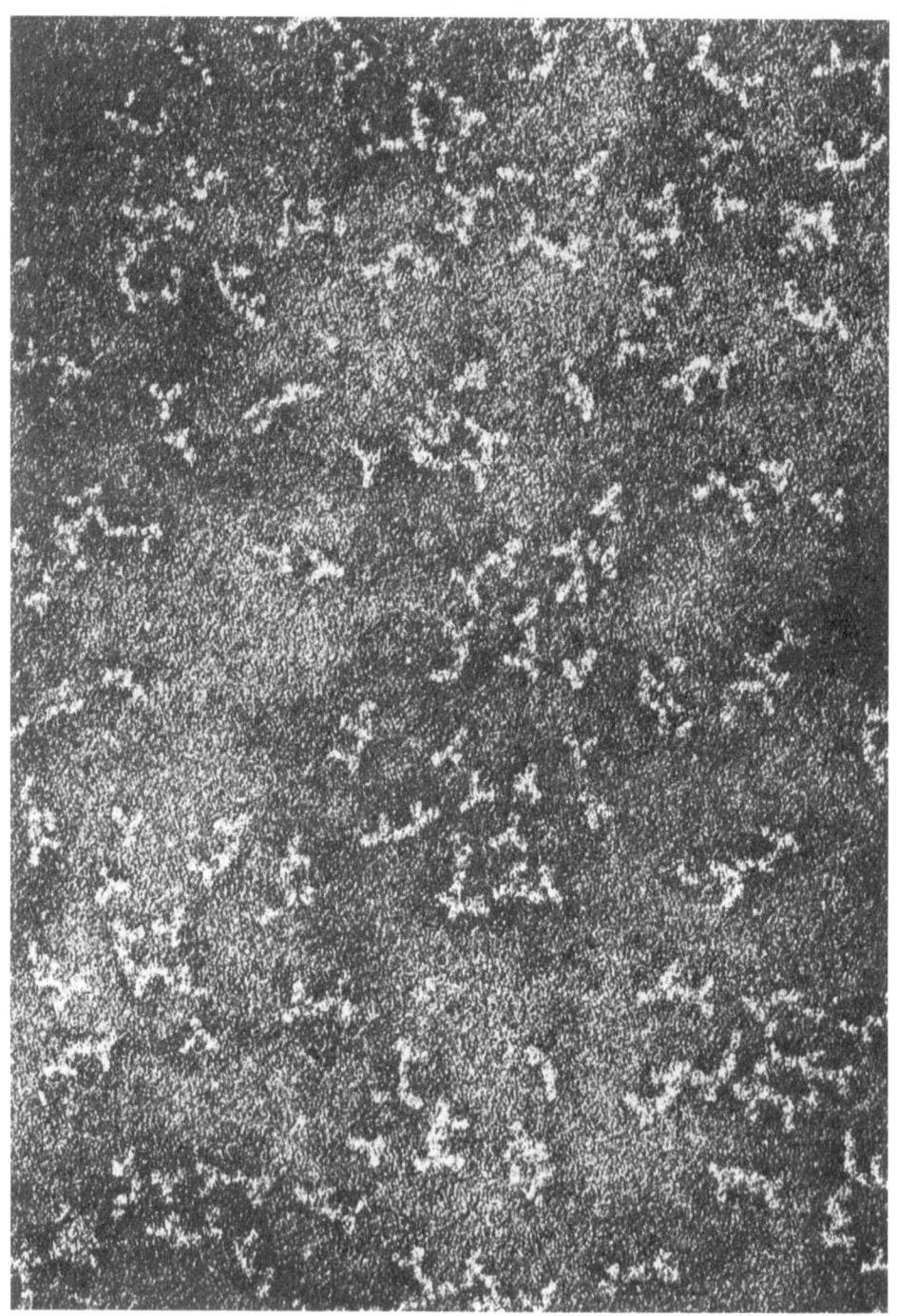

Figure 13. Electron micrograph of murine myeloma MOPC 315 IgA. Both monomers and dimers are visible. Courtesy of R. Dourmashkin and Academic Press, Inc.

probably domains, and forked projections at the four corners of the bar. Reduction of the dimeric IgA to monomer and subsequent binding of the same haptens gave double bars without the projections at the corners. One model that both laboratories proposed consists of a collapsed structure in which two pairs of parallel Fab fragments are joined end to end by two molecules of bivalent hapten (see Figure 14). Side-by-side aggregation through Fab regions would yield the central bar; the forked structures at the corners would then consist of the second monomer in each

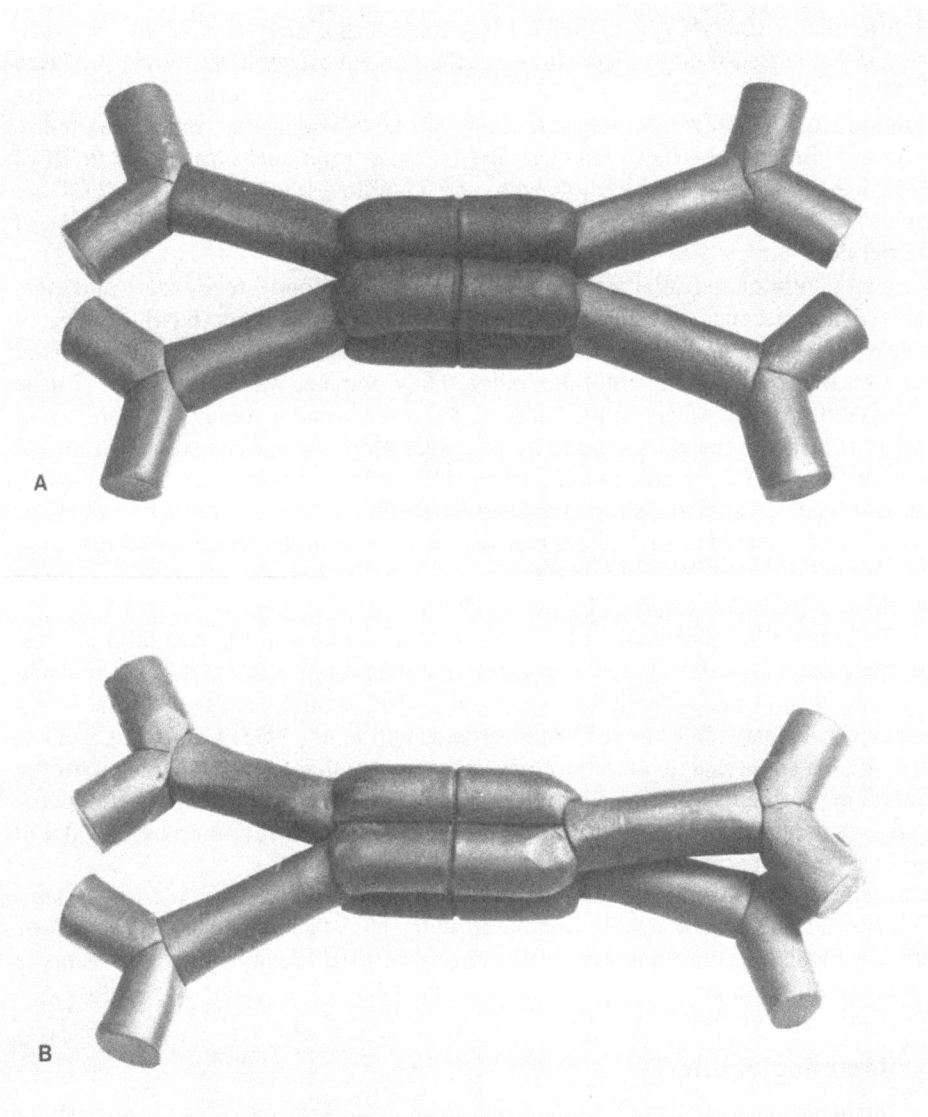

Figure 14. Two possible models for the polymers of MOPC 315 (dimer) with the bis-DNP hapten. A. Side-by-side aggregation of two linked dimers. B. Tetramer in which all four molecules are linked by hapten. Adapted from Green *et al.* (1971).

dimer that were apparently unlinked by hapten. Recent support for this model is given by sedimentation studies of the same types of complex by Wilder *et al.* (1975). Such a model requires a large conformational change in IgA from the open Y structure of the Fab regions to the collapsed structure in which the angle between adjacent Fabs is effectively zero. This structure is partly stabilized by protein–protein interactions, however, and may not be typical of other IgA molecules.

4.2. Flexibility

The evidence for segmental flexibility in IgA is equivocal. On the other hand, electron micrographs of serum dimeric IgA suggest that there is flexibility between Fab and Fc, since different dispositions of the Fab can be seen, as shown in Figure 13 (Munn *et al.*, 1971; Dourmashkin *et al.*, 1971). In a recent series of steady-state fluorescence depolarization measurements of DNS-conjugated myeloma monomeric and dimeric IgA (both subclass IgA1), mean rotational correlation times of 26–32 nsec were obtained (Zagyansky and Gavrilova, 1974). These values are similar to those obtained for Fabα fragments, and thus also suggest the presence of internal flexibility.

On the other hand, Weltman and Davis (1970) made both steady-state and time-resolved fluorescence depolarization measurements on another DNS-conjugated IgA myeloma with a sedimentation coefficient of 10.4 S, of the IgA1 subclass, and found no evidence of segmental flexibility. They obtained values of $\bar{\phi} = 147$ nsec (steady-state) and a single value of $\phi = 493$ nsec (time-resolved), which are in marked contrast to the values found by Zagyansky and Gavrilova (1974) for IgA and by others for IgG (Yguerabide *et al.*, 1970). The difference between $\bar{\phi}$ and ϕ for IgA was attributed to rapid and short-lived depolarization of the covalently bound DNS, which would contribute to $\bar{\phi}$ and which was also seen in the nanosecond emission experiments as an initial and fast component with an apparent correlation time of less than 15 nsec (Weltman and Davis, 1970).

To explain the discrepancy between results obtained in the two laboratories, Zagyansky and Gavrilova (1974) suggested that the protein studied by Weltman and Davis might have had a deleted hinge region, which would have resulted in a rigid molecule. Such molecules have been observed (Fett *et al.*, 1973; Lopes and Steiner, 1973). Results obtained in our laboratory suggest a possible additional reason for the discrepancy; because of the initial rapid depolarization of covalently linked fluorophore, correlation times of intermediate value (i.e., ≈ 30 nsec) may be masked in time-resolved experiments (Chan and Cathou, unpublished).

Ideally, nanosecond depolarization experiments should be made on an anti-DNS IgA so that results can be compared with those already obtained for IgG or with IgA to which a chromophore with a longer intrinsic lifetime, such as pyrene, is noncovalently absorbed.

5. Immunoglobulin D

IgD is normally present in serum at low concentrations (approximately 60 μg/ml or less). Leslie *et al.* (1975) measured the circulating IgD levels in a population of children and adults and found that while neonates have no measurable IgD, levels steadily increase from 2 μg/ml in children 1–6 months old to about 58 μg/ml in adults. The role of serum IgD has remained enigmatic, although there is increasing evidence that IgD antibody may be most commonly directed against chronically presented antigens (Lertora *et al.*, 1975). Recently, it was observed that IgD can fix complement by the alternate pathway (Konno *et al.*, 1975).

In the last few years, however, a considerable amount of evidence has accumulated that suggests that the primary role of IgD may be as a lymphocyte surface Ig. In the human newborn, IgD is the most frequently detected surface Ig (Rowe *et al.*, 1973), in contrast to the low concentration in serum, and a large fraction of adult human peripheral blood lymphocytes also bear IgD (van Boxel *et al.*, 1972). Lymphoid cell lines grown in continuous *in vitro* culture bear IgD and Ig's of other classes, so that the same cell is capable of synthesizing several Ig's, even though only one class is normally secreted (van Boxel and Buell, 1974). Recently, an Ig thought to be a homologue of human IgD was demonstrated on the surface of murine lymphocytes (Melcher *et al.*, 1974). The role of membrane-bound IgD is still unknown.

Luckily, a number of myeloma proteins in the IgD class have been observed, so that structural studies have been possible. Curiously, these proteins have all contained λ L chains.

5.1. Conformation

5.1.1. Covalent Structure

The IgD molecule has an architecture similar to that of IgG: it contains two H (δ) chains and two L chains. A single disulfide bond connects the δ chains (Perry and Milstein, 1970; Spiegelberg *et al.*, 1970). The amino acid sequence around the bridge is (Perry and Milstein, 1970): Thr-Pro-Glu-Cys-Pro-Ser-His-Thr-Gln-Pro-Leu-Gly-Val.

The molecular weight of the polypeptide portion of the δ chain has been variously reported as 61,000 (Leslie *et al.*, 1975) and as 50,000 (Spiegelberg *et al.*, 1970; Goyert *et al.*, 1976). The higher molecular weight would suggest a fourth constant-homology domain, as is found in μ chains, while the lower molecular weight has been interpreted in terms of an extended hinge region. It is to be hoped that the complete amino acid sequence of several δ chains will be available in the near future to resolve this discrepancy.

The IgD-like molecule on the surface of murine splenocytes is a four-chain structure just like the secreted myeloma proteins (Melcher and Uhr, 1976). Some comparisons of mobility of membrane δ and μ chains were made by sodium dodecyl sulfate–polyacrylamide gel electrophoresis (SDS-PAGE) (Finkelman *et al.*, 1976). Both human membrane δ and μ chains exhibit similar mobilities, an observation that points out the necessity of additional criteria for identifying a given chain. On the other hand, the murine homologue of δ chain has a faster mobility than the μ chain. Thus, the molecular weight or the oligosaccharide content, or both, of the mouse "δ" chain could be different from that of the human chain. Interestingly, the molecular weight of the murine "δ" chain is 65,800 (Melcher and Uhr, 1976), which falls about midway between the molecular weights reported for human δ chain: 69,700 (Leslie *et al.*, 1975) and 60,000 (Spiegelberg *et al.*, 1970) (no corrections made for oligosaccharide content).

5.1.2. Conformation

Few studies have been made on the conformation of IgD. Measurement of the CD spectra of several IgD myeloma proteins showed negative bands at 217 nm and fine structure in the 250–300 nm region; one protein had a positive band at 232 nm (Johnson *et al.*, 1975). These features are similar to those observed in the CD spectra of other Ig's, so that no unusual features can be discerned (Cathou and Dorrington, 1975).

IgD does, however, exhibit a very unusual feature in another respect: it is extremely labile to enzymatic proteolysis. Exposure for 2 min to trypsin at 56°C results in the complete disappearance of the intact molecule (Wolcott *et al.*, 1975). After 4 min of digestion, several fragments could be isolated: an Fab-like fragment with a molecular weight of 48,000, Fc with a molecular weight of 64,000 in 80–85% yield, a small quantity of material with a molecular weight greater than 100,000 with both H- and L-chain antigenic determinants, and a small fragment with a molecular weight of 18,000 with neither H- nor L-chain determinants. The Fab-like fragment was not homogeneous, and was susceptible to further digestion. The Fc fragment, on the other hand, was homogeneous by several criteria: *N*-terminal amino acid analysis (Thr), SDS-PAGE, immunoelectrophoresis, and ultracentrifugation. This fragment, then, is suitable for primary structure analysis. The lability to proteolysis has also been noted for the murine cell-surface IgD-like molecule (Melcher and Uhr, 1976). It was tentatively ascribed to an extended or more exposed hinge region on the basis of hydrodynamic measurements (Griffiths and Gleich, 1972). The frictional coefficient ratios f/f_{min} of intact IgD and of the Fc fragment are considerably higher than those of other Ig's (Griffiths and Gleich, 1972). For example, $f/f_{min} = 1.80$ for IgD and its Fc fragment (mol. wt. 58,000), whereas $f/f_{min} = 1.47$ for IgG and 1.21 for its Fc fragment (Noelken *et al.*, 1965) and 1.69 for IgMs (Miller and Metzger, 1965). Since hydration of carbohydrate residues would increase the value of f/f_{min}, a comparison between the values obtained for IgD and IgMs is more meaningful than for IgD and IgG. It can be seen that the f/f_{min} of IgD is larger. Thus, Griffiths and Gleich suggested that IgD and its Fc fragment may have a less compact conformation.

5.2. Flexibility

No measurements of the flexibility of IgD have been reported. With, however, the increased interest in IgD due to its presence on lymphocyte membranes, more information should be available in the near future.

6. Immunoglobulin E

6.1. Conformation

IgE represents an important class of Ig's that is synthesized primarily in respiratory and gastrointestinal mucosa and regional lymph nodes, but is generally present in only very low concentrations of serum (for reviews, see Ishizaka, 1970; Bennich and Johansson, 1971). IgE is present in man and higher primates, and has been identified in several mammals. Most IgE is found bound to skin mast cells and basophils; its primary functions appear to be stimulation of target cells to release histamine, slow-reacting substance of anaphylaxis (Ishizaka, 1972), and a chemotactic factor of eosinophils (Kay and Austen, 1971). Because the serum concentrations are generally in the nanograms-per-milliliter range (Bennich and Johansson, 1971), much of our present knowledge on the structure, conformation, and flexibility of IgE has been obtained from studies on several myeloma proteins (Johansson and Bennich, 1967; Ogawa *et al.*, 1969; Nezlin *et al.*, 1973).

6.1.1. Covalent Structure

The IgE molecule consists of two L and two H (ϵ) chains linked by interchain disulfides (Bennich and Johansson, 1971). The intact molecule has a molecular weight of 188,100 and a sedimentation coefficient of $S^\circ_{20,w} = 8.20$ (Bennich and Johansson, 1971). Total carbohydrate content is about 12% (Bennich and Johansson, 1971; Kochwa *et al.*, 1971; Nezlin *et al.*, 1973). There are most likely two antigen-combining sites per IgE molecule, since antibodies against ragweed antigen were found to agglutinate red cells coated with this antigen (Ishizaka, 1970). The molecular weight of the ϵ chain is 72,500, and when corrected for carbohydrate content, is about 60,000 (Bennich and Dorrington, 1972), so that the ϵ chain contains five homology domains similar to the μ chain.

The ϵ chain of protein ND was sequenced recently (Bennich and von Bahr-Lindström, 1974) and the positions of intra- and interchain disulfides located. IgE is unique among the Ig's in that the Cϵ2 domains are flanked on either side by the two inter-ϵ-chain disulfides at Cys 231 and Cys 318 (Bennich and von Bahr-Lindström, 1974). The L chain is bonded to the adjacent H chain via a cysteine at position 128 or 129. There is also an additional intrachain disulfide between Cys 128 and Cys 129 (the one not involved in the L–H disulfide) and Cys 215 that is quite labile to reduction. The arrangement of these latter bonds is similar to that found in rabbit IgG (O'Donnell *et al.*, 1970).

6.1.2. Proteolytic Fragmentation

The action of several proteolytic enzymes on IgE (ND) has been extensively studied. Digestion for 2 hr by papain produces a mixture of Fab and Fc, as well as a small fragment designated Fc″ and a fragment of the L chain, C$_\lambda$ (Bennich and Johansson, 1971). Two sizes of Fab are produced, one with carbohydrate and a molecular weight of 50,000 and another without carbohydrate and a molecular weight of 40,000. The Fc fragment exhibits a molecular weight of 95,000 and contains the Cϵ2, Cϵ3, and Cϵ4 domains. Fc″ has a molecular weight of 38,000, contains 20% carbohydrate, and is a covalently linked dimer of the Cϵ2 domains. After 16 hr of digestion, the only identifiable fragments are Fc, Fc″, and C$_\lambda$, so that the Fab moieties are quite labile. Trypsin digestion, on the other hand, produces primarily (Fab′)$_2$ (mol. wt. 103,000) and Fc″, while pepsin produces a larger (Fab′)$_2$ fragment (mol. wt. 140,000) and, in low yield, a fragment designated pFc, which was identified as a covalently linked dimer of Cϵ4 (mol. wt. 30,000) (Bennich and Johansson, 1971). No fragment consisting of just Cϵ3 and Cϵ4 has been recovered from any of these digests. Of all these fragments, only the intact Fc (Cϵ2–4) possesses cytotropic activity, and since Fc″ does not, this activity must reside in either or both of Cϵ3 and Cϵ4 (Bennich and Dorrington, 1972). The isolated Cϵ4-domain fragment, pFc, does not possess cytotropic activity, so that either or both

Cε3 and Cε4 contribute directly to the cell-fixation site, or both domains are necessary for conformational stability of the relevant domain (Dorrington and Bennich, 1973).

6.1.3. Secondary and Tertiary Structure and Lability of Domains

The CD spectra of IgE (ND) and IgE (PS) both exhibit bands at 217 nm, a common feature of all Ig's that has been attributed to peptide bonds in the β conformation (Dorrington and Bennich, 1973). Both proteins also exhibit numerous bonds that can be attributed to aromatic amino acid residues. The CD spectra of the (Fab')$_2$, Fc″, and Fc fragments of IgE (ND) also show these features, so that the basic immunoglobulin fold is probably present in all domains. An exception may be pFc, which corresponds to the Cε4 domain and is partially unfolded when isolated (Dorrington and Bennich, 1973).

On being heated at 56°C for 4 hr, IgE antibodies lose their skin-sensitizing activity as well as class-specific antigenic determinants in the Fc portion, although antigen-binding activity remains (Ishizaka et al., 1967). Dorrington and Bennich (1973) showed that heating at 56°C for 30 min causes irreversible conformational changes in Fc, but not in (Fab')$_2$ or Fc′, so that these changes must be associated with the Cε3 and Cε4 domains.

Reduction of disulfide bonds also causes loss of skin-sensitizing activity (Stanworth et al., 1970; Ishizaka, 1972), which appears to be associated with reduction of the extra intrachain disulfide in Cε1 and the inter-ε disulfide in Cε1 and the inter-ε disulfide at Cys 318 (Kehoe and Lundkvist, 1974). The L–H disulfide is the most labile, being reduced by 1.0 mM dithiothreitol in less than 25 min (Bennich and Dorrington, 1972; Kochwa et al., 1971); however, no changes in CD are produced and reduction of the L–H bond probably does not lead to changes in cytotropic activity (Bennich and Dorrington, 1972).

The conformation of the Cε2 domain appears to be rather different from that of the homologous Cμ2 domain. Cε2 is stable to proteolytic digestion (Bennich and Johansson, 1971), and any conformational transitions caused by heating at 56°C are reversible and do not lead to loss of antigenic determinants (Dorrington and Bennich, 1973). These properties are in marked contrast to those of Cμ2, which is very sensitive to degradation and irreversible conformational changes (see Section 3.2.2).

6.1.4. Gross Conformation

No information is available at present on the topological arrangement of the domains in IgE.

6.2. Flexibility

All studies of segmental flexibility have been performed on the two IgE myeloma proteins, ND and Yu. Steady-state fluorescence polarization, ESR, and time-resolved fluorescence depolarization measurements have been made; in all cases, the probe was covalently attached to the protein. The results suggest that IgE exhibits much less flexibility in the nanosecond time range than IgG or IgM does.

6.2.1. Fluorescence Polarization

75

SOLUTION
CONFORMATION
AND SEGMENTAL
FLEXIBILITY OF
IMMUNOGLOBULINS

The mean rotational correlation time obtained for DNS-IgE (Yu) from steady-state measurements was 55 nsec (Nezlin *et al.*, 1973). This value is higher than that found for IgG in the same study ($\bar{\phi} = 21$ nsec), and suggests that IgE as a whole is more rigid. The value obtained for $(Fab')_2\epsilon$ was 49 nsec, so that removal of the $C\epsilon 3$ and $C\epsilon 4$ domains had little effect on $\bar{\phi}$ Since the calculated values of ϕ_0 (spherical molecule) for both $(Fab')_2\epsilon$ and IgG are similar, i.e., about 68 nsec, the higher value of $\bar{\phi}$ for $(Fab')_2\epsilon$ also suggests that $(Fab')_2\epsilon$ is a more rigid or more asymmetrical molecule than is IgG.

Time-resolved fluorescence depolarization measurements of the $(Fab')_2\epsilon$ fragment of IgE (ND) with 1,8-N-(aminoethyl)-8-naphthylamine-1-sulfonic acid covalently and randomly attached (*not* at reduced cystines), with excitation at a wavelength that minimized excitation of freely rotating dye, gave an anisotropy decay curve that could be fit either by a single value of $\phi = 120$ nsec or by two exponential components with values of $f_s = 0.2$, $\phi_s = 37$ nsec, $f_L = 0.8$, and $\phi_L = 150$ nsec (Chan *et al.*, unpublished). The average difference in statistical error of these two solutions, with two separate preparations, was 11%, which makes it difficult to choose between them. A value of $\phi_s = 37$ nsec could represent rotation of an Fab moiety. If so, a weighting factor of 0.2 suggests little contribution from this type of motion. Results on whole IgE showed an even smaller contribution of segmental flexibility; in this case, $f_s = 0.08$, $\phi_s = 45$ nsec, $f_L = 0.92$, $\phi_L = 210$ nsec.

Thus, both steady-state and time-resolved fluorescence measurements show that IgE is more rigid than IgG, at least on a nanosecond time scale.

6.2.2. ESR Studies

Both IgE (Yu) and IgE (ND) have been labeled with a spin probe (Nezlin *et al.*, 1973; Käiväräinen and Nezlin, 1976). With both proteins, the ESR spectra showed contributions from spin label in two states that were ascribed to the presence of two conformers in equilibrium with each other, as in the case of IgG (see Section 2.2.5). The transition time between conformers must be slow, with a mean lifetime of each conformer of greater than 100 nsec, in order to resolve them by ESR. In IgE, however, in contrast to IgG, the more compact conformer appears to predominate. Mean rotational correlation times of the IgE conformers were also larger than those of the IgG conformers (see Table 4). $\bar{\phi}_1$ and $\bar{\phi}_2$ of IgE must thus represent either or both the motion of a larger molecular fragment than Fab [$(Fab')_2$?] and a larger contribution from rotation of the whole molecule than in the case of IgG. In any case, these ESR results also suggest that IgE is more rigid than IgG. More data are

TABLE 4. Mean Rotational Correlation
Times of Spin-Labeled IgG and IgE[a]

Immunoglobulin	$\bar{\phi}_1$ (nsec)	$\bar{\phi}_2$ (nsec)
IgG	35	23
IgE (Yu)	60	43

[a]From Nezlin *et al.* (1973).

clearly needed to describe the internal motions, if any, of IgE, and it would be most helpful to make measurements on antibodies with probe bound in the combining sites.

7. Concluding Remarks

With the advent of more sensitive physicochemical techniques, considerable interest has been rekindled in the possible role of conformational changes in triggering immunological events on molecular and cellular levels and the importance of measurements of dynamic structure of Ig's. One of the benefits of X-ray diffraction studies has been to define clearly the tertiary structures of domains and to show that the simple classic models of protein structure, i.e., ellipsoids, cylinders, and spheres, may not be entirely appropriate as the best descriptions of shape. It is to be hoped that this realization will inspire the development of more rigorous mathematical models to refine the interpretation of physicochemical results.

A number of basic questions remain unanswered. For example: (1) What is the nature of the conformational changes that occur on binding of antibody and antigen, and how do such changes lead to complement fixation (if they do at all)? (2) Does Fab exist in more than one quaternary structure conformation in solution, and is there interconversion triggered by antigen? (3) What is the conformation of antigen receptor IgMs, and what is the nature of any conformational changes that might lead to B-memory-cell differentiation? (4) What are the dynamic structures of IgD and IgE? (5) What is the structure of T-cell Ig's? Finally, a number of problems, although partially answered, still need more precise solutions, i.e., a comparison of gross conformation and flexibility of IgG in the absence and presence of antigen. Immunochemistry does not appear to be in any danger of an early death.

References

Amzel, L. M., Poljak, R. J., Saul, F., Varga, J. M., and Richards, F. F., 1974, The three-dimensional structure of a combining region–ligand complex of immunoglobulin New at 3.5-Å resolution, *Proc. Natl. Acad. Sci. U.S.A.* **71**:1427–1430.

Appella, E., Roholt, O. A., Chersi, A., Radziminski, G. and Pressman, D., 1973, Amino acid sequence of the light chain derived from a rabbit anti-*p*-azobenzoate antibody of restricted heterogeneity, *Biochem. Biophys. Res. Commun.* **53**:1122–1129.

Ashman, R. F., Kaplan, A. P., and Metzger, H., 1971, A search for conformational change on ligand binding in a human γ M macroglobulin. I. Circular dichroism and hydrogen exchange, *Immunochemistry* **8**:627–641.

Beale, D., 1974, Fragmentation and reduction of porcine 19S immunoglobulin M, *FEBS Lett.* **44**:236–239.

Beale, D., and Feinstein, A., 1969, Studies on the reduction of a human 19S immunoglobulin M, *Biochem. J.* **112**:187–194.

Bennich, H., and Dorrington, K. J., 1972, Structure and conformation of immunoglobulin E, in: *The Biological Role of the Immunoglobulin E System*, Proceedings of a conference held June 4–7, 1972 (K. Ishizaka and D. H. Dayton, Jr., eds.), pp. 19–32, U.S. Department of Health, Education and Welfare, Washington, D.C.

Bennich, H., and Johansson, S. G. O., 1971, Structure and function of human immunoglobulin E, *Adv. Immunol.* **13**:1–55.

Bennich, H., and von Bahr-Lindström, H., 1974, Structure of immunoblobulin E (IgE), in: *Progress in Immunology II*, Vol. 1 (L. Brent and J. Holborow, eds.), pp. 49–58, North-Holland, Amsterdam.

Bjork, I., and Tanford, C., 1971, Recovery of native conformation of rabbit immunoglobulin G upon recombination of separately renatured heavy and light chains at near-neutral pH, *Biochemistry* **10**:1289–1295.

Bjork, I., Karlsson, F. A., and Berggård, I., 1971, Independent folding of the variable and constant halves of a lambda immunoglobulin light chain, *Proc. Natl. Acad. Sci. U.S.A.* **68**:1707–1710.

Brochon, J.-C., and Wahl, P., 1972, Measures des declins de L'anisotropie de fluorescence de la γ-globuline et des ses fragments Fab, Fc et F(ab)₂ marques avec le 1-sulfonyl-5-dimethyl-aminonaphtalène, *Eur. J. Biochem.* **25**:20–32.

Brown, J. C., and Koshland, M. E., 1975, Activation of antibody Fc function by antigen-induced conformational changes, *Proc. Natl. Acad. Sci. U.S.A.* **72**:5111–5115.

Bunting, J. R., and Cathou, R. E., 1973, Energy transfer distance measurements in immunoglobulins. II. Localization of the hapten binding sites and the interheavy chain disulfide bond in rabbit antibody, *J. Mol. Biol.* **77**:223–235.

Bunting, J. R., and Cathou, R. E., 1974, Energy transfer distance measurements in immunoglobulins. III. Location of the light–heavy interchain disulfide bond in rabbit immunoglobulin G antibody, *J. Mol. Biol.* **87**:329–338.

Cathou, R. E., and Dorrington, K. J., 1975, The conformation, interaction, and biological roles of immunoglobulin subunits, in: *Subunits in Biological Systems,* Part C (S. N. Timasheff and Fasman, G. D., eds.), pp. 91–223, M. Dekker, New York.

Cathou, R. E., and O'Konski, C. T., 1970, A transient electric birefringence study of the structure of specific IgG antibody, *J. Mol. Biol.* **48**:125–131.

Cathou, R. E., Kulczycki, A., Jr., and Haber, E., 1968, Structural features of γ-immunoglobulin, antibody, and their fragments: Circular dichroism studies, *Biochemistry* **7**:3958–3964.

Cathou, R. E., Holowka, D. A., and Chan, L. M., 1974, Conformation and flexibility of immunoglobulins, in: *Progress in Immunology II,* Vol. 1 (L. Brent and J. Holborow, eds.), pp. 63–73, North-Holland, Amsterdam.

Chan, L. M., and Cathou, R. E., 1977, The role of the inter-heavy chain disulfide bond in modulating the flexibility of immunoglobulin G antibody, *J. Mol. Biol.* **112**:653–656.

Chapuis, R. M., and Koshland, M. E., 1974, Mechanism of IgM polymerization, *Proc. Natl. Acad. Sci. U.S.A.* **71**:657–661.

Colman, P. M., Deisenhofer, J., Huber, R., and Palm, W., 1976, Structure of the human antibody molecule Kol (immunologlobulin G1): An electron density Map at 5 Å resolution, *J. Mol. Biol.* **100**:257–282.

Crothers, D. M., and Metzger, H., 1972, The influence of polyvalency on the binding properties of antibodies, *Immunochemistry* **9**:341–357.

Cunniff, R. V. H., Cole, H. H., and Stollar, B. D., 1968, Properties of 19S antibodies in complement fixation. II. Selective inactivation of a complement-fixing site by urea, *J. Immunol.* **101**:695–701.

Dale, R., and Eisinger, J., 1975, Polarized excitation energy transfer, in: *Biochemical Fluorescence Concepts,* Vol. 1 (R. F. Chen and H. Edelhoch, eds.), pp. 115–284, Marcel Dekker, New York.

Deisenhofer, J., Colman, P. M., Huber, R., Haupt, H., and Schwick, G., 1976, Crystallographic structural studies of a human Fc-fragment. I. An electron-density map at 4 Å resolution and a partial model, *Hoppe-Seyler's Z. Physiol. Chem.* **357**:435–445.

Deutsch, G., and Amiraian, K., 1968, A study of the complement fixing properties of equine antisera, *Immunology* **15**:623–632.

Dorrington, K. J., and Bennich, H., 1973, Thermally induced structural changes in immunoglobulin E, *J. Biol. Chem.* **248**:8378–8384.

Dorrington, K. J., and Mihaesco, C., 1970, Subunit structure of human γM-globulins, *Immunochemistry* **7**:651–660.

Dorrington, K. J., and Painter, R. H., 1974, Functional domains of immunoglobulin G, in: *Progress in Immunology II,* Vol. 1 (L. Brent and J. Holborow, eds.), pp. 75–84, North-Holland, Amsterdam.

Dorrington, K. J., and Smith, B. R., 1972, Conformational changes accompanying the dissociation and association of immunoglobulin-G subunits, *Biochim. Biophys. Acta* **263**:70–81.

Dorrington, K. J., and Tanford, C., 1968, The optical rotatory dispersion of human γM-immunoglobulins and their subunits, *J. Biol. Chem.* **243**:4745–4749.

Dorrington, K. J., and Tanford, C., 1970, Molecular size and conformation of immunoglobulins, *Adv. Immunol.* **12**:333–381.

Dourmashkin, R. B., Virella, G., and Parkhouse, R. M. E., 1971, Electron microscopy of human and mouse myeloma serum IgA, *J. Mol. Biol.* **56**:207–208.

Dwek, R. A., Givol, D., Jones, R., McLaughlin, A. C., Wain-Hobson, S., White, A. I., and Wright, C., 1976, Interactions of the lanthanide and hapten binding sites in the Fv fragment from the myeloma protein MOPC 315, *Biochem. J.* **155**:37–53.

Edelman, G. M., Cunningham, B. A., Gall, W. E., Gottlieb, P. D., Rutishauser, U., and Waxdal, M. J., 1969, The covalent structure of an entire γG immunoglobulin molecule, *Proc. Natl. Acad. Sci. U.S.A.* **63**:78–85.

Epp, O., Colman, P., Fehlhammer, H., Bode, W., Schiffer, M., and Huber, R., 1974, Crystal and molecular structure of a dimer composed of the variable portions of the Bence–Jones protein Rei, *Eur. J. Biochem.* **45**:513–524.

Fanger, M. W., and Smyth, D. G., 1972, The oligosaccharide units of rabbit immunoglobulin G, *Biochem. J.* **127**:757–765.

Feinstein, A., and Munn, E. A., 1969, Conformation of the free and antigen-bound IgM antibody molecules, *Nature (London)* **224**:1307–1309.

Feinstein, A., and Rowe, A. J., 1967, Molecular mechanism of formation of an antigen–antibody complex, *Nature (London)* **205**:147–149.

Feinstein, A., Munn, E. A., and Richardson, N. E., 1971, The three-dimensional conformation of γM and γA globulin molecules, *Ann. N. Y. Acad. Sci.* **190**:104–121.

Fett, J. W., Deutsch, H. F., and Smithies, O., 1973, Hinge-region deletion localized in the IgG1-globulin Mcg, *Immunochemistry* **10**:115–118.

Finkelman, F. D., van Boxel, J. A., Asofsky, R., and Paul, W. E., 1976, Cell membrane IgD: Demonstration of IgD on human lymphocytes by enzyme-catalyzed iodination and comparison with cell surface Ig of mouse, guinea pig, and rabbit, *J. Immunol.* **116**:1173–1181.

Frangione, B., Milstein, C., and Pink, J. R. L., 1969, Structural studies of immunoglobulin G, *Nature (London)* **221**:145–148.

Frangione, B., Prelli, F., Mihaesco, C., Wolfenstein, C., Mihaesco, E., and Franklin, E. C., 1971, Structural studies of immunoglobulin G, M and A heavy chains, *Ann. N. Y. Acad. Sci.* **190**:71–82.

Froese, A., and Sehon, A., 1965, Kinetic and equilibrium studies of the reaction between anti-*p*-nitrophenyl antibodies and a homologous hapten, *Immunochemistry* **2**:135–143.

Ghose, A. C., 1971, Comparative conformational studies on the tryptic digestion fragments of human immunoglobulins M and G, *Biochem. Biophys. Res. Commun.* **45**:1144–1150.

Givol, D., and DeLorenzo, F., 1968, The position of various cleavages of rabbit immunoglobulin G, *J. Biol. Chem.* **243**:1886–1891.

Gopalakrishnan, P. V., and Karush, F., 1974, Antibody affinity. VI. Synthesis of bivalent lactosyl haptens and their interaction with anti-lactosyl antibodies, *Immunochemistry* **11**:279–283.

Goyert, S. M., Hugh, T. E., Meinke, G. C., and Speigelberg, H. L., 1976, Structural studies of IgD, *Fed. Proc. Fed. Am. Soc. Exp. Biol.* **35**:313 (Abstract).

Green, N. M., 1969, Electron microscopy of the immunoglobulins, *Adv. Immunol.* **11**:1–30.

Green, N. M., Dourmashkin, R. B., and Parkhouse, R. M. E., 1971, Electron microscopy of complexes between IgA (MOPC 315) and a bifunctional hapten, *J. Mol. Biol.* **56**:203–206.

Griffiths, R. W., and Gleich, G. J., 1972, Proteolytic degradation of IgD and its relation to molecular conformation, *J. Biol. Chem.* **247**:4543–4548.

Grossberg, A. L., Marcus, G., and Pressman, D., 1965, Change in antibody conformation induced by hapten, *Proc. Natl. Acad. Sci. U.S.A.* **54**:942–945.

Halpern, M. S., and Koshland, M. E., 1973, The stoichiometry of J chain in human secretory IgA, *J. Immunol.* **111**:1653–1660.

Haselkorn, D., Friedman, S., Givol, D., and Pecht, I., 1974, Kinetic mapping of the antibody combining site by chemical relaxation spectrometry, *Biochemistry* **13**:2210–2222.

Heidelberger, M., and Pedersen, K. O., 1937, The molecular weight of antibodies, *J. Exp. Med.* **65**:393–414.

Hester, R. B., Mole, J. E., and Schrohenloher, R. E., 1975, Evidence for the absence of non-covalent bonds in the Fc region of IgM, *J. Immunol.* **114**:487–491.

Hochman, J., Inbar, D., and Givol, D., 1973, An active antibody fragment (Fv) composed of the variable portions of heavy and light chains, *Biochemistry* **12**:1130–1135.

Holowka, D. A., 1975, Nanosecond fluorescence depolarization studies of segmental flexibility in IgM, Ph.D. thesis, Tufts University, Medford, Massachusetts.

Holowka, D. A., and Cathou, R. E., 1974, Evolution of conformational flexibility of immunoglobulin M, in: *Advances in Experimental Medicine and Biology,* Vol. 64 (W. H. Hildemann and A. A. Benedict, eds.), pp. 207–215, Plenum, New York.

Holowka, D. A., and Cathou, R. E. 1976a, The conformation of IgM. I. Characterization of anti-DNS IgM antibodies from horse, pig and shark, *Biochemistry* **15**:3373–3379.

Holowka, D. A., and Cathou, R. E., 1976b, The conformation of IgM. II. Nanosecond fluorescence depolarization analysis of segmental flexibility in anti-DNS IgM from horse, pig and shark, *Biochemistry* **15**:3379–3390.

Holowka, D. A., Strosberg, A. D., Kimball, J. W., Haber, E., and Cathou, R. E., 1972, Changes in intrinsic circular dichroism of several homogeneous anti-Type III pneumococcal antibodies on binding of a small hapten, *Proc. Natl. Acad. Sci. U.S.A.* **69**:3399–3403.

Hornick, C. L., and Karush, F., 1972, Antibody affinity. III. The role of multivalence, *Immunochemistry* **9**:325–340.

Hurst, M. M., Volanakis, J. E., Hester, R. B., Stroud, R. M., and Bennett, J. C., 1974, The structural basis for binding of complement by immunoglobulin M, *J. Exp. Med.* **140**:1117–1121.

Inbar, D., Hochman, J., and Givol, D., 1972, Localization of antibody-combining sites within the variable portions of heavy and light chains, *Proc. Natl. Acad. Sci. U.S.A.* **69**:2659–2662.

Isenman, D. E., Dorrington, K. J., and Painter, R. H., 1975, The structure and function of immunoglobulin domains. II. The importance of interchain disulfide bonds and the possible role of molecular flexibility in the interaction between immunoglobulin G and complement, *J. Immunol.* **114**:1726–1729.

Ishizaka, K., 1970, Human reaginic antibodies, *Annu. Rev. Med.* **21**:187–200.

Ishizaka, K., 1972, Historical aspects of immunoglobulin E, in: *The Biological Role of the Immunoglobulin E System,* Proceedings of a conference held June 4–7, 1972 (K. Ishizaka and D. H. Dayton, Jr., eds.), pp. 3–16, U.S. Department of Health, Education and Welfare, Washington, D.C.

Ishizaka, K., Ishizaka, T., and Menzel, A. E. O., 1967, Physicochemical properties of reaginic antibodies. VI. Effect of heat on γE, γG, and γA antibodies in the sera of ragweed sensitive patients, *J. Immunol.* **99**:610–618.

Jaton, J.-C., Huser, H., Blatt, Y., and Pecht, I., 1975a, Circular dichroism and fluorescence studies of homogeneous antibodies to Type III pneumococcal polysaccharide, *Biochemistry* **14**:5308–5311.

Jaton, J.-C., Huser, H., Braun, D. G., Givol, D., Pecht, I., and Schlessinger, J., 1975b, Conformational changes induced in a homogeneous anti-type III pneumococcal antibody by oligosaccharides of increasing size, *Biochemistry* **14**:5312-5315.

Jaton, J.-C., Huser, H., Riesen, W. F., Schlessinger, J., and Givol, D., 1976, The binding of complement by complexes formed between a rabbit antibody and oligosaccharides of increasing size, *J. Immunol.* **116**:1363–1366.

Johansson, S. G. O., and Bennich, H., 1967, Immunological studies of an atypical (myeloma) immunoglobulin, *Immunology* **13**:381–394.

Johnson, P. M., Howard, A., and Scopes, P. M., 1975, The conformation of human immunoglobulin D. *FEBS Lett.* **49**:310–313.

Käiväräinen, A. I., and Nezlin, R. S., 1976, Evidence for mobility of immunoglobulin domains obtained by spin-label method, *Biochem. Biophys. Res. Commun.* **68**:270–276.

Käiväräinen, A. I., Nezlin, R. S., Lichtenstein, H. I., Misharin, A. U., and Volkenstein, M. V., 1973, Conformational changes of spin-labeled antibodies and antigens during formation of specific complexes, *Mol. Biol. (USSR)* **7**:760–768.

Käiväräinen, A. I., Nezlin, R. S., and Volkenstein, M. V., 1974, Distances between iminoxyl radicals in antibody binding sites and the relative freedom of rotation of antibody subunits, *Mol. Biol. (USSR)* **8**:816–823.

Kay, A. B., and Austen, K. F., 1971, The IgE-mediated release of an eosinophil leukocyte chemotactic factor from human lung, *J. Immunol.* **107**:899–902.

Kehoe, J. M., and Lundkvist, U., 1974, Structure and biology of IgE, in: *Progress in Immunology II,* Vol. 1 (L. Brent and J. Holborow, eds.), pp. 276–279, North-Holland, Amsterdam.

Kim, Y. D., and Karush, F., 1973, Equine anti-hapten antibody. VII. Antilactoside antibody induced by a bacterial vaccine. *Immunochemistry* **10**:365–371.

Kishimoto, T., Onoue, K., and Yamamura, Y., 1968, Structure of human immunoglobulin M. III. Pepsin fragmentation of IgM, *J. Immunol.* **100**:1032–1040.

Klapper, D. G., Clem, L. W., and Small, P. A. Jr., 1971, Proteolytic fragmentation of elasmobranch immunoglobulins, *Biochemistry* **10**:645–652.

Knopp, J. A., and Weber, G., 1969, Fluorescence polarization of pyrenebutyric–bovine serum albumin and pyrenebutyric–human macroglobulin conjugates, *J. Biol. Chem.* **244**:6309–6315.

Kochwa, S., Terry, W. D., Capra, J. D., and Yang, N. L., 1971, Structural studies of immunoglobulin E. I. Physicochemical studies of the IgE molecule, *Ann. N. Y. Acad. Sci.* **190**:49–70.

Konno, T., Hirai, H., and Inai, S., 1975, Studies in IgD. I. Complement fixing activities of IgD myeloma proteins, *Immunochemistry* **12**:773–777.

Koshland, M. E., 1975, Structure and function of the J chain, *Adv. Immunol.* **20**:41–69.

Lertora, J. J. L., Gomez-Perez, F. J., and Leslie, G. A., 1975, Structure and biological functions of human IgD. V. Insulin antibodies of the IgD class in sera from some diabetic patients, *Int. Arch. Allergy Appl. Immunol.* **49**:597–606.

Leslie, G. A., Correa, R. H. L., and Holmes, J. N., 1975, Structure and biological functions of human IgD. IV. Ontogeny of human serum immunoglobulins D (IgD) as related to IgG, IgA and IgM, *Int. Arch. Allergy Appl. Immunol.* **49**:350–357.

Liberti, P. A., Stylos, W. A., and Maurer, P. H., 1972, Conformational change(s) induced in sheep calcium-dependent antibody upon interaction with homologous polypeptide antigen. I. Hydrogen-exchange studies of immunoglobulin G and (Fab')$_2$ fragment, *Biochemistry* **11**:3312–3320.

Lopes, A. D., and Steiner, L. A., 1973, A structural defect in a crystallizable myeloma protein, *Fed. Proc. Fed. Am. Soc. Exp. Biol.* **32**:1003 (Abstract).

Lovejoy, C., Holowka, D. A., and Cathou, R. E., 1975, Nanosecond fluorometry of anti-pyrene antibody, *Fed. Proc. Fed. Am. Soc. Exp. Biol.* **34**:44A.

Lovejoy, C., Holowka, D. A., and Cathou, R. E., 1977, Nanosecond fluorescence spectroscopy of pyrene butyrate-antipyrene antibody complexes, *Biochemistry* **16**:3668–3672.

Marchalonis, J. J., 1975, Lymphocyte surface immunoglobulins, *Science* **190**:20–29.

Melcher, U., and Uhr, J. W., 1976, Cell surface immunoglobulin. XVI. Polypeptide chain structure of mouse IgM and IgD-like molecule, *J. Immunol.* **116**:409–415.

Melcher, U., Vitetta, E. S., McWilliams, M., Lamm, M. E., Philips-Quagliata, J. M., and Uhr, J. W., 1974, Cell surface immunoglobulin. X. Identification of an IgD-like molecule on the surface of murine splenocytes, *J. Exp. Med.* **140**:1427–1431.

Mestecky, J., and Schrohenloher, R. E., 1974, Site of attachment of J chain to human immunoglobulin M, *Nature (London)* **249**:650–652.

Mestecky, J., Schrohenloher, R. E., Kulhavy, R., Wright, G. P., and Tomana, M., 1974, Site of J chain attachment to human polymeric IgA, *Proc. Natl. Acad. Sci. U.S.A.* **71**:544–548.

Metzger, H., 1970, Structure and function of γM macroglobulins, *Adv. Immunol.* **12**:57–116.

Metzger, H., Perlman, R. L., and Edelhoch, H., 1966, Characterization of a human macroglobulin. IV. Studies of its conformation by fluorescence polarization, *J. Biol. Chem.* **241**:1741–1744.

Miller, F., and Metzger, H., 1965, Characterization of a human macroglobulin. I. The molecular weight of its subunit, *J. Biol. Chem.* **240**:3325–3333.

Miller, F., and Metzger, H., 1966, Characterization of a human macroglobulin. IV. The products of tryptic digestion, *J. Biol. Chem.* **241**:1732–1740.

Milstein, C. P., Richardson, N. E., Deverson, E. V., and Feinstein, A., 1975, Interchain disulphide bridges of mouse immunoglobulin M. *Biochem. J.* **151**:615–624.

Morris, D. H., Williams, R. E., and Young, N. M., 1974, Comparison of three phosphorylcholine-binding mouse myeloma proteins by circular dichroism, *Biochem. Biophys. Res. Commun.* **61**:1167–1173.

Morris, J. E., and Inman, F. P., 1968, Isolation of the monomeric subunit of immunoglobulin M with its interchain disulfide bonds intact, *Biochemistry* **7**:2851–2857.

Müller-Eberhard, H. J., 1974, Patterns of complement activation, in: *Progress in Immunology II*, Vol. 1 (L. Brent and J. Holborow, eds.), pp. 173–182, North-Holland, Amsterdam.

Munn, E. A., Feinstein, A. and Munroe, A. J., 1971, Electron microscope examination of free IgA molecules, and of their complexes with antigen, *Nature (London)* **231**:527–529.

Nezlin, R. S., Zagyansky, Y. A., Käiväräinen, A. I., and Stefani, D. V., 1973, Properties of myeloma immunoglobulin E (Yu): Chemical, fluorescence polarization and spin-labeled studies, *Immunochemistry* **10**:681–688.

Nisonoff, A., Wissler, F. C., Lipman, L. N., and Woernley, D. L., 1960, Separation of univalent fragments from the bivalent rabbit antibody molecule by reduction of disulfide bonds, *Arch. Biochem. Biophys.* **89**:230–244.

Noelken, M. E., Nelson, C. A. Buckley, C. E., and Tanford, C., 1965, Gross conformation of rabbit 7S γ-immunoglobulin and its papain-cleaved fragments, *J. Biol. Chem.* **240**:218–224.

O'Donnell, I. J., Frangione, B., and Porter, R. R., 1970, The disulphide bonds of the heavy chain of rabbit immunoglobulin G, *Biochem. J.* **116**:261–268.

Ogawa, M., Kochwa, S., Smith, C., Ishizaka, K., and McIntyre, O. P., 1969, Clinical aspects of IgE myeloma, *N. Engl. J. Med.* **281**:1217–1220.

Onoue, K., Kishimoto, T., and Yamamura, Y., 1968, Structure of human immunoglobulin M. II. Isolation of a high molecular weight Fc fragment of IgM composed of several Fc subunits, *J. Immunol.* **100**:238–244.

Parkhouse, R. M. E., 1974, Non-covalent association of IgM subunits produced by reduction and alkylation, *Immunology* **27**:1063–1071.

Parkhouse, R. M. E., Askonas, B. A., and Dourmashkin, R. R., 1970, Electron microscopic studies of mouse immunoglobulin M: Structure and reconstitution following reduction, *Immunology* **18**:575–584.

Percy, M. E., and Percy, J. R., 1975, The immunoglobulin M molecule: Isomeric forms of the monomer subunit, *Can. J. Biochem.* **53**:923–929.

Perry, M. B., and Milstein, C., 1970, Interchain bridges of human IgD, *Nature (London)* **228**:934–935.

Pilz, I., Puchwein, G., Kratky, O., Herbst, M., Haager, O., Gall, W. E., and Edelman, G. M., 1970, Small angle X-ray scattering of a homogeneous γG1 immunoglobulin, *Biochemistry* **9**:211–219.

Pilz, I., Kratky, O., Licht, A. and Sela, M., 1973, Shape and volume of anti-poly(D-alanyl) antibodies in the presence and absence of tetra-D-alanine as followed by small-angle X-ray scattering, *Biochemistry* **12**:4998–5005.

Pilz, I., Kratky, O., and Karush, F., 1974, Changes of the conformation of rabbit IgG antibody caused by the specific binding of a hapten, *Eur. J. Biochem.* **41**:91–96.

Pilz, I., Kratky, O., Licht, A., and Sela, M., 1975, Shape and volume of fragments Fab' and (Fab')₂ of anti-poly(D-alanyl) antibodies in the presence and absence of tetra-D-alanine as determined by small-angle X-ray scattering, *Biochemistry* **14**:1326–1333.

Plaut, A. G., and Tomasi, T. B., Jr., 1970, Immunoglobulin M: Pentameric Fcμ fragments released by trypsin at higher temperatures, *Proc. Natl. Acad. Sci. U.S.A.* **65**:318–322.

Poljak, R. J., Amzel, L. M., Avey, H. P., Chen, B. L., Phizackerley, R. P., and Saul, F., 1973, Three-dimensional structure of the Fab' fragment of a human immunoglobulin at 2.8 Å resolution, *Proc. Natl. Acad. Sci. U.S.A.* **70**:3305–3310.

Porter, R. R., 1958, Separation and isolation of fractions of rabbit gamma-globulin containing the antibody and antigenic combining sites, *Nature (London)* 670–671.

Poulsen, K., Fraser, K. J., and Haber, E., 1972, An active derivative of rabbit antibody light chain composed of the constant and the variable domains held together only by a native disulfide bond, *Proc. Natl. Acad. Sci. U.S.A.* **69**:2495–2499.

Prahl, D. G., Mandy, W. J., and Todd, C. W., 1970, The molecular determinants of the A11 and A12 allotypic specificities in rabbit immunoglobulin, *Biochemistry* **8**:4935–4940.

Putnam, F. W., Florent, G., Paul, C., Shinoda, T., and Shimizu, A., 1973, Complete amino acid sequence of the mu heavy chain of a human IgM immunoglobulin, *Science* **182**:287–291.

Riesen, W., Rudikoff, S., Oriol, R., and Potter, M., 1975, An IgM Waldenström with specificity against phosphorylcholine, *Biochemistry* **14**:1052–1057.

Rowe, D. S., Hug, K., Faulk, W. P., McCormick, J. N., and Gerber, H., 1973, IgD on the surface of Peripheral blood lymphocytes of the human newborn, *Nature (London) New Biol.* **242**:155–157.

Sarma, V. R., Silverton, E. W., Davies, D. R., and Terry, W. D., 1971, The three-dimensional structure at 6 Å resolution of a human γG1 immunoglobulin molecule, *J. Biol. Chem.* **246**:3753–3759.

Schiffer, M., Girling, R. L., Ely, K. R., and Edmundson, A. B., 1973, Structure of a λ-type Bence–Jones protein at 3.5 Å resolution, *Biochemistry* **12**:4620–4631.

Schlessinger, J., Steinberg, I. Z., Givol, D., Hochman, J., and Pecht, I., 1975, Antigen-induced conformational changes in antibodies and their Fab fragments studies by circular polarization of fluorescence, *Proc. Natl. Acad. Sci. U.S.A.* **72**:2775–2779.

Schur, P. H., and Christian, G. D., 1964, The role of disulfide bonds in the complement-fixing and precipitating properties of 7S rabbit and sheep antibodies, *J. Exp. Med.* **120**:531–545.

Segal, D. M., Padlan, E. A., Cohen, G. H., Rudikoff, S., Potter, M., and Davies, D. R., 1974, The three-dimensional structure of a phosphorylcholine-binding mouse immunoglobulin Fab and the nature of the antigen binding site, *Proc. Natl. Acad. Sci. U.S.A.* **71**:4298–4302.

Sharon, J., and Givol, D., 1976, Preparation of Fv fragment from the mouse myeloma XRPC-25 immunoglobulin possessing anti-dinitrophenyl activity, *Biochemistry* **15**:1591–1594.

Shelton, E., and McIntire, K. R., 1970, Ultrastructure of the γM immunoglobulin molecule, *J. Mol. Biol.* **47**:595–597.

Shimizu, A., Watanabe, S., Yamamura, Y., and Putnam, F. W., 1974, Tryptic digestion of immunoglobulin M in urea: Conformational lability of the middle part of the IgM molecule, *Immunochemistry* **11**:719–727.

Sledge, C. R., and Bing, D. H., 1973, Binding properties of the human complement protein C1q, *J. Biol. Chem.* **248**:2818–2823.

Smyth, D. S., and Utsumi, S., 1967, Structure at the hinge region in rabbit immunoglobulin-G, *Nature (London)* **216**:332–335.

Spiegelberg, H. L., Prahl, J. W., and Grey, H. M., 1970, Structural studies of human γD myeloma protein, *Biochemistry* **9**:2115–2122.

Stanworth, D. R., Housley, J., Bennich, H., and Johansson, S. G. O., 1970, Effect of reduction upon the PCA-blocking activity of immunoglobulin E, *Immunochemistry* **7**:321–325.

Steiner, L. A., and Lowey, S., 1966, Optical rotatory dispersion studies of rabbit γG-immunoglobulin and its papain fragments, *J. Biol. Chem.* **241**:231–240.

Stollar, B. D., Stadecker, M. J., and Morecki, S., 1976, Comparison of the inactivation of IgM and IgG complement fixation sites by acid and base, *J. Immunol.* **117**:1387–1391.

Stryer, L.. 1968, Fluorescence spectroscopy of proteins, *Science* **162**:526–533.

Svehag, S. E., and Bloth, B., 1970, Ultrastructure of secretory and high-polymer serum immunoglobulin A of human and rabbit origin, *Science* **168**:847–849.

Tao, T., 1969, Time-dependent fluorescence depolarization and Brownian rotational diffusion coefficients of macromolecules, *Biopolymers* **8**:609–632.

Tischendorf, G. W., Zeichhardt, H., and Stoffler, G., 1975, Architecture of the *Escherichia coli* ribosome as determined by immune electron microscopy, *Proc. Natl. Acad. Sci. U.S.A.* **72**:4820–4824.

Tomasi, T. B., Jr., 1973, Production of a noncovalently bonded pentamer of immunoglobulin M: Relationship to J chain, *Proc. Natl. Acad. Sci. U.S.A.* **70**:3410–3414.

Tumerman, L. A., Nezlin, R. S., and Zagyansky, Y. A., 1972, Increase of the rotational relaxation time of antibody molecule after complex formation with dansyl-hapten, *FEBS Lett.* **19**:290–292.

Underdown, B. J., and Dorrington, K. J., 1974, Studies on the structural and conformational basis for the relative resistance of serum and secretory immunoglobulin A to proteolysis, *J. Immunol.* **112**:949–959.

Valentine, R. C., and Green, N. M., 1967, Electron microscopy of an antibody–hapten complex, *J. Mol. Biol.* **27**:615–617.

Van Boxel, J. A., and Buell, D. N., 1974, IgD on cell membranes of human lymphoid cell lines with multiple immunoglobulin classes, *Nature (London)* **251**:443–444.

van Boxel, J. A., Paul, W. E., Terry, W. D., and Green, I., 1972, IgD-bearing human lymphocytes, *J. Immunol.* **109**:648–651.

Vitetta, E. S., and Uhr, J. W., 1975, Immunoglobulin receptors revisited, *Science* **189**:964–969.

Warner, C., and Schumaker, V. N., 1970, Detection of a conformational change in an antihapten–antibody system upon interaction with divalent hapten, *Biochemistry* **9**:451–459.

Warner, C., Schumaker, V., and Karush, F., 1970, The detection of a conformational change in the antibody molecule upon interaction with hapten, *Biochem. Biophys. Res. Commun.* **38**:125–128.

Watanabe, S., Barnikol, H. V., Horn, J., and Hilschmann, N., 1973, Die Primärstruktur eines monoklonalen IgM-Immunoglobulins (Makroglobulin Ga1.). II. Die Aminosäuresequenz der H-Kette (μ-typ, Subgruppe III), Struktur des Gesamten IgM-Moleküls, *Hoppe-Seyler's Z. Physiol. Chem.* **354**:1505–1509.

Weber, G., 1952, Polarization of the fluorescence of marcromolecules, I. Theory and experimental method, *Biochem. J.* **51**:145–155.

Weber, G., 1953, Rotational Brownian motion and polarization of the fluorescence of solutions, *Adv. Protein Chem.* **8**:415–459.

Weltman, J., and Davis, R. P., 1970, Fluorescence polarization study of a human IgA myeloma protein: absence of segmental flexibility, *J. Mol. Biol.* **54**:177–185.

Weltman, J. K., and Edelman, G. M., 1967, Fluorescence polarization of human γG-immunoglobulins, *Biochemistry* **6**:1437–1447.

Werner, T. C., Bunting, J. R., and Cathou, R. E., 1972, The shape of immunoglobulin G molecules in solution, *Proc. Natl. Acad. Sci. U.S.A.* **69**:795–799.

Wilder, R. L., Green, B., and Schumaker, V. N., 1975, Bivalent hapten–antibody interactions. III. Formation of an unusual polymer by IgA (MOPC 315) upon binding a bivalent hapten, *Immunochemistry* **12**:55–60.

Wittman, H. G., 1976, Structure, function, and evolution of ribosomes, *Eur. J. Biochem.* **61**:1–13.

Wolcott, M., Freeman, D. G., Schrohenloher, R. E., Hammack, W., and Bennett, J. C., 1975, Tryptic cleavage of IgD at elevated temperature and isolation of a Fc-like fragment in high yield, *Immunochemistry* **12**:685–689.

Wu, C., and Stryer, L., 1972, Proximity relationships in rhodopsin, *Proc. Natl. Acad. Sci. U.S.A.* **69**:1104–1108.

Yguerabide, J., 1972, Nanosecond fluorescence spectroscopy of macromolecules, *Methods in Enzymology,* Vol. XXVI, Part C, (C. H. W. Hirs and S. N. Timasheff, eds.), pp. 498–578, Academic Press, New York.

Yguerabide, J., Epstein, H. F., and Stryer, L., 1970, Segmental flexibility in an antibody molecule, *J. Mol. Biol.* **51**:573–590.

Zagyansky, Y. A., and Gavrilova, E. M., 1974, Segmental flexibility of human myeloma immunoglobulins A, *Immunochemistry* **11**:681–682.

Zagyansky, Y. A., and Ivannikova, E. I., 1974, The general structure of shark *(Squalis acantias)* and hen *(Galus domesticus)* immunoglobulins, *Mol. Biol. Rept.* **1**:301–304.

Zagyansky, Y. A., Nezlin, R. S., and Tumerman, L. A., 1969, Flexibility of immunoglobulin G molecules as established by fluorescent polarization measurements, *Immunochemistry* **6**:787–800.

Zagyansky, Y. A., Tumerman, L. A., and Egorov, A. M., 1972, Segmental flexibility of immunoglobulin M molecules, *Immunochemistry* **9**:91–94.

Zikán, J., and Bennett, J. C., 1973, Isolation of F(c)$_5\mu$ and Fabμ fragments of human IgM, *Eur. J. Immunol.* **3**:415–419.

3

The Affinity of Antibody: Range, Variability, and the Role of Multivalence

FRED KARUSH

1. Introduction

During the past decade, the concept of antibody affinity has been increasingly employed in the analysis of immunological phenomena, and it is now generally understood to be an essential element in developing molecular interpretations of immunological processes. Consequently, there has been increased attention to a number of distinctive features of antibody affinity, particularly its variability and regulation, the role of antibody multivalence, and the biological concomitants of these properties. In an earlier discussion of the affinity of antibody (Karush, 1962), the main emphasis was placed on the nature and quantitative significance of the intermolecular forces involved and on some thermodynamic aspects of the reversible reaction of antibody and ligand. This analysis differs in its focus because it is based on experimental studies concerned with the variability of affinity ("the maturation process") as well as the range of affinity, the kinetic features of the rapid antibody–ligand interaction, and the contribution of multivalence to the effective affinity of the antibody molecule. The information now available in these areas stems from the introduction of new experimental methods into immunological research. These methods include (1) the techniques of stop-flow and temperature jump for evaluating the kinetic parameters of the formation of antibody–ligand complexes; (2) the inhibition of hemolytic plaques, formed by suspensions of antibody-secreting cells, by soluble ligands to estimate relative affinities; and (3) the neutralization of hapten-conjugated bacteriophage with antihapten antibody to measure rates of binding of antibody to large ligands and to evaluate the quantitative effects of multivalent interaction.

FRED KARUSH • Department of Microbiology, University of Pennsylvania School of Medicine, Philadelphia, Pennsylvania 19104.

The effective use of the concept of affinity in contemporary immunological discussion has been compromised by an inadequate perception of its molecular and thermodynamic meaning. In an attempt to provide some rectification of this shortcoming, we will first turn our attention to a consideration of the distinction between intrinsic and functional affinity and to a discussion of the relationship of affinity to the concepts of specificity and selectivity.

1.1. Intrinsic Affinity and Functional Affinity

The recognition of the multivalent interactions of antibody has led in recent years to the use of the term *avidity* in place of the conventional and thermodynamically defined quantity *affinity*. The compulsion for this substitution is apparently the desire to emphasize the significance of multivalent interaction for the stabilization of antibody–antigen complexes involved in biological systems. "Avidity," however, has rarely been defined precisely and in thermodynamic terms, although the reversibility of the formation of multivalently linked complexes provides an adequate basis for a precise thermodynamic characterization. Rather, over the years, the meanings assigned to "avidity" have been variable, often obscure, and frequently unrelated to experimental operations. It appears to me that the conceptual clarity of immunological analysis would benefit greatly from the abandonment of this term.

As an alternative concept, I shall employ the term *functional affinity* (Karush, 1970) to characterize those systems involving multivalent linkages. The use of this term implies, of course, a distinction between "intrinsic affinity" and "functional affinity." Both terms refer to formally identical reversible processes, as follows:

$$F_1 + L_1 \rightleftharpoons 1 : 1 \text{ complex (monovalent)}$$

$$Ab_n + L_m \rightleftharpoons 1 : 1 \text{ complex (multivalent)}$$

where F_1 is a monovalent antibody fragment, L_1 a monovalent ligand, Ab_n a multivalent antibody, and L_m a multivalent ligand with m identical groups. In each instance, two kinetic units combine reversibly to form one unit, and each process can, in principle, be characterized by an association constant. Since the association constant is a measure of the thermodynamic affinity, both processes can be assigned quantitative values of the affinity.

The utility of the distinction between "intrinsic affinity" and "functional affinity" arises from the different emphasis involved in each. The former is most useful when the structural relationship between the antibody-combining site and the complementary region of the ligand is under scrutiny or when the kinetic mechanisms of the specific interaction are under investigation. The latter is particularly significant when the quantitative measurement of the enhancement of affinity is being examined or when this enhancement is relevant to a biological process, such as viral neutralization and cell stimulation.

1.2. Specificity and Selectivity

Although the terms *specificity* and *selectivity* may appear to be synonymous when applied to antibody–ligand interactions, a useful distinction may be made between them in the analysis of the binding of structurally similar molecules. At the conceptual level, immunological specificity is related to the degree of chemical and steric complementarity between the combining region of the antibody and the interacting ligand. The complementarity is measured by the extent of van der Waals' contact between the reactants and by the chemical matching of the groups in close proximity. This matching provides stabilizing noncovalent interactions involving, particularly, hydrophobic and ionic contributions as well as hydrogen bonding. The nature, and example *par excellence,* of this kind of complementarity is most clearly seen in organic crystals. In these structures, any particular internal organic molecule can be regarded as the ligand, and the combining site would be defined by the array of the nearest-neighbor molecules (Marrack, 1938; Karush, 1962).

This conception of specificity implies that in the comparison between two interacting ligands, the one with the more extensive complementarity will exhibit the higher affinity. Thus, at the experimental level, specificity can be quantitated by measuring the difference of free energy (i.e., the ratio of intrinsic association constants) for the binding of two appropriate ligands, one of which is usually homologous with the inducing antigenic determinant. An example of such a comparison is the binding of dinitrophenyl (DNP)-Lys and trinitrophenyl (TNP)-Lys by anti-DNP antibody. Since the comparison of the specificity of different antibody populations is often the point of interest, as in the case of different monoclonal populations induced with the same antigen, such populations may be compared by measuring the ratio of binding constants for a homologous and appropriate heterologous ligand for each population. Differences in these ratios would generally reflect structural differences of the combining regions of the antibody. In the case of monoclonal populations, such measurable differences could be used for clonal phenotypic characterization.

Although specificity can thus be assigned an operational meaning and evaluated quantitatively, an ambiguity arises when the term specificity is used in experimental situations concerned with the discriminatory capacity of antibody. A preferable term for this phenomenon is *selectivity,* because the matter of interest here is usually the ability of an antibody to react with the homologous ligand, not with a closely related molecule. Thus, for example, high-affinity anti-DNP antibody can give both *in vitro* and *in vivo* reactions with a TNP ligand. On the other hand, anticarbohydrate antibodies fail to react with ligands involving minimal structural variation. This phenomenon may be seen in the failure of antilactose antibody to show reactivity with cellobiose antigens.

The difference in the discriminatory behavior of anti-DNP antibody (high-affinity) and antilactose antibody (low-affinity) does not reflect a difference of specificity in the sense described above. It derives, rather, from the large difference in the intrinsic affinities for homologous ligands. Since anti-DNP antibody can bind its homologous ligands with a K_0 as high as 1×10^9 M^{-1}, the binding of a TNP ligand with a 100-fold lower K_0, namely, 1×10^7 M^{-1}, is nevertheless adequate to give a variety of *in vitro* reactions, such as precipitation, as well as *in vivo* reactions. On the other hand, reduction of K_0 by 100-fold for the binding of a cellobiose ligand by antilactose antibody would yield a K_0 of 1×10^3 to 1×10^4 M^{-1}. These values are generally insufficient to lead to observable interactions. Thus, the low-affinity antilactose antibody would, in effect, be more selective in its interaction and exhibit finer recognition of structural variation. It may be suggested from this comparison that low-affinity antibody is biologically advantageous where cross-reactivity with self-constituents might otherwise occur.

2. Affinity for Monovalent Ligands

2.1. Range of Intrinsic Affinity

The immune response is characterized not only by an immense variety of combining site structures that can be induced and distinguished, such as receptors and humoral antibody, but also by a wide range of intrinsic association constants. The accumulation of reliable affinity measurements to date is probably sufficient to establish the upper limits of affinity for different types of antigens (Table 1).

The highest levels of affinity have generally been observed with a variety of antigens and carrier-conjugated ligands in which a sufficient volume or hydrophobicity, or both, of the ligands have been utilized for immunogenesis. This conclusion is based on the values of K_0 listed in Table 1 for the first group of antigens. Except for SLAC-ALME* these values exceed 1×10^9 M^{-1} and approach the value of 1×10^{11} M^{-1}. It may be inferred that the latter value is probably the maximum figure for the intrinsic affinity that can be achieved by the combining site of the antibody molecule. An apparent exception to this conclusion was recently provided by the fluorescein–antifluroescein system (Portmann *et al.*, 1975). The relatively large hydrophobic volume of this hapten can lead to the production, under appropriate conditions of induction, of rabbit IgG antibody with an intrinsic affinity of approximately 5×10^{11} M^{-1}.

The inclusion of SLAC-ALME in the first group is intended to demonstrate the substantial enhancement in affinity that the noncarbohydrate portion of the molecule has provided. Although the lactosyl moiety is the immunodominant group (Gopalakrishnan *et al.*, 1973), it would probably exhibit a value of K_0 not more than 1×10^5 M^{-1} (Ghose and Karush, 1973). More than a 1000-fold increase of K_0 can therefore be attributed to the additional portion of the ligand containing both hydrophobic and polar substituents.

The other extreme of the affinity scale is found with anticarbohydrate antibodies, which exhibit a maximum K_0 of the order of magnitude of 10^5 M^{-1} (Table 1). Particular significance attaches to the results with the homologous hexasaccharide derived from the pneumococcal polysaccharide S III and the octasaccharide derived from S VIII. In these cases, it is likely that the entire binding site is occupied by the ligand, based on our current knowledge of the size of the combining region (Kabat, 1966). A caveat should be noted here because of the manner in which the antibodies were induced. In both cases, immunization was carried out by intravenous injection of bacterial vaccines. Induction of tolerance of high-affinity B lymphocytes may have precluded the expression of the full affinity potential. Nevertheless, the chemical nature of the immunogen as well as other investigations involving antibody induction with protein-conjugated carbohydrates (Karush, 1957) provide substantial support for the conclusion that a value for K_0 of 1×10^6 M^{-1} constitutes a maximum for anticarbohydrate antibodies.

In this connection, it is of interest to note that lactose itself can be bound with a K_0 of 1×10^5 M^{-1} at 25° by rabbit antibody induced with a bacterial vaccine (*Str. faecalis*, strain N) (Table 1) (Ghose and Karush, 1973). This result emphasizes again

---

*N^ϵ-SLAC,N^α-acetyl-L-lysine methylester where SLAC is lactosyl-β-ϕ-N=N-ϕ-NH-CO-CH$_2$-S-CH$_2$-CO.

the major energetic contribution made by the appropriate disaccharide in the response to a polysaccharide antigen. A parallel observation was described for the antidextran system (Kabat, 1966).

For protein antigens, the values of K_0 shown in Table 1 encompass the entire range already noted with the immunogens that are smaller or simpler, or both. This observation is not unexpected in view of the chemical variety of the amino acid residues found in proteins. It may be inferred that the antigenic determinants of proteins include clusters of hydrophobic residues, polar and ionic residues, and, perhaps, mixtures of these two types (Atassi, 1975).

The most persuasive demonstration of the formation of an antibody with high intrinsic affinity for a single antigenic determinant of protein is the study of antibody to staphylococcal nuclease (Sachs et al., 1972a). The antibody employed was specific for an antigenic determinant associated with amino acid residues 99–126, and was separated from antibodies directed against other portions of the single polypeptide chain containing 149 residues (Sachs et al., 1972b). Since the selected antibody was induced by immunization with the intact enzyme, its binding to the enzyme represented a homologous reaction involving the formation of a 1 : 1

TABLE 1. Intrinsic Affinities of 7-S-Induced Antibodies for Different Types of Antigens

Antigen or ligand	K_0 (M^{-1})	T (°C)	Species	Ref. No. [a]
Gastrin (12,514) [b]	2.7×10^{11}	4	Guinea pig	1
Fluorescein (332) [b]	6×10^{10}	22	Rabbit	2
Digoxin (781) [b]	1.7×10^{10}	24	Rabbit	3
Vasopressin (1083) [b]	4.5×10^{9}	4	Rabbit	4
Angiotensin (1030) [b]	4.3×10^{9}	25	Rabbit	5
N^ϵ-DNP-Lys (312) [b]	3×10^{9}	25	Rabbit	6
SLAC-ALME [c] (871) [b]	2.2×10^{8}	25	Horse	7
Hexasaccharide (S III) [d]	3.2×10^{5}	4	Rabbit	8
Octasaccharide (S VIII) [e]	1.25×10^{5}	25	Rabbit	9
Lactose [f]	0.97×10^{5}	25	Rabbit	10
Insulin	1.7×10^{10}	37	Human	11
Staphylococcal nuclease	8.3×10^{8}	25	Goat	12
Ovalbumin	2×10^{8}	1.5	Rabbit	13
TMV [c] protein	2.8×10^{5}	26	Rabbit	14
Lysozyme (57–107) [f]	1.6×10^{5}	10	Sheep	15
Lysozyme (1–27, 122–129) [h]	8.0×10^{5}	10	Sheep	15
Lysozyme "loop" peptide	3.0×10^{6}	4	Goat	16

[a] References: (1) Goldenberg et al. (1974); (2) Portmann et al. (1971); (3) Smith et al. (1970); (4) H.-H. Wu and Rockey (1969); (5) Worobec et al. (1972); (6) Haber et al. (1967); (7) Gopalakrishnan et al. (1973); (3) Katz and Pappenheimer (1969); (9) Pappenheimer et al. (1968); (10) Ghose and Karush (1973); (11) Berson and Yalow (1959); (12) Sachs et al. (1972a); (13) Dandliker and Levison (1968); (14) Mamet-Bratley (1966); (15) Sakato et al. (1971); (16) Pecht et al. (1971).

[b] The number in parentheses is the molecular weight.

[c] (SLAC-ALME) N^ϵ-SLAC, N^α-acetyl-L-lysine methylester, where SLAC is lactosyl-β-ϕ-N $=$N-ϕ-NH-CO-CH$_2$-S-CH$_2$-CO; (TMV) tobacco mosaic virus.

[d] Hexasaccharide derived from type III pneumococcal polysaccharide. The antiserum was prepared against type III pneumococcal vaccine.

[e] Octasaccharide derived from Type VIII pneumococcal polysaccharide. The antiserum was prepared against Type VIII pneumococcal vaccine.

[f] The antiserum was prepared against a vaccine of Streptococcus faecalis, strain N.

[g] Lysozyme peptide containing residues 57–107.

[h] Lysozyme peptide containing residues 1–27 and 122–129.

complex. Furthermore, because the enzyme could be assayed at low concentrations ($\approx 10^{-9}$ M) by the inhibition of nuclease activity due to complex formation, appropriately low concentrations of antibody could be employed. The K_0 value of 8.3×10^8 M^{-1} suggests that the antigenic determinant is largely constituted of hydrophobic residues.

The formation of high-affinity antiprotein antibody was also demonstrated in another system by kinetic measurements with fluorescein-labeled ovalbumin and rabbit antiovalbumin antibody (Dandliker and Levison, 1968). The antiserum was shown to contain a population of antibody with a K_0 of 2×10^8 M^{-1} at 1.5°C (Table 1). This result is in agreement with earlier equilibrium measurements of the system based on fluorescence polarization (Dandliker *et al.*, 1964).

The highest reported value of K_0 for an antiprotein antibody was provided by Berson and Yalow (1959) in their pioneering and meticulous study of human antiinsulin antibody. The value of 1.7×10^{10} M^{-1} (Table 1) is near the maximum capability of the antibody molecule, as surmised above, and suggests again a predominance of hydrophobic residues in the relevant antigenic determinant. It should be noted that in this system, the insulin monomer behaved as a monovalent antigen; i.e., it formed complexes that contained only one antibody molecule. Because of the low concentrations of insulin employed in the binding studies, the investigators concluded that there was no significant quantity of dimers, trimers, or other oligomers. This conclusion would appear to rule out an enhancement of intrinsic affinity due to bivalent interaction between an insulin dimer and the bivalent antibody.

The occurrence of antiprotein antibodies with K_0's at the low end of the affinity range is illustrated by lysozyme and the coat protein of tobacco mosaic virus (TMV) (Table 1). In the latter instance, the interaction of the Fab fragment derived from purified antibody was studied by ultracentrifugation with the TMV particle. The mixture was initially equilibrated and the concentration of the free Fab measured by supernatant analysis after ultracentrifugation. The K_0 of 2.8×10^5 M^{-1} is in satisfactory agreement with the value of 3.8×10^5 M^{-1} obtained previously (Rappaport, 1959). In the earlier study, free antibody in the equilibrium mixture was assayed by the viral inactivation procedure.

Antibodies against restricted regions of the lysozyme molecule were obtained from rabbit (Fujio *et al.*, 1971) and sheep (Sakato *et al.*, 1971) antisera to hen egg-white lysozyme. These antisera were isolated by adsorption to an immunoadsorbent coupled with a peptide containing residues 57–107 or a peptide with residues 1–27 and 122–129. Binding measurements were carried out by equilibrium dialysis with the ^{125}I-labeled lysozyme. Thus, the values for sheep antibody of 1.6×10^5 M^{-1} and 8.0×10^5 M^{-1} for K_0 (Table 1) measure the affinity for homologous reactions.

The result shown for the "loop" peptide of lysozyme in Table 1 measures the affinity of the reaction of antibody induced against the peptide, consisting of residues 60–83 including a disulfide bridge, with the peptide labeled with the dansyl group at the amino terminal residue. Since it was shown (Pecht *et al.*, 1971) that the intact lysozyme was equally effective in inhibition, on a molar basis, as a nondansylated "loop" peptide, the structure of the antigenic determinant of the peptide must be very similar to the corresponding determinant of the intact protein. We may therefore consider the K_0 value of 3.0×10^6 M^{-1} as representing the affinity for the homologous reaction of an antiprotein antibody.

Recent elaboration of the antigenic reactive regions of proteins, particularly of sperm whale myoglobin, demonstrates the variety of amino acid residues that can participate in antigenic determinants. In the case of myoglobin, all the antigenic reactive regions of the native protein have been identified (Atassi, 1975). These are five in number, and each consists of six or seven residues. Every region contains one or more charged residues, polar residues, and hydrophobic residues, such as lysyl, seryl, and leucyl, respectively. Affinity measurements of the binding by site-specific antibodies of the native protein would be valuable for understanding the energetic significance of the involved residues. It may be anticipated that the association constants would fall in the intermediate portion of the range seen in Table 1 for protein antigens.

2.2. Kinetic Aspects of Antibody–Ligand Interaction

Since the formation of an antibody–ligand complex is a reversible process, the stability of the complex, i.e., its association constant, is governed by the ratio of the rate constant for association to the rate constant for dissociation. Because of the rapidity of formation of the initial complex, special techniques, such as the stopped-flow or temperature-jump procedures, or special assays, such as viral neutralization, that allow experimentation with concentrations of antibody less than 1×10^{-9} M, must be employed to yield quantitative values for the association rates. Most kinetic studies have involved complex formation between antihapten antibody and a low-molecular-weight ligand, with the predominant use of DNP ligands. The bulk of the quantitative information available to date for such systems is given in Table 2. In addition, a few investigations with antiprotein antibody have been done in which the interaction was limited to the formation of 1 : 1 complexes and from which reliable rate constants could be obtained. These results are also included in Table 2. The most striking feature of the results in Table 2 is the consistently high values of the rate constants for the association process. Since this property favors maximum association constants, it is appropriate for the biological function of antibody. It allows minimal concentration of antibody and antigen to form biologically effective complexes such as would be involved in viral neutralization and cell stimulation. The disparity in association constants would thus arise from a much greater variation in the rate constants for dissociation. That this is apparently the case was surmised by Froese (1968), who found in his studies with antihapten systems that the stability of antibody–hapten complexes depended mainly on the dissociation rate constant of the complex.

The predominant role of the dissociation process for anti-DNP antibody and antibody for two other hydrophobic haptens is clearly seen in Table 2. The rate constants for association fall in the 10-fold range of 10^7 to 10^8 M^{-1} sec^{-1}, in contrast to a 1000-fold range of the dissociation rate constants. The corresponding range of K_0 for the homologous hydrophobic ligands is more than 1000-fold.

Although the association rate constants reach values as high as 5×10^8 M^{-1} sec^{-1}, this process does not appear to be diffusion-limited (Haselkorn *et al.*, 1974). In addition to the role of the diffusion coefficients of the reactants and the steric requirements for a successful encounter, the detailed and penetrating investigation by Haselkorn *et al.* (1974) revealed that several interactions with the ligand involving subsites of the binding region of the antibody are involved in the forma-

TABLE 2. Rate Constants for the Formation of Antibody–Ligand Complexes

Ligand	Antibody	Species	T (°C)	k_a (M⁻¹sec⁻¹)[a]	k_d (sec⁻¹)[a]	K (M⁻¹)[a]	Ref. No.[b]
N^ϵ-DNP-Lys	Anti-DNP	Rabbit	25	8×10^7	1	7.7×10^7	1
N-R'[c]	Anti-phenylarsonate	Rabbit	25	2×10^7	50	—	2
DHNDS-NP[c]	Anti-p-nitrophenyl	Rabbit	25	1.8×10^8	7.6×10^2	5.8×10^5	3
1N-2, 5S-4DNP[c]	Anti-DNP	Rabbit	23	1.7×10^7	70	2.4×10^5	4
1N-2, 5S-pNP[c]	Anti-DNP	Rabbit	23	1.4×10^7	410	$\approx 1 \times 10^4$	4
1N-2, 5S-4DNP[c]	Anti-DNP	Rabbit	25	0.9×10^7	76	1.5×10^5	5
N^ϵ-DNP-lys	Anti-DNP	Rabbit	25	1.1×10^7	(0.51)	1.1×10^7	5
2,4-Dinitroaniline	IgA myeloma (MOPC 315)	Mouse	21	4.8×10^8	927	3.00×10^5	6
N-DNP-ethylenediamine	IgA myeloma (MOPC 315)	Mouse	21	6.5×10^7	735	1.3×10^5	6
N^ϵ-DNP-aminocaproic acid	Anti-DNP	Rabbit	25	0.74×10^8	8.7	4.37×10^7	7
N^ϵ-TNP-aminocaproic acid	Anti-TNP	Rabbit	25	1.0×10^8	1.6	7.24×10^8	7
Fluorescein-labeled ovalbumin	Anti-ovalbumin	Rabbit	1.5	2×10^5	1×10^{-3}	(2×10^8)	8
Hemoglobin S	Site-specific anti-HbS (Fab)	Rabbit	2.0	5.8×10^5	2.67×10^{-5}	2.1×10^{10}	9
Staphylococcal nuclease	Region-specific anti-nuclease	Goat	25	4.1×10^5	(4.9×10^{-4})	8.3×10^8	10
Lactoside-conjugated ØX174	Anti lactoside	Rabbit	25	9.4×10^5	8.0×10^{-4}	6.7×10^9	11
Acetyl-EK[c]	IgM Fab anti lactose	Horse	25	1.8×10^6	4	3.5×10^5	12
DNP-conjugated ØX174	Anti-DNP	Rabbit	25	6×10^6	3.3×10^{-4}	3.7×10^{10}	13

[a] Values in parentheses are calculated.

[b] References: (1) Day et al. (1963); (2) Froese et al. (1962); (3) Froese and Sehon (1965); (4) Froese (1968); (5) Kelly et al. (1971); (6) Haselkorn et al. (1974); (7) Barisas et al. (1975); (8) Dandliker and Levison (1968); (9) Noble et al. (1972); (10) Sachs et al. (1972a); (11) Gopalakrishnan and Karush (1974b); (12) Blatt et al. (1972); (13) Hornick and Karush (unpublished); (13) Hornick and Karush (1972).

[c] (N-R') 1-Naphthol-4[4-(4'-azobenzeneazo) phenylarsonic acid]; (DHNDS-NP) 4,5-dihydroxy-3-(p-nitrophenylazo)-2,7-naphthalene disulfonate; (1N-2, 5S-4DNP) 1-hydroxy-4-(2,4-dinitrophenylazo)-2,5-naphthalene disulfonate; (1N-2, 5S-pNP) 1-hydroxy-4-(4-nitrophenylazo)-2,5-napththalene disulfonate; (Acetyl-EK) N-(Nᵃ-acetyl,Nᵉ-DNP-L-lysyl)-p-aminophenyl-β-lactoside.

tion of the complex. To account for the dependence of the forward rate constant on fine structural variations of the bound ligands, they proposed a two-step mechanism for the reaction. This mechanism involves, first, the formation of a hypothetical diffusion-controlled "encounter" complex, followed by a unimolecular transformation step to yield the stable complex. The finding of only one relaxation time in their temperature-jump experiments is attributed to the relatively low equilibrium concentration of the initial complex.

The restriction in the published studies of the kinetics of antibody–hapten interaction to hydrophobic ligands leaves uncertain the generality of the range of 10^7 to 10^8 M^{-1} sec^{-1} for such interaction. The one system involving antilactose antibody and a lactose-containing ligand that was recently studied (Blatt *et al.*, unpublished) (Table 2) produced the significantly lower value of 1.8×10^6 M^{-1} sec^{-1} for the forward rate constant. Additional studies with this system and with other anticarbohydrate antibodies would provide important information.

The formation of 1 : 1 complexes between a protein antigen and antiprotein antibody in three cases (Table 2) is characterized by an association rate constant at 25°C of approximately 5×10^5 M^{-1} sec^{-1}. The consistency of the three reported values indicates that values close to this figure may be characteristic for protein antigens and related to the fact that their antigenic determinants consist of clusters of amino acid residues. The availability of site-specific antibodies to protein antigens (Noble *et al.*, 1972; Sachs *et al.*, 1972a,b) provides the opportunity for important kinetic investigation of their interaction.

The minor role played by the size of the interacting components is evident from the forward rate constants for the interaction of antihapten antibody with the critical site of hapten-conjugated bacteriophage (ØX174) (Table 2). It should be pointed out that although the bacteriophage was extensively conjugated, the experimentally observed neutralization reaction obeyed single-site kinetics, at least approximately (Hornick and Karush, 1972; Gopalakrishnan and Karush, 1974b). Two points may be made regarding the forward rate constants involving anti-DNP and antilactoside antibody. The value for the former (6×10^6 M^{-1} sec^{-1}) is virtually within the range previously noted for anti-DNP antibody forming complexes with small ligands. The lower value for the latter antibody (9.4×10^5 M^{-1} sec^{-1}) may, as noted above, reflect distinctive features of the hydrophilic determinant for which the antibody site is specific.

2.3. Selective Limitation of Intrinsic Affinity of IgM Antibody

Although the variety of IgM antibodies for which affinity measurements have been made compared with 7 S antibody is limited, the general impression has emerged that IgM antibodies are restricted in their affinity relative to their 7 S counterparts. This observation has been related to the process of maturation of affinity (discussed in Section 2.4) involving the inability of IgM antibody to change with time in contrast to the temporal dynamics of the 7 S response. There is little doubt that the intrinsic affinity of IgM is subject to a severe and selective limitation. The most persuasive evidence for this conclusion is summarized in the discussion that follows.

The initial observations were made with serum antibody, and almost all measurements with IgM antibody involved hydrophobic ligands, especially the popular DNP ligands. It was reported by Voss and Eisen (1968) that the binding of DNP-Lys by rabbit and equine anti-DNP antibody was characterized by K_0 values of 1×10^5 and 6×10^5 M^{-1}, respectively, and that no increase with time was noted. These constants are to be contrasted with values of the magnitude of 10^8 M^{-1} exhibited by IgG antibodies after appropriate duration (Table 2). A direct comparison of 7 S and 18 S anti-DNP antibodies in the nurse shark was made by Voss and Sigel (1972). Whereas the maximum value of K_0 for the binding of DNP-Lys by 7 S antibody was 2×10^7 M^{-1}, the K_0 for the 18 S antibody did not exceed 2×10^5 M^{-1}. A less striking, but nevertheless significant, demonstration of this difference was given by Mäkelä et al. (1970) using rabbit antisera containing IgG and IgM anti-NIP (5-nitro-3-iodo-4-hydroxyphenylacetic acid) antibody separated into 7 S and 19 S fractions. The bleedings were made 14 days after one administration of antigen, but the antibodies were not specifically purified to avoid selection based on affinity. On the average, the value of K_0 (2×10^6 M^{-1}) for the binding of NIP-ϵ-aminocaproic acid by IgG antibody was 4-fold higher than that for IgM antibody.

An alternative approach to the evaluation of the comparative affinities of IgG and IgM antibodies is the inhibition by soluble ligands of the formation of hemolytic plaques by antibody-secreting cells (Andersson, 1970). This method suffers from some theoretical ambiguities (DeLisi and Goldstein, 1974), and at best provides only a measure of relative affinities. It was used by Huchet and Feldmann (1973) to compare the affinities of IgG and IgM anti-DNP antibody secreted by plaque-forming cells in the mouse. This was done on the basis of the difference in the concentrations of DNP-Lys required to give 50% inhibition of the direct (IgM-producing) plaques and the indirect (IgG-producing) plaques from the same sample of splenic cells. It was concluded that during the primary response (28 days), the IgM binding constant averaged about 10-fold lower than that for IgG.

Further confirmation of the restricted affinity of IgM antibody and support for its generality was obtained with equine antilactose antibody (Kim and Karush, 1974). Binding measurements were carried out with a lactose-containing ligand (Lac dye) using isoelectric fractions of purified and separated preparations of IgM and 7 S antibody. The maximum value of K_0, exhibited by a functionally homogeneous fraction of IgM, was 4×10^5 M^{-1}, compared with a plateau value of 2.5×10^6 M^{-1} for the 7 S fractions.

The selective limitations of the intrinsic affinity of the IgM antibody pose a difficulty for the notion of an IgM–7 S switch, i.e., the conversion of an IgM-producing cell to a 7-S-producing cell. This notion implies that the transcription of the gene specifying the constant region of the μ chain is halted and an alternate gene, e.g., a γ gene, specifying the constant (C) region of a different heavy (H) chain is activated. Since the particular variable (V)-region genes of the cell undergoing the conversion are presumed to remain active, the intrinsic affinity of the 7 S product should be identical to that of the parent IgM antibody. It is clear from the observed differences in intrinsic affinity, however, that clones that are responsible for the synthesis of the bulk of 7 S antibody cannot have arisen from the major clones for IgM synthesis without some further modification or replacement of the V-region genes during a proliferative phase. An alternative model that retains the IgM-7 S conversion as an essential feature of the immune response utilizes the concept of a selective conversion. In this view, that minor fraction of IgM clones leading to a high-affinity IgM molecule would be selectively stimulated to convert by interaction of antigen with the receptor molecule. It is implied thereby that the higher affinity of this interaction would generate the distinctive signal required for the transcriptional substitution. Unfortunately, these speculative alternatives do not readily lend themselves to experimental scrutiny.

2.4. Temporal Variation of IgG Affinity

2.4.1. Studies with Serum Antibody

There are now available a number of studies of the IgG response to defined antigenic structures in which a temporal increase of average intrinsic affinity has been observed. The variety of specificities and species for which this phenomenon, commonly referred to as *maturation of the immune response,* has been demonstrated is shown by the systems listed in Table 3. Also listed are the time span following initial immunization over which measurements of the association constants were made, the maximum value at the end of this interval, and the factor by which the association constant increased during this interval.

The generality of the phenomenon may be inferred with reasonable confidence from the results in Table 3. Its demonstration in the five species listed and other, less direct studies, e.g., in the mouse (Davie and Paul, 1972; Claflin *et al.,* 1973) suggest that it is a general feature of the immune response. With respect to the variety of antigens examined, the hydrophobic haptens, particularly DNP, have been employed in the large majority of the studies (Table 3), but the occurrence of the phenomenon with antibodies to β-galactosidase and lactose indicates that it is not essentially dependent on the nature of the antigen. The quantitative significance of the effect does probably depend, however, on the maximum affinity that can be exhibited by antibody of a particular specificity. This maximum would, of course,

TABLE 3. Temporal Variation of Intrinsic Affinity of Serum 7 S Antibody

Specificity	Ligand	Species	Time interval	Final K_0	Increase (−fold)	Ref. No. [a]
Anti-DNP	DNP-Lys	Rabbit	2–8 wk	2.5×10^8	250	1
Anti-SUP	p-(p-aminobenzeneazo)hippurate	Rabbit	2–10 wk	3.4×10^7	29	2
Anti-dansyl	Dansyl-Lys	Rabbit	6 wk–8 mo	3×10^8	15	3
Anti-DNP	DNP-Lys	Rat	11–21 days	4.2×10^7	21	4
Anti-DNP	DNP-Lys	Guinea pig	2 wk–2 mo	1.7×10^9	10^4	5
Anti-β-D-galactosidase[b]	Defective β-D-galactosidase	Rabbit	11–31 days	1×10^8	400	6
Antifluorescein	Fluorescein	Rabbit	1–12 mo	5×10^{11}	4×10^3	7
Antilactose	Lac dye	Horse	5–21 wk	3.6×10^5	20	8
Antilactose	Lac dye	Rabbit	13–27 wk	2×10^6	100	9
Anti-DNP	DNP-Lys	Nurse shark	10–30 mo	2×10^7	100	10
Antivasopressin	Vasopressin	Rabbit	92–377 days	2×10^9	None	11
Anti-DNP	DNP-Lys	Rabbit	2½ wk–7 mo	2×10^8	None	12

[a]References: (1) Eisen and Siskind (1964); (2) Fujio and Karush (1966); (3) Parker *et al.* (1967); (4) Lamelin and Paul (1971); (5) Goidl *et al.* (1968); (6) Macario *et al.* (1972); (7) Portmann *et al.* (1975); (8) Chua *et al.* (1975); (9) Ghose and Karush (1973); (10) Voss and Sigel (1972); (11) H.-H. Wu and Rockey (1969); (12) Richards and Haber (1967).
[b]In fragment culture of lymph nodes from primed animals.

reflect the chemical nature of the antigenic determinant. Thus, as seen in Table 3, the large increases in the association constant of 10^4-fold and 4×10^3-fold occur with anti-DNP and antifluorescein, respectively. With antilactose, on the other hand, the increase was not more than 100-fold.

The maturation of affinity is not always an observed concomitant of the immune response, as is evident from the last two studies listed in Table 3. In the case of antivasopressin, the large K_0 of 2×10^9 M^{-1} found initially at 92 days after immunization was unchanged for an additional period of 285 days. With DNP conjugated to a nonimmunogenic carrier, the initial antibody, at 2½ weeks, was high-affinity ($K_0 = 2 \times 10^8$ M^{-1}) and remained unchanged for a total interval of 7 months. This is a particularly significant case because it emphasizes that the process of affinity development can be substantially abbreviated or bypassed by appropriate conditions of immunogenic stimulation.

The occurrence of cellular processes that may lead to the modulation and reversal of increase in affinity with time was inferred from studies with anti-DNP (Werblin et al., 1973), antigalactosidase (Macario and Conway de Macario, 1973), and antilactose antibodies (Ghose and Karush, 1973). In the case of anti-DNP (Werblin et al., 1973), rabbits immunized with different quantities of antigen (0.05–50 mg DNP-BGG in Freund's adjuvant) required different periods, ranging from 42 to 180 days, to attain the maximum affinity. Beyond these periods, the average affinity decreased together with the antibody concentration. The decline in antibody level was relatively greater for the high-affinity fraction, however, than for the remainder of the population. It was evident from the analysis of the heterogeneity of the affinity that low-affinity antibody persisted throughout the period of observation, and was even detectable in the serum at the time the maximum average affinity was achieved.

The studies with the antigalactosidase system (Macario and Conway de Macario, 1973) were especially striking in that the antibody affinity exhibited an oscillatory behavior with multiple cycles. These observations were made using an in vitro culture system containing multiple lymph node microfragments from a rabbit primed with β-D-galactosidase 1 year earlier. The fragment cultures were initially exposed to 5 μg of the enzyme for 30 min, and the antibody, accumulated over a few days in the supernatant, was studied serially for a period of several months. The activation of a defective β-D-galactosidase enzyme by antibody provided a sensitive and quantitative assay of the affinity of the activating antibody (Macario et al., 1972). During the 105-day period of observation three cycles of modulation of antibody affinity were discerned associated with a minimum K_0 of 5×10^5 to a maximum of 74×10^5 M^{-1} (Figure 1). Although this cyclical behavior may be evident only under the special condition of the in vitro culture, it appears to reveal an important and complex feature of the clonal dynamics of the immune response.

In the antilactose study (Ghose and Karush, 1973), the modulation of the maturation process was revealed by following the affinity of purified rabbit antibody over a period of about 1 year. In addition, the fractionation of the purified antibody by preparative isoelectric focusing provided evidence of temporal changes in the distribution of the antibody-producing clones (Figure 2). After a period of 13 weeks involving multiple administration of a bacterial vaccine (Str. faecalis, strain N), the purified antilactose antibody was heterogeneous with respect to affinity with a K_0

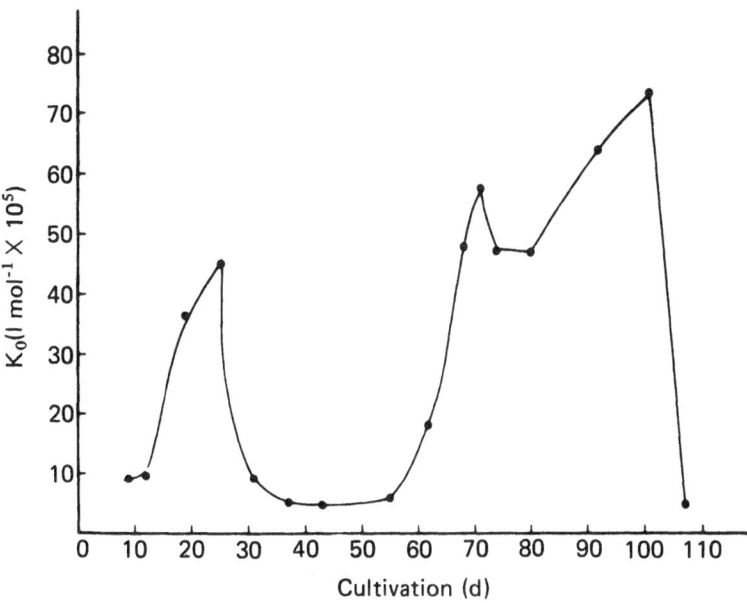

Figure 1. Sequential changes in the association constant of the anti-β-D-galactosidase-activating antibodies during the immune response *in vitro*. Reproduced from Macario and Conway de Macario (1973) with permission.

value of 2.2×10^4 M^{-1}. This population exhibited 13 or 14 bands in isoelectric focusing, demonstrating, together with the heterogeneity of affinity, that multiple clones were involved. Continued immunization led at 27 weeks to a functionally homogeneous antibody and a highly restricted isoelectric profile consistent with a monoclonal product. The K_0 value had increased 100-fold to 2.07×10^6 M^{-1}. In the following 21 weeks, which included a 12-week rest period during which the antibody content was virtually zero, restimulation led to a heterogeneous antibody population, after a total interval of 48 weeks, with the intermediate K_0 value of 2.09×10^5 M^{-1}. In addition, all the isoelectric bands initially found reappeared, but with a quantitative redistribution favoring the high-affinity fractions, in accord with the 10-fold higher value of K_0, compared with the 13-week population.

An important implication could be drawn from the recurrence after 48 weeks of the same isoelectric fractions detected at 13 weeks: that memory cells associated with the clones initially producing low-affinity antibody were continuously present in the animal, even during the period when such antibody was not being synthesized. Furthermore, it was inferred that no somatic diversification, i.e., emergence of new clones, was involved between the 13th and 48th weeks. The survival of low-affinity memory cells is in accord with the continued production in the case of anti-DNP antibody of a low-affinity fraction during the maturation process (Werblin *et al.*, 1973). The same conclusion was reached independently by Macario *et al.* (1973) using the microfragment culture described above. In this case, microfragments were obtained from a rabbit immunized 9 months previously and containing in its serum functionally homogeneous activating antibody with a K_0 of 2.7×10^6 M^{-1}. The early

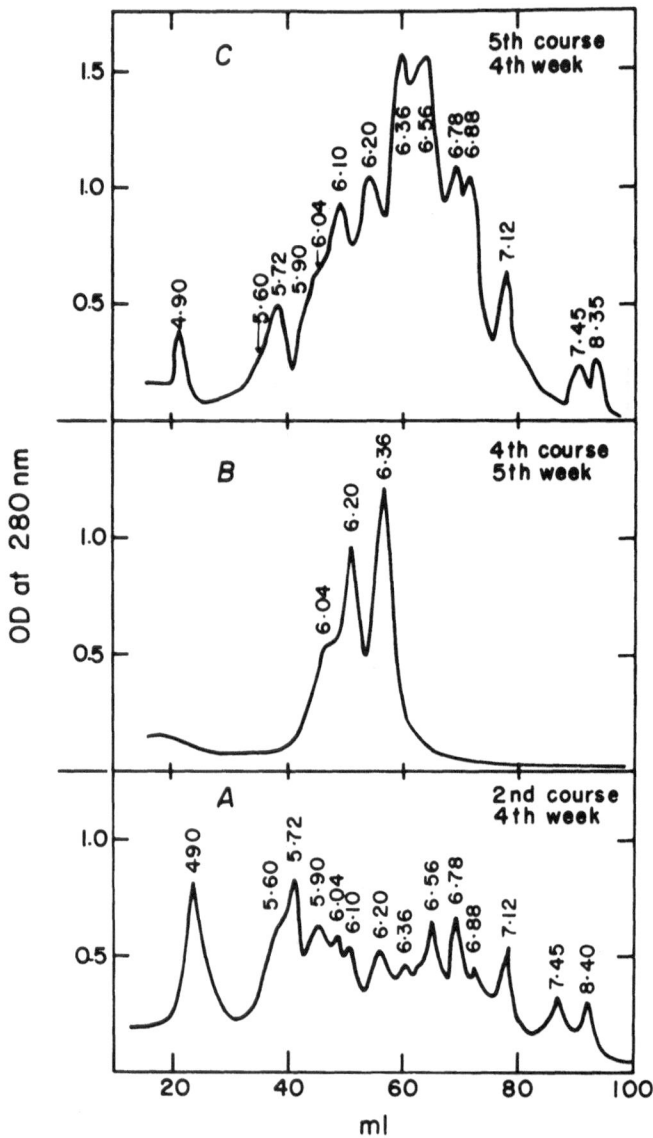

Figure 2. Liquid isoelectric focusing elution profiles of purified antilactose antibodies in the pH range 5–8. The different isoelectric bands and shoulders are characterized by the average isoelectric pH values shown at the top. Reproduced from Ghose and Karush (1973) with permission.

secondary response of the microfragments produced antibody in the positive culture supernatants with K_0's ranging from 2×10^4 to 2×10^7 M^{-1}. This concordance of findings for the antilactose and anti-β-D-galactosidase systems indicates that the persistence of low-affinity memory cells is probably not T-cell-dependent, since the production of antilactose antibody in response to a vaccine immunogen probably does not involve T-cell collaboration (Howard et al., 1971).

The maturation phenomenon has generally been interpreted as the result of selective interaction of antigen with high-affinity receptors on the precursors of antibody-forming cells (Siskind and Benacerraf, 1969). This hypothesis is attractive because of its parsimonious theme and reasonable because it is based on a sound physicochemical principle, namely, the law of mass action. Clearly, it does not provide explicitly for the persistence of low-affinity clones of memory cells or account for the occasional reversal in time of a high-affinity-dominated population to a low-affinity-dominated population. The regulatory process underlying these complex features of the immune response are unclear, but biological utility may be their consequence (Macario *et al.*, 1973).

2.4.2. Cellular Studies

The clonal distribution and dynamics of antibody-forming cells, antigen-sensitive cells, and memory cells were further clarified by studies based on the inhibition by soluble ligands of the formation of hemolytic plaques due to individual antibody-secreting cells (Andersson, 1970). The general advantage of the method involving plaque-forming cells (PFC) is that each antibody-secreting cell can be examined with respect to the nature and quantity of the secreted antibody. The supplementary advantage afforded by the inhibition of plaque formation through competitive binding of soluble ligands is the capability to estimate relative affinities (DeLisi and Goldstein, 1974). Thus, different PFC populations can be compared in terms of their relative average affinities. Of particular value is the fact that the distribution of the cell population with respect to antibody affinity can be evaluated. Furthermore, the presence of minor subpopulations secreting antibody of affinity much greater or less than the average value can be recognized and estimated.

Several studies involving anti-DNP PFC have been made to demonstrate the maturation phenomenon at the cellular level. In the investigation by Davie and Paul (1972), serum samples and lymph node cell suspensions were obtained at different intervals from guinea pigs immunized with DNP-guinea pig alumbin in complete Freund's adjuvant. Measurement of the affinity for the binding of DNP-Lys by serum anti-DNP IgG antibody showed a 25- to 50-fold increase from a K_0 value of $2 \times 10^6 \ M^{-1}$ at day 12 after immunization to that found at day 30. A parallel change in the average relative affinities of the antibody secreted by the PFC sampled at the same times was inferred. This conclusion was based on the observation that the concentration of DNP-Lys required to give 50% inhibition of plaque formation decreased from $7 \times 10^{-6} \ M$ at day 12 to $3 \times 10^{-8} \ M$ at day 30. Further insight into the cellular dynamics of the maturation process was secured from the affinity profiles of the population of PFC obtained at different intervals after immunization. The profiles were established by measuring the extent of plaque inhibition as the inhibiting ligand was increased in 10-fold steps from 10^{-7} to $10^{-4} \ M$. The change in the profiles suggested that high-affinity precursor cells were present before immunization, and that somatic diversification following antigenic stimulation was therefore not necessary for the generation of high-affinity clones. Furthermore, the increase in affinity of serum IgG antibody was attributed to the persistence of clones secreting antibody of high affinity accompanied by the loss of clones producing antibody of lower affinity.

Similar investigations were carried out by Claflin *et al.* (1973) in the mouse (BALB/c) with an enlarged DNP hapten, *N*-(2,4-dinitrophenyl)-β-alanylglycylglycine (DNP-AGG), conjugated to hemocyanin. The intrinsic affinity for the binding of DNP-β-alanine by IgG serum antibody increased 64-fold from a value for K_0 of 1.4×10^6 M^{-1} at day 10 after immunization to 8.7×10^7 M^{-1} at day 30. The affinity characteristics of the IgG antibody secreted by PFC obtained from lymph node samples were established by plaque inhibition with the monovalent ligand DNP-AGG-t-Boc hydrazide. A parallel change was found by this assay consisting of a 32-fold decrease in the concentration of ligand giving 50% inhibition, from 5.0×10^{-6} M at day 6 to 1.6×10^{-7} M at day 26. An analysis of the affinity profile of PFC was made by incremental inhibition measurements, as noted above. The essential findings were (1) that the entire range of affinity was expressed in the heterogeneous population of IgG-secreting cells present 6 days after primary immunization, the earliest point at which a reliable profile could be established; and (2) that the subsequent maturation consisted of a relative decline of low-affinity PFC and a consequent dominance by high-affinity PFC. Thus, it was not necessary to invoke the notion of continued, antigen-driven somatic diversification establishing new precursor cells to account for the rise in average affinity of serum antibody and maintenance at a plateau level. It should be noted, however, that in the absence of idiotypic analysis or other genetic characterization, the clonal identity of the initial high-affinity PFC and those found after full maturation can only be presumed.

In a further elaboration of the system described above, Claflin and Merchant (1973) attempted to establish the earliest appearance of the PFC subpopulation secreting antibody of the maximum affinity. Experimental limitation allowed its detection no earlier than 4.5 days following the primary immunization. It was found that despite procedures favoring development of a PFC population of maximum affinity, this maximum did not exceed the affinity of subpopulations present in the earliest response. It was inferred that the precursor clones of the PFC induced by the DNP-AGG-conjugated antigen exist prior to the immunization process.

Concordant results were obtained by Huchet and Feldmann (1973) in their study of CBA mice immunized with DNP antigens. In this case, the maturation of memory cells as well as changes in the PFC were evaluated from the inhibition of plaque formation by DNP-Lys. Measurement of the concentration of ligand required for 50% inhibition of PFC in the primary response showed a 10-fold decrease between days 5 and 18. The maturation of memory cells was clearly shown by the results obtained with PFC produced by secondary stimulation following a primary immunization 5 months earlier. The maturation process observed in the early part of the primary response evidently continued beyond the period of detection and was manifested in the secondary response. Thus, under optimum conditions, there was an overall 600-fold increase in the relative average affinity of secreted anti-DNP antibody when DNP-fowl γ-globulin (DNP-FGG) was the antigen. With DNP-flagellin (DNP-Fla), the corresponding increase was about 100-fold. The use of these protein carriers is of particular relevance with respect to the role of T cells in the maturation phenomenon. Whereas DNP-FGG requires T-cell cooperation for an observable immune response and DNP-Fla does not (Feldmann and Basten, 1971), T-cell participation is not essential to the maturation process. This conclusion is in accord with the affinity increase of antilactose antibody described above involving an immunogen (bacterial vaccine) that, presumably, is T-cell-independent (Howard *et al.*, 1971).

The studies we have summarized above involving the properties of antibody secreted by PFC provide a partial view of the cellular dynamics responsible for the maturation of affinity of serum antibody. Furthermore, the modulation of this process can be related to the demonstration of the persistence of low-affinity clones, probably memory cells, available for subsequent proliferation or differentiation or both. The picture that has emerged thus far is subject, however, to a potentially important qualification arising from the almost exclusive concentration on anti-DNP antibody. The DNP group can apparently stimulate thousands of clones (Kreth and Williamson, 1973) as a result, undoubtedly, of its distinctive chemical structure, and this number is probably much larger than the normal range of clones responsive to naturally occurring determinants, such as those associated with proteins and poly-saccharides. The consequence of this difference might be a distorted pattern of cellular dynamics for anti-DNP, if not, indeed, an anomalous one. The extension of the cellular analysis of the maturation process to other chemical types of determi-nants merits serious attention.

101

THE AFFINITY OF
ANTIBODY: RANGE,
VARIABILITY, AND
THE ROLE OF
MULTIVALENCE

2.5. Temporal Variation of IgM Affinity

We have previously discussed the selective limitation of the intrinsic affinity of IgM antibody and noted that the cellular basis of this restriction may be the inability of IgM precursor cells to undergo the antigen-directed maturation process. The available evidence does indeed demonstrate that IgM maturation is severely limited in its duration and in the associated increase of intrinsic affinity, in comparison with the corresponding features of IgG maturation.

2.5.1. Studies with Serum Antibody

Investigations of temporal changes in the affinity of IgM antibody present in serum have been limited to a few cases. The main difficulty has been that in most instances, production of IgM antibody is relatively transient and sufficient levels for affinity measurement are available only for a restricted time interval. In the early study of Voss and Eisen (1968), there was no significant increase of affinity with time of rabbit and equine anti-DNP IgM antibody in its interaction with DNP-Lys. The equine antibody was studied over a 3-month period. A parallel result was reported by Sarvas and Mäkelä (1970) with rabbit anti-NIP IgM. In this study, a bacteriophage neutralization assay was used to evaluate the antibody affinity. No maturation was evident during the period from 6 to 34 days after primary immuniza-tion, in striking contrast to the changes in the affinity of the IgG anti-NIP antibody.

The maturation process was also examined in two instances in which a sustained IgM response could be maintained. In an interesting study of a nonmam-malian response, anti-DNP IgM antibodies induced in the nurse shark with DNP-hemocyanin were examined at 10 and at 30 months after initial immunization (Voss and Sigel, 1972). The binding of DNP-Lys, measured by equilibrium dialysis, showed a relatively low value of K_0 (1×10^5 M^{-1}), and was not significantly greater when measured after an additional period of 20 months with booster immunizations. This finding contrasted with the behavior of the 7 S antibody, which showed a 100-fold increase during this period to a K_0 value of 2×10^7 M^{-1}.

A different type of immunogen, containing lactose as the immunodominant moiety, was used in the study of equine IgM antilactose antibody (Kim and Karush, 1974). Isoelectric fractions of purified IgM antibody were isolated at 6, 10, and 14 weeks after initial immunization and intrinsic affinities measured by equilibrium dialysis. The dominant fraction had a K_0 value of 4×10^5 M^{-1} and showed functional homogeneity at 6 weeks. Some heterogeneity was evident in the later two bleedings, but no change in K_0 was apparent. Three other, minor isoelectric fractions exhibited somewhat lower K_0 values ($\approx 2 \times 10^5$ M^{-1}) with, possibly, a slight increase in K_0, less than 2-fold, during an 8-week period. During the same period, it should be emphasized, the 7 S antibody population reached an average K_0 about 6-fold higher than the maximum for IgM antibody. In a subsequent study (Chua *et al.*, 1975), IgM antilactose antibody from a group of horses was studied during the period between 5 and 44 weeks after initial immunization. Although some indication of an early maturation was suggested, the results clearly showed the absence of a clear-cut and consistent increase of affinity with time.*

2.5.2. Cellular Studies†

The maturation of IgM-secreting cells has also been examined by the hemolytic plaque method. In most cases, the inhibition by multivalent ligand has been used as a quantitative assay to evaluate relative association constants of the secreted IgM antibody.

The observation that when BALB/c mice are immunized with type III pneumococcal polysaccharide (S III) only IgM antibody-producing cells are detectable was used by Barker *et al.* (1971) to study time-dependent changes in the secreted antibody. In this report, the use of polysaccharide to inhibit formation of hemolytic plaques means that the effectiveness of the ligand (S III) was dependent on the functional affinity of its interaction with antibody and was reflected in the concentration of ligand required for 50% inhibition. The relevant finding for our purpose was the invariance of this required concentration of ligand for the IgM-secreting cells obtained between 5 and 17 days following primary immunization. It was evident, therefore, that no detectable change of functional affinity—or, presumably, of intrinsic affinity—had taken place in the intervening 12 days. As implied by the authors, however, the large value of the functional affinity might obscure actual changes in intrinsic affinity. On the basis of the bivalent binding of antilactose IgG antibody (Gopalakrishnan and Karush, 1974b) we would estimate that the functional association constant exceeded 10^{10} M^{-1}.

Turning to a hydrophobic type of hapten, namely, TNP, we find that the IgM response to a TNP antigen in BALB/c is characterized by a rapid and significant increase of intrinsic affinity (Claflin and Merchant, 1972). The concentration of a monovalent TNP-containing ligand, *N*-TNP-aminocaproic acid, required for 50% plaque inhibition was determined for splenic IgM-secreting cells. Cells were sampled prior to immunization and periodically over a period of 98 days. A 6-fold decrease in concentration of ligand was found for the 50% end point between day 0 and day 4. No further change occurred even following secondary immunization. In

---

*In contrast to the findings summarized above, Oriol and Rousset (1974) have identified a presumed 19 S fraction of rat anti-Dnp antibody which followed the same maturation process as the corresponding 7 S antibody. It was not clearly established, however, that this high-molecular-weight fraction was IgM.

†It has recently been pointed out by DeLisi (1976) that the optimum conditions for the detection of changes in affinity using the hemolytic plaque inhibition technique are significantly different for IgM antibody from those appropriate for IgG antibody. He has argued that the disparity in the results of studies on IgM maturation can be attributed to differences in assay conditions.

addition the maturation process appeared to consist of a modified distribution of secreting cells expressing a broad range of affinity. It was inferred, therefore, that maturation did not require the generation of new clones subsequent to immunization, but rather could be accounted for by a selective proliferation of precursor clones present prior to administration of antigen.

This type of cellular analysis was extended by Claflin *et al.* (1973) to IgM production in BALB/c mice immunized with an enlarged DNP hapten, DNP-AGG. Substantially the same observations were made as already described for the TNP antibody, namely, reduction in the concentration of ligand for 50% inhibition from day 0 to day 9 and an apparent selective stimulation of high-affinity precursor clones present before immunization.

The anti-DNP IgM response on the cellular level was also analyzed in the mouse (CBA) by Huchet and Feldmann (1973) using the concentration for 50% inhibition by DNP-Lys as a measure of relative affinity. Their findings, though more restricted with respect to time interval, were in agreement with the other DNP and TNP studies. That is, over the period of 4–28 days following primary immmunization with DNP-conjugated proteins, no increase was detectable in the average affinity of the IgM antibody secreted by PFC.

A cellular analysis was also carried out with lymph node cells from rabbits immunized with proteins coupled to *p*-azobenzenearsonic acid (Wu, C. Y., and Cinader, 1972). Mono-(*p*-azobenzenearsonic acid)-L-tyrosine was used as a monovalent inhibitor for plaque formation. Measurements at 5 and 15 days after primary immunization exhibited 3- to 10-fold decreases of ligand concentrations for 50% inhibition. The extent of the increase in intrinsic affinity that is implied by these values was primarily dependent on the antigen dose, with the largest increase associated with the lower doses.

2.6. Genetic Control of IgM

The quantitative evaluations summarized above of the intrinsic affinity of IgG and IgM antibody and its temporal dependence clearly establish two essential differences between these classes of immunoglobulin. In the first place, there is a selective limitation of affinity for IgM antibody such that the maximum value of K_0 for IgG antibody may exceed that for IgM by more than 1000-fold, as in the case of anti-DNP. With low-affinity systems, such as antilactose, the ratio is probably no more than 10-fold. The second difference, which provides the cellular basis for this selective limitation of affinity, relates to the restricted potentiality for maturation of IgM production. With IgG antibody, maturation may proceed for weeks and months with increases in K_0 of several-hundred-fold, whereas IgM maturation, when detectable at all, occurs only during the first few days after antigenic stimulation and exhibits only a several fold increase in K_0. It appears that there is no selection at the lower end of the affinity range; i.e., IgM and IgG antibody may exhibit the same relatively low values of K_0. The lower limits are probably set by the experimental restrictions involved in measuring values of K_0 of less than 10^4 M^{-1}. It may also be noted that there is substantial evidence that the IgM response involves the stimulation of precursor clones present prior to administration of antigen. The evidence on this point for IgG production is less direct but also indicative of a heterogeneous population of preexisting precursor clones potentially capable of expressing the full range of affinity as seen in the measured K_0 values of secreted antibody.

The interpretation of affinity and maturation differences between IgG and IgM in terms of differential genetic expression implies that the pool of V-region genes available for the IgM antibody is a subclass of those available for expression in the IgG product. With respect to the V regions of the H chains, the notion of a subclass of V_H genes is supported by the fact that the same set of prototype sequences has been identified for the μ and γ chains (Kohler *et al.*, 1970). Thus, the identification of the V_H genes expressed in the μ and γ chains with common prototype sequences provides a simple, conceptual basis for the proposed subclass relationship. A similar argument can be made for the utilization of a subclass of V_L genes in the expression of IgM antibody.

Although the nature of the subclass of V genes, i.e., the principle of its selection, cannot be inferred from the established differences in the properties of IgG and IgM antibody, one attractive, and verifiable, hypothesis may be advanced. It is based on the assumption that the substantial number of V genes transmitted by inheritance (Cohn, 1974) undergoes somatic diversification, perhaps only during ontogeny. In this way, a natural subclass relationship is established in which the germ-line V genes constitute the members of the subclass. The essential notion in the hypothesis, then, is that IgM production utilizes entirely, or primarily, germ-line genes, whereas IgG synthesis expresses not only these genes but also their somatic derivatives. It may further be suggested that the expression as receptors of these somatically derived genes in clones of relatively small numbers of cells would account qualitatively for the affinity and maturation differences noted above. With respect to the higher affinity acquired by IgG antibody, the increased number of precursor clones available for stimulation would provide a larger number with high affinity. The more extended maturation period for IgG would be the consequence of the initially small size of the precursor clones somatically generated.

The proposed utilization of germ-line V genes for IgM synthesis is open to experimental analysis. This analysis would involve the preparation of purified IgM antibody against a defined determinant and the fractionation of its heavy or light chains, or both, by isoelectric focusing. Comparison of the patterns from different animals would be informative but not conclusive, since isoelectric fractions with the same isoelectric point are not necessarily identical in amino acid sequence. Such fractions would have to be compared further by sequence analysis or peptide mapping. A consistent pattern of identity among several animals would provide substantial support for the proposed thesis.*

3. Role of Multivalence

The evolutionary development of the architecture of the antibody molecule has provided in its contemporary form a distinctive structure superbly suited for multivalent interaction. In addition to multivalence, the general occurrence of multiple and identical antigenic determinants on the surfaces of infectious agents and neoplastic cells has led to the emergence of two further structural features.

---

*Claflin and Rudikoff (1976) have studied the antiphosphorylcholine antibody from 18 inbred strains of mice by quantitative idiotypic analysis, analytical isoelectric focusing of L chains, and limited sequence analysis of H and L chains. From the close similarities among the antibody populations produced in the several strains it was concluded that these populations are specified by germ-line structural genes. It is of considerable interest to note that this was IgM antibody in view of our discussion above.

These, indeed, are required for the effective utilization of the multivalence of antibody. They comprise the property of intramolecular structural symmetry, i.e., identical subunits, resulting in the identity of the antigen-binding sites of the antibody, and the segmental flexibility of the Fab portions of the molecule. The conjunctive effect of these properties is the capacity of the antibody molecule to adjust the separation and relative orientation of its binding sites to the generally fixed distances between the identical complementary groups of the complex ligand. The biological utility of the resulting multivalent interaction is undoubtedly linked to the enhanced affinity that is associated with multivalent binding.

The concept of the enhancement of intrinsic affinity by virtue of multiple attachment has become widely recognized among immunologists only within the past decade, although its possible significance was pointed out as early as 1937 (Burnet et al., 1937) and the bivalence of 7 S antibody was clearly demonstrated in 1949 (Eisen and Karush, 1949). The quantitative description of the enhancement is usefully specified as a factor that represents the multiple by which the intrinsic affinity, expressed as an association constant, is increased by virtue of multivalent interaction. Operationally, the enhancement factor is evaluated by the ratio of affinities for the interaction of a particular antibody population with a monovalent ligand and a multivalent one. The ligands should, of course, possess as nearly identical reactive groups as is chemically feasible. The occasional reference in the immunological literature to the notion that multivalent interaction involves nonspecific factors, in implied contrast to monovalent binding, is misleading since, obviously, both interactions are dependent on such factors as temperature, pH, and ionic strength.

The quantitative evaluation of the enhancement factor has been possible for only a few systems. The main difficulties in the determination are the selection of a system in which multivalent binding does not proceed beyond the formation of the 1:1 complex and the measurement of association constants in excess of 10^9 M^{-1}. A further restriction has emerged since 1972 from the recognition that the distance of closest approach between the binding sites of a 7 S antibody is about 9 nm (Werner et al., 1972). This geometrical limitation requires, therefore, that on multivalent ligands one or more pairs of reactive groups exist with a separation between members of the pair that falls within 9 to approximately 20 nm. The failure of several bivalent lactose-containing ligands to exhibit enhanced binding with 7 S antilactose antibody (Gopalakrishnan and Karush, 1974a) demonstrated the significance of this requirement.

3.1. Studies with Bivalent Antibody

Several studies have been concerned with the functional affinity of the interaction of bivalent antibody with multivalent ligand. The earliest of these studies that provided an estimate of the enhancement factor was that of Greenbury et al. (1965), who studied the interaction of bivalent (7 S and 5 S) rabbit antibody and monovalent (5 S and 3.5 S) antibody specific for blood group A with human A_1 cells. Although association constants of these interactions were not obtained, the relative values of K_0 were estimated from the difference in the quantity of red cells required to bind 50% of the labeled antibody. On this basis, it was estimated that the enhancement factor for this system ranged between 150 and 450.

Another experimental approach for the analysis of multivalent interaction is based on viral neutralization. This method provides the advantage that the multivalent ligand, i.e., the virus, can be used at extremely low concentrations (10^{-17} M) and the extent of neutralization of the virus quantitatively assessed. It carries the additional simplification that the concentration of uncombined antibody remains perceptibly unchanged in the course of the reaction. The earliest studies of viral neutralization with antiviral antibody revealed a substantial loss of neutralizing capacity when bivalent antibody was converted to monovalent fragments (Klinman et al., 1967). It was not possible, however, to determine association constants for the formation of the neutralized complexes. Subsequently, the utility of viral neutralization for the quantitative evaluation of the multivalent interaction of antihapten antibody with hapten conjugated to bacteriophage emerged from the demonstration that hapten-conjugated bacteriophage was subject to neutralization by antihapten antibody (Haimovich and Sela, 1966; Mäkelä, 1966). This method has been the most fruitful one to date in providing a quantitative measure of the enhancement factor.

The first application of this method for the measurement of functional affinity and for the evaluation of the enhancement factor in bivalent interaction ("monogamous bivalency") was made with rabbit anti-DNP IgG antibody and DNP-conjugated ØX174 (Hornick and Karush, 1969). In this system, it was possible to determine the association constant both by equilibrium measurements and by the evaluation of the rate constants for neutralization and reactivation. The measurement of the reactivation kinetics was feasible because the antibody that dissociated from the bacteriophage was rendered inactive by the presence of a relatively high concentration of DNP-Lys. The equilibrium value of 3.5×10^{11} M^{-1} (37°C) was in excellent agreement with the calculated value of 1.1×10^{11} M^{-1} (37°C) from the rate constants (3.7×10^7 M^{-1} $sec^{-1}/3.4 \times 10^{-4}$ sec^{-1}). The association constant for the binding of DNP-Lys was measured by equilibrium dialysis at 37°C to yield a K_0 of 6×10^6 M^{-1}. The enhancement factor for this system was thus found to lie between 2×10^4 and 6×10^4. The decisive element responsible for this striking value is, as would be expected for bivalent binding, the decreased rate of dissociation compared with monovalent binding. The value of 3.7×10^7 M^{-1} sec^{-1} for the rate of association is comparable to that found with monovalent ligands, but the dissociation rate constant is several orders of magnitude lower (see Table 2).

In a later study with anti-DNP antibody, the interaction with rabbit 7 S antibody was compared with that of bivalent 5 S antibody and 7 S and 3.5 S monovalent antibody at 25°C (Hornick and Karush, 1972). The purified preparation of rabbit anti-DNP IgG in this case gave an enhancement factor of about 10^3, with a K_0 for the intrinsic affinity of approximately 1×10^7 M^{-1}. The 5 S fragment prepared by peptic digestion of the 7 S antibody gave the same values for functional and intrinsic affinity as the parent preparation. On the other hand, the monovalent 3.5 S fragment and the monovalent hybrid 7 S sample exhibited a greatly reduced K_0 for the neutralization reaction, as anticipated. In both instances, however, there was a 10-fold disparity between the K_0 measured by equilibrium dialysis and that determined by bacteriophage neutralization. For the 7 S monovalent antibody, the values were 3.3×10^7 and 3.3×10^8 M^{-1}, respectively. Since the antibody concentration was many fold higher than the bacteriophage concentration (10^{-9} vs. 10^{-17} M), it is quite likely that the apparent discrepancy was due to a secondary equilibrium involving the preferential binding of high-affinity molecules. The gener-

107

THE AFFINITY OF
ANTIBODY: RANGE,
VARIABILITY, AND
THE ROLE OF
MULTIVALENCE

ally heterogeneous nature of the anti-DNP response would provide the basis for such selective interaction. A similar reequilibration reaction appears to have been involved in the study by Blank *et al.* (1972) of the neutralization of DNP-T$_4$ bacteriophage with anti-DNP antibody. Although this system did not permit quantitative measurement of functional affinity, and therefore of the enhancement factor, the wide variation in the apparent neutralization rate constants was in accord with a decisive role for multivalent interaction.

The uncertainty of interpretation arising from the heterogeneous nature of the anti-DNP populations was avoided in a later study with antilactoside antibody (Gopalakrishnan and Karush, 1974b). In addition, the latter system served to confirm the energetic importance of multivalent interaction for antibodies in general. In this study, multiple lactoside groups were conjugated to $\emptyset$X174 to render the bacteriophage susceptible to neutralization with antilactoside antibody. Purified antibody was obtained from a rabbit immunized with a vaccine prepared by conjugating the R36A strain of pneumococcus with *p*-aminophenyl-β-lactoside (PAPL). The antibody was fractionated by preparative isoelectric focusing to yield one, and possibly a second, functionally homogeneous population. Binding measurements with a monovalent ligand, *N*-acetyl-*p*-aminophenyl-β-lactoside (*N*-acetyl-PAPL), were made at 25° by equilibrium dialysis. The neutralization reaction was studied at 25°C with an antibody concentration varying between 2.5×10^{-10} and 5×10^{-10} M. The values for the intrinsic and functional association constants are shown in Table 4 together with the second-order rate constants for the neutralization reaction. The value of the intrinsic association constant (2×10^5 M^{-1}) is at least 30-fold smaller than the K_0's for the anti-DNP antibody preparations used in the earlier neutralization studies. Since the K_0's for the functional affinity exceed 2×10^9 M^{-1}, it can be concluded that the enhancement factor for this system is of the order of 10^4. In the light of the similar, but not identical, results from the anti-DNP studies, a reasonable generalization for the enhancement due to bivalent interaction is a factor of the order of magnitude of 10^4.

3.2. Studies with IgM Antibody

It is a common observation that IgM antibody is more effective on a molar basis than IgG antibody in such assays as neutralization (Finkelstein and Uhr, 1966) and hemagglutination (Onoue *et al.*, 1965), a difference that is attributed to the

TABLE 4. **Equilibrium and Rate Constants for Neutralization Reaction and Ligand-Binding at 25°C with Anti-PAPL Antibody**[a]

Preparation	Antibody concentration in neutralization mixture (M)	Rate constant for neutralization, k_t (M^{-1} sec^{-1})	Association constant for neutralization (M^{-1})	Association constant for ligand-binding (M^{-1})
IgG antibody	4.3×10^{-10}	7.1×10^5	8.7×10^9	2.4×10^5
Fraction I	5.9×10^{-10}	9.4×10^5	6.7×10^9	2.4×10^5
Fraction I	2.5×10^{-10}	4.3×10^5	2.3×10^9	2.4×10^5
Fraction II	4.0×10^{-10}	1.26×10^6	1.22×10^{10}	1.6×10^5

[a]Adapted from Gopalakrishnan and Karush (1974b) with permission. The ligand was *N*-acetyl-PAPL.

higher valence of the IgM antibody. The quantitative measurement of the functional affinity of IgM antibody and the determination of the enhancement factor has apparently been reported only in the study of anti-DNP IgM antibody by Hornick and Karush (1972). In an earlier investigation, Onoue *et al.* (1965) compared rabbit IgM and IgG anti-*p*-azobenzenearsonate antibody. It was observed that although the intrinsic affinities of these classes of antibody were approximately the same, the IgM antibody was more effective on a molar basis in hemolytic and hemagglutinating reactions than the IgG antibody by a factor of 60–180. This difference was attributed to the greater opportunity for multivalent attachment and enhanced affinity.

In the study of IgM anti-DNP antibody (Hornick and Karush, 1972), both the intrinsic and functional association constants were measured. The latter were obtained by equilibrium measurements of the extent of neutralization of DNP-$\emptyset$X174 at known concentrations of purified antibody. Four antibody preparations from three species were evaluated, and the relevant results are summarized in Table 5. The intrinsic association constants for the binding of DNP-Lys were relatively low in comparison with those for IgG antibody and in accordance with the selective limitation of IgM affinity. On the other hand, the functional association constants reached a level of 2×10^{11} M^{-1}, a value equal to the highest exhibited by IgG antibody. The enhancement factor in the case of IgM appears to range between 10^6 and 10^7. This exceeds the enhancement factor of the bivalent IgG antibody by a factor of at least 100-fold. It would thus appear that in the neutralization of DNP-$\emptyset$X174, the IgM antibody molecule utilizes at least three of its combining sites for attachment to DNP groups on the surface of the bacteriophage. In this connection, it should be noted that an additional factor contributes to enhanced affinity for IgM binding beyond the use of more than two binding sites. This factor is a statistical one arising from the number of ways in which the 10 sites of the IgM molecule can be used to form n linkages. Undoubtedly, however, severe topological restraints are involved in the actual expression of these alternatives. It is evident that in interactions permitting a larger number of sites to be occuped, the process would appear to be virtually irreversible. Except for the chicken IgM preparation used at a concentration of 1×10^{-9} M, the second-order rate constants for the neutralization reaction were similar to those for IgG antibody, namely, about 10^7 M^{-1} sec^{-1}. This value emphasizes again that the increased enhancement factor is due primarily to a reduced rate of dissociation.

TABLE 5.   A Comparison of Multivalent and Monovalent Affinities at 25°C of Anti-DNP IgM Preparations[a]

Preparation	Antibody concentration in neutralization mixture (M)	Association constant for neutralization (M^{-1})	Association constant for ligand-binding (M^{-1})
Rabbit IgM	5×10^{-12}	2.4×10^{11}	$< 10^6$
Chicken (M) IgM	1×10^{-9}	4.6×10^9	$< 10^4$
Chicken (H) IgM	2×10^{-11}	8.1×10^{10}	4×10^4
Shark IgM	9×10^{-12}	1.7×10^{11}	$\approx 1 \times 10^4$

[a] Adapted from Hornick and Karush (1972) with permission.

109

THE AFFINITY OF
ANTIBODY: RANGE,
VARIABILITY, AND
THE ROLE OF
MULTIVALENCE

An interesting example of a nonantibody multivalent interaction showing enhancement of affinity was described by Hammarström (1973). The invertebrate agglutinin *Helix pomatia* A hemagglutinin agglutinates human A erythrocytes. It is a hexavalent molecule with a K_0 for the appropriate monovalent ligand of 5×10^3 M^{-1} at 25°C. The binding of the hexavalent molecule to A erythrocytes was studied with the ^{125}I-labeled agglutinin and characterized by a functional association constant of the order of 10^{10} M^{-1}. The approximate enhancement factor of 10^6 is strikingly similar to the corresponding value for IgM antibody. Furthermore, the binding of bivalent subunits showed a reduced K_0 value of about 5×10^7 M^{-1}. In this instance also, the enhancement factor of 10^4 is in accord with the IgG results.

3.3. Theoretical Analysis

The theoretical calculation of quantitative values for the enhancement factor is a complex and unsolved problem even for bivalent antibody. Several attempts have been made to develop theoretical equations from which estimates can be made of the enhancement (Greenbury *et al.*, 1965; Crothers and Metzger, 1972; Schumaker *et al.*, 1973). The simplest system to consider is the formation of a bivalently linked complex between bivalent antibody and a bivalent ligand, a process that may be formulated as follows:

$$
\begin{array}{ccccc}
\text{L}\rule{1.5cm}{0.4pt}\text{L} & \rightleftharpoons & \begin{array}{c}\text{L}\rule{1.5cm}{0.4pt}\text{L} \\ | \\ \text{S}\rule{1.5cm}{0.4pt}\text{S}\end{array} & \rightleftharpoons & \begin{array}{c}\text{L}\rule{1.5cm}{0.4pt}\text{L} \\ | \qquad | \\ \text{S}\rule{1.5cm}{0.4pt}\text{S}\end{array} \\
\text{S}\rule{1.5cm}{0.4pt}\text{S} & & \text{Complex I} & & \text{Complex II}
\end{array}
$$

The formation of complex I is a second-order process involving the loss of one kinetic unit. The association constant for this reaction is measured, at least approximately, by the intrinsic affinity for complex formation between the corresponding monovalent antibody and monovalent ligand. In addition, there is a small favorable statistical factor (4) adding to the stability of complex I. The analysis of the stabilization achieved in complex II by the formation of a second S–L linkage requires attention to several additional considerations. Since the conversion from complex I to complex II is a first-order process, the free-energy difference between these forms does not include a decrease in the entropy of mixing (Karush, 1962). On the other hand, since association constants for the binding of monovalent ligand almost invariably use molar concentrations, this entropy loss is a significant factor in the quantitative value of K_0 and in the corresponding value of the standard free energy. This value of the standard free energy, without appropriate correction, is therefore not the proper value to use as a first approximation to the free-energy change resulting from the formation of the second linkage of complex II.

Beyond the proper value for this required starting point in all the theoretical analyses, the formation of complex II involves other contributions to the free-energy change. From a topological point of view, it is clear that the accessibility of a second specific group and the number available enter directly into consideration. These factors and related structural aspects can be formulated in terms of (1) the loss of internal degrees of freedom of both the bivalent antibody and the bivalent ligand, (2) the strain or distortion of intramolecular linkages introduced into each of the two molecules, and (3) the statistical factors associated with the multiplicity of accessible ligand groups in the case of multivalent antigens, e.g., cell surfaces. It may be noted also that with IgM antibody, additional statistical enhancement is provided by the decavalence of this molecule.

In the earliest and most simplified attempt at a mathematical formulation of the enhancement effect, Greenbury *et al.* (1965) assumed that the forward rate constant for the formation of complex I was equal to the rate constant for the formation of complex II, and that the corresponding rate constants for dissociation were equal. With these questionable assumptions, the enhancement factor was given by the product of the intrinsic association constant and a factor representing the concentration of membrane groups available to the free site of the monovalently linked antibody. With reasonable estimates of the parameters determining the value of this concentration factor a crude approximation to the observed enhancement values was obtained.

The theoretical analysis of Crothers and Metzger (1972) includes both statistical–mechanical and structural considerations. It represents a more sophisticated version of the earlier model employed by Greenbury *et al.* (1965) and avoids the questionable assumptions of the latter. The form of the approximate equations for the calculation of the enhancement factor is, however, the same in both cases. The primary difference in the equations is the separation assumed most probable of the combining sites of the bivalent antibody. Greenbury and co-workers used a distance of 25 nm based on the model of a rod-shaped molecule with one site at each end. Crothers and Metzger calculated a most probable distance of 8.7 nm, taking into account the dimensions of the Fab fragment but assuming complete flexibility between the Fab arms. In both cases, the enhancement factor is given by a product that includes the intrinsic association constant and the distance between antibody sites.

There remains an unresolved difficulty associated with the use of the intrinsic association constant in this calculation. The problem arises from the fact that the intrinsic constant includes a contribution from the loss of translational and rotational entropy due to the conversion of two kinetic units into one. Although there may also be some loss of entropy arising from constraints generated in the bivalently linked complex, this loss is likely to be much smaller (Jencks, 1975). The result is that the intrinsic association constant is not the appropriate quantity for the calculation of the enhancement factor. Further application and, perhaps, a more critical test of the utility of the formulation of Crothers and Metzger will be possible when studies are done with well-defined bivalent ligands and homogeneous bivalent antibody.

The analysis of the interaction of bivalent antibody and bivalent ligand by Schumaker *et al.* (1973) was made strictly in thermodynamic terms. The basic equation relating the association constants for the variety of possible complexes to the thermodynamic and statistical parameters is

$$K(m,n) = S(m,n)e^{-[b\delta F + \xi(m,n)]/RT}$$

where $K(m,n)$ is the equilibrium constant for the formation of a complex ($HmAn$) containing m bivalent ligands denoted H and n bivalent antibody molecules denoted A, and is related to the free concentrations as follows:

$$(HmAn) = K(m,n)(H)^m(A)^n$$

where (H) and (A) represent the free concentrations of ligand and antibody,

111

THE AFFINITY OF
ANTIBODY: RANGE,
VARIABILITY, AND
THE ROLE OF
MULTIVALENCE

respectively. $S(m,n)$ is the statistical factor equal to the number of distinct ways of assembling the complex divided by the number of distinct ways of taking it apart (V. N. Schumaker, personal communication). All the free-energy contributions arising from steric restrictions, loss of internal degree of freedom, loss of translational entropy, and other changes that make the total free energy of interaction different from $b\delta F$ are included in the term $\xi(m,n)$. The number of occupied antibody sites is b and δF, in effect, is the intrinsic affinity. The value of δF is obtained by setting $\xi(2,1)$ equal to zero, i.e., assigning zero strain to the complex $H2A1$ and using the following relationship, including the statistical factor of 4 for this complex:

$$2\delta F = -RT\ln[K(2,1)/4]$$

With the aid of a computer program and judicious choices of the thermodynamic parameters δF and $\xi(m,n)$ guided by available experimental data, the distribution of antibody and ligand among various complexes can be calculated as a function of concentration of reactants and the selected thermodynamic quantities. One of the distinctive features of this analysis is that it provides explicitly for the existence of circular (i.e., closed) complexes as well as linear ones. It is of particular interest that in the absence of strain, the 1 : 1 closed complex, i.e., bivalently linked, is 1000-fold more stable than the next most stable form, which is the closed dimer, the 2 : 2 complex, with all sites occupied. The approach used by Schumaker and co-workers will probably find fruitful application when suitable experimental systems are developed.

An alternative version of the formulation of Schumaker and co-workers may be suggested in which the contribution of the entropy of mixing is explicitly included rather than contained in the strain term $\xi(m,n)$. Since this contribution is simply statistical and dependent on the composition of the complex, its separation from $\xi(m,n)$ would relate the latter directly to the structural properties of the reactants.

The correction for the entropy of mixing (ΔS_{mix}) depends on the standard states chosen for the reactants and products, i.e., the concentration units. For the formation of the complex ($HmAn$), the value of ΔS_{mix} may be expressed by

$$\Delta S_{\text{mix}} = -R\ln(f/f^m f^n)$$

where f is the factor required to convert the concentration unit used to define the standard state to mole fraction. For the usual case of dilute solutions in which the concentration of the solutes is expressed in mol per liter, the factor f is 1/55.6 and ΔS_{mix} is given by

$$\Delta S_{\text{mix}} = -(m + n - 1)R\ln 55.6$$

The modified equation for obtaining δF is given by

$$2\,\delta F = -RT\ln[K(2,1)/4] - 2RT\ln 55.6$$

The value of δF given by the equation above is the unitary free energy (Kauzmann, 1959). It is calculated from the value of the equilibrium constant $K(2,1)$ with concentrations expressed in moles per liter. The corresponding modification required in the general equation is as follows:

$$K(m,n) = S(m,n)\frac{e^{-[b\delta F + \xi(m,n)]/RT}}{(55.6)^{m+n-1}}$$

In the computation of $K(m,n)$, the unitary free energy (δF) must be used, and the value of $K(m,n)$ would be given in units of (mol/liter)$^{1-m-n}$.

4. Structural Analysis of Combining Sites

Important developments have recently taken place in the structural analysis of antibody-combining sites by X-ray analysis of crystalline antibody–ligand complexes (Amzel *et al.*, 1974; Padlan *et al.*, 1973; Segal *et al.*, 1974). These studies have generated the possibility of relating the affinity of such complexes to specific intermolecular interactions between individual contact amino acid residues and adjacent groups of the ligand molecule.

One study was carried out with the Fab' fragment derived from a human IgG myeloma protein that binds the γ-hydroxy derivative of vitamin K$_1$ with a K_0 of 1.7 $\times$ 10^5 M^{-1} (Amzel *et al.*, 1974). The active site consists of a shallow groove with approximate dimensions of 16 Å $\times$ 7 Å and a depth of 6 Å. The site is defined by amino acid residues located in the hypervariable regions of variable portions of both the H and L chains. It appears that the H chain contributes the predominant number of residues to the site (Poljak *et al.*, 1974). The number of residues that make contact with the ligand is estimated at a minimum of 10–12. This figure falls within the range of 10–20 that was estimated in 1962 as the number required to make contact with an antigenic determinant (Karush, 1962). The number of hypervariable residues available for selection of contact residues, however, is much greater (Poljak *et al.*, 1974). From the 3.5-Å structure of the complex (Amzel *et al.*, 1974) and the 2.8-Å structure of Fab' (Poljak *et al.*, 1974), it was seen that the methyl-naphthoquinone ring makes contact with, among others, the phenolic ring of L-chain tyrosine 90 and with H-chain residue 104. In addition, the phytyl tail of the ligand makes close contacts with L-chain residues 29 and 30 (Gly and Asn, respectively), with H-chain residue 104, and with the side chains of H-chain residues 54, 57, and 63. Not all the contact residues have been established, but the relatively weak binding of the quinone portion of the ligand ($K_0 = 1 \times 10^3$ M^{-1}) shows that the phytyl tail contributes significantly to the association constant. It has not been excluded, however, that its contribution is due to a nonspecific hydrophobic interaction.

The expected variety in the structure of the combining site is evident from the study at 3.1-Å resolution of the phosphorylcholine-binding Fab fragment obtained from a mouse myeloma IgA (Segal *et al.*, 1974). In contrast to the site defined above for the vitamin ligand, the site in this case is a large wedge-shaped cavity. It is approximately 12 Å deep, 15 Å wide at the mouth, and 20 Å long. The walls of this cavity are lined exclusively with residues located in hypervariable regions L1, L3, H1, H2, and H3. The phosphoryl ligand is bound to a small part of the cavity and makes contact predominantly with H-chain residues. Electrostatic interaction and hydrogen bonding are involved in the interaction, as shown by the hydrogen bonds between the phosphate group and H-chain residues Tyr 33 and Arg 52, and the proximity of Arg 52 to the negative phosphate. H-chain Lys 54 also apparently provides an electrostatic contribution, since it lies in the immediate vicinity of the negative charge of the ligand. In addition, the positively charged nitrogen of choline is about 5 Å away from H-chain Glu 35, and probably also makes a significant contribution. Finally, the entire ligand is in van der Waals' contact with H-chain Tyr 33. Further refinement of the two systems studied to date, including binding studies with structural analogues and extension of the structural analysis to homogeneous induced antibody, would provide a greatly improved basis for relating the structure of the ligand–site complex to the affinity of the interaction.

113

THE AFFINITY OF
ANTIBODY: RANGE,
VARIABILITY, AND
THE ROLE OF
MULTIVALENCE

5. Closing Statement

Further analysis of the significance of antibody affinity in immunological processes should include emphasis on the interaction of antibody and antigen with cell-surface reactants. The interaction of antigen with immunoglobulin receptors on B lymphocytes, for example, and the consequent signals for proliferation and differentiation may depend critically on the functional binding affinity. This may, in turn, involve the density and mobility of the cell-surface receptors. These parameters may be variable features of the cell surface and differ, for example, between virgin and memory cells (Klinman, 1972).

Examination of the dependence of affinity on these properties will require advances in experimental techniques. The use of optical probes with fluorescent-labeled antigen or receptors or both will undoubtedly be incorporated in the new technology.

ACKNOWLEDGMENT

The author is recipient of a Public Health Service research career award from the National Institute of Allergy and Infectious Diseases.

References

Amzel, L. M., Poljak, R. J., Saul, F., Varga, J. M., and Richards, F. F., 1974, The three dimensional structure of a combining region–ligand complex of immunoglobulin New at 3.5-Å resolution, *Proc. Natl. Acad. Sci. U.S.A.* **71**:1427–1430.

Andersson, B., 1970, Studies on the regulation of avidity at the level of the single antibody-forming cell, *J. Exp. Med.* **132**:77–88.

Atassi, M. Z., 1975, Antigenic structure of myoglobin: The complete immunochemical anatomy of a protein and conclusions relating to antigenic structures of proteins, *Immunochemistry* **12**:423–438.

Barisas, B. G., Singer, S. J., and Sturtevant, J. M., 1975, Kinetics of binding of 2,4-dinitrophenyl and 2,4,6-trinitrophenyl haptens to homologous and heterologous rabbit antibodies, *Immunochemistry* **12**:411–421.

Barker, P. J., Prescott, B., Stashal, P. W., and Amsbaugh, D. F., 1971, Characterization of the antibody response to type III pneumococcal polysaccharide at the cellular level. III. Studies on the average avidity of the antibody produced by specific plaque-forming cells, *J. Immunol.* **107**:719–724.

Berson, S. A., and Yalow, R. S., 1959, Quantitative aspects of the reaction between insulin and insulin-binding antibody, *J. Clin. Invest.* **38**:1996–2016.

Blank, S. E., Leslie, G. A., and Clem, L. W., 1972, Antibody affinity and valence in viral neutralization, *J. Immunol.* **108**:665–673.

Burnet, F. M., Keogh, E. V., and Lush, D., 1937, Immunological reactions of filterable viruses, *Aust. J. Exp. Biol. Med. Sci. (Sup.)* **15**:231–368.

Chua, M.-M., Morgan, D. O., and Karush, F., 1975, Equine anti-hapten antibody. IX. IgM anti-lactose antibodies, *J. Immunol.* **114**:99–101.

Claflin, L., and Merchant, B., 1972, Restricted maturation of antibody-binding characteristics for hapten-specific IgM-plaque-forming cells in mice, *Cell. Immunol.* **5**:209–220.

Claflin, L., and Merchant, B., 1973, Antibody binding characteristics at the cellular level. II. Presence of cells secreting high-affinity IgG antibody at the outset of the immune response, *J. Immunol.* **110**:252–261.

Claflin, L., and Rudikoff, S., 1976, Uniformity in a clonal repertoire: a case for a germ-line basis of antibody diversity, *Cold Spring Harbor Symp. Quant. Biol.* **41**:725–734.

Claflin, L., Merchant, B., and Inman, J., 1973, Antibody-binding characteristics at the cellular level. I. Comparative maturation of hapten-specific IgM and IgG plaque-forming cell populations, *J. Immunol.* **110**:241–251.

Cohn, M., 1974, A rationale for ordering the data on antibody diversification, in: *Progress in Immunology II,* Vol. 2 (L. Brent and J. Holborow, eds.), pp. 261–284, North-Holland, Amsterdam.

Crothers, D. M., and Metzger, H., 1972, The influence of polyvalency on the binding properties of antibodies, *Immunochemistry* **9**:341–357.

Dandliker, W. B., and Levison, S. A., 1968, Investigation of antigen–antibody kinetics by fluorescence polarization, *Immunochemistry* **5**:171–183.

Dandliker, W. B., Shapiro, H. S., Meduski, J. W., Alonso, R., Feigen, G. A., and Hamrick, J. R., 1964, Application of fluorescence polarization to the antigen–antibody reaction: Theory and experimental method, *Immunochemistry* **1**:165–191.

Davie, J. M., and Paul, W. E., 1972, Receptors on immunocompetent cells. V. Cellular correlates of the "maturation" of the immune response, *J. Exp. Med.* **135**:660–674.

Day, L. A., Sturtevant, J. M., and Singer, S. J., 1963, The kinetics of the reactions between antibodies to the 2,4-dinitrophenyl group and specific haptens, *Ann. N. Y. Acad. Sci.* **103**:611–625.

DeLisi, C., 1976, Hemolytic plaque inhibition: the physical chemical limits on its use as an affinity assay, *J. Immunol.* **117**:2249–2257.

DeLisi, C., and Goldstein, B., 1974, On the mechanism of hemolytic plaque inhibition, *Immunochemistry* **11**:661–665.

Eisen, H. N., and Karush, F., 1949, The interaction of purified antibody with homologous hapten: Antibody valence and binding constant, *J. Am. Chem. Soc.* **71**:363–364.

Eisen, H. N., and Siskind, G. W., 1964, Variations in affinities of antibodies during the immune response, *Biochemistry* **3**:996–1008.

Feldmann, M., and Basten, A., 1971, The relationship between antigenic structure and the requirement for thymus-derived cells in the immune response, *J. Exp. Med.* **134**:103–119.

Finkelstein, M. S., and Uhr, J. W., 1966, Antibody formation. V. The avidity of γM and γG guinea pig antibodies to bacteriophage ØX 174, *J. Immunol.* **97**:565–576.

Froese, A., Sehon, A. H., and Eigen, M., 1962, Kinetic studies of protein–dye and antibody-hapten interactions with the temperature-jump method, *Can. J. Chem.* **40**:1786–1797.

Froese, A., and Sehon, A. H., 1965, Kinetic and equilibrium studies of the reaction between anti-*p*-nitrophenyl antibodies and a homologous hapten, *Immunochemistry* **2**:135–143.

Froese, A., 1968, Kinetic and equilibrium studies on 2,4-dinitrophenyl hapten–antibody systems, *Immunochemistry* **5**:253–264.

Fujio, H., and Karush, F., 1966, Antibody affinity. II. Effect of immunization interval on anti-hapten antibody in the rabbit, *Biochemistry* **5**:1856–1863.

Fujio, H., Sakato, N., and Amano, T., 1971, The immunological properties of region specific antibodies directed to hen egg-white lysozyme, *Biken J.* **14**:395–404.

Ghose, A. C., and Karush, F., 1973, Fractions of anti-lactose antibody and their temporal variation, *Biochemistry* **12**:2437–2443.

Goidl, E. W., Paul, G. W., Siskind, G. W., and Benacerraf, B., 1968, The effect of antigen dose and time after immunization on the amount and affinity of anti-hapten antibody, *J. Immunol.* **100**:371–375.

Goldenberg, K., Berkowitz, J. M., and Praissman, M., 1974, Methods in the quantitation of antigen–antibody reactions measured by radioimmunoassay: Application to the gastrin system revealing large and restricted binding energies, *J. Immunol.* **112**:1008–1018.

Gopalakrishnan, P. V., and Karush, F., 1974a, Antibody affinity. VI. Synthesis of bivalent lactosyl antibodies, *Immunochemistry* **11**:279–283.

Gopalakrishnan, P. V., and Karush, F., 1974b, Antibody affinity. VII. Multivalent interaction of anti-lactoside antibody, *J. Immunol.* **113**:769–778.

Gopalakrishnan, P. V., Hughes, W. S., Kim, Y., and Karush, F., 1973, Antibody affinity. IV. The synthesis and immunogenicity of a large β-lactoside hapten, *Immunochemistry* **10**:191–196.

Greenbury, C. L., Moore, D. H., and Nunn, L. A. C., 1965, The reaction with red cells of 7 S rabbit antibody, its subunits and their recombinants, *Immunology* **8**:420–431.

Haber, E., Richards, F. F., Spragg, J., Austen, K. F., Vallotton, M., and Page, L. B., 1967, Modification in the heterogeneity of the antibody response, *Cold Spring Harbor Symp. Quant. Biol.* **32**:299–310.

Haimovich, J., and Sela, M., 1969, Inactivation of bacteriophage T4, poly-D-alanyl bacteriophage and of penicilloyl bacteriophage by immunospecifically isolated IgM and IgG antibodies, *J. Immunol.* **103**:45–55.

115

THE AFFINITY OF
ANTIBODY: RANGE,
VARIABILITY, AND
THE ROLE OF
MULTIVALENCE

Hammarström, S., 1973, Binding of *Helix Pomatia* A hemagglutinin to human erythrocytes and their cells. Influence of multivalent interaction on affinity, *Scand. J. Immunol.* **2**:53–66.

Haselkorn, D., Friedman, S., Givol, D., and Pecht, I., 1974, Kinetic mapping of the antibody combining site by chemical relaxation spectrometry, *Biochemistry* **13**:2210–2222.

Hornick, C. L., and Karush, F., 1969, The interaction of hapten-coupled bacteriophage ØX174 with antihapten antibody, *Isr. J. Med. Sci.* **5**:163–170.

Hornick, C. L., and Karush, F., 1972, Antibody affinity. III. The role of multivalence, *Immunochemistry* **9**:325–340.

Howard, J. G., Christie, G. H., Courtenay, B. M., Leuchars, E., and Davies, A. J. S., 1971, Studies on immunologic paralysis. VI. Thymic-independences of tolerance and immunity to type III pneumococcal polysaccharide, *Cell. Immunol.* **2**:614–626.

Huchet, R., and Feldmann, M., 1973, Studies on antibody affinity in mice, *Eur. J. Immunol.* **3**:49–55.

Jencks, W. P., 1975, The Circe effect, *Adv. Enzymol.* **43**:219–410.

Kabat, E. A., 1966, The nature of an antigenic determinant, *J. Immunol.* **97**:1–11.

Karush, F., 1957, The interaction of purified anti-beta-lactoside antibody with haptens, *J. Am. Chem. Soc.* **79**:3380–3384.

Karush, F., 1962, Immunologic specificity and molecular structure, *Adv. Immunol.* **2**:1–40.

Karush, F., 1970, Affinity and the immune response, *Ann. N. Y. Acad. Sci.* **169**:56–64.

Katz, M., and Pappenheimer, A. M., Jr., 1969, Quantitative studies on the specificity of anti-pneumococcal antibodies, types III and VIII. IV. Binding of labeled hexasaccharides derived from S3 and anti-S3 antibodies and their Fab fragments, *J. Immunol.* **103**:491–495.

Kauzmann, W., 1959, Some factors in the interpretation of protein denaturation, *Adv. in Prot. Chem.* **14**:1–63.

Kelly, K. A., Sehon, A. H., and Froese, A., 1971, Kinetic studies, on antibody–hapten reactions. I. Reactions with antibodies and their univalent Fab' fragments, *Immunochemistry* **8**:613–625.

Kim, Y. D., and Karush, F., 1974, Equine anti-hapten antibody. VIII. Isoelectric fractions of IgM and 7 S anti-lactose antibody. *Immunochemistry* **11**:147–152.

Klinman, N., 1972, The mechanism of antigenic stimulation of primary and secondary clonal precursor cells, *J. Exp. Med.* **136**:241–260.

Klinman, N. R., Long, C., and Karush, F., 1967, The role of antibody bivalence in the neutralization of bacteriophage, *J. Immunol.* **99**:1128–1133.

Kohler, H., Shimizu, A., Pau, C., Moore, V., and Putnam, F. W., 1970, Three variable-gene pools common to IgM, IgG and IgA immunoglobulins, *Nature (London)* **227**:1318–1320.

Kreth, H. W., and Williamson, A. W., 1973, The extent of diversity of anti-hapten antibodies in inbred mice: Anti-NIP(4-hydroxy-5-iodo-3-nitro-phenacetyl) antibodies in CBA/H mice, *Eur. J. Immunol.* **3**:141–147.

Lamelin, J.-P., and Paul, W. E., 1971, Rate of increase of antibody affinity in different rat strains, *Int. Arch. Allergy* **40**:351–360.

Macario, A. J. L., and Conway de Macario, E., 1973, Low and high affinity antibodies can alternate during the immune response, *Nature (London)* **245**:263–264.

Macario, A. J. L., Conway de Macario, E., Franceshi, C., and Celada, F., 1972, Maturation of the immune response *in vitro*: Focal fluctuation and changes in affinity of anti-β-D-galactosidase activating antibody, *J. Exp. Med.* **136**:353–368.

Macario, A. J. L., Conway de Macario, E., and Celada, F., 1973, Rabbit memory cells are not restricted to the affinity of circulating antibodies, *Nature (London) New Biol.* **241**:22–24.

Mäkelä, O., 1966, Assay of anti-hapten antibody with the aid of hapten-coupled bacteriophage, *Immunology* **10**:81–86.

Mäkelä, O., Ruoslahti, E., and Seppälä, I. J. T., 1970, Affinity of IgM and IgG antibodies, *Immunochemistry* **7**:917–932.

Mamet-Bratley, M. D., 1966, Evidence concerning the homogeneity of the combining site of purified antibody, *Immunochemistry* **3**:155–162.

Marrack, J. R., 1938, *The Chemistry of Antigens and Antibodies,* Report No. 230, Medical Research Council, pp. 116–118, Her Majesty's Stationery Office, London.

Noble, R. W., Reichlin, M., and Schreiber, R. D., 1972, Studies on antibodies directed toward single antigenic sites on globular proteins, *Biochemistry* **11**:3326–3332.

Onoue, K., Tanigaki, N., Yagi, Y., and Pressman, D., 1965, IgM and IgG anti-hapten antibody: Hemolytic, hemagglutinating and precipitating activity, *Pro. Soc. Exp. Biol. Med.* **120**:340–346.

Oriol, R., and Rousset, M., 1974, The IgM antibody site. I. Increase of binding affinity of rat 19 S and 7 S anti-dinitrophenyl antibodies during the course of the immune response, *J. Immunol.* **112**:2227–2234.

Padlan, E. A., Segal, D. M., Spande, T. F., Davies, D. R., Rudikoff, S., and Potter, M., 1973, Structure at 4.5 Å resolution of a phosphorylcholine-binding Fab, *Nature (London) New Biol.* **245**:165–167.

Pappenheimer, A. M., Jr., Reed, W. P., and Brown, R., 1968, Quantitative studies of the specificity of anti-pneumococcal polysaccharide antibodies, types III and VIII. III. Binding of a labeled oligosaccharide derived from S8 by anti-S8 antibodies, *J. Immunol.* **100**:1237–1244.

Parker, C. W., Gott, S. M., and Johnson, M. C., 1967, Fluorescent probes for the study of the antibody–hapten reaction. II. Variation in the antibody combining site during the immune response, *Biochemistry* **6**:3417–3427.

Pecht, I., Maron, E., Arnon, R., and Sela, M., 1971, Specific excitation energy transfer from antibodies to dansyl-labeled antigen: Studies with the "loop" peptide, *Eur. J. Biochem.* **19**:368–371.

Poljak, R. J., Amzel, L. M., Chen, B. L., Phizackerley, R. P., and Saul, F. 1974, The three-dimensional structure of the Fab' fragment of a human myeloma immunoglobulin at 2.0-Å resolution, *Proc. Natl. Acad. Sci. U.S.A.* **71**:3440–3444.

Portmann, A. J., Levison, S. A., and Dandliker, W. B., 1971, Anti-fluorescein antibody of high affinity and restricted heterogeneity as characterized by fluorescence polarization and quenching equilibrium techniques, *Biochem. Biophys. Res. Commun.* **43**:207–212.

Portmann, A. J., Levison, S. A., and Dandliker, W. B., 1975, Equilibrium binding studies on antifluorescein antibody during various stages of the immune response, *Immunochemistry* **12**:461–466.

Rappaport, I., 1959, The reversibility of the reaction between rabbit antibody and tobacco mosaic virus, *J. Immunol.* **82**:526–534.

Richards, F. F., and Haber, E., 1967, An approach to an homogeneous antigen. II. Some properties of antibodies directed against a hapten located in a relatively homogeneous environment, *Fed. Proc. Fed. Am. Soc. Exp. Biol.* **26**:311.

Sachs, D. H., Schechter, A. N., Eastlake, A., and Anfinsen, C. B., 1972a, Inactivation of staphylococcal nuclease by the binding of antibodies to a distinct antigenic determinant, *Biochemistry* **11**:4268–4273.

Sachs, D. H., Schechter, A. N., Eastlake, A., and Anfinsen, C. B., 1972b, Antibodies to a distinct antigenic determinant of staphylococcal nuclease, *J. Immunol.* **109**:1300–1310.

Sakato, N., Fujio, H., and Amano, T., 1971, The electric charges of antibodies directed to unique regions of hen egg-white lysozyme, *Biken J.* **14**:405–411.

Sarvas H., and Mäkelä, O., 1970, Haptenated bacteriophage in the assay of antibody quantity and affinity: Maturation of an immune response, *Immunochemistry* **7**:933–943.

Schumaker, V. N., Green, G., and Wilder, R. L., 1973, A theory of bivalent antibody–bivalent hapten interactions, *Immunochemistry* **10**:521–528.

Segal, D. M., Padlan, E. A., Cohen, G. H., Rudikoff, S., Potter, M., and Davies, D. R., 1974, The three-dimensional structure of a phosphorylcholine-binding mouse immunoglobulin Fab and the nature of the antigen binding site, *Proc. Natl. Acad. Sci. U.S.A.* **71**:4298–4302.

Siskind, G. W., and Benacerraf, B., 1969, Cell selection by antigen in the immune response, *Adv. Immunol.* **10**:1–50.

Smith, T. W., Butler, V. P., Jr., and Haber, E., 1970, Characterization of antibodies of high affinity and specificity for the digitalis glycoside digoxin, *Biochemistry* **9**:331–337.

Voss, E. W., Jr., and Eisen, H. N., 1968, Valence and affinity of IgM antibodies to the 2,4-dinitrophenyl (DNP) group, *Fed. Proc. Fed. Am Soc. Exp. Biol.* **27**:684.

Voss, E. W., and Sigel, M. M., 1972, Valence and temporal change in affinity of purified 7 S and 18 S nurse shark anti-2,4-dinitrophenyl antibodies, *J. Immunol.* **109**:665–673.

Werblin, T. P., Kim, Y. T., Quabiata, F., and Siskind, G. W., 1973, Studies on the control of antibody synthesis. III. Changes in heterogeneity of antibody affinity during the course of the immune response, *Immunology* **24**:477–492.

Werner, T. C., Bunting, J. R., and Cathou, R. E., 1972, The shape of immunoglobulin G molecules in solution, *Proc. Natl. Acad. Sci. U.S.A.* **69**:795–799.

Worobec, R. B., Wallace, J. H., and Huggins, C. G., 1972, Angiotensin–antibody interactions. II. Thermodynamic and activation parameters, *Immunochemistry* **9**:239–251.

Wu, C.-Y., and Cinader, B., 1972, Dose- and time-dependent changes in the binding capacity of IgM antibody, *Eur. J. Immunol.* **2**:398–405.

Wu, H.-H., and Rockey, J. H., 1969, Antivasopressin antibody: Characterization of high-affinity rabbit antibody with limited association constant heterogeneity, *Biochemistry* **8**:2719–2728.

4

Antibody Combining Regions

FRANK F. RICHARDS, ROBERT W. ROSENSTEIN,
JANOS M. VARGA, and WILLIAM H. KONIGSBERG

1. Background

1.1. Complementarity and Specificity

An immune serum usually consists of a very heterogeneous population of immuno-globulins (Ig's) the appearance of which in the serum has been induced by antigen. The antigen-ligating function of the Ig molecule (see Figure 1) is confined to the combining regions, which are two symmetrical areas at the solvent-exposed ends of the Fab arms of the Y-shaped Ig molecules. The combining region is situated in the variable (V-region) domain, a compact region consisting of the N-terminal half of the light (L) chain and the N-terminal quarter of the heavy (H) chain that is linked by sulfhydryl bonds. Between the areas of this domain occupied by the L- and H-chain V regions is a cleft exposed to the solvent. Antigens have been shown to bind in, or close to, this cleft (Amzel *et al.*, 1974). An induced antibody population is said to be *specific* because it usually binds most strongly to the immunizing antigen and with lesser binding energies to certain compounds that resemble the immunogen in structure. Heteroclitic antibodies may be induced that bind more strongly to some determinant other than the immunogen (Mäkelä, 1965). In general, antibody popula-tions show a high degree of specificity, in that they are able to discriminate among chemical compounds differing by as little as a single functional group, between stereoisomers, or between two proteins differing by as little as a single amino acid residue (Reichlin, 1974).

FRANK F. RICHARDS and ROBERT W. ROSENSTEIN • Department of Medicine, Yale Univer-sity School of Medicine.   JANOS M. VARGA • Department of Dermatology, Yale University School of Medicine.   WILLIAM H. KONIGSBERG • Department of Molecular Biophysics and Biochemistry and of Human Genetics, Yale University, New Haven, Connecticut.

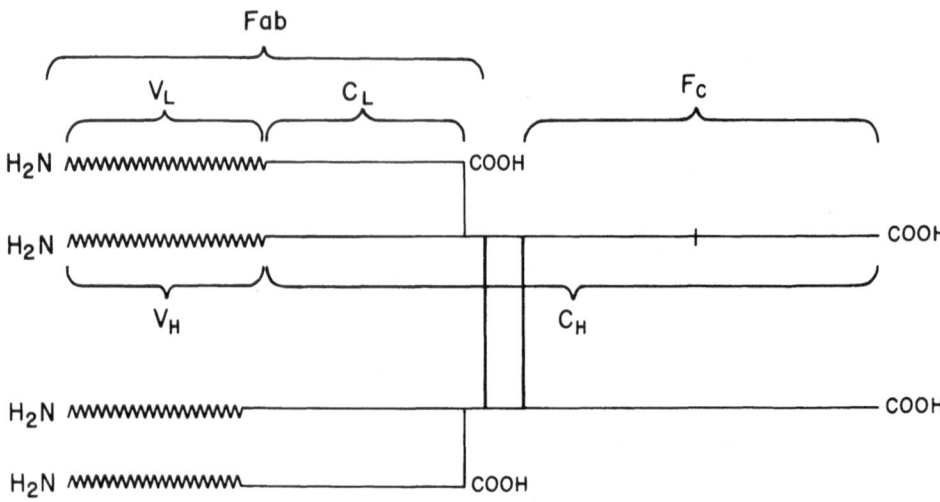

Figure 1. A conceptualization of the four-chain structure of Ig. V_L and V_H are the variable (V) regions of the light (L) and heavy (H) chains. C_L and C_H are the constant (C) regions. The antigen-binding sites, one per each H–L-chain pair, are made up of amino acid residues from the V regions. Fab and Fc are the fragments produced by papain digestion of Ig.

1.2. Immunoglobulin Heterogeneity

The number of individual Ig's in an immune serum may be quite large. It is not unusual to see as many as 50 protein bands on isoelectric focusing, all of which are capable of binding the immunogen. Such a population of Ig's does not behave uniformly with respect to ligand binding; in fact, subpopulations can be identified that bind ligand over a wide range of intrinsic binding constants (K_a) (Eisen and Siskind, 1964; Eisen, 1964a). This, in turn, suggests that the antigen-combining sites also show corresponding variations of structure. This structural heterogeneity is further complicated by a degree of temporal heterogeneity, since during the immune response, the composition of the antibody population does not remain constant (Steiner and Eisen, 1966, 1967a,b; Macario and Conway de Macario, 1975). New antibodies appear while others disappear, suggesting that the antibodies expressed at any one moment during the immune response are only a small proportion of the total number of antibodies with complementarity to the immunizing antigen that the animal is capable of producing. Thus, the immune response is at once very heterogeneous, but when viewed as a population, also highly specific with respect to antigen-binding. This chapter will explore the structural basis of antibody specificity and the associated biology of antibody heterogeneity.

1.3. How Many Antigens and Antibodies Exist?

Most biological macromolecules, such as proteins, peptides, polysaccharides, complex lipids, and nucleic acids, are immunogenic. In addition, an extremely large number of smaller organic and inorganic compounds attached as haptenic groupings to macromolecular carriers will elicit specific complementary antibodies (Karush, 1962). For instance, approximately 6 million organic ring compounds have been catalogued (Wiswesser, 1973). A reasonable estimate might put the number of organic ring compound haptens at perhaps 1–2 million. Clearly, the number of potential haptens is very large.

Several research groups have attempted to estimate the number of antibody-producing cell clones that, in a single mouse, produce antibody that is complementary to a single small haptenic determinant. Since one cannot do this directly, various sampling techniques have been tried. Kreth and Williamson (Williamson, 1973) assumed that the spleen cells from a mouse immunized with the determinant 4-hydroxy-3-iodo-5-nitrophenyl (NIP) coupled to a protein carrier contained all the potential antibody-producing cells. Such cells in very high dilution were injected into irradiated recipient mice, so that one or two anti-NIP cell clones multiplied in each host mouse when the host was challenged with NIP. The host antibodies were subjected to isoelectric focusing (IEF), and the bands representing single anti-NIP antibodies were detected with radioactive NIP. Since the Ig products of single clones have both characteristic IEF band patterns and characteristic isoelectric points, it is possible to count the number of times a pattern repeats itself. When 337 IEF patterns from four donor mice were examined, five "repeats" were seen. The number of repeats expected is inversely proportional to the number of different antibody-producing cell clones. It is possible to calculate that within 90% confidence limits, not fewer than 3000 and not more than 16,000 different Ig's in one mouse bind the NIP determinant. Using similar logic, Quattrochi *et al.* (1969) examined the tryptic peptides from 100 different mouse myeloma tumor L chains. They looked for identity of pattern by two-dimensional peptide-mapping analysis, but were unable to find any identical patterns. They concluded that at least 1000 different L chains must exist to account for their results. It is not known, however, whether the distribution of myeloma L chains resembles the distribution of L chains in nonneoplastic cells. It is possible that the inducing chemical irritant, and possibly the virus that may be involved in myeloma induction, may have some selective influence and do not provide an unbiased sample of antibody-producing cells (Potter, 1972; Warner *et al.,* 1974). Other investigators have estimated the number of antibodies that are induced by trinitrophenyl (TNP) and that also bind dinitrophenyl (DNP) as being approximately 500 (Pink and Askonas, 1974), suggesting that even when these somewhat more rigid binding criteria are invoked, the subpopulation of clones able to meet these requirements may still be quite large.

1.4. Restricted Antibody Populations

The general impression from these experiments and others not quoted here is that the population of different antibody molecules having specificity for a single antigenic determinant may be very large, consisting of as many as 10^3–10^4 antibodies. On the other hand, some antigens and some modes of antigenic stimulation may give rise to very restricted responses in which perhaps only 1–10 different clones of antibody-producing cells participate. Over the last decade, we have learned how to induce a number of such restricted responses *in vivo*. There appear to be two groups of mechanisms: It is possible to select antigens that are very rigid in their binding requirements. Thus, an isolated antigenic determinant on a relatively nonantigenic carrier may bind to very few V regions on cell-surface antibody receptors with sufficient energy of interaction to induce the immune response. It seems likely that the defined sequence antigen of Richards *et al.* (1967), DNP gramicidin (Montgomery *et al.*, 1972), and the compound substituted phospholipid antigens of Uėmara *et al.* (1975) belong to this group. Sometimes antigens that occupy a large proportion of the combining region may have complicated binding requirements needing multipoint contacts over a wide area to generate sufficient binding energy. Thus, relatively restricted responses are seen, for instance, with the peptides, bradykinin, and vasopressin (Haber *et al.*, 1967), and the mouse antidextran response. Since dextran induces antibodies with λ L chains and the mouse has mainly κ and very few λ chains, a restricted response results (Cesari and Weigert, 1973).

The second general mechanism for producing restricted responses has been called *clonal dominance*. When rabbits are hyperimmunized with streptococcal or staphylococcal antigens, a small percentage of rabbits show a change from the normal complex antibody patterns to a restricted pattern, in which the Ig products of one or a few clones become dominant in quantity (Krause, 1970; Haber *et al.*, 1975). It is suspected, but not proved, that this may be a suppression phenomenon perhaps related to the suppression of normal antibodies observed during the rapid growth of a myelomatous clone of cells. It is certainly tempting to classify the monoclonal "M" spikes of Ig occurring occasionally in man during chronic infectious processes as a phenomenon of this type, although at present there is no evidence to sustain this.

1.5. Factors That Modify Combining-Region Heterogeneity

The number of potential antigens is very large, probably numbering in the millions. The number of different antibodies complementary to a single determinant at any one time may vary from one to several thousand, although at any one time, it is usual to find complex IEF patterns that suggest that as many as 100 antibodies are directed against the antigen. Further, it is known that the antibody populations themselves alter in composition with time. Much of the earlier thinking on the origin of combining-region diversity was based on the assumption that since antibody populations were apparently highly specific in their binding, individual antibodies comprising such populations would also show a single specificity and bind only to one type of chemical structure and its close relatives. This would mean that to compute the number of potential antibodies, one would need to multiply I, the number of immunogenic determinants, by M, the average number of Ig molecules complementary to a single immunological determinant. There would thus have to be 10^8–10^{12} distinct antibodies. Hence, much effort has been devoted to suggest means whereby a relatively smaller amount of genetic information, coding perhaps for fewer than a hundred germ-line genes, was inherited, and how this number of genes could be amplified and diversified.

Talmage, however, had already pointed out in 1959, that a high degree of specificity in component Ig's was not a requisite for a highly specific immune serum (Talmage, 1959). In the last five years, evidence has accumulated that Ig's do bind a number of structurally dissimilar antigens to a single combining region (Rosenstein *et al.*, 1972; Cameron and Erlanger, 1976; Tolleshaug and Hannestad, 1975; Secher, 1977) and that such binding is physiologically functional, i.e., that when, for instance, two dissimilar antigens bind to one Ig, both antigens will induce the production of that Ig (Varga *et al.*, 1973). Thus, if each individual antibody were capable of binding n different antigens, the total antibody repertoire of an animal would be reduced by a factor equal to n. The crucial question is: how large is n?

This question cannot be answered without considering the energy of interaction between antigen and combining site. Testing of Ig's with banks of antigens has shown that low-energy interactions with intrinsic binding constants (K_a) of the order of 1×10^3 liters/mole or less are extremely common, occurring with an approximate frequency of 1 per 20–25 compounds tested (4–5%) (Varga *et al.*, 1974a; Freedman *et al.*, 1976). Interactions with a K_a of 1×10^5 liters/mole are far less common, occurring only once in approximately 140 compounds tested (0.7%) (Varga *et al.*, 1974a). Since it is difficult to select compounds for testing in a random fashion, these figures to some extent reflect the bias of the experimenter. The main point is, however, that the ability to bind some antigens with relatively low affinity is probably widely distributed (Parker and Osterland, 1969; Glazer, 1970), while high-affinity binding is relatively infrequent (Varga *et al.*, 1974a; Eisen *et al.*, 1967).

There is ample evidence that certain L chains may be associated with more than one H chain. It seems likely that recombination of L and H chains can give rise to new combining regions. Although it is possible that there might be some degree of restriction between completely free L- and H-chain recombination, nevertheless the genetic recombination between L and H chains seems to have contributed to antibody diversity (Edelman and Gall, 1969).

1.6. Physiological Significance of Binding Energies

There has been considerable discussion about the binding energy that should be considered "physiologically significant." It has been suggested that below a certain cutoff value for K_a, binding of antigen to the cell-surface receptor is insignificant (Eisen *et al.*, 1967), and no immune response is obtained. With each antigen, however, it is possible to determine experimentally the K_a for the least avid antibody fractions that are induced by the antigen. With aromatic haptens such as the DNP group, early antibody populations with average intrinsic K_a of around 1×10^5 liters/mole are produced, and such populations include subpopulations with average K_a as low as 1×10^3 to 1×10^4 liters/mole (Eisen and Siskind, 1964). Carbohydrate antigens have generally a rather low average K_a, and subpopulations with K_a in the range of 1×10^3 to 10^4 liters/mole exist. It must be remembered that one IgG has two binding regions, and in IgA and IgM, up to ten binding regions are found on the same molecule. The actual rate of dissociation of the Ig molecule attached to antigen is proportional to the number of combining regions by which the antibody molecule is attached to antigen, so that complexes may be much harder to dissociate than simple equilibrium considerations of the binding constant for a monovalent hapten would suggest (Eisen, 1964a; Crothers and Metzger, 1974).

In summary, it is certain that there is a large number of potential antigens, and that the average population of antibodies directed against each determinant is large. Such populations may not be specific only for one determinant, however, but will include subpopulations binding other, structurally dissimilar determinants. The degree of overlap of subpopulations is small though significant when binding constants of higher interaction energy are considered, but may be substantial at lower K_a. The intrinsic binding constant is by itself not the only important index of antigen ligation; the multiplicity of antigenic determinants and combining regions is also important.

2. Structural Properties of Antibody Combining Regions

2.1. Location and Properties of Antibody Combining Regions

The first quantitative assessments of the number of antigen and antibody molecules in antigen–antibody complexes suggested that 7 S antibody molecules were bivalent (Porter and Press, 1962). This conclusion was reinforced by ultracentrifugal studies (Nisonoff and Thorbecke, 1964), and when accurate molecular weights of antibody molecules became available, the dimeric nature of the binding units confirmed the hypothesis (Cohen and Porter, 1964).

Both H and L chains are necessary for optimal binding. Experiments testing isolated L or H chains for their ability to ligate hapten showed that isolated L chains had little ability to bind, although with sensitive methods, low-affinity binding of haptens could be detected (Yoo *et al.*, 1967; Painter *et al.*, 1972). Isolated H chains were generally insoluble, although when made soluble, 1 mole of H chain generally bound 1 mole of antigen. The binding affinity was greatly reduced (Utsumi and Karush, 1964), however, even though the ability to discriminate among related antigens was retained by isolated H chains (Haber and Richards, 1967).

Experiments in Porter's laboratory showed that papain digestion of the IgG molecule produced Fab fragments containing the whole L chain and the *N*-terminal half of the H chain. These Fab fragments were shown to bind antigen with a valence of 1 (Porter, 1958). Pepsin digestion under controlled conditions in some myeloma Ig's gave a fragment that consists of the *N*-terminal half [or, in Konigsberg's and Edelman's nomenclature, the first domain (Edelman *et al.*, 1969; Waxdal *et al.*, 1968)] of the Fab fragment (Inbar *et al.*, 1972). It contains the variable *N*-terminal half of the L chain and the *N*-terminal variable quarter of the H chain. This Fv fragment retains the binding function of the Fab fragment and carries the idiotype (or combining-region-related) antigenic determinants of the Ig molecule.

These studies show that the 7 S unit of Ig's has two combining regions located at the *N*-terminal ends of the Fab fragments and that both the L and H chains are necessary for maximal antigen-binding.

On the basis of fluorescence polarization studies, Edelman originally proposed that the combining regions were situated at either end of a long, rodlike molecule (Weltman and Edelman, 1967), but the electron micrographs of Feinstein and Rowe (1965), followed by the detailed pictures of bivalent hapten–antigen complexes by Valentine and Green (Valentine and Green, 1967; Green, 1969), left little doubt that the molecule was in fact Y-shaped, with the combining regions occupying the ends of the two Fab arms of the Y. In addition, the Valentine–Green experiments showed that the site at which DNP bound was at some distance below the surface of the molecule, since bivalent DNP antigens, in which the two DNP groups were connected by a short spacer moiety, failed to form head-to-head Ig polymers. This finding supported earlier observations indicating a hydrophobic environment for the DNP-binding site, which suggested that the site was located below the surface (Little and Eisen, 1967). Other experiments, not detailed here, had indicated that the Fab arms were movable with respect to each other and the Fc fragment (Yguerabide *et al.*, 1970; Cathou *et al.*, 1974). Thus, prior to X-ray crystallographic analysis, a speculative picture had emerged of a combining region located at the ends of the movable Fab arms, containing a cleft or cavity, surrounded by both L- and H-chain V regions. It is remarkable how accurately the antigen probe methods were able to foresee the probable size and shape of the combining region, which were substantiated by X-ray crystallographic findings.

2.2. Serological Probes for the Antibody Combining Region

The antibody molecule itself is antigenic both when injected into heterologous species (Brient *et al.*, 1971) and when introduced into mice of the same inbred strain from which the immunizing antibody was derived (Sirisinha and Eisen, 1971). In heterologous immunization, the quantatively dominant immunogenic region is the Fc fragment of the molecule. For instance, a sheep antirabbit serum has most of its binding activity directed against rabbit Fc regions. When homogenous Ig's are introduced into a syngeneic inbred mouse line, i.e., when a mouse myeloma tumor Ig derived from a BALB/c mouse is injected repeatedly into other BALB/c mice, antibodies to the Fc region are relatively lower in titer, and antibodies appear that react with Fab fragments. These antibodies were believed to recognize only the inducing myeloma protein, and were therefore called *antiidiotypic* antibodies (Nisonoff *et al.*, 1975). A characteristic of a proportion of the early "antiidiotype" sera was that the "idiotype–antiidiotype" interaction was inhibited to some extent by antigen (Brient *et al.*, 1971). Inbar and his colleagues (1972) showed that the Fv region of a mouse myeloma IgA molecule (derived from tumor MOPC 315) was able to adsorb the "antiidiotypic" activity of a mouse serum induced by immunizing with protein 315, and that it therefore contained all the "idiotypic" determinants. The Fv fragment had previously been shown to contain one V region of the L chain and the whole V region of the H chain. Comparative sequence analysis by Wu and Kabat (1970) and Capra and Kehoe (1975) had identified three groups of amino acid residues within the V region of both the L and H chains that were more variable than other residues in this region. These "hypervariable" residues were shown by X-ray diffraction analysis to be located on the outside of six polypeptide loops on the free distal region of the *N*-terminal domain that are accessible to solvent and that surround the antibody-combining region (Poljak *et al.*, 1974; Padlan *et al.*, 1974). Isolated L and H chains are capable of inhibiting the "idiotype–antiidiotype" interaction (Hoessli *et al.*, 1976). From these data, it seems reasonable to deduce that antiidiotypic sera are directed against the solvent-accessible regions and hypervariable loops of the *N*-terminal domain. Since whole L chains may be common to two different antibodies, and since sequence data suggest that whole hypervariable loops may have structures that resemble each other, antiidiotypic sera are clearly not antiidiotypic in the sense that they can characterize only one combining region. The lack of "idiotypy" in these determinants has also been recognized experimentally, and the literature abounds in terms such as "shared idiotypic specificities" that have been recognized not only among mouse strains (Kuettner *et al.*, 1972), but also among different species (Varga *et al.*, 1974b). Antiidiotype antibodies are therefore not antibodies that define a unique set on V-region structures. In this chapter, the term *antibodies to V regions* will henceforth be used.

The relationship between the antigen-binding capacity of a single V region and the antibodies raised against the V region has been studied in detail (Potter and Lieberman, 1970; Lieberman *et al.*, 1975). These extensive studies can be summarized as follows: Antibodies may be prepared complementary to a region of a myeloma protein binding some determinant such as phosphorylcholine. These antibodies cross-react with some, but generally not with all, myeloma V regions binding the same antigenic determinant. Those myeloma proteins that cross-react with the same anti-V-region serum generally show the same "fine specificity"; i.e., they all bind a series of haptens related to the antigenic determinant. Thus, it appears that there may be several families of antibodies complementary to a single antigen, and that such families may be distinguished from each other by anti-V-region sera. Similar considerations also apply to antibodies elicited by antigens (Lieberman *et al.*, 1974).

Antibodies to V regions are inhibited by antigens to a different extent, and this can be understood if it is remembered that bound antigens may encroach on different solvent-exposed loops to varying degrees, and that anti-V-region sera are not necessarily directed against all loops to the same degree. An interesting method was developed by Claflin and his associates (Claflin and Davie, 1975). Antibodies to V regions are bound to affinity columns containing the requisite V regions attached to the solid support. The bound antibodies are eluted with haptens, thus displacing only those Ig's that are directed against loops in close apposition to the hapten binding site. By exploiting the multiple binding potential of a single binding region, it should be possible to produce serological probes directed against individual peptides within the combining region, a potentially very useful tool for probing the structure of the combining region.

Since antibodies to V regions may bind in the same general area as antigens, they appear to be able to mimic some of the physiological consequences of antigen-binding and induce a limited immune response (Cosenza and Kohler, 1972). Also, they can blanket the combining region, prevent the access of antigen, and thereby inhibit the immune response. For this reason, control or suppression of certain antibodies by anti-V-region antibodies has been considered recently. The bimodal nature of the reaction of antibodies to V regions has suggested to some workers that antibodies to the second or third (or perhaps nth) degree may form a network controlling the immune response (Jerne, 1974). Whether or not this theoretical web is firmly anchored remains to be determined. Among the more recent practical uses of anti-V-region antibodies is the detection of idiotypic determinants present on, or close to, the antigen-recognition site of thymus-derived lymphocytes (Binz *et al.*, 1973, 1974. This suggests that a recognition mechanism having some common features with Ig V regions is also present on the T cell. This area is at present under extensive investigation.

2.3. Polymeric Ligand Probes

An important method that accurately predicted the size of the combining region was originally devised by Kabat (1960): If there is point-to-point contact with antigen in the antibody-combining region, one should be able to raise antibodies to homopolymers of the type $(X)_n$, where n is a large number. Monomers, dimers, trimers, tetramers, and oligomers of X can be prepared and their ability to inhibit the reaction between the X polymer and the antibody can be determined. It was reasoned that on a molar basis, the inhibition of the oligomers should increase until the combining region is completely filled. After that, increasing the size of competing molecules should have no further effect on the inhibition. In his original experiments, Kabat used dextran for immunization and found that polysaccharide units containing up to five or six glucose units inhibited maximally, and that thereafter, increasing length did not increase inhibition. From these data, he suggested that the combining region could be as large as 34 × 12 × 7 Å, the extended measurement of the isomaltohexaose unit. Kabat also noted that there was evidence of heterogeneity in the type of contact that was made. With some sera, the isomaltotriose unit was almost as efficient an inhibitor as the isomaltohexaose (Kabat, 1960).

Numerous laboratories repeated these studies using other homopolymers such as polyamino acids, and polynucleotides, as well as random amino acid copolymers. The combined conclusions of these studies were that the size of the site was compatible with binding extended polymers of the size range 25–36 × 10–17 × 6–7 Å and that, most recently, careful quantitative studies by Schechter *et al.* (1970) with polyalanine and by Moreno and Kabat (1969) with antibodies to blood group A substance, inhibited by various polysaccharides, have substantiated that binding energy is incremental with each added unit and that antibody–antigen contact in these complexes must extend over a relatively large area. Similar methods have been used to determine whether there is a change in the average size of the combining region during the changes in antibody population that occur during maturation of the immune response. Polyasparagine was used as antigen, and it was concluded that there was some increase in average site dimensions during maturation (Murphy and Sage, 1970).

2.4. Affinity and Photoaffinity Probes

A chemically reactive ligand, which initially is bound by noncovalent interactions at the binding site of a ligating protein, can be induced to react with the protein with the formation of covalent bonds. If these bonds are sufficiently stable, the protein may be digested chemically or enzymatically into peptides, and the location in the primary amino acid sequence of the amino acid residues modified with the affinity reagent may be determined. This method was introduced into immunology by Wofsy *et al.* (1962), and has been used extensively to study the combining regions of both myeloma proteins and whole antibody populations directed against antigenic determinants (Singer and Doolittle, 1966; Knowles, 1972; Givol, 1974).

Affinity reagents consist of chemically reactive moieties either attached to, or an integral part of, a haptenic determinant. Such reagents depend entirely on the higher concentrations of the reagents at, or near, the combining region for differential labeling. Unlike the situation with regard to the serine proteases, we have no evidence of special reactivity of a single amino acid residue side chain within the Ig combining region. Since concentration differences are a crucial factor in affinity labeling, high affinity of the Ig for the hapten and a low molar ratio of ligand to Ig combining region favor site-related labeling. At higher ligand concentrations, local ligand concentrations in regions of the protein not related to the high-affinity site are likely to increase and modify the protein in these regions. "Protection" of the combining region by the hapten itself is used as an index of "site-directed" labeling. When there is a considerable difference in K_a between hapten and the hapten-based affinity reagents, however, the question is raised of the possible nonequivalence of the two binding processes.

In practice, only two types of reactive groups have been used as affinity reagents with Ig's. Wofsy *et al.* (1962) used diazonium fluoroborate for the purpose of labeling antibody combining regions. These are relatively stable salts, which react with amino groups of proteins, the amino groups of the lysine side chain, and the phenolic ring of tyrosine. Reaction of this diazonium salt with histidine was also reported (Wofsy and Parker, 1967). The stability and ease of synthesis recommend this reagent. The limited reactivity may mean, however, that the contact site itself may not be labeled, but rather that reaction occurs at the nearest or most reactive tyrosine, lysine, or histidine residue.

The haloketone compounds employed as affinity reagents by Givol, Eisen, and their associates have similar strengths and weaknesses (Givol, 1974; Haimovich *et al.*, 1970, 1972; Eisen, 1971). Their spectrum of reactivity with amino acid residues resembles that of the diazonium salts. Since all affinity reagents are introduced into the aqueous solvent and enter the combining site by diffusion, the rate of hydrolysis of such reagents must be low, and this requirement in turn limits both the spectrum of reactivity and the concentrations in which the reagent may be used.

If a nonreactive labeling reagent can be placed in the combining site, and if within the combining site the reagent can be activated to produce a moiety capable of forming covalent bonds with the antibody protein, some, but by no means all, of the difficulties associated with affinity reagents may be ameliorated. Converse and Richards (1968, 1969) synthesized a DNP-based diazoketone reagent of the type described earlier by Vaughn and Westheimer (1969) that may be photoactivated to a carbene or a ketene and showed that it reacted with anti-DNP antibodies. Fleet *et al.* (1969) introduced another light-activated compound, an aromatic azide, for the same purpose (Fisher and Press, 1974). It is possible to isolate antibody–reagent complexes and activate them specifically, although to do so requires a relatively high binding energy for the hapten–antibody complex. The major advantage, however, is that some molecules of these reagents are in contact with the protein very shortly after they are generated and do not first pass through the solvent. Most reagents that are highly reactive with protein will also react with aqueous solvents. By generating highly reactive reagents *in situ,* it is possible to specifically label amino acid residue side chains. For instance, the activated carbenes are potentially capable of inserting into any carbon–heteroatomic linkage, and it is probable that the nitrenes generated by light from the aromatic azido compounds have a similar broad range of reactivity. It must be remembered, however, that light will activate not only those molecules of labeling reagent held immobile in the site, but also those in the vicinity of the site. Moreover, if the chemical half-life of the activated species is sufficiently long, migration of the activated species may occur (Yoshioka *et al.,* 1973; Hew *et al.,* 1973; Lifter *et al.,* 1974; Richards *et al.,* 1974). Ruoho *et al.* (1973) suggested that scavenger molecules should be employed to deal with the wandering activated photoaffinity label molecules. Such molecules, however, may react with activated reagent bound at the site, and since scavenger molecules may themselves undergo low-affinity interactions with the protein, there is at least a possibility that an already complex system will become even more complex with such corrective measures. A second approach has been to synthesize photoaffinity reagents with shorter chemical half-lives, such as the azulene reagents (Smith and Knowles, 1973).

The chemistry of affinity and photoaffinity reagents has been introduced in some detail, since it is difficult to interpret results of the exploration of antibody-combining regions without this knowledge. Although it is probable that no single affinity or photoaffinity reagent is ideal, the hope has been expressed that a consensus of the labeling information will give us some understanding of the binding properties of Ig's. No easy, general conclusions are possible. Perhaps the following points can be made: In general, modifications occur at, or near, some of the hypervariable regions. There are, however, two reports of labeling outside the accepted hypervariable regions (Richards *et al.*, 1974; Franek, 1973). Some residues, i.e., the tyrosine at position 33 or 34 in the L chain, are modified in a number of different experiments. There is, however, reasonable doubt whether this is a contact amino acid residue. It is a constant residue within a hypervariable region. Modification of this residue reduces the strength of binding, but does not affect the number of DNP groups that can be bound (Goetzl and Metzger, 1970). The same residue is modified both by nitrophenol affinity reagents in anti-DNP Ig's and by a phosphorylcholine-based affinity reagent in a phosphorylcholine-binding myeloma protein. Also, in labeling experiments on myeloma protein 460, the modified residues may well be so far apart as to make it likely that these residues could not have been modified by a reagent binding to only a single site within each Fab fragment.

To summarize, it seems likely that affinity reagents do modify amino acid residues in the general combining region. It may be that in some instances they modify contact amino acids of a single major binding site. In other instances, a number of different binding sites (perhaps of a wide range of binding affinities) are modified. There is no *a priori* reason why only one binding site of high binding constant should be modified (Richards *et al.*, 1974, 1977) if others of lower affinity are also present (Haselkorn *et al.*, 1974). While the original expectations of affinity labeling may have been unduly simplistic, affinity and photoaffinity labeling methods may still be valuable tools for studying the complex geometry of hapten ligation to antibodies.

2.5. Physicochemical Probes of Antibody Combining Regions

The properties of all molecules are affected by their environment. With certain molecules, such changes in property between the molecule in solution and the molecule bound to an Ig combining region may be observed directly. Such observable physical and chemical alterations on binding may include differences in ionization (Albertson and Phillipson, 1960) or solubility properties (Day, L. A., *et al.*, 1963), increases or decreases of fluorescence either of the protein or of the ligand (Velick *et al.*, 1960), or in the rotatory dispersion of light, in the circular dichroism (CD) of polarized light, and in the CD of polarized emitted fluorescent light (Steinberg, 1974). The magnetic properties of the nucleus as well as the electron spin resonance (ESR) of ligand and ligating molecule may be affected by binding (Dwek *et al.*, 1975a). Sensitive calometric methods can measure changes in enthalpy and indirectly of entropy during antibody–antigen interaction (Johnston *et al.*, 1974). Changes in the rotatory behavior of whole Ig molecules on binding large antigens can be monitored by depolarization of emitted fluorescence, and even changes in specific molar volume have been observed (Ohta *et al.*, 1970). More recently, the internal patterns of movement of macromolecules—the concerted breaking and re-formation of hydrogen bonds that has been described as the "breathing" of the molecule and that may affect ligand-binding—has become accessible to observation. This wealth of physicochemical information cannot be reviewed in detail here; it is covered by specialized reviews (Cathou *et al.*, 1974; Day, E. D., 1972). It is perhaps disappointing how little direct information on combining-region structure and function this work has yielded in comparison with that yielded by X-ray diffraction analysis. It seems likely that, as with other proteins, the largest and most important contributions these methods will make are yet to come. It is in the fine analysis of mechanism in macromolecules the overall anatomy of which is understood that these methods are most powerful.

The areas in which physicochemical probes have given the most information about the combining region have been the depth and hydrophobicity of the combining sites, the involvement of L and H chains in ligand-binding, and the unexpected degree to which small ligands stabilize L- and H-chain interaction. Physicochemical methods have also been a mainstay in the assessment of possible conformational changes secondary to antigen-binding.

X-ray crystallographic studies quoted elsewhere in this chapter show that in the two antibody V regions so far examined, both the small ligand phosphorylcholine and a larger one, vitamin K_1OH, appear to make contact with both the L and the H chain. Nevertheless, the area of contact of phosphorylcholine with the L chain is small. It is known, however, that L–H chain contacts in the V and C_1 domains of the Fab fragment are extensive, involving many amino acid residues. It is therefore somewhat surprising that small ligands such as the DNP moiety should stabilize L–H chain interaction to a considerable degree. L and H chains may be isolated from reduced and alkylated IgG in dissociating solvents by gel filtration. Metzger and Singer (1963) found that L- and H-chain yields were considerably reduced when the small DNP antigen was present in the mixture. CD studies by Cathou and colleagues (Cathou and Haber, 1967; Cathou and Werner, 1970) showed that the presence of the DNP hapten also greatly retarded the unfolding of antibody molecules in the dissociating agent, guanidine hydrochloride. Thus, antibody without the DNP ligand unfolds in the presence of 2 N guanidine hydrochloride, while in the presence of the ligand, binding activity is still intact in the presence of 4 N guanidine hydrochloride. Yet isolated H chains derived from DNP antibodies still show binding activity, albeit with a greatly reduced K_a, which may be due to the presence of new structures resembling combining regions formed from H-chain dimers (Stevenson, 1973).

When tryptophan is excited by ultraviolet light at 280 nm, it emits fluorescent light of 345-nm wavelength. Such tryptophan residues are found in close association with the combining region. Introduction of a DNP group or a folic acid group into the combining region will usually absorb emitted tryptophan fluorescence. The quenching of fluorescence has been used both as a structural tool and as an indication of hapten-binding. The wavelength of maximum absorptivity of incident light exhibited by ligands such as DNP may also be red-shifted by binding to the protein (Eisen, 1964b). The observed spectral changes have suggested to some workers that charge-transfer complexes may be found between aromatic ligands and residues such as tryptophan, but convincing evidence for the presence of charge-transfer complexes remains elusive (Rubinstein and Little, 1970). It is now well recognized that a large number of different V regions may bind small ligands such as DNP with K_0 ranging from 1×10^{-4} to 1×10^{-10} M. It is unlikely that such a wide range of binding energies can be consistent with one type of DNP-binding site.

Optical spectrophotometric evidence for conformational changes secondary to antigen binding has been dealt with elsewhere. The introduction of ESR probes (Stryer and Griffith, 1965; Hsia and Piette, 1969; Piette *et al.*, 1972) has added an additional tool for the study of combining regions. Both groups of workers used haptens that had been linked to moieties containing the nitroxide spin label. When the hapten is attached to the nitroxide spin label, it can be shown that it is firmly bound. By producing molecules in which the hapten and the spin label are separated by chemical spacer groups of various lengths, the degree of rotational freedom of the spin label can be estimated as a function of spacer length. Some information on the size or depth of the combining region can be extrapolated from this information. The lanthanide element series bind to both the Fc and the Fv region of antibody molecules. In rabbit IgG, the Fc binding constant is around 5×10^{-6} M, while those in the combining region are with K_0 around 10^{-4} M for gadolinum. It has been shown that in the DNP-binding IgA myeloma protein, the gadolinum (Gd III)-binding site is close to the DNP-binding site and that DNP-binding weakens the attachment of lanthanide (Dwek *et al.*, 1975b; Dower *et al.*, 1975). Using Piette's technique, the same workers also showed that the portion of the combining region binding DNP probably measures $11 \times 9 \times 6$ Å based on nitroxide spin labels. Proton nuclear magnetic resonance spectroscopy at 270 MHz gives a paramagnetic difference spectrum that suggests that about 30 aliphatic and 30 aromatic residues are involved around the DNP combining site.

2.6. Electron-Microscopic Probes

Although early biophysical studies had suggested that the viscosity of the IgG molecule was consistent with the interpretation that is composed of three independently moving units of molecular weight approximately 50,000 each (Noellsen *et al.*, 1965), the first convincing demonstration that it was in fact Y-shaped, and that the two combining regions were located at the ends of the two movable arms of the Y, came from electron microscopy (EM). The studies of Almeida and Waterson (1969) and Lafferty and Oertelis (1963) showed viruses with threadlike structures forming U-shaped bands on the viral surface, while Feinstein and Rowe (1965) demonstrated ferritin molecules held together by thin, angled molecules. Valentine and Green (1967) used bifunctional DNP haptens that were separated from each other by carbon skeletons of various lengths. With the bifunctional antigen (DNP-NH[CH$_2$]$_8$NH-DNP), containing an eight-carbon skeleton, excellent cross-linked complexes were obtained in which the combining region of one molecule was joined head to head with the combining region of the next molecule (see Chapter 1, Figure 2). The EM field at ×400,000 magnification showed predominantly ring-shaped structures of various sizes with knobs protruding outward. These rings were composed of two, three, four, or more molecules of IgG joined by their combining regions and held together by the bifunctional antigen. The knobs could be removed with pepsin, an enzyme known to cleave the Fc fragment from the dimeric Fab^2 fragment. When bifunctional DNP antigens with a carbon skeleton of five or fewer carbons were tested with protein 315, an anti-DNP mouse IgA myeloma protein, no ring structures were produced. These eloquent electron micrographs showed that (1) the IgG and IgA molecules were Y-shaped and (2) the arms were movable about a hingelike region. Unlike previous studies, deformation of the molecule due to fixation on the carbon grid could not be invoked to explain the different angles that Fab segments exhibited with respect to each other. The circular structures had clearly closed prior to fixation on the grid, demonstrating that flexibility of the Fab fragments with respect to each other was a functional feature of the molecule. The failure to form circular structures with short bifunctional haptens suggested that the DNP-binding site was at least 15 Å below the surface of the protein, and that a cleft or cavity was probably present at the free end of the Fab fragment (Green, 1969). The major dimensions of the molecule could be measured from the EM photographs: the Fab fragment containing the combining region was estimated as 60 Å long and 35 Å broad. Careful examination of the IgA protein 315 molecules and of the IgG molecules showed that each Fab region was composed of two compact round structures, giving visual evidence of the Ig sulfhydryl-linked molecule domains that had been proposed on structural grounds by Edelman, Konigsberg, and their collaborators (Waxdal *et al.*, 1968). Later, electron micrographs of a human IgG₁ myeloma protein crystal using an optical averaging method confirmed the Y-shaped structure of the whole molecule and the dimensions of the Fab fragment (Labaw and Davies, 1971).

2.7. X-Ray Crystallography of Combining Regions

Northrop described the first crystalline preparation derived from trypsin-treated antibody in 1942 (Northrop, 1942), and a number of investigators subsequently reported crystalline antibodies or antibody fragments (Nisonoff *et al.*, 1967; Hochman *et al.*, 1973). The first Fab fragment crystals that had potential for high-resolution X-ray analysis became available, however, only in the late 1960's. A human IgG1 myeloma protein, New, was analyzed at 2-Å resolution by Roberto Poljak and his collaborators at Johns Hopkins Medical School (Poljak *et al.*, 1974), and a mouse IgA myeloma protein, derived from the McPc 603 tumor, was studied by David Davies' group at the National Institutes of Health at a resolution of 2 Å (Segal *et al.*, 1974). A third myeloma protein was studied extensively at the Argonne National Laboratories by Edmundson, Schiffer, and their collaborators. This is a λ L-chain dimer associated with the McG human myeloma protein (Schiffer *et al.*, 1973; Edmundson *et al.*, 1974). In addition, a group of researchers from Munich and the Argonne National Laboratories compared the structure at 2-Å resolution of two κ L-chain dimers, Au and Rei, that differ in structure by only 16 amino acid residues (Fehlhammer *et al.*, 1975; Epp *et al.*, 1975).

At the time of writing, there is available detailed information on the antigen–combining region complex of one human IgG myeloma (New), on one mouse λIgA combining region–antigen complex (McPc 603), and on three L-chain dimer models of the combining region (from McG, Au, and Rei).

Knowledge of the three-dimensional structure of the combining region has answered or can potentially answer a number of questions about antibody specificity: (1) What is the extent of the region complementary to antigen? (2) Can several diverse antigen-binding sites be demonstrated in the combining region? (3) The V region has a common folding pattern associated with areas of conserved amino acid sequence. Depsite this, it shows very large variation of antigen-binding specificity.

By what mechanism is structural variation in binding sites created? (4) Why does antigen bind predominantly to the combining region? What physical characteristics found in this region, but not elsewhere on the molecule, facilitate binding? (5) What are the structural consequences of antigen ligation? Are physiologically important conformational changes found secondary to antigen-binding? If so, are these conformational signals transmitted to the Fc region, or does some other mechanism obtain?

A comparison of the structure of the V domain shows more striking similarities between proteins New and 603 (Poljak, 1975). First, the basic immunoglobulin fold of the V-region polypeptides is essentially the same in both proteins, the same fold being found in the L-chain V region and the H-chain V region. The only difference is that the second L-chain hypervariable region is absent in New and the polypeptide backbone bridges across the base of the loop. A single S–S bond links cysteine residues at loci equivalent to positions 26 and 85 on the L chain. The polypeptide backbone is principally in parallel folds in the form of β-pleated sheets. There are no substantial α-helical segments. There are two sets of loops at either end of the V region of each chain (Figure 2) (see also Chapter 1, Figure 13). One set of loops makes contact with the first C domain; the other set is free in the sense that it is exposed to solvent. These three solvent-exposed loops correspond approximately to the hypervariable regions. Hypervariable regions center on residues 25–30, 50, and 95–100 in the L chain and residues 30, 55–60, and 105–110 in the H chain. It must be remembered that these are not rigidly bounded areas. The extent of hypervariability will depend on whether all L chains, κ or λ or chains within each κ or λ subgroup, are compared; the greater the difference between the groups and subgroups, the more extensive the region of hypervariability. While hypervariable residues in mouse and man occur in the combining-region area, there is no evidence to suggest that these are obligatory contact residues for antigens. The X-ray evidence shows that some hypervariable residues are in contact with antigen, others are close, and others do not make contact. Contact is also made by antigen with regions other than the hypervariable ones (Poljak, 1975). In the rabbit, the relationship between hypervariability and antigen contact is even less certain (Haber *et al.*, 1975). It is distinctly possible that hypervariability does not reflect only the variation in amino acid sequence needed to bind directly to antigen. Compensatory sequence changes in regions away from the contact residues may also give rise to hypervariability. The predictions made from analysis of variability have proved very valuable in showing the general area in which antigen-binding takes place.

In other regions of the backbone polypeptide fold, the side chains of residues are involved in H–L chain interactions. These include residues 35, 37, 42, 43, 86, and 99 in the V_L and residues 37, 39, 43, 45, 47, 95, and 108 in the V_H region of protein New (Poljak, 1975).

These interacting residues are mainly, although not exclusively, hydrophobic, and their presence does not appear to correlate with Y- or L-chain subgroup or L-chain class, suggesting that there is no very rigid restriction on recombination of H and L chains. The V_L and V_H regions are essentially similar in shape. On association, they interact in the manner of a Chinese puzzle to form a roughly spherical domain. The solvent-exposed distal end forms an approximately flat plate fringed by the hypervariable loops. Between the areas occupied by the L and H chain on this plate runs a cleft that is approximately 15–17 Å long. In protein New, this cleft is

FRANK F. RICHARDS
ET AL.

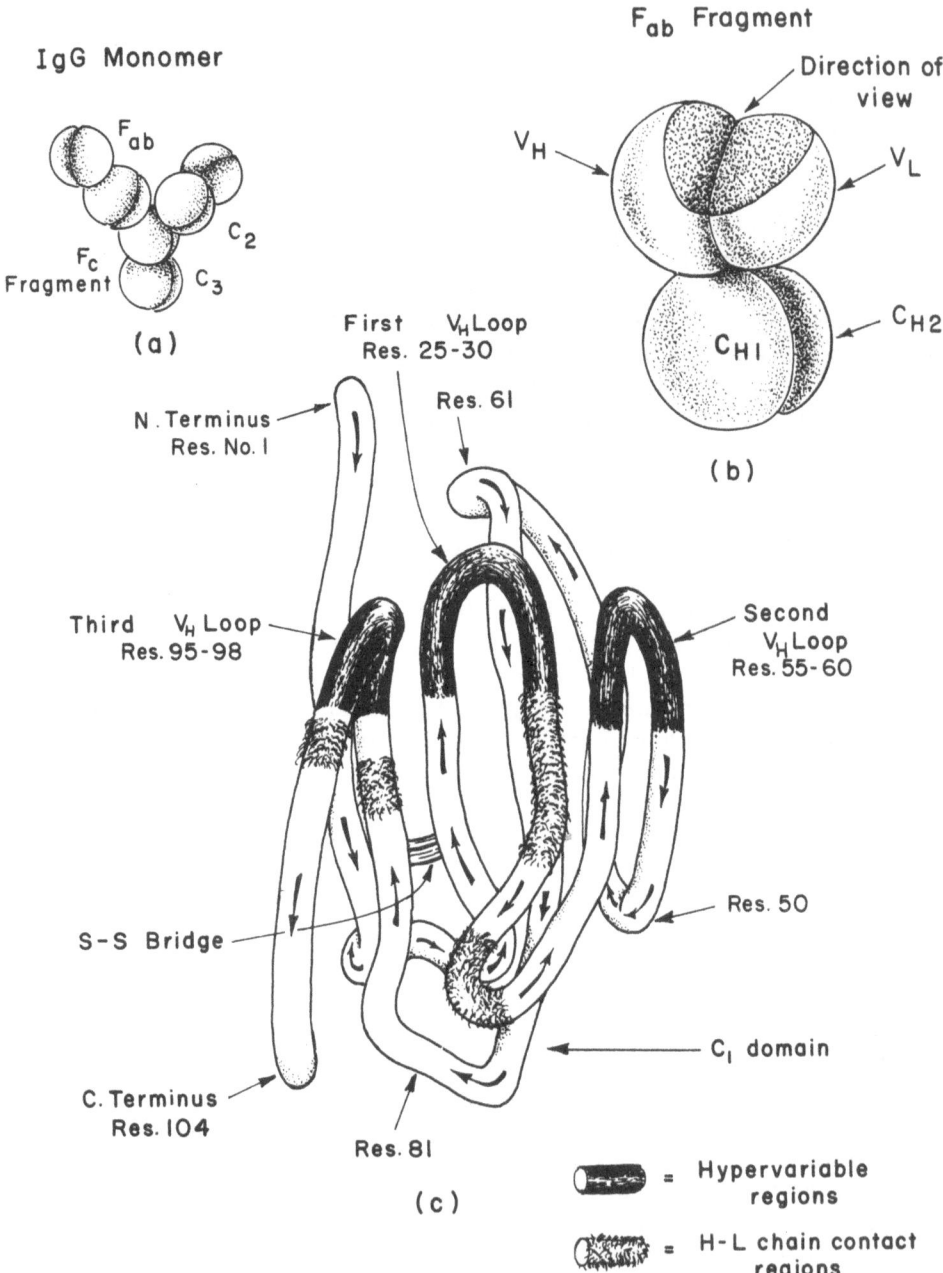

IgG Monomer

F_{ab}

F_C Fragment

C_2

C_3

(a)

F_{ab} Fragment

Direction of view

V_H

V_L

C_{H1}

C_{H2}

(b)

First V_H Loop Res. 25-30

Res. 61

N. Terminus Res. No. 1

Third V_H Loop Res. 95-98

Second V_H Loop Res. 55-60

Res. 50

S-S Bridge

C_1 domain

C. Terminus Res. 104

Res. 81

(c)

= Hypervariable regions

= H-L chain contact regions

Figure 2. (a) Arrangement of the six domains of the antibody molecule with respect to each other. (b) Exploded diagram of the V domain showing the V_L–V_H contact surface that is drawn in (c). (c) Polypeptide backbone fold of the H chain indicating the areas in contact with the L chain and the approximate location of the hypervariable regions. Redrawn from data on the New Ig molecule from Poljak *et al.* (1973) and Poljak (1975).

shallow (Figure 3), perhaps 5–6 Å deep, while in protein 603, its is 12 Å deep, 15 Å wide, and 20 Å long (Poljak *et al.*, 1974). The L chain of protein 603 is of the κ type and has an insertion of six residues at, or close to, the first hypervariable region. This has the effect of "forcing apart" the V_L and V_H regions and increasing the depth and width of the cleft. In the λ L-chain dimer studied, one L chain takes on a rotational position corresponding to the "H" chain; the other takes the L-chain position (Schiffer *et al.*, 1973; Edmundson *et al.*, 1974). The cleft in these dimers is much deeper, forming a funnel with a cavity at the bottom the floor of which is approximately 16–17 Å below the entrance to the cleft. The κ-chain dimers Au and Rei also have a large cavity between the L- and H-chain regions. An important difference in this region is the presence in Au of tryptophan at position 96 in place of the tyrosine residue found in Rei. The indole ring of tryptophan 96 protrudes into the cavity and looks as though it might impede access to a considerable part of the cavity by a moderately large presumptive hapten (Epp *et al.*, 1975; Fehlhammer *et al.*, 1975).

The mouse IgA myeloma, protein 603, binds the small molecule phosphoryl-choline approximately in the middle of the cleft. The phosphate moiety touches only the H chain at tyrosine residue 33 and arginine 52 of the H chain. The choline moiety lies at the bottom of the cleft, making contact with residues 102–103 of H and residues 91–94 of the L chain; the contact region seems to be predominantly composed of H chain, and it is of interest that phosphorylcholine-binding myeloma proteins that do not share the TEPC 15 idiotype may have L chains that have little resemblance to those found on protein 603 (Poljak, 1975). This suggests that conditions for binding of this small determinant may be relatively nonstringent, and that binding is not dependent on a particular L chain, whereas some larger antigens making substantial contact with both L and H chains might show a considerable degree of stringency. It is noteworthy that the hypervariable loops form a very extensive region that frames the site of hapten attachment. The third hypervariable region of the H chain and the second hypervariable region of the L chain do not make contact with the hapten.

The human IgG myeloma protein New binds a γ-hydroxyl derivative of vitamin K_1 (see Chapter 1, Figure 13) with K_a of 1.7×10^5 liters/mole. Fab¹ fragment–ligand complexes were crystallized and analyzed by Fourier difference maps (Amzel *et al.*, 1974; Poljak *et al.*, 1974). Vitamin K_1OH is a large molecule consisting of a naphthoquinone moiety and a long hydrophobic phytyl side chain. The whole molecule is nestled in the cleft, almost completely filling it. The naphthoquinone residue lies obliquely on the floor of the cleft, making contact with tyrosine residue

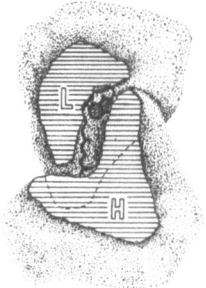

Figure 3. Scheme of the combining region of protein New looking into the long axis of the Fab fragment. The areas labeled L and H are occupied by the L and H chain, respectively. Between lies a depression approximately 5–6 Å deep in which the γ-hydroxy-vitamin K_1 molecule is located.

90 of the L chain and with the backbone and side chain of H-chain residue 104 and with L-chain residues 29 and 30. When 2-methyl, 1:4 naphthoquinone, which is the vitamin K molecule without the phytyl tail, is bound to protein New, it occupies a site identical to that occupied when vitamin K_1OH is bound. Of the total binding energy (approximately 7.2 kcal/mol at 20°C), the naphthoquinone rings provide approximately 4.2 kcal/mol, and it is estimated by difference that the phytyl tail provides 3.0 kcal/mol. The phytyl tail loops upward and around, making close contact with the L chain at Gly 29 and Asn 30. It then proceeds downward and superficially, making contact with the L chain at residues 93 and 94, and with the H chain at residue 104. At the free end of the chain, contact is made with a constant H-chain tryptophan residue, 54. Approximately 10–12 amino acids make contact with the antigen, and contact is made extensively with both H and L chains over a maximum dimension of perhaps 15 Å (Amzel *et al.*, 1974; Poljak *et al.*, 1974).

The McG λ L-chain dimer appears to have at least three distinct binding sites. One is located on the rim of the funnel-shaped cleft; a second is at the constriction between funnel and cavity, and a third is at the bottom of the cavity. These sites bind a whole range of compounds including ε-dansyl lysine, colchicine, 1,10-phenanthroline, methadone, morphine, meperidine, 5-acetyl uracil, caffeine, theophylline, menadione, triacetin, and other compounds (Schiffer *et al.*, 1973).

2.8. Conclusions from X-Ray Crystallography and Remaining Problems

Certain general principles are beginning to emerge from the studies so far carried out. These answer, in part, the questions set out at the beginning of this section. It is, however, distinctly possible that further structure elucidation could modify these conclusions:

(1) Antigen-binding so far observed occurs in the solvent channel between the L- and H-chain areas of the V domain. Since only two antigens have been mapped so far in actual combining regions, we do not yet know whether or not antigen-binding is confined to the channel or can extend outside. Certainly the L-chain dimer model of the combining region suggests that very deep hapten-binding clefts and cavities might exist in some antibodies. More mapping with antibody–antigen complexes will be required before we can define all the region involved in ligation of antigen.

(2) Analysis of the protein Fab New–vitamin K_1OH complex suggests strongly that antigen-binding is not confined to one small localized contact point, but consists of multipoint contact over an extensive region of the Ig molecule, an observation consistent with the existence of multiple binding sites. If the McG model of the Ig combining region resembles L–H chain combining regions, the clustering of binding sites may also be found in antibodies.

(3) It is now clear that both the L and H V regions as well as the C regions all have a common polypeptide fold. Each L and each H folded unit has a relatively flat surface that makes contact with the other unit. On assembly, each unit makes an angle with the other; i.e., the two units are not completely symmetrical, but show one dyad axis. At the free end of the Fv domain, the H and L chains are not in contact, creating a solvent-filled channel. Antigens have been shown to bind to the walls of this channel. The walls of the cleft are composed of six loops (five in protein New), the tips of which bear hypervariable residues. The nature of the insertions or deletions of amino acid sequence apparently alter the depth of the cleft; for

instance, the "insertion" of six amino acid residues in the first hypervariable loop in κ L chain of the McPc 603 protein "forces apart" the H- and L-chain regions and gives rise to a deeper cleft. From the three-dimensional models, it has been predicted that variations in the length of the third hypervariable loop (around residue 105) would have the same effect. The pattern of amino acid residue variability found at the tips of the loops resembles the pattern of variable or 'permissive" residues found when cytochromes from different species are compared. Here also, the loci of greatest variation are found at the tips of outside polypeptide loops. This variability may be permissive in the sense that compensatory changes for differences in cleft structure are visible here. It is equally likely, however, that residues at the tips of the loops have some direct functional significance. Haptens appear to bind along the walls of the cleft, and not only at the hypervariable residues. The present scanty evidence does not rule out that the binding region could be much more extensive. It appears that the depth of the cleft can be modulated, exposing new binding sites, and that this may be one method of introducing variability in antigen-binding. The L-chain dimers show an extremely wide and deep cleft at which a very large number of determinants bind. L-chain dimers found in human myelomas not infrequently show strong affinity for tissue components, infiltrating tissues in the form of amyloid deposits. This effect may be directly related to the large number of combining sites exposed.

(4) It is quite unclear why antigen-binding occurs primarily at the Fab combining region, or why most of the ligand-binding observed, for example, in an enzyme molecule such as lysozyme, should occur in the cleft in which the substrate binds. Since we know that deep cavities are not required for ligand-binding in Ig's, a number of crevices, folds, and channels elsewhere in the molecule might be thought to serve equally well. Frederic Richards addressed himself to a similar problem with ribonuclease (Richards, 1974). He calculated that the atomic packing densities within the substrate combining cleft are considerably less than at other solvent-exposed regions of the molecules. This suggests that the vibratory modes of various functional groups in the combining region could occur with greater degrees of freedom, and that this may be associated with greater ligating potential. Similar studies carried out with the Ig molecule would be of great potential interest.

3. Structural and Functional Correlates of Antigen-Binding

3.1. Relationship between Primary Amino Acid Sequence and Antigen-Binding Specificity

Antibodies of different ligand-binding specificities may have large regions of the primary sequence in common. It is therefore reasonable to suggest that in these antibodies, those regions that show amino acid sequence variability are the regions that are concerned with binding antigens. It does *not* follow from this proposition, however, that those amino acid residues that show the greatest sequence variability are necessarily the contact residues at which antigens bind. Wu and Kabat (1970) analyzed L-chain sequences for variability. They plotted variability at each amino acid position vs. position and obtained a graph showing three regions of greatest sequence variability. They termed these *hypervariable* regions. Capra and Kehoe (1976) performed a similar analysis on H-chain V-region sequences and were also able to demonstrate "hypervariable" regions.

3.2. Variable-Region Groups and Subgroups

Early studies comparing partial amino acid sequences of different myeloma Ig's showed that if one made an attempt to maximize amino acid residue homology, the V regions of both the κ and λ L-chain groups could be divided into a number of subgroups. Five human λ (V_λ 1–5) and three human κ (V_κ 1–3) subgroups have been described (Smith *et al.*, 1971). In the V regions of human H chains, three analogous subgroups V_H 1–3 have been delineated. Similar analyses of mouse κ chains show that the number of subgroups and sub-subgroups is rather large (Hood *et al.*, 1973).

With each group or subgroup, there are amino acid residues that are subgroup-specific (e.g., found only in the V_κ1 subgroup), group-specific (e.g., found only in κ chains), chain-specific (e.g., found only in L chains), and species-specific (e.g., found only in dog L chains).

3.3. Hapten Contact Residues and Hypervariable Regions

Several groups of research workers have compared both monoclonal Ig's and antibody populations of known specificity to see whether the amino acid sequence in the hypervariable regions can be correlated with antigen-binding specificity. Cebra and his colleagues at Johns Hopkins University compared the amino acid sequence in the hypervariable regions of guinea pig anti-DNP and antiarsonate antibodies. These workers use purified antibodies from strain 13 guinea pigs. The hypervariable regions are additionally identified by attachment of radioactive affinity reagents. It is found that distinct sequences occur in the hypervariable regions that correlate with DNP-binding and other sequences that correlate with the ability to bind arsonate (Cebra *et al.*, 1974).

Capra *et al.* (1971) examined the L chains from some homogeneous antibodies derived from patients with hypergammaglobulinemic purpura. All these had IgG-ligating activity. The amino acid residue sequence was identical in some up to residue 40; among others, there were only infrequent amino acid differences. The hypervariable regions of most of these proteins closely resembled each other.

In contrast to the observations of workers who were able to correlate primary sequence and specificity is the work of Haber and his colleagues. Rabbits were hyperimmunized with Type VIII staphylococcal polysaccharide. A percentage of such rabbits show the clonal dominance phenomenon, in which the normally heterogeneous antibody response becomes highly restricted or monoclonal. Using this phenomenon, a large number of homogeneous rabbit antibodies having specificity for the Type VIII staphylococcal polysaccharide were isolated. These antibodies show the normal variations in binding constants for the antigen. The primary structure of a number of V_L and some V_H regions from these monoclonal Ig's was determined (Margolies *et al.*, 1975).

Cluster analysis was carried out using both the specific antistaphylococcal antibodies and control monoclonal antibodies. The computer searched the sequences for groups or clusters of amino acid residues that were both internally consistent within the experimental (anti-Type VIII polysaccharide) group and different from these sequences in the control group. No such clusters could be demonstrated, suggesting that in the rabbit system, many different combining regions contribute to the binding or staphylococcal polysaccharide (Haber *et al.,* 1977).

These results are by no means mutually incompatible. If one considers a set of Ig's on neighboring branches of an evolutionary tree, these will have diverged from each other by only a few residues. Among the multiple specificities represented in the combining region, it is quite likely that one function will not have been altered by the few amino acid replacements in the V region. Neighboring branches on such a genetic tree will have a set of proteins with V-region structures that closely resemble each other and that have a common antigen-binding specificity.

Since other sets of contact amino acids may also bind the same antigen, however, several dissimilar sets of Ig's will be widely distributed over nonadjacent branches of the tree, since they have no necessary close evolutionary kinship. Depending on the method used for selecting the Ig's, either sets of Ig's with similar V regions or sets with dissimilar V regions can be obtained. It is also conceivable that some antigens may be so stringent in their binding requirements that only one set of evolutionarily related clones on adjacent branches may be able to bind the antigen. In brief, it is a logical fallacy to believe that because antibodies with similar V regions bind a common antigen, this antigen can be bound *only* by that type of V region.

3.4. Conservation of Variable Regions

When initital comparisons were made between partial L-chain amino acid sequences in mouse and man, it was noted that there was more sequence homology between certain mouse and human L chains than between certain V_L-region sequences of two L chains within the species (Smith, 1973). Later work showed great similarity in structure between V regions of inbred and outbred animals of the same species and between the V regions of similar specificity raised in guinea pigs and mice (Capra and Kehoe, 1975). This similarity is not surprising. It may represent, for instance, the *retention* of certain sequences that ligate some persisting pathogens and thus be subject to selective pressure. Alternatively, they may represent an example of parallel evolution, or the development of the same ligating sequence from two originally different sequences under the selective pressure exerted by, perhaps, a common pathogen.

3.5. Relationship between Structure and Function in Antibody Combining Regions

The relationship between primary amino acid sequence in the V region and antibody specificity is on the one hand very simple: related structures share specificities. On the other hand, it is very complex, since many different unrelated V regions may bind a single antigenic determinant with different degrees of avidity. It is probably naïve to expect to find some common structural feature in the V regions of all antibodies to some small determinant "X." There may be several anti-X families. The families need bear little resemblance to each other, although within each family, the family members will have close similarities, sharing idiotypes and perhaps the ability to bind other antigens. The ability to bind "X" by itself alone is a poor indicator of "consanguinity," since it is the property of many families of antibodies. A large, site-filling antigen that requires interaction at several points and demands stringent binding conditions is more likely to select a smaller set of antibody-producing cell clones, perhaps only one family or even only one clone, that is able to meet these conditions. Again, nonstringent selection conditions that select for binding of a small determinant over a wide range of binding energies will select a relatively large heterogeneous collection of antibody-producing cell clones that are able to meet these nonstringent conditions.

3.6. Kinetics of Antigen-Binding

In the ideal case, the binding of a univalent antigen (hapten) to a single antibody-binding site can be represented by the law of mass action, such that at equilibrium

$$S + L \rightleftharpoons S \times L$$

where S represents the concentration of antibody-binding sites and L represents the concentration of univalent ligand. If 1 mole of sites and 1 mole of ligand are mixed and form x moles of complex $S \times L$, then at equilibrium, there will be $(1 - x)$ moles of sites free and $(1 - x)$ moles of ligand free, with x moles of each in the form $S \cdot L$. The binding constant for this equilibrium can be defined as

$$K_a = \frac{(S \times L)}{(S)_{free} \times (L)_{free}}$$

From this relationship, it can be seen that if 50% of the available antibody-binding sites were associated with ligand

$$(S)_{free} = (S \times L) \text{ and } K_a = \frac{1}{(L)_{free}}$$

Thus, the binding constant is defined as the reciprocal of the free or unbound ligand concentration resulting in 50% of the available binding sites associated with ligand. It should be noted that the K_a is *independent* of the antibody concentration. The relationship between bound sites and free sites or between bound ligand and free ligand is not linear, but hyperbolic. A linear relationship can be derived from this general equation. Let us define the following terms:

(1) Let $(L)_{free} = C$

(2) Let $r = \dfrac{\text{moles of ligand bound}}{\text{moles of antibody}}$

    so that $r = \dfrac{(L)_{bound}}{(Ab)}$

    and $(L)_{bound} = r \times (Ab)$

    also $(L)_{bound} = (S \times L)$

(3) Let the number of binding sites per antibody be n, so the total site concentration is $n \times (Ab)$.

(4) It follows from (2) and (3) that the free site concentration, $(S)_{free} = n(Ab) - (L)_{bound}$,

$$K_a = \frac{(S \times L)}{(S)_f \times (L)_f} = \frac{(L)_{bound}}{(S)_{free} \times (L)_{free}} = \frac{r(Ab)}{[n(Ab) - (L)_b] \times C}$$

Dividing top and bottom by (Ab), we obtain

$$K = \frac{r}{[n - (L)_b/AB](C)} = \frac{r}{(n - r)(c)}$$

Hence, $(K \times C \times n) - (K \times C \times r) = r$ and $r/c = nK - rK$, which is a linear relationship between r/c and r, the slope is $-K_a$ and the y intercept of which is nK_a.

This useful relationship is known as a Scatchard plot (Scatchard, 1949). From it, both the equilibrium binding constant K_a and the number of binding sites per antibody, n, can be determined. Since an antibody has a finite number of binding sites, as C increases, r/c tends to 0. When C is very large, all the antibody-binding sites are saturated with ligand and $r/c = 0$. Thus, the line extrapolates to $r = n$ at $r/c = 0$. Knowing K_a for a particular antibody–ligand interaction enables one to calculate the free-energy change associated with binding:

$$\Delta F = -2.303 \, RT \log K_a$$

where R is the gas constant and T is the temperature in degrees Kelvin. The free-energy change associated with binding is composed of two thermodynamic components, enthalpy (heat) and entropy (order):

$$\Delta F = \Delta H - T\Delta S$$

where ΔH is the heat component and ΔS is the order component. Either or both of these components can be the driving force for the formation of the site–ligand complex. The ΔH contribution can be determined experimentally, either by sensitive calorimetry measurements (Johnston *et al.*, 1974) or by observing the K_a at several different temperatures, since ΔH and K_a are related:

$$\Delta H = \frac{2.303 \, R \log (K2/K1)}{1/T1 - 1/T2}$$

If ΔH is 0, then $K2 = K1$ and the binding constant is independent of temperature. In this case, the driving force for binding is entropy, or ΔS.

For the interaction of small haptenic groups such as 2,4-DNP amino acids and their corresponding antibodies, K_a is temperature-dependent.

Homogeneous and Heterogeneous Binding. The treatment outlined above is for the ideal case: homogeneous population of binding sites, each with an identical K_a. These results would obtain for a myeloma protein or a pure enzyme. Naturally raised antibodies are generally not homogeneous species, however, but consist of populations of proteins, each having a distinct K_a for the test ligand. In such a case, a Scatchard binding plot would not be a straight line, but would be a curve, as is shown in Figure 4.

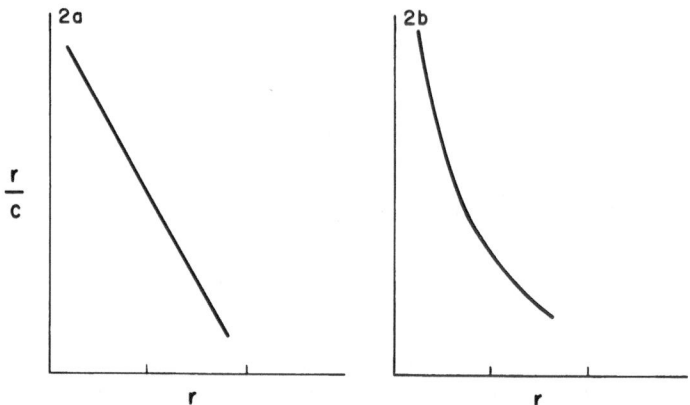

Figure 4. Scatchard plots of the binding of a small ligand to antibody. (2a) Binding of the ligand to homogeneous binding sites. (2b) Binding of the ligand to a population of heterogeneous (with respect to binding constant, K_a) binding sites.

At low r values, i.e., when ligand concentrations are low, only the binding sites with the highest K_a's will start to fill with ligand. Hence, the slope of the plot at these values is steep. As ligand concentration increases and r starts to approach n, the number of binding sites, the lower and lower affinity sites begin to fill and the slope of the plot decreases. The curve still extrapolates to $r = n$ at $r/c = 0$. An average K_a for the population can be calculated by observing the slope at which r is 50% of saturation.

It is possible to obtain information about the distribution of binding constants, also called the *degree of heterogeneity,* by using the Sips distribution function (Nisonoff and Pressman, 1958a,b), relating the fractional saturation of the binding sites to the concentration of ligand.

Since we have already derived the relationship $r = nK_aC - CK_ar$, terms can be rearranged to yield

$$r = K_a \times C(n - r)$$

and

$$\frac{r}{n - r} = K_a \times C$$

Taking the log of this equation:

$$\log\left(\frac{r}{n - r}\right) = \log K_a + \log C$$

A plot of log $[r/(n - r)]$ against log C will yield a straight line of slope $= 1$, and $[r/(n - r)]$ axis intercept of log K_a.

If a population of naturally raised antihapten antibodies is subjected to this analysis, the plot will actually have a slope considerably less than 1. This slope is called the *heterogeneity index,* and modifies the equation

$$\log \left(\frac{r}{n - r} \right) = a \log K_a + a \log C$$

This relationship is truly valid only for a Gaussian type of distribution of binding constants around the mean K_a for the population, and no conclusions can be drawn from the heterogeneity index about the number of antibodies present when the index is less than 1.0. Due to the imprecision of the measurement, even when the index is 1.0 or close to that figure, more than one antibody may be present (Pincus *et al.,* 1968).

The binding equilibrium between antibody-binding site and ligand is composed of two rate reactions: a forward reaction, the velocity V_1 of which is

$$V_1 = k_1 (S) \times (L)$$

where k_1 is the forward rate constant (dimensions, sec $^{-1}M^{-1}$) and a reverse reaction, the velocity V_{-1} of which is

$$V_{-1} = k_{-1} (S \times L)$$

where k_{-1} is the reverse direction rate constant (dimensions, sec $^{-1}$). At equilibrium, $V_1 = V_{-1}$ and $k_1 (S) \times (L) = k_{-1} (SL)$. Therefore

$$\frac{(SL)}{(S) \times (L)} = \frac{k_1}{k - 1} = K_a$$

The ratio of the forward and reverse rate constants equals the equilibrium binding constant. Experimentally, with the stopped-flow technique, it is easier to determine the forward rate constant. By also determining the equilibrium binding constant K_a, the reverse rate constant can then be calculated. With relaxation techniques such as temperature-jump, both rate constants can be experimentally derived. Using such a method, Pecht (1974) studied in detail the on and off rates for a series of DNP ligands binding to protein 315, an IgA_2 mouse myeloma protein. The DNP ligands were synthesized with various modifications in the ring, different alkyl tail lengths, and various degrees of side-chain branching. He found a range of forward and reverse rate constants depending on what changes were made in the various parts of the ligand. All the forward rates were fast, on the order of 1 to 5 $\times$ $10^8 m^{-1}$ sec^{-1}. The off rates were much slower, varying from 40 to 1300 sec^{-1}. His conclusion was that DNP ligands interacted with the binding site of protein 315 at four subsites:

S_1 concerned the nature of the ring; S_2 depended on the degree and nature of branching of the side chain; S_3 was a hydrophobic site near the end of the ligand; and S_4 interacted with the charge at the end of the molecule.

Thus, even a hapten such as DNP attached to an aliphatic side chain interacts with the binding site of an antibody over a considerable distance, involving several points of interaction.

4. Biological Significance of Antigen-Binding

4.1. Polyfunctional Antibody Combining Regions

In recent years, two lines of evidence have suggested that a single Ig may be complementary to several structurally dissimilar antigens. Haimovich and DuPasquier (1973) showed that the tadpole has approximately 1×10^6 lymphocytes, yet is able to mount a specific humoral response directed against the DNP determinant (anti-DNP). The response to single haptens is usually heterogeneous, involving many different clones of cells that produce anti-DNP antibody. In order that the antibody reach detectable levels, the number of cells involved in this specific anti-DNP response must be a very considerable proportion of the total. There is no doubt that the tadpole can respond to many antigens. Thus, there seem to be too few cells at any one time to account for the range of immune responses observed. The clonal dilution studies that indicated the presence of many antibodies complementary to one antigenic determinant were summarized earlier by Williamson (1973). All these studies may be summarized by stating that if there is only one antihapten specificity per antibody molecule (or per cell), there do not appear to be enough lymphoid cells to account for the number of antigenic specificities. Reciprocally, there appears to be a very large number of clones involved in the production of antibodies against a single haptenic determinant. Over the last decade, homogeneous myeloma proteins that bind antigens have become available. An early finding was that a number of these myeloma proteins bound more than one haptenic determinant. This binding was competitive, and since only one determinant could be bound at a time to a single combining region, it was usually assumed that there were common structural features in the competing determinants that were bound to a single locus on the protein.

Rosenstein and his co-workers examined the combining region of protein 460, a mouse γA myeloma protein that binds competitively the haptens DNP and menadione (Eisen *et al.*, 1970):

DNP   Menadione

These workers found an –SH group in relation to the combining region (Rosenstein *et al.*, 1972; Jackson and Richards, 1974). When this –SH group was substituted with a bulky reagent, the ability of protein 460 to bind menadione was impaired, while the ability to bind DNP remained intact. When the protein was partially denatured with 4.3 M guanidine HCl and then allowed to refold partially, the ability to bind DNP was ablated, while menadione-binding remained intact. Other methods for differentiating affecting one binding activity were also described. This work suggested, but did not prove, that there were spatially separated sites within the combining region. Later work on the same protein using the technique of fluorescent energy transfer between donor fluorescent probes placed on the –SH groups and the DNP and menadione molecules bound to their sites showed that there was a minimum separation of 12–14 Å between the DNP- and the menadione-binding site (Manjula *et al.*, 1976). To support these findings, dextran-bead–spacer–DNP and dextran-bead-spacer–menadione columns were constructed with spacer molecules of varying length. The shortest spacer–determinant combination needed to hold protein 460 to the column was determined for both the DNP and menadione determinants. The difference in length between the two shortest molecules was 12.5 Å, a finding consistent with the separation distance calculated from the energy-transfer experiments (Rosenstein and Richards, 1976). There appears to be reasonable evidence that there is substantial spatial separation between two combining sites within the antibody-combining region, making it probable that the combining region is in fact a mosaic of determinant-binding sites.

Even though an individual antibody-combining region may bind diverse determinant at different sites, this is not by itself proof that multiple binding is physiologically significant; it is possible, for instance, that binding at only one subsite of the V-region cell-surface receptor induces cell proliferation and antibody production. Experiments have shown, however, that this objection does not appear to be true. In rabbits (Varga *et al.*, 1973) and in mice (Varga *et al.*, 1974b), IEF can pick out individual Ig bands that bind two dissimilar haptens. In the same animal, the same double-binding bands can be induced by either of the two antigens (Figure 5), showing that the binding of both antigens induces cell proliferation and antibody production within the cell clone that binds both antigens (Varga *et al.*, 1973).

Double-binding myeloma proteins appear to have V regions that resemble those of some of the induced antibodies binding the same antigens. Antiidiotypic sera raised against determinants in the V regions of myeloma proteins cross-react with their naturally induced counterparts. They will even do this occasionally when the double-binding myeloma proteins arise in one species and the "natural" double-binding antibodies are induced in another species (Varga *et al.*, 1974b), stressing that there is considerable conservation of the V region between species, or perhaps that parallel evolution has occurred in the combining region.

It is not yet clear how many different antigens are complementary to a single combining region. It has been estimated that when "random" antigens are screened, interactions with a K_0 of approximately 1×10^5 liters/mole occur once in about 140 compounds screened, while weaker interactions in the range of 1×10^3 liters/mole occur much more frequently (1 in 20 compounds screened). Clearly, these figures are only approximate, since the choice of antigens can never be really random. Nevertheless, the general principle is clear: the higher the interaction energy, the less frequently cross-reactions are found (Inman, 1974). It is also intuitively clear that if high-energy cross-reactions were very common, antibody populations would be like glue, sticking together all biological structures and showing no population specificity.

4.2. Specificity of Immune Sera

The high degree of specificity of an immune serum was discussed earlier. It has been a frequently made assumption that if a population of antibodies has apparently exclusive specificity for one antigen, the individual antibodies constituting that

FRANK F. RICHARDS
ET AL.

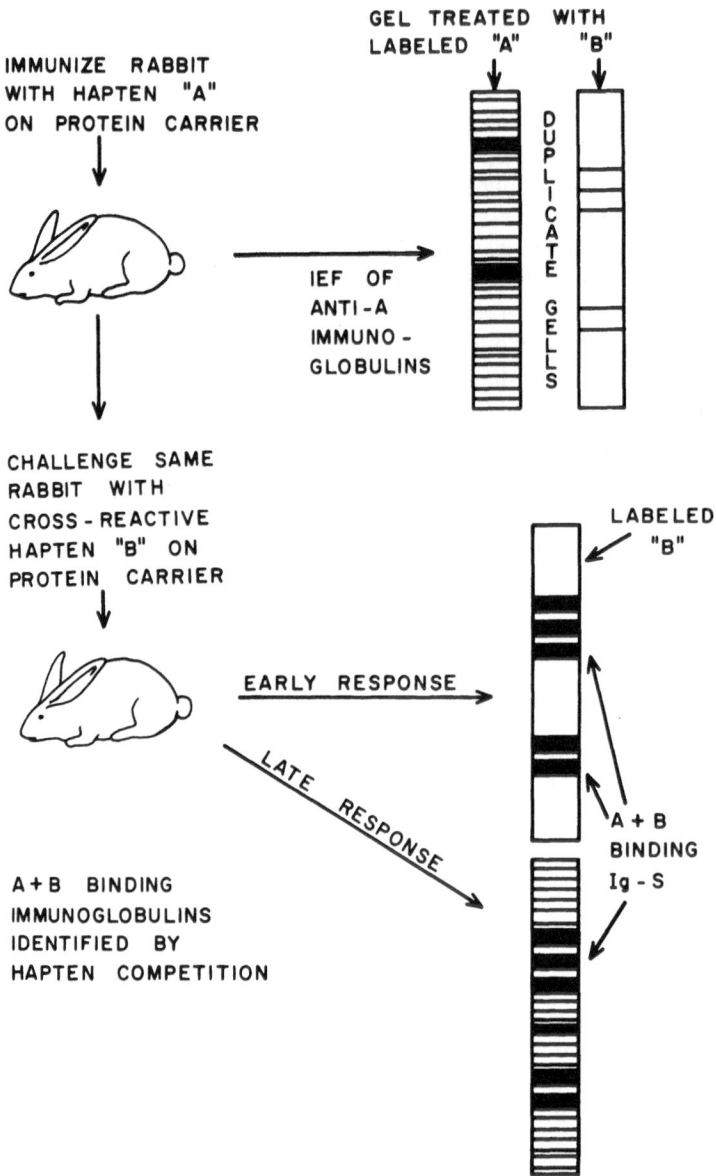

Figure 5. Experimental protocol for determining the presence of Ig's with polyfunctional combining regions in antihapten antisera.

population must show the same exclusive specificity. In a perceptive article published in 1959, Talmage (1959) showed that this need not be true and that an apparently highly specific population could be derived from members having different specificities. We now know that in myeloma proteins, individual hapten combining sites have, in fact, a high degree of specificity and will, for instance, distinguish DNP from mononitrophenols and trinitrophenols (Haimovich and DuPasquier,

1973). At the same time, protein 460 will bind a number of unrelated haptens at other sites within the combining region. The consequences of this, however, are exactly as Talmage first suggested. Let us suppose that a single V region may bind 100 different determinants. If the animal is immunized with determinant A, all those cells producing A-binding Ig's of sufficient affinity will respond to the antigenic stimulus by cell proliferation and antibody production. Thus, all antibody species produced bind A. Each antibody will also bind 99 other determinants, but these *need not be the same* for each antibody, and such ligating activity will be present only at a lower level (i.e., 1%) in the antibody population and will be diluted out. Thus, antibody specificity is, in essence, a *population phenomenon,* an average characteristic, rather than the property of each member of the population (see Figure 6).

4.3. Epidemiological Considerations

There would be advantages to the animal if a single V region had specificity to more than one antigenic determinant. Thus, a single determinant may ensure

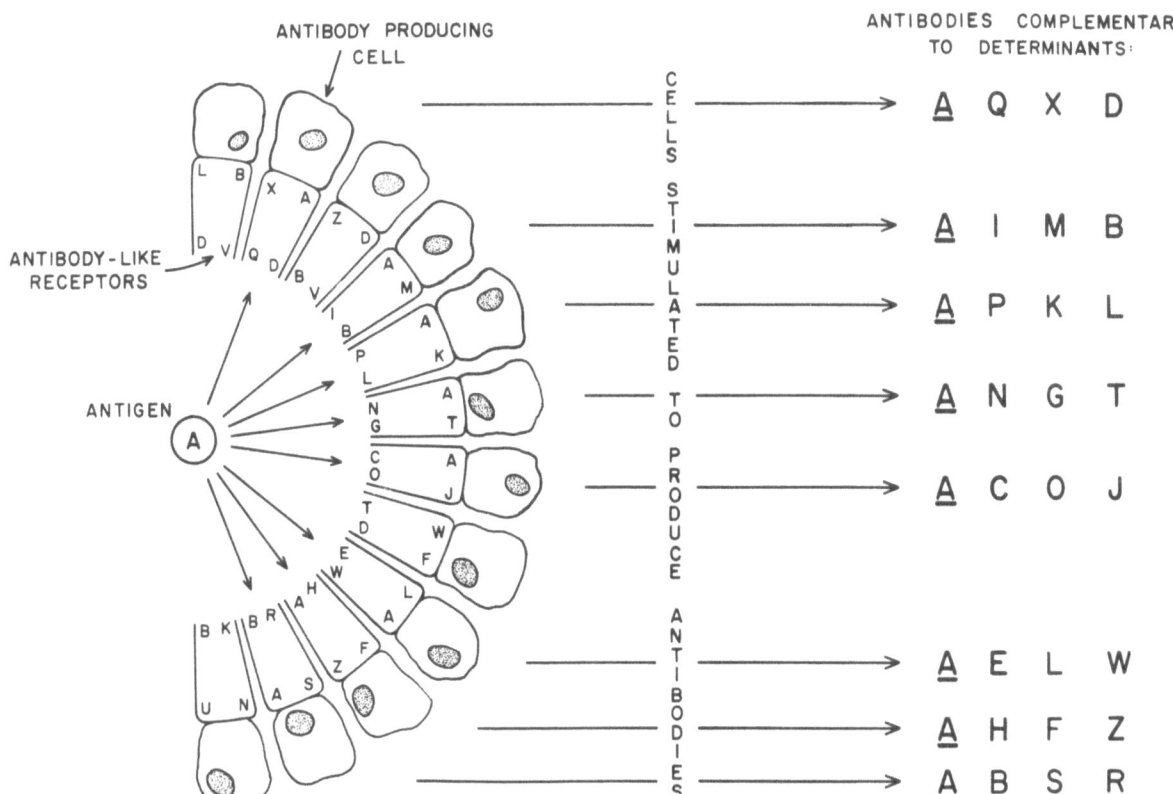

Figure 6. Immune serum specificity as a population phenomenon. Individual B-cell receptors are shown as having properties similar to Ig combining regions. For illustrative purposes, these receptors are drawn as being each complementary to four different antigens; we suppose that this figure is in fact much larger. Stimulation by antigen A causes the cells with A specificity to divide and produce antibodies directed against A. The immune serum produced will therefore react in high titer with antigen A. Each Ig also has other specificities, but because these specificities need not be the same in every molecule, the other specificities B–Z will be diluted out and will react only in low titer.

survival of antibodies complementary to a large number of unrelated antigenic determinants even if those determinants are no longer represented in the environment. "Memory" for a specific antibody to some pathogen may be retained by the presence of a quite different infective agent that need have no common antigenic determinants. This type of "linked" immune response was first recorded many years ago by Weil and Felix (1916), who observed during World War I that many of the German soldiers under their care who had previously been exposed to typhoid fever *(Salmonella typhi)* showed a highly specific increase in antibodies to *Sal. typhi* when they contracted an infection with *Rickettsia prowazekii,* an entirely unrelated organism having no detectable common antigenic determinants. There is a close relationship between this phenomenon and "original antigenic sin" (Francis, 1953; Fazekas and Webster, 1966), the power of a "related" antigen to induce production of antibodies to an antigen introduced long before. This phenomenon may occur both where there are truly "common" determinants and where there are "linked specificities." Since there would appear to be advantage in retaining the capacity for multiple binding, it may well be that the combining region has evolved structurally in such a way as to maximize the determinant-binding potential of the structure.

4.4. Maturation of Antibody Specificity

Early in the immune response to haptens, the antibody population often shows a lower average intrinsic binding constant for the immunizing antigen than later in the response. One classic pattern of antibody maturation of this type was described by Eisen and Siskind (1964). There is much evidence to suggest that the increase in antibodies of higher average affinity is an active process of recruitment of new antibodies, and is not due to selective removal of either high- or low-affinity antibodies (Steiner and Eisen, 1966, 1967a,b). Siskind and Benacerraf (1969) suggested that early in the immune response when antigen levels are high, effective stimulation of cells producing both low- and high-affinity antibodies will occur. Later in the immune response, when the antigen levels are low, only those cells with high-affinity receptors on their surface, producing high-affinity antibodies, will be stimulated, with an increased production of high-affinity antibodies. Segre and Segre (1973) tried to obtain direct confirmation in tissue culture for the role of antigen concentration as the driving force in this process, but were unable to do so. It must be emphasized that added antigen *per se* may also not reflect antigen concentration at the receptor site. Since combination of antigen with the cell-surface-receptor V region is a reversible reaction, there can be little doubt that the antigen concentration near the receptor must influence the immune response. It probably is not, however, the only influence on antibody maturation.

"Polyfunctional" combining regions may play a role in the phenomenon of antibody maturation. When an animal is sensitized to antigen A, a small proportion of the antibodies produced will also bind an unrelated antigen B. Since the antibodies produced were "selected" by antigen A, those Ig's that also bind B will do so on the average with low affinity. When primed with antigen A and then challenged with antigen B, the early anti-B antibodies produced after challenge will be predominantly of the double-binding type that have low average affinity for B. Only later will anti-B antibodies be produced that were "selected" by antigen B and have a higher average binding for this antigen. Hence, the antibodies to antigen B will exhibit an increase in the average binding constant with time. The primary challenge with antigen A would have its natural counterpart in the fact that experimental animals are not immunologically virgin and have been subjected to immunological priming by ubiquitous microflora and perhaps also by "self" antigens.

Many examples have now been described of antigens that do not produce classic antibody-maturation patterns (Wu and Rockey, 1969; Haber and Stone, 1969; Montgomery *et al.*, 1972; Gopalakrishnan and Karush, 1974; Steward and Petty, 1972; Steward and Voller, 1973). Decreases in the average intrinsic binding constants late in the immune response seem to be a common occurrence, and examples of cyclical changes in antibody affinity have also been described (Macario and Conway de Macario, 1975). Moreover, not only the type and quantity of antigen used, but also the mode of administration, the kinetics of cell replication, the antigen carrier, the T-cell controlling mechanism, genetic and infective factors, and the previous immunological history of the host, appear to influence the alteration of the antibody population produced. Thus, the patterns of antibody maturation are probably the results of many interacting factors, and while they often result in antibody populations of higher affinity late in the immune response, many variations on this theme as well as complete absence of maturation may at times be encountered.

5. Summary

It seems likely that Ig combining regions have evolved from some archetypal molecule and those forms that are useful to the animal have been retained. It is the entire population of antibody-combining regions that forms the antigen-recognition repertoire of the humoral immune system, and in such a system, not only the properties of individual antibody-combining regions, but also the properties of the multiprotein system as a whole, are important for the defenses of the body against pathogens.

Antibody-combining sites may bind a disparate set of structurally related and unrelated ligands. This *multispecificity* can be biologically meaningful: the same clone can be stimulated by different antigens. The most significant impact of the multispecificity is: (1) It reduces the number of V-genes necessary to code for the total number of combining sites. (2) The cross-stimulation of clones by structurally related and unrelated antigens may be instrumental in the normal maintenance of immune responsiveness, and in addition, it may explain the ability to respond to unusual and less ubiquitous antigens. (3) The antigenic history of the animal may contribute to the maturation of the immune response by cross-stimulation of preselected clones of antigen-binding cells.

ACKNOWLEDGMENTS

The authors would like to thank the U.S. Public Health Service, the National Science Foundation, and the American Heart Association for their support of this work. This chapter was completed while F.F.R. was a Senior Faculty Fellow of the Josiah Macy Foundation at Glasgow University, Scotland. Most of all, our thanks are due to Mrs. Valerie Vishno, whose skill and patience in putting together this manuscript are acknowledged with much gratitude.

FRANK F. RICHARDS
ET AL.

Albertson, P., and Phillipson, L., 1960, Antigen–antibody in liquid two-phase systems: A method for studying immunological reactions, *Nature (London)* **185**:38–40.

Almeida, J. D., and Waterson, A. P., 1969, Morphology of virus–antibody interaction, *Adv. Virus Res.* **15**:307–338.

Amzel, L. M., Poljak, R. J., Saul, F., Varga, J. M., and Richards, F. F., 1974, The three-dimensional structure of a combining region–ligand complex of immunoglobulin New at 3.5 Å resolution, *Proc. Natl. Acad. Sci. U.S.A.* **71**:1427–1430.

Bell, G. I., 1974, Model for the binding of multivalent antigen to cells, *Nature (London)* **248**:430–431.

Binz, H., Lindemann, J., and Wigzell, H., 1973, Inhibition of local graft-versus-host reaction by anti-alloantibodies, *Nature (London)* **246**:146–148.

Binz, H., Lindemann, J., and Wigzell, H., 1974, Idiotypic receptors for alloantigens on T-cells, in: *The Immune System: Genes, Receptors, Signals* (E. E. Sercarz, A. R. Williamson, and C. F. Fox, eds.), pp. 533–552, Academic Press, New York.

Brient, B. W., Haimovich, J., and Nisonoff, A., 1971, Reaction of anti-idiotypic antibody with the hapten-binding site of a myeloma protein, *Proc. Natl. Acad. Sci. U.S.A.* **68**:3136–3139.

Cameron, D. J., and Erlanger, B. F., 1976, Nucleic acid-reactive antibodies of restricted heterogeneity, *Immunochemistry* **13**:263–269.

Capra, J. D., and Kehoe, J. M., 1974, Structure of antibodies with shared idiotypy: The complete sequence of the heavy chain of two immunoglobulin M anti-gamma globulins, *Proc. Natl. Acad. Sci. U.S.A.* **71**:4032–4036.

Capra, J. D. and Kehoe, J. M., 1975, Hypervariable regions, idiotypy, and the antibody binding site, *Adv. Immunol.* **20**:1–40.

Capra, J. D., Winchester, R. J., and Kunkel, H. G., 1971, Hypergammaglobulinemic purpura, *Medicine (Baltimore)* **50**:125–138.

Cathou, R. E., and Haber, E., 1967, Structure of the antibody combining site. I. Hapten stabilization of antibody conformation, *Biochemistry* **6**:513–517.

Cathou, R. E., and Werner, T. C., 1970, Hapten stabilization of antibody conformation, *Biochemistry* **9**:3149–3154.

Cathou, R. E., Holowka, D. A., and Chan, L. M., 1974, Confirmation and flexibility of immunoglobulins, in: *Progress in Immunology II,* Vol. 1 (L. Brent and Holbrown, eds.) p. 63, North-Holland, Amsterdam.

Cebra, J. J., Koo, P. H., and Ray, A., 1974, Specificity of antibodies: Primary structural basis of hapten binding, *Science* **186**:263–265.

Cesari, I. M., and Weigert, M. G., 1973, Mouse lambda-chain sequences, *Proc. Natl. Acad. Sci. U.S.A.* **70**:2112–2116.

Claflin, J. L., and Davie, J. M., 1975, Specific isolation and characterization of antibody to binding site antigenic determinants, *J. Immunol.* **114**:70–75.

Cohen, S., and Porter, R. R., 1964, Structural and biological activity of immunoglobulins, *Adv. Immunol.* **4**:287–349.

Converse, C. A., and Richards, F. F., 1968, Two-stage active site labeling of antibody by photolysis of an unreactive diazoketone hapten to a reactive carbene within the combining site, *Fed. Proc. Fed. Am. Soc. Exp. Biol.* **27**:683.

Converse, C. A., and Richards, F. F., 1969, Two-stage photosensitive label for antibody combining sites, *Biochemistry* **8**:4431–4436.

Cosenza, H., and Kohler, H., 1972, Specific suppression of the antibody response by antibodies to receptors, *Proc. Natl. Acad. Sci. U.S.A.* **69**:2701–2705.

Cramer, M., and Braun, D. G., 1974, Cross-stimulation of monoclonal antibodies in anamnestic responses, *J. Exp. Med.* **138**:1533–1544.

Crothers, D. M., and Metzger, H., 1974, The influence of polyvalency on the binding properties of antibodies, *Immunochemistry* **9**:341–357.

Day, E. D., 1972, *Advanced Immunochemistry,* 1st Ed. Williams and Wilkins, Baltimore.

Day, L. A., Sturtevant, J. M., and Singer S. J., 1963, The kinetics of the reactions between antibodies to the 2,4-dinitrophenyl group and specific haptens, *Ann. N.Y. Acad. Sci.* **103**:611–625.

Dower, S. K., Dwek, R. A., McLaughlin, A. C., Mole, L. M., Press, E. M., and Sunderland, C. A., 1975, The binding of lanthanides to non-immune rabbit IgG and its fragments, *Biochem. J.* **149**:73–82.

Dwek, R. A., Jones, R., Marsh, D., McLaughlin, A. C., Press, E. M., Price, N. C., and White, A. I., 1975a, Antibody–hapten interactions in solution, *Philos. Trans. R. Soc. London Ser. B* **272**:53–74.

Dwek, R. A., Knott, J. C. A., Marsh, D., McLaughlin, A. C., Press, E. M., Price, N. C., and White, A. I., 1975b, Structural studies on the combining region of the myeloma protein MOPC 315, *Eur. J. Biochem.* **53**:25–39.

Edelman, G. M., and Gall, W. E., 1969, The antibody problem, *Annu. Rev. Biochem.* **38**:415–456.

Edelman, G. M., Cunningham, B. A., Gottlieb, P. D., Rutishauser, U., and Waxdal, M. J., 1969, The covalent structure of an entire γG immunoglobulin molecule, *Proc. Natl. Acad. Sci. U.S.A.* **63**:78–85.

Edmundson, A. B., Ely, K. R., Girling, R. L., Abola, E. E., Schiffer, M., Westholm, F. A., Fausch, M. D., and Deutsch, H. F., 1974, Binding of 2,4-dinitrophenyl compounds and other small molecules to a crystalline λ-type Bence-Jones dimer, *Biochemistry* **13**:3816–3827.

Eisen, H. N., 1964a, Antibody–antigen reactions, in: *Immunology,* 2nd Ed., Chapter 15, p. 359, Harper and Row, Hagerstown, Maryland.

Eisen, H. N., 1964b, Determination of antibody affinity for haptens and antigens by means of fluorescent quenching, in: *Methods in Medical Research,* Vol. 10, pp. 115–121, Year Book Medical Publishers, Chicago.

Eisen, H. N., 1971, Combining sites of anti-2,4-dinitrophenyl antibodies, in: *Progress in Immunology,* pp. 243–251, Academic Press, New York.

Eisen, H. N., and Siskind, G. W., 1964, Variations in the affinity of antibodies during the immune response, *Biochemistry* **3**:996–1008.

Eisen, H. N., Little, J. R., Osterland, C. K., and Simms, E. S., 1967, A myeloma protein with antibody activity, *Cold Spring Harbor Symp. Quant. Biol.* **32**:75–81.

Eisen, H. N., Michaelides, M. C., Underdown, B. J., Schulenburg, E. P., and Simms, E. S., 1970, Myeloma proteins with anti-hapten antibody activity, *Fed. Proc.* **29**:78–84.

Epp, O., Lattman, E. E., Schiffer, M., Huber, R., and Palm, W., 1975, The molecular structure of a dimer composed of the variable portions of the Bence Jones protein Rei refined at 2.0 Å resolution, *Biochemistry* **14**:4943–4952.

Fazekas, D., and Webster, R. G., 1966, Disquisition on original antigenic sin, I. Evidence in man, *J. Exp. Med.* **124**:331–345.

Fehlhammer, H., Schiffer, M., Epp, O., Colman, P. M., Lattman, E. E., Schwager, P., Steigemann, W., and Schramm, H. J., 1975, The structure determination of the variable portion of the Bence–Jones protein Au, *Biophys. Struct. Mechanism* **1**:139–146.

Feinstein, A., and Rowe, A. J., 1965, Molecular mechanism of formation of an antigen–antibody complex, *Nature (London)* **205**:147–149.

Fisher, C. E., and Press, E. M., 1974, Affinity labeling of the antibody combining site, *Biochem. J.* **139**:135–149.

Fleet, G. W., Knowles, J. R., and Porter, R. R., 1969, Affinity labeling of antibodies with an aryl nitrene reactive group, *Nature (London)* **224**:511–512.

Francis, T., 1953, Influenza—the new acquaintance, *Ann. Intern. Med.* **39**:203–221.

Franek, F., 1973, Affinity labeling by m-nitro benzenediazonium fluoroborate of porcine anti-dinitrophenol antibodies, *Eur. J. Biochem.* **33**:59–66.

Freedman, M., Merret, T. R., and Pruzanski, W., 1976, Human monoclonal immunoglobulins with antibody-like activity, *Immunochemistry* **13**:193–202.

Givol, D., 1974, Affinity labeling and topology of the antibody combining site, *Essays Biochem.* **10**:73–103.

Glazer, A. N., 1970, On the prevalence of "nonspecific" binding at the specific binding sites of globular proteins, *Proc. Natl. Acad. Sci. U.S.A.* **65**:1057–1063.

Goetzl, E. J., and Metzger, H., 1970, Affinity labeling of a mouse myeloma protein which binds nitrophenyl ligands: Sequence and position of a labeled tryptic peptide, *Biochemistry* **9**:3826–3871.

Gopalakrishnan, P. V., and Karush, F., 1974, Antibody affinity. VII. Multivalent interaction of anti-lactoside antibody, *J. Immunol.* **113**:769–778.

Green, N. M., 1969, Electron microscopy of the immunoglobulins, *Adv. Immunol.* **11**:1–30.

Haber, E., and Richards, F. F., 1967, The specificity of antigenic recognition of antibody heavy chains, *Proc. R. Soc. Lond.* **166**:176–187.

Haber, E., and Stone, M., 1969, Characteristics of antibody to a limited antigenic stimulus, *Isr. J. Med. Sci.* **5**:332–337.

Haber, E., Richards, F. F., Spragg, J., Austen, K. F., Valloton, M., and Page, L. B., 1967, Modification in the heterogeneity of the antibody response, *Cold Spring Harbor Symp. Quant. Biol.* **32**:299–310.

Haber, E., Margolies, M. N., Cannon, L. E., and Rosenblatt, M. S., 1975, Restricted clonal responses—a tool in understanding antibody specificity, in: *Molecular Approaches to Immunology*, Miami Winter Symposia, Vol. 9 (E. E. Smith and D. W. Ribbons, eds.), pp. 303–338, Academic Press, New York.

Haber, E., Margolies, M. N., and Cannon, L. E., 1977, Structure of the framework and complementarity regions of elicited antibodies, in: *Antibodies in Human Diagnosis and Therapy* (E. Haber and R. M. Krouse, eds.), pp. 45–78, Raven Press, New York.

Haimovich, J., and DuPasquier, L., 1973, Specificity of antibodies in amphibian larvae possessing a small number of lymphocytes, *Proc. Natl. Acad. Sci. U.S.A.* **70**:1898–1902.

Haimovich, J., Givol, D., and Eisen, H. N., 1970, Affinity labeling of the heavy and light chains of a myeloma protein with anti-2-4 dinitrophenyl activity, *Proc. Natl. Acad. Sci. U.S.A.* **67**:1656–1661.

Haimovich, J., Eisen, H. N., Hurwitz, E., and Givol, D., 1972, Localization of affinity labeled residues on the heavy and light chains of two myeloma proteins with anti-hapten activity, *Biochemistry* **11**:2389–2398.

Haselkorn, D., Friedman, S., Givol, D., and Pecht, I., 1974, Kinetic mapping of the antibody combining site by chemical relaxation spectrometry, *Biochemistry* **13**:2210–2222.

Hew, C.-L., Lifter, J., Yoshioka, M., Richards, F. F., and Konigsberg, W. H., 1973, Affinity-labeled peptides obtained from the combining region of protein 460: Light chain labeling patterns using dinitrophenyl-based photoaffinity labels, *Biochemistry* **12**:4685–4689.

Hochman, J., Inbar, D., and Givol, D., 1973, An active fragment (Fv) composed of the variable portions of heavy and light chains, *Biochemistry* **12**:1131–1135.

Hoessli, D., Olander, J., and Little, J. R., 1976, Heterologous recombination between mouse myeloma 315 heavy chains and rabbit antibody light chains: Structural and functional properties of the hybrid molecules, *J. Immunol.* **113**:1024–1032.

Hood, L., McKean, D., Farnsworth, V., and Potter, M., 1973, Mouse immunoglobulin chains: A survey of the amino-terminal sequences of λ chains, *Biochemistry* **12**:741–749.

Hsia, J. C., and Piette, L. H., 1969, Spin-labeling as a general method in studying antibody active site, *Arch. Biochem. Biophys.* **129**:296–307.

Inbar, D., Hochman, J., and Givol, D., 1972, Localization of the antibody combining site within the variable portions of the heavy and light chains, *Proc. Natl. Acad. Sci. U.S.A.* **69**:2659–2662.

Inman, J. K., 1974, Multispecificity of the antibody combining region and antibody diversity, in: *The Immune System: Genes, Receptors, Signals* (E. E. Sercarz, A. R. Williamson, and C. F. Fox, eds.), pp. 19–52, Academic Press, New York.

Jackson, P., and Richards, F. F., 1974, The hapten-binding region of protein 460: Sequence of a sulfhydryl containing peptide which affects menadione binding, *J. Immunol.* **112**:96–100.

Jaton, J.-C., Huser, H., Riesen, W. F., Schlessinger, J., and Givol, D., 1976, The binding of complement by complexes formed between a rabbit antibody and oligosaccharides of increasing size, *J. Immunol.* **116**:1363–1366.

Jerne, N. K., 1974, Towards a network theory of the immune system, *Ann. Immunol. (Paris)* **125c**:373–389.

Johnston, M. F. M., Barisas, B. G., and Sturtevant, J. M., 1974, Thermodynamics of hapten binding to MOPC 315 and MOPC 460 mouse myeloma proteins, *Biochemistry* **13**:390–396.

Kabat, E. A., 1960, The upper limit for the size of the human anti-dextran combining site, *J. Immunol.* **84**:82–85.

Kabat, E. A., 1966, The nature of an antigenic determinant, *J. Immunol.* **97**:1–11.

Karush, F., 1962, Immunologic specificity and molecular structure, *Adv. Immunol.* **2**:1–40.

Knowles, J. R., 1972, Photogenerated reagents for biological receptor-site labeling, *Acc. Chem. Res.* **5**:155–160.

Krause, R. M., 1970, The search for antibodies with molecular uniformity, *Adv. Immunol.* **12**:1–65.

Kuettner, M. C., Wang, A. L., and Nisonoff, A., 1972, Quantitative investigations of idiotypic antibody, *J. Exp. Med.* **135**:579–595.

Labaw, L. W., and Davies, D. R., 1971, An electron microscopic study of human γ G₁ immunoglobulin crystals, *J. Biol. Chem.* **246**:3760–3762.

Lafferty, K. J., and Oertelis, S., 1963, The interaction between virus and antibody, *Virology* **21**:91–99.

Lieberman, R., Potter, M., Mushinski, E. B., Humphrey, W., Jr., and Rudikoff, S., 1974, Genetics of a new IgV$_H$ (T 15 idiotype) marker in the mouse regulating natural antibody to phosphoryl choline, *J. Exp. Med.* **139**:983–1001.

Lieberman, R., Potter, M., Humphrey, W., Mushinski, E. B., and Vrana, M., 1975, Multiple individual and cross-specific idiotypes on 13 levan-binding myeloma proteins of BALB/c mice, *J. Exp. Med.* **142**:106–119.

Lifter, J., Hew, C.-L., Yoshioka, M., Richards, F. F., and Konigsberg, W. H., 1974, Affinity-labeled peptides obtained from the combining region of myeloma protein 460, *Biochemistry* **13**:3567–3571.

Little, J. R., and Eisen, H. N., 1967, Evidence for tryptophan in the active sites of antibodies to polynitrobenzenes, *Biochemistry* **6**:3119–3215.

Macario, A. J. L., and Conway De Macario, E., 1975, Antigen-binding properties of antibody molecules, in: *Current Topics in Microbiology and Immunology*, Vol. 71, pp. 125–170, Springer-Verlag, New York.

Mäkelä, O., 1965, Single lymph node cells producing heteroclitic bacteriophage antibody, *J. Immunol.* **95**:378–381.

Manjula, B. N., Richards, F. F., and Rosenstein, R. W., 1976, The distance between the contact sites for DNP and menadione ligands in the combining region of myeloma proteins binding both haptens. I. Estimation of distance using fluorescent energy transfer in protein 460, *Immunochemistry* **13**:929–937.

Margolies, M. N., Cannon, L. E., III, Strosberg, A. D., and Haber, E., 1975, Diversity of light chain variable region sequences among rabbit antibodies elicited by the same antigens, *Proc. Natl. Acad. Sci. U.S.A.* **72**:2180–2184.

Metzger, H., 1970, The antigen receptor problem, *Annu. Rev. Biochem.* **39**:889–928.

Metzger, H., and Singer, S. J., 1963, Binding capacity of reductively fragmented antibodies to the 2,4-dinitrophenyl group. *Science* **142**:674–676.

Montgomery, P. C., Rockey, J. H., and Williamson, A. R., 1972, Homogeneous antibody elicited with dinitrophenyl gramicidin-S, *Proc. Natl. Acad. Sci. U.S.A.* **69**:228–232.

Moreno, C., and Kabat, E. A., 1969, Studies on human antibodies, *J. Exp. Med.* **129**:871–896.

Murphy, P. D., and Sage, H. J., 1970, Variation in the size of antibody sites for the poly L aspartate hapten during the immune response, *J. Immunol.* **105**:460–470.

Nisonoff, A., and Pressman, D., 1958a, Heterogeneity and average combining constants of antibodies from individual rabbits, *J. Immunol.* **80**:417–428.

Nisonoff, A., and Pressman, D., 1958b, Heterogeneity of antibody sites in their relative combining affinities for structurally related haptens, *J. Immunol.* **81**:126–135.

Nisonoff, A., and Thorbecke, G. J., 1964, Immunochemistry, *Annu. Rev. Biochem.* **33**:355–402.

Nisonoff, A., Zappacosta, S., and Jureziz, R., 1967, Properties of crystallized rabbit anti *p*-azobenzoate antibody, *Cold Spring Harbor Symp. Quant. Biol.* **32**:89–93.

Nisonoff, A., Hopper, J. E., and Spring, S. B., 1975, Idiotypic specificities in human monoclonal proteins, in: *The Antibody Molecule*, Chapter II, pp. 448–492, Academic Press, New York.

Noellsen, M. E., Nelson, C. A., III, and Tanford, C., 1965, Gross conformation of rabbit 7S γ-immunoglobulin and its papain-cleaved fragments, *J. Biol. Chem.* **240**:218–224.

Northrop, J. A., 1942, Purification and crystallization of diphtheria antitoxin, *J. Gen. Physiol.* **25**:465–485.

Ohta, Y., Gill, T. J., III, and Leung, C. S., 1970, Volume changes accompanying the antibody–antigen reaction, *Biochemistry* **9**:2708–2712.

Padlan, E. A., Segal, D. M., Cohen, G. A., and Davis, D. R., 1974, The three dimensional structure of the antigen binding site of McPc protein, in: *The Immune System, Genes, Receptors, Signals*, (E. E. Sercarz, A. R. Williamson, and C. F. Fox, eds.), pp. 7–14, Academic Press, New York.

Painter, R. G., Sage, H. J., and Tanford, C., 1972, Contributions of heavy and light chains of rabbit immunoglobulin G to antibody activity, *Biochemistry* **11**:1327–1337.

Parker, C. W., and Osterland, C. K., 1969, Hydrophobic binding sites on immunoglobulins, *Biochemistry* **9**:1074–1081.

Pecht, I., 1974, Kinetic mapping of antibody binding sites, in: *The Immune System: Genes, Receptors, Signals* (E. E. Sercarz, A. R. Williamson, and C. F. Fox, eds.), pp. 15–35, Academic Press, New York.

Piette, L. H., Kiefer, E. F., Grossberg, A. L., and Pressman, D., 1972, Spin-label studies of combining sites in antibodies to charged haptens, *Immunochemistry* **9**:17–22.

Pincus, J. H., Haber, E., Katz, M., and Pappenheimer, A. M., Jr., 1968, Antibodies to pneumococcal polysaccharides: Relation between binding and electrophoretic heterogeneity, *Science* **162**:667–668.

Pink, J. R. L., and Askonas, B. A., 1974, Diversity of antibodies to cross-reacting nitrophenyl haptens in inbred mice, *Eur. J. Immunol.* **4**:426–430.

Poljak, R. J., 1975, The three-dimensional structure, function and genetic control of immunoglobulins, *Nature (London)* **256**:373–376.

Poljak, R. J., Amzel, L. M., Avey, H. P., Chen, B. L: Phizackerley, R. P., and Saul, F., 1973, Three dimensional structure of the Fab fragment of a human immunoglobulin at 2.8 Å resolution, *Proc. Natl. Acad. Sci. U.S.A.* **70**:3305–3310.

Poljak, R. J., Amzel, L. M., Chen, B. L., Phizackerley, R. P., and Saul, F., 1974, The three dimensional structure of the Fab^l fragment of a human myeloma immunoglobulin at 2.0 Å resolution, *Proc. Natl. Acad. Sci. U.S.A.* **71**:3440–3444.

Porter, R. R., 1958, Separation and isolation of fractions of rabbit γ globulin containing the antibody and the antigenic combining sites, *Nature (London)* **182**:670–671.

Porter, R. R., and Press, E. M., 1972, Immunochemistry, *Annu. Rev. Biochem.* **31**:621–652.

Potter, M., 1972, Immunoglobulin producing tumors and myeloma tumors in mice, *Physiol. Rev.* **52**:631–719.

Potter, M., and Lieberman, R., 1970, Common individual antigenic determinants in five of eight BALB/c IgA myeloma proteins that bind phosphorylcholine, *J. Exp. Med.* **132**:737–751.

Quattrochi, R., Cioli, D., and Baglioni, C., 1969, A study of immunoglobulin structure, *J. Exp. Med.* **130**:401–415.

Reichlin, M., 1974, Quantitative immunological studies on single amino acid substitution in human hemoglobin: Demonstration of specific antibodies to multiple sites, *Immunochemistry* **11**:21–27.

Richards, F. M., 1974, The interpretation of protein structures, total volume, group volume distributions and packing densities, *J. Mol. Biol.* **82**:1–14.

Richards, F. F., and Konigsberg, W. H., 1977 ,DNP-based diazoketones and azides, in: *Methods in Enzymology*, Vol. 46 (W. B. Jakoby and M. Wilchek, eds.), pp. 508–515, Academic Press, New York.

Richards, F. F., Sloane, R. W., Jr., and Haber, E., 1967, The synthesis and antigenic properties of a macromolecular peptide of defined sequence bearing the dinitrophenyl hapten, *Biochemistry* **6**:476–484.

Richards, F. F., Lifter, J., Hew, C. -L., Yoshioka, M., and Konigsberg, W. H., 1974, Photoaffinity labeling of the combining region of myeloma protein 460. II. An interpretation of the labeling patterns, *Biochemistry* **13**:3572–3575.

Richards, F. F., Konigsberg, W. H., Rosenstein, R. W., and Varga, J. M., 1975, On the specificity of antibodies, *Science* **187**:130–137.

Rosenstein, R. W., and Richards, F. F., 1976, The distance between the contact sites for DNP and menadione ligands in the combining region of myeloma protein binding both haptens. II. Estimation of distance using haptenic probes with variable length spacers, *Immunochemistry* **13**:939–943.

Rosenstein, R. W., Musson, R. A., Armstrong, M. Y. K., Konigsberg, W. H., and Richards, F. F., 1972, Contact regions for dinitrophenyl and menadione haptens in an immunoglobulin binding more than one antigen, *Proc. Natl. Acad. Sci. U.S.A.* **69**:877–881.

Rubinstein, W. A., and Little, J. R., 1970, Properties of the active sites of antibodies specific for folic acid, *Biochemistry* **9**:2106–2114.

Ruoho, A. E., Kiefer, H., Roeder, P. E., and Singer, S. J., 1973, The mechanism of photoaffinity labeling, *Proc. Natl. Acad. Sci. U.S.A.* **70**:2567–2571.

Scatchard, G., 1949, The attractions of proteins for small molecules and ions, *Ann. N. Y. Acad. Sci.* **51**:660–672.

Schechter, B., Schechter, I., and Sela, M., 1970, Antibody combining sites to a series of peptide determinants of increasing size and defined structure, *J. Biol. Chem.* **245**:1438–1457.

Schiffer, M., Girling, R. L., Ely, K. R., and Edmundson, A. B., 1973, Structure of a λ-type Bence Jones protein at 3.5 Å resolution, *Biochemistry* **12**:4620–4631.

Schlessinger, J., Steinberg, I. Z., Givol, D., Hochman, J., and Pecht, I., 1975, Antigen-induced conformational changes in antibodies and their Fab fragments studied by circular polarization of fluorescence, *Proc. Natl. Acad. Sci. U.S.A.* **72**:2775–2779.

Schubert, D., Jobe, A., and Cohn, M., 1968, Mouse myelomas producing precipitating antibody to nucleic acid bases and/or nitrophenyl derivatives, *Nature (London)* **220**:882.

Secher, D., 1977, Multispecific antibodies, *Nature* **268**:689–690.

Segal, D., Padlan, E. A., Cohen, G. H., Rudikoff, S., Potter, M., and Davies, D. R., 1974, The three dimensional structure of a phosphoryl choline-binding mouse immunoglobulin Fab and the nature of the antigen binding site, *Proc. Natl. Acad. Sci. U.S.A.* **71**:4298–4302.

Segre, D., and Segre, M., 1973, Failure of limiting antigen doses to selectively stimulate high-avidity memory cells, *Science* **181**:851–853.

Singer, S. J., and Doolittle, R. F., 1966, Antibody active sites and immunoglobulin molecules, *Science* **153**:13–25.

Sirisinha, S., and Eisen, H. N., 1971, Autoimmune-like antibodies to the ligand-binding sites of myeloma proteins, *Proc. Natl. Acad. Sci. U.S.A.* **68**:3130–3135.

Siskind, G. W., and Benacerraf, B., 1969, Cell selection by antigen in the immune response, *Adv. Immunol.* **10**:1–50.

Smith, G. P., 1973, *The Variation and Adaptive Expression of Antibodies,* Harvard University Press, Cambridge, Massachusetts.

Smith, G. P., Hood, L., and Fitch, W. M., 1971, Antibody diversity, *Annu. Rev. Biochem.* **40**:969–1012.

Smith, R. A. G., and Knowles, J. R., 1973, Aryldiazirines. Potential reagents for photolabeling of biological receptor sites, *J. Am. Chem. Soc.* **95**:5072–5073.

Steinberg, J. Z., 1974, in: *Concepts in Biochemical Fluorescence* (R. Chen and H. Edelhoch, eds.), Marcel Dekker, New York.

Steiner, L. A., and Eisen, H. N., 1966, Variations in the immune response to a simple determinant, *Bacteriol. Rev.* **30**:383–396.

Steiner, L. A., and Eisen, H. N., 1967a, Sequential changes in the relative affinity of antibodies synthesized during the immune response, *J. Exp. Med.* **126**:1161–1184.

Steiner, L. A., and Eisen, H. N., 1967b, The relative affinity of antibodies synthesized in the secondary response, *J. Exp. Med.* **126**:1185–1205.

Stevenson, G. T., 1973, The binding of haptens by the polypeptide chains of rabbit antibody molecules, *Biochem. J.* **133**:827–836.

Steward, M. W., and Petty, R. E., 1972, The antigen binding characteristics of antibody pools of different relative affinity, *Immunology* **23**:881–887.

Steward, M. W., and Voller, A., 1973, The effect of malaria on the relative affinity of mouse antiprotein antibody, *Br. J. Exp. Pathol.* **54**:198–202.

Stryer, L., and Griffith, O. H., 1965, A spin-labeled hapten, *Proc. Natl. Acad. Sci. U.S.A.* **54**:1785–1791.

Talmage, D. W., 1959, Immunological specificity, *Science* **129**:1643–1648.

Tolleshaug, H., and Hannestad, K., 1975, Binding of ligands to a monoclonal IgM macroglobulin with multiple specificity, *Immunochemistry* **12**:173–182.

Uemara, K.-I., Claflin, J. L., Davie, J. M., and Kinsky, S. C., 1975, Immune responses to lysosomal model membranes, *J. Immunol.* **114**:958–961.

Utsumi, S., and Karush, F., 1964, The sub-units of purified rabbit antibody, *Biochemistry* **3**:1329–1338.

Valentine, R. C., and Green, N. M., 1967, Electron microscopy of an antibody–hapten complex, *J. Mol. Biol.* **27**:615–617.

Varga, J. M., Konigsberg, W. H., and Richards, F. F., 1973, Antibodies with multiple binding functions: Induction of single immunoglobulin species with structurally dissimilar haptens, *Proc. Natl. Acad. Sci. U.S.A.* **70**:3269–3274.

Varga, J. M., Lande, S., and Richards, F. F., 1974a, Immunoglobulins with multiple binding functions. II, The use of nylon–polyserine whisker discs in screening myeloma immunoglobulins for binding activity, *J. Immunol.* **112**:1565–1570.

Varga, J. M., Rosenstein, R. W., and Richards, F. F., 1974b, Antibodies with multiple binding functions: Anti-idiotypic sera directed against a mouse myeloma protein binding two structurally diverse haptens also precipitate elicited rabbit antibody molecules binding the same two haptens, *Fed. Proc. Fed. Am. Soc. Exp. Biol.* **33**:810 (abstract).

Vaughan, R. J., and Westheimer, F. H., 1969, A method for marking the hydrophobic binding sites of enzymes: An insertion into the methyl group of an alanine residue of trypsin, *J. Am. Chem. Soc.* **91**:217–218.

Velick, S. F., Parker, C. W., and Eisen, H. N., 1960, Excitation energy transfer and the quantitative study of antibody–hapten reaction, *Proc. Natl. Acad. Sci. U.S.A.* **46**:1470–1482.

Warner, N. L., Potter, M., and Metcalf, D. (eds.), 1974, *Multiple Myeloma and Related Immunoglobulin-Producing Neoplasms,* pp. 1–40, Workshop No. 1, International Union Against Cancer, Geneva.

Waxdal, M. J., Konigsberg, W. H., and Edelman, G. M., 1968, The covalent structure of human γ G globulin, *Biochemistry* **7**:1967–1972.

Weil, E., and Felix, A., 1916, *Wien, Klin. Wochenschr.* **29**:974–992.

Weltman, J. K., and Edelman, G. M., 1967, Fluorescence polarization of human γ G-immunoglobulins, *Biochemistry* **6**:1437–1447.

Williamson, A. R., 1973, Extent and control of antibody diversity, *Biochem. J.* **130**:325–333.

Wiswesser, W. J., 1973, Editorial, *Aldrichim. Acta* **6**:41–42.

Wofsy, L., and Parker, D. A., 1967, Comparative studies of antibody active sites, *Cold Spring Harbor Symp. Quant. Biol.* **32**:111–116.

Wofsy, L., Metzger, H., and Singer, S. J., 1962, Affinity labeling—a general method for labeling the active sites of antibody and enzyme molecules, *Biochemistry* **1**:1031–1039.

Wu, T. T., and Kabat, E. A., 1970, An analysis of the sequences of the variable regions of Bence-Jones proteins and myeloma light chains and their implications for antibody complementarity, *J. Exp. Med.* **132**:211–250.

Wu, W. H., and Rockey, J. H., 1969, Anti-vasopressin antibody: Characterization of high-affinity rabbit antibody with limited association constant heterogeneity, *Biochemistry* **8**:2719–2728.

Yguerabide, J., Epstein, H. F., and Stryer, L., 1970, Segmental flexibility in an antibody molecule, *J. Mol. Biol.* **51**:573–590.

Yoo, T. J., Roholt, O. A., and Pressman, D., 1967, Specific binding activity of isolated light chains of antibodies, *Science* **157**:707–709.

Yoshioka, M., Lifter, J., Hew, C.-L., Converse, C. A., Armstrong, M. Y. K., Konigsberg, W. H., and Richards, F. F., 1973, Studies on the combining region of protein 460, a mouse γA immunoglobulin which binds several haptens: Binding and reactivity of two types of photoaffinity labeling reagents, *Biochemistry* **12**:4679–4684.

5

The Secretory Component and the J Chain

CHARLOTTE CUNNINGHAM-RUNDLES

1. Introduction

There are two unique polypeptide chains that may be found in covalent association with immunoglobulins A and M (IgA and IgM). These polypeptides are called the *secretory component* (SC) and the J *chain*. While the SC, a large glycoprotein secreted by the lining epithelium of exocrine glands, is the primary distinguishing feature between serum and secretory IgA, the J chain is a small acidic polypeptide that is secreted by the immunocyte itself. The J chain is a characteristic feature of dimeric IgA or polymeric IgM wherever these Ig's may appear. Although the exact role of the SC and J chain is still obscure, it appears that these polypeptides may serve in the three-dimensional organization or in the transport and distribution of the resulting Ig complexes. Because of the importance of these biological functions, the chemical nature of the SC and J chain and their cooperative interactions with IgA and IgM have been the subject of a number of research investigations. This chapter summarizes the physicochemical data that have been compiled concerning these two unique polypeptides and discusses current understanding regarding their molecular associations with IgA and IgM.

2. The Secretory Component

The SC was first described by Tomasi (1965), who observed that secretory IgA had an extra antigenic determinant in comparison with serum IgA. In addition to this form of the SC, which is bound to secretory IgA (BSC), the SC also exists free in exocrine secretions (FSC), and it is present even if IgA is deficient or absent (South *et al.*, 1966; Hurliman *et al.*, 1969). In man, the majority of the IgA-associated SC is disulfide-bonded, but the degree of covalent bonding varies in

CHARLOTTE CUNNINGHAM-RUNDLES • Memorial Sloan-Kettering Cancer Center, New York, New York 10021.

other species; e.g., in the rabbit, only noncovalent forces exist between IgA and SC (Cebra and Robbins, 1966; Tomasi and Grey, 1972).

2.1. Physicochemical Data

2.1.1. Molecular Weight

Table 1 shows estimates of molecular weight of BSC and FSC as determined by ultracentrifugation, gel filtration, SDS-PAGE, and disc electrophoresis. Several species are included for comparison.

TABLE 1. Molecular Weights of the Bound and the Free Secretory Component

Secretory component	Molecular weight	Method	References
Human			
BSC	50,000	Ultracentrifugation	Hong et al. (1966)
BSC	58,000	Ultracentrifugation	Tomasi and Bienenstock (1968)
BSC	76,000	Gel filtration	Newcomb et al. (1968)
BSC	54,000	Gel filtration	Hurliman et al. (1969)
BSC	60,000	Gel filtration	Tomasi and Calvanico (1968)
FSC	80,000	Gel filtration	Brandtzaeg (1970)
FSC	85,000	SDS-PAGE[a]	Mach (1970)
FSC	74,000	SDS-PAGE	van Munster et al. (1971)
FSC	75,000	SDS-PAGE	Kobayashi (1971)
FSC	80,000	Gel filtration	Kobayashi (1971)
BSC	90,000–97,000	Disc electrophoresis	Mestecky et al. (1972a)
BSC	1,000	Ultracentrifugation	Lamm and Greenberg (1972)
BSC	88,000	SDS-PAGE	Lamm and Greenberg (1972)
FSC	80,000	SDS-PAGE	Lamm and Greenberg (1972)
FSC	75,000	SDS-PAGE	Björk and Lindh (1974)
Canine			
BSC	50,000	Gel filtration	Reynolds and Johnson (1971)
FSC	77,500 ± 6500	SDS-PAGE	Thompson et al. (1975)
BSC			
Bovine			
FSC	46,000	Gel filtration	Butler et al. (1970)
FSC	75,000	SDS-PAGE	Mach (1970)
FSC	69,000–75,000	Gel filtration	Butler (1971)
FSC	86,000	Ultracentrifugation	Butler (1971)
Ovine FSC	85,000	Ultracentrifugation	Pahud and Mach (1972)
Goat FSC	85,000	Ultracentrifugation	Pahud and Mach (1970)
Equine FSC	80,000	Gel filtration	Pahud and Mach (1972)
Porcine			
FSC	4 S	Ultracentrifugation	Porter and Allen (1970)
BSC	4.3 S	Ultracentrifugation	Bourne (1974)
Rabbit			
FSC	60,000	Ultracentrifugation	O'Daly and Cebra (1971)
BSC	64,000–70,000	SDS-PAGE	Halpern and Koshland (1970)
FSC	64,000	SDS-PAGE	Halpern and Koshland (1970)
Mouse FSC	4 S	Ultracentrifugation	Asofsky and Hylton (1968)
Guinea pig			
FSC	88,000	SDS-PAGE	Vaerman et al. (1975)

[a]Sodium dodecyl sulfate–polyacrylamide gel electrophoresis.

2.1.2. Carbohydrate Composition

Collected figures for SC carbohydrate analyses are given in Table 2. Estimates of total carbohydrate content vary from 15.9 to 22.8% by weight. On the basis of the absence of N-acetylgalactosamine, Svensson et al. (1977) proposed that the carbohydrate–peptide bond probably exists between N-acetylglucosamine and the asparagine residues of the SC. Isolation of the individual glycopeptides and subsequent structural analyses must be completed to verify this proposal.

2.1.3. Amino Acid Composition

The amino acid composition of human FSC compiled from a number of sources is given in Table 3. Also included are analyses obtained from rabbit, canine, and bovine FSC. There are few analyses for the BSC, but the data of Lamm and Greenberg (1972) are similar to those shown for the FSC.

2.1.4. Peptide Maps

The BSC and FSC have very similar tryptic-peptide maps, with the exception of two additional peptides that were found for the BSC. In each map, 40–50 ninhydrin-positive peptides were found, which agrees with the combined lysine and arginine content of the SC. A mixture of BSC and FSC produced a map that was the same as the FSC protein digest mapped alone, with the exception of the two additional peptides evidently contributed from the BSC. The compositions of the two extra peptides have not been determined, nor is it clear whether these two peptides represent real differences between the FSC and the BSC or differences due to methods of preparation (Cunningham-Rundles et al., 1974a,b).

2.1.5. NH_2-Terminal Sequences

Several authors have now reported NH_2-terminal amino acid sequences for the SC. Table 4 is a composite of the sequences reported to date. Canine, bovine, and human sequences are clearly quite similar. Comparing human and bovine material,

TABLE 2. Carbohydrate Composition of the Secretory Component[a]

	Human				Canine FSC
	BSC	FSC			
Carbohydrate	Lamm and Greenberg (1972)	Kobayashi (1971)	Sletten et al. (1975)	Svensson et al. (in press)	Thompson et al. (1975)
Galactose		3.1	4.1	4.6	
Mannose	10.7	4.0	3.6	4.3	5.9
Fucose		2.3	2.1	4.5	
N-Acetylglucosamine	8.7	4.4	4.8	6.5	6.4
N-Acetylgalactosamine			Traces	0	6.6
Sialic acid	—	1.9	4.0	2.9	—
Totals:	19.4	15.7	18.6	22.8	18.9

[a]Expressed as weight percent.

CHARLOTTE
CUNNINGHAM-RUNDLES

TABLE 3. Amino Acid Composition of the Free Secretory Component[a]

Amino acid	Human					Rabbit	Bovine	Canine
	Kobayashi (1971)	Lamm and Greenberg (1972)	Mestecky et al. (1972b)	van Munster et al. (1971)	Sletten et al. (1975)	O'Daly and Cebra (1971)	Tomasi and Grey (1972)	Thompson et al. (1975)
Lys	57	62	45	56	55	56	56	69
His	10	10	16	9	9	21	13	14
Arg	50	38	41	47	49	37	47	37
Asx	105	94	82	106	107	95	109	118
Thr	54	53	88	59	56	61	67	60
Ser	72	120	114	81	80	92	94	85
Glx	106	113	102	103	110	120	107	105
Pro	50	42	75	48	53	67	45	51
Gly	98	110	89	94	98	98	88	93
Ala	56	57	66	61	61	52	62	42
Val	83	81	78	81	87	84	93	84
Met	0	0.5	8	< 0.06	0	4	4	12
Ile	34	29	20	36	39	30	3	40
Leu	97	80	89	87	91	81	72	75
Tyr	42	37	30	36	40	28	39	40
Phe	33	31	31	31	32	38	34	43
Cys	32	24	29	35	33	37	22	49

[a]Composition is given in moles per 1000 moles.

there appear to be deletions of positions 7 and 8 and a single base change at position 9. Human and canine material differs by a single base change at position 12. Antigenic cross-reactivities were demonstrated between human and bovine FSC using a bovine antiserum (Tomasi and Capra, 1974), but human and canine material has not yet been shown to cross-react despite similarities in NH_2-terminal sequence.

Some evidence has been presented to show that allotypic differences may occur in rabbit SC, but such differences have not yet been demonstrated for the SC of any other species (Knight *et al.*, 1974). The amino acid sequence differences presumably responsible for these antigenic differences are not yet known.

2.2. Integration of the Secretory Component with Immunoglobulin A

The secretory component is not actually visible in electron micrographs of secretory IgA (SIgA), but a possible location may be inferred from these studies. Two main configurations of SIgA are found. One resembles the Y form that IgG appears to have in electron micrographs, but is more electron dense; the other appears as a double Y (>—<) (Svehag and Bloth, 1970; Bloth and Svehag, 1971). From such pictures, it was proposed that SIgA may have both a folded configuration, in which the two IgA molecules are stacked on top of each other, and a more prevalent, extended form, in which the two IgA molecules are joined together at their Fc ends. The SC could be present in either configuration if it had a linear form and could lie parallel to the heavy (H) chains (Svehag and Bloth, 1970; Bloth and Svehag, 1971). For this model to be correct, it must be assumed that a generous degree of flexibility is maintained at the junctions of these Fc regions, and that the insertion of the SC does not hinder what appears to be rather free rotation at this point. Recent optical rotary dispersion and circular dichroism data do appear to show that human SC itself has a linear conformation that would be requisite to the positioning in the IgA dimer described above (Björk and Lindh, 1974).

Where the SC is covalently attached to IgA is still a matter of conjecture, but taking several kinds of evidence into consideration, it appears most probable that it is bonded to some point within the Fc region of the α chain. [While the SC is occasionally found in secretions in association with IgM if IgA is deficient, the bonding mechanism in this latter instance appears to be exclusively *non*covalent (Weicker and Underdown, 1975; Lindh and Björk, 1976b) and will not be further considered here.]

TABLE 4. NH_2-Terminal Amino Acid Sequences of the Secretory Component from Several Species

Protein	Species	1 2 3 4 5 6 7 8 9 10 11 12 13 14 15 16	References
FSC	Human	Lys-Ser-Pro-Ile-Phe-Gly-Pro-Glu-Glu-Val-Asp-Ser-Val-Glu-Gly-Gly-	Cunningham-Rundles *et al.* (1974b)
BSC	Human	Lys-Ser-Pro-Ile-Phe-Gly-Pro-Glu-Glu-Val-Asp-Ser-Val-Glu-	Cunningham-Rundles *et al.* (1974b)
FSC	Human	Lys- ? -Pro-Ile-Phe-Gly-Pro-Glu-Glu-Val-	Sletten *et al.* (1975)
FSC	Bovine	Lys-Ser-Pro-Ile-Phe-Gly——— -Asp-Val-Asp-Ser-Val-Asp-Gly-	Tomasi and Capra (1974)
BSC	Rabbit	PCA-Ser-Ser-	Johnstone and Mole (1975)
FSC	Canine	Lys-Ser-Pro-Ile-Phe-Gly-Pro-Glu-Glu-Val-Asn-Ile (Val-Glu-Gly)-	Thompson *et al.* (1975)

Experimental evidence for an α-chain attachment for the SC was first given by Hurliman *et al.* (1969), who showed that gel filtration of denatured salivary IgA produced three fractions: intact SIgA, SC attached to two α chains, and light (L) chain dimers. The dissociated SIgA probably derived from the IgA2 $Am_2(+)$ allotype, which lacks H–L chain disulfide bonds (Grey *et al.*, 1968). The bonding between the SC and the dissociated α chains was shown to be covalent, reduction being required to release the individual components.

Experiments of Jerry *et al.* (1972) confirmed this view. In these experiments, *in vitro* recombination of the SC with a myeloma IgA2 was shown to prevent this denaturant-dissociable myeloma from separating into dimer H- and dimer L-chains in guanidine. This "stabilization" was based on covalent bonding, since subsequent reduction allowed the usual dissociation to occur. This was demonstrated also in a pepsin-treated IgA2 myeloma that retained the hinge but no Fc determinants. These authors concluded that the location of the covalent bonding between the SC and IgA2 may be in the hinge region of the α chain. Similar conclusions were reached by Mehta *et al.* (1973) from experiments in which a microbial enzyme isolated from human feces was used to split human SIgA into Fab and Fc fragments. After gel filtration, the Fc, which included the hinge region, was found associated with the SC. The position of this covalent bond, however, was not localized.

From the observations described above, it appears clear that the SC is covalently bonded to the α chain, but the C_H3 region of the α chain is clearly not linked to the SC by a disulfide bond, since cyanogen bromide treatment of whole SIgA followed by gel filtration effectively removes the COOH-terminal 100 amino acids of each IgA monomer, while the SC remains covalently attached to the remainder of the molecule (Cunningham-Rundles, 1974; Mestecky *et al.*, 1974a). It appears, therefore, that while the SC is probably attached to the Fc region of the α chain, it must be in the C_H1, C_H2, or hinge region.

Despite uncertainty about the exact points of attachment on the α chain, it was recently shown that the SC is probably bonded to IgA through two disulfide bridges. This bonding was shown in two different laboratories. The first observation (Cunningham-Rundles and Lamm, 1975) was based on calculations of specific activity of partially reduced and radioalkylated preparations of BSC that were isolated from pooled human SIgA. Confirmation of this observation was obtained by Lindh and Björk (1976a) from experiments with recombined FSC and myeloma IgA1. Next to be considered is whether the SC is then bonded to one or to both monomeric IgA subunits. From analysis of the molecular weights of the cyanogen-bromide-produced fragments of SIgA, Underdown (1975) and Mestecky *et al.* (in press) concluded that the SC cannot be bound to both IgA monomers of SIgA, but must be bound to only one of them. It appears, therefore, that the SC is disulfide-linked to the two α chains of one IgA monomer.

The two SC peptides containing these half-cystines were isolated from the FSC and sequenced (Cunningham-Rundles and Lamm, 1974, 1975). While it was found technically impractical to isolate these same peptides from the BSC, on autoradiographs of peptide maps of ^{14}C-alkylated peptides of the BSC and FSC, the radioactive peptides of both forms of SC had identical mobility and were presumed to be the same (Cunningham-Rundles *et al.*, 1974a,b). Subsequently, the two radioalkylated peptides isolated from the FSC were found on diagonal mapping to be joined into one disulfide bridge in the native molecule (Cunningham-Rundles and

Lamm, 1975). Since no free sulfhydryl groups were detected in the FSC (Cunningham-Rundles and Lamm, 1975; Lindh and Björk, 1976a) and no interchain disulfides are present, the isolated peptides must form an *intra*chain disulfide bridge in native FSC.

These results suggested that the single reactive intrachain disulfide bridge of the FSC forms two interchain disulfide bridges when the FSC is covalently joined to dimeric IgA during the assembly of the secretory IgA molecule. This reaction presumably takes place by a disulfide-exchange reaction catalyzed within the exocrine gland. Figure 1 shows the sequences of the half-cystine peptides and illustrates the presumptive mechanism involved.

With the use of this sequence information for the two labile half-cystines of the SC, attempts were made to locate the point of attachment of the SC to the α chain, using diagonal mapping of hinge-region peptides of SIgA. The hinge region was chosen because it is readily identified by amino acid composition, having large amounts of proline and cysteine, and for the very reason that many cysteic acid residues of uncertain function lie in this region. Some 70 peptides were isolated and analyzed from the hinge region, but SC peptides were not detected (Cunningham-Rundles and Lamm, unpublished). Whether this is evidence against a hinge-region attachment for SC, or whether SC peptides are technically difficult to locate by this means, remains uncertain. If the former is true, C_H1 or C_H2 attachment is to be expected.

2.3. Physiological Role of the Secretory Component

The SC is produced by the mucosal epithelial cells of all exocrine glands and is secreted into the spaces surrounding these cells and into the glandular lumen

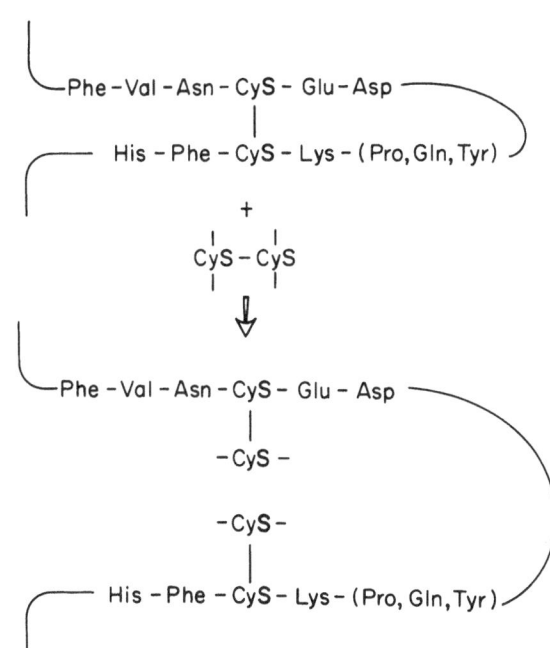

Figure 1. Proposed mechanism of formation of the secretory IgA molecule. The reactive half-cystines of the FSC are joined in one intrachain bridge in this molecule, but are broken and reformed into two new disulfide bridges with the α chain.

(Tomasi, 1965; South *et al.*, 1966; Lawton *et al.*, 1970). A current model of assembly of SIgA proposes that IgA is produced by local plasma cells and migrates through the epithelial cell where it is covalently attached to the SC, presumably by a disulfide-exchange reaction catalyzed by a cytoplasmic enzyme (Poger and Lamm, 1974; Brandtzaeg, 1974). The point at which IgA is dimerized still remains uncertain.

A number of different kinds of experiments have shown that the resulting SIgA complex is more resistant to proteolytic degradation than dimeric serum-type IgA. In one type of experiment, progressive amounts of the SC were removed from rabbit or human SIgA, and the susceptibility to proteolysis was related to the content of SC remaining (Ghetie and Mota, 1973). Another approach was to study enhanced resistance to enzymes as the SC was progressively reassociated with dimeric IgA (Lindh, 1975). Both kinds of studies demonstrated that the presence of attached SC promotes resistance to enzymatic cleavage. Whether this is a nonspecific effect, resulting from shielding of otherwise susceptible α-chain cleavage points, or a "true" physiological function, would be difficult to determine.

An interesting point to consider in this regard is the known stabilization of IgA2 $Am_2(+)$ molecules by the SC, which prevents dissociation by denaturants. This could lead to a selective advantage for this IgA2 species, and it may explain the rather remarkable enrichment of the IgA2 subclass in secretions as compared with serum (Grey *et al.*, 1968).

An early proposal was that the SC may serve in the transport of IgA into the secretions (Tomasi, 1965; South *et al.*, 1966), but this has been difficult to prove. More recently, Brandtzaeg (1974) suggested that the SC may serve as a receptor for IgA, directing its transport through the epithelial cells of the mucosal membrane.

3. The J Chain

The presence of this component was first noted in human colostral IgA by Rejnek *et al.* (1966) and Cederblad *et al.* (1966), and has since been detected in association with the Ig's of a large number of diverse species. Several recent reviews have dealt with the isolation, physical characteristics, and synthesis of this small protein (see Koshland, 1975; Inman and Mestecky, 1974). Unlike the SC, the J chain is synthesized by the same cells that secrete Ig's (Parkhouse, 1972; Halpern and Coffman, 1972), but it is clearly a distinctly different protein from the various classes of Ig H and L chains, as judged from its antigenic determinants, amino acid composition, and peptide maps (Mestecky *et al.*, 1971, 1972b).

3.1. Physicochemical Data

3.1.1. Molecular Weight

The original estimates of molecular weight for the J chain ranged from 23,000 to 27,000, using gel filtration or SDS-PAGE (Halpern and Koshland, 1970; Morrison and Koshland, 1972). Ultracentrifugation in denaturants, however, shows the J chain to have a molecular weight of 14,000–15,000 (see Table 5). These discrepancies appear to be due to the remarkably linear shape of the J chain, which produces an increase in effective volume in gel filtration or SDS-PAGE, as discussed by Koshland (1975). Another factor is the tendency of the J chain to form dimers that

Molecular weight	Method	Source	References
23,000	Gel filtration	Human SIgA	Halpern and Koshland (1970)
26,500	Gel filtration	Human IgM	Mestecky et al. (1971)
48,000	Gel filtration	Human IgM	Kownatzki (1971)
25,400	SDS-PAGE	Human IgM	Kownatzki (1971)
26,000	SDS-PAGE	Human SIgA	Mestecky et al. (1972a)
24,500	Gel filtration	Human myeloma IgA, SIgA, and IgM	Morrison and Koshland (1972)
24,000 ± 1200	SDS-PAGE	Human SIgA	Kobayashi et al. (1973)
25,700	SDS-PAGE	Human SIgA	Mestecky et al. (1972a)
24,500	SDS-PAGE	Human myeloma IgA	Mendez et al. (1973a)
22,000	Gel filtration	Human myeloma IgA	Mestecky et al. (1972a)
15,000 ± 200	Ultracentrifugation	Human myeloma IgA	Schrohenloher et al. (1973)
15,000 ± 500	Ultracentrifugation	Human myeloma IgA	Wilde and Koshland (1973)
25,000	SDS-PAGE	Human myeloma IgA	Wilde and Koshland (1973)
15,000	Ultracentrifugation	Human myeloma IgA and IgM	Tomasi and Hauptman (1974)
27,000	SDS-PAGE	Human IgM	Ricardo et al. (1974)
14,500	SDS-PAGE after 21 days in guanidine HCl	Human IgM	Ricardo et al. (1974)
15,200	Ultracentrifugation after 14 days in guanidine HCl	Human IgM	Ricardo et al. (1974)
13,300–17,700 6,400–11,500	Ultracentrifugation	Human IgA SIgA and IgM	Kang et al. (1974)
22,500	SDS-PAGE	Rabbit SIgA	O'Daly and Cebra (1971)
15,000	Ultracentrifugation	Rabbit SIgA	O'Daly and Cebra (1971)
16,000	SDS-PAGE	Mouse myeloma IgA and IgM	Parkhouse and Della Corte (1973)
25,200	SDS-PAGE	Mouse myeloma IgA	Mosmann and Baumal (1975)
20,000–24,000	SDS-PAGE	Mouse myeloma IgM	Barger and Inman (1976)
15,756	Ultracentrifugation	Mouse myeloma IgM	Barger and Inman (1976)

are held together by strong noncovalent forces. Some of the most accurate values of molecular weight for human J chain were determined from protein samples that had been exposed to 5 M guanidine HCl for a period of some days (Ricardo and Inman, 1974).

3.1.2. Carbohydrate Composition

Recently, it was shown that the catfish J-chain counterpart has a carbohydrate composition similar to that of the human (Table 6).

3.1.3. Amino Acid Composition

Table 7 lists amino acid composition analyses for the J chains of human and animal Ig's. As would be expected, the J chains isolated from human IgA and IgM have very similar, if not identical, analyses. Studies on the composition of the J-chain analogues of other species have been remarkable in their similarity to that of

TABLE 6. Carbohydrate Composition of the J
Chain[a]

Carbohydrate	Human (mol %)	Catfish (mol %)
Fucose	0.34	0.3
Mannose	2.13	2.03
Galactose	1.27	0.87
Glucosamine	2.72	1.99
Galactosamine	0	0
Sialic acid	1.11	1.39

[a]From Mestecky et al. (1975).

the human J chain, and it is striking that human and catfish J-chain amino acid compositions are so similar (see Table 7). The J chains that have been isolated have a rapid anodal migration that is easily understood considering the large amounts of aspartic, glutamic, and cysteic acids that are present. Tryptophan is evidently absent, as based upon two experiments in which it was sought. Two analyses of mouse J chain are included; these agree poorly, but the analysis of Barger and Inman (1976) appears more consistent with results obtained from other mammalian J chains. Since mouse and mammalian J chains are antigenically cross-reactive (see Section 3.2), this latter analysis would appear to be more nearly correct.

3.2. Species Cross-Reactions

As might be expected from the similarities of amino acid composition of J chains isolated from different animals, there are numerous antigenic cross-reactions that can be demonstrated with rabbit antisera raised against human J chain. More surprisingly, antisera to human and rabbit J chains have also shown reactivity toward an acidic polypeptide isolated from several birds, amphibians, and fish. Table 8 lists species for which data are available, and the method by which the J-chain candidate was identified. A strong tendency toward amino acid sequence preservation, at least for a few key areas, must underlie these observations. This extensive amino acid homology may be a prime reason for the relatively poor antigenicity exhibited by the J chain, and the fact that only reduced and alkylated samples will stimulate antibody production. This problem has been discussed by Kunkel (1974) and Inman and Mestecky (1974).

3.3. J-Chain Attachment

Since the J chain is normally found in covalent association with either polymeric IgA or IgM, some distinctive feature of these Ig's has been sought as a point of attachment. Both the α and the μ chains were known to have an additional 19 amino acids at the COOH-terminus in comparison with other H chains, and the sequences of these additional amino acids were found to be quite similar for α and μ chains (Chuang et al., 1973). It was subsequently shown by several laboratories that the J chain is, in fact, disulfide-bonded to the α and μ chains in this region. For both H chains, the half-cystine involved was found to be the penultimate residue; this was shown for α chain by Mendez et al. (1973) and for μ chain by Mestecky and

TABLE 7. Amino Acid Composition of the J Chain[a]

Amino acid	Human — Morrison and Koshland (1972) — Myeloma IgA	Human — Mestecky et al. (1972b) — Secretory IgA	Mestecky (1974) — Myeloma IgM	Pig — Zikan (1973) — Secretory IgA	Rabbit — O'Daly and Cebra (1971) — Secretory IgA	Dog — Kehoe et al. (1972) — Myeloma IgA	Mouse — Rosenstein and Jackson (1973) — Myeloma IgA	Mouse — Barger and Inman (1976) — Myeloma IgM	Catfish — Mestecky et al. (1975) — IgM
Lys	42.8	48.2	41.3	56.9	43.4	24	76	45.3	47.2
His	7.4	10.2	8.3	18.2	13.8	8	29.6	18.8	16.7
Arg	72.0	74.2	78.7	49.4	56.6	68	35.5	53.3	26.3
Asp	168.2	149.4	160.5	168.4	144.1	168	88.8	182.2	88.0
Thr	96.1	81.2	87.6	83.2	97.9	84	59.2	95.5	74.5
Ser	57.7	52.1	52.5	64.7	84.5	76	82.8	66.0	130.1
Glu	112.0	112.9	109.2	127.2	99.8	128	142.0	111.4	111.9
Pro	60.0	72.3	71.7	40.9	70.5	60	53.3	64.0	64.8
Gly	16.0	21.8	21.0	19.7	47.7	40	82.8	46.1	70.3
Ala	43.4	48.4	47.7	45.4	44.5	48	88.8	37.4	50.6
Val	75.6	75.7	79.6	61.3	58.0	88	53.3	76.4	78.9
Met	5.6	9.6	7.2	8.4	7.4	20	11.8	3.8	0
Ile	66.9	67.4	65.2	62.4	53.4	48	29.6	43.4	27.6
Leu	60.4	68.0	64.2	80.9	70.4	60	88.8	50.2	88.5
Tyr	45.2	46.1	44.8	36.3	40.6	28	35.5	33.8	32.8
Phe	10.1	11.8	9.8	22.1	22.7	8	41.4	12.7	37.7
Cm-Cys[b]	60.2	ND[c]	50.6	53.6	47.1	44	ND	ND	ND
Cysteic acid	ND	50.7	ND	ND	ND	ND	ND	60.0	54.1
Try	0	ND	ND	ND	ND	ND	ND	ND	ND

[a] Composition is given in residues per 1000.
[b] Cm-Cys = carboxymethyl cysteine.
[c] ND = Not done.

TABLE 8. Detection of J Chain in Human Material and in Other Species

Source	Detected	Methods	References
Human serum polymeric IgA	+	Physicochemical data, antigenic cross-reaction	Halpern and Koshland (1970)
			Mestecky et al. (1971)
			Morrison and Koshland (1972)
Human secretory IgA	+	Physicochemical data, antigenic cross-reaction	Morrison and Koshland (1972)
Human serum IgM	+	Physicochemical data, antigenic cross-reaction	Morrison and Koshland (1972)
Human Waldenström IgM	+	Physicochemical data, antigenic cross-reaction	Morrison and Koshland (1972)
Human 7 S IgA	0	Physicochemical data, antigenic cross-reaction	Niedermeier et al. (1972)
Human 7 S IgG	0	Physicochemical data, antigenic cross-reaction	Niedermeier et al. (1972)
Human 7 S IgD	0	Physicochemical data, antigenic cross-reaction	Niedermeier et al. (1972)
Human 7 S IgE	0	Physicochemical data, antigenic cross-reaction	Niedermeier et al. (1972)
Human urine containing Bence Jones protein	Trace in 2/100 urine samples	Physicochemical data, antigenic cross-reaction	Meinke and Spiegelberg (1974)
Dog IgA and IgM	+	Physicochemical data, antigenic cross-reaction	Hurvitz et al. (1971), Kehoe et al. (1972)
Rabbit IgA	+	Physicochemical data, antigenic cross-reaction	Halpern and Koshland (1970)
Mouse IgA	+	Physicochemical data, antigenic cross-reaction	Parkhouse (1972), Halpern and Coffman (1972)
Horse SIgA and IgM	+	Antigenic cross-reaction	Kobayashi (1971)
Pig SIgA	+	Physicochemical data, antigenic cross-reaction	Zikan (1973)
Sheep (mixture of SIgA and IgM)	+	Electrophoretic mobility	Heimer et al. (1969)
Hedgehog (mixture of SIgA and IgM)	+	Antigenic cross-reaction	Kobayashi et al. (1973)
Guinea pig SIgA and IgM	+	Antigenic cross-reaction	Kobayashi et al. (1973)
Rat IgA and IgM	+	Antigenic cross-section	Kobayashi et al. (1973)
Cow SIgA and IgM	+	Molecular weight, antigenic cross-reaction	Butler (1971), Kobayashi et al. (1973)

(Continued)

TABLE 8. (*Continued*)

167

THE SECRETORY
COMPONENT AND
THE J CHAIN

Source	Detected	Methods	References
Cat (mixture of IgA and IgM)	+	Molecular weight anti-genic cross-reaction	Kobayashi *et al.* (1973)
Goat SIgA and IgM	+	Antigenic cross-reaction	Kobayashi *et al.* (1973)
Pheasant macroglobulin	+	Electrophoretic mobility	Weinheimer *et al.* (1971)
Chicken macroglobulin	+	Antigen cross-reaction	Kobayashi *et al.* (1973)
Marine toad macroglobulin	+	Electrophoretic mobility	Weinheimer *et al.* (1971)
Catfish macroglobulin	+	Electrophoretic mobility	Weinheimer *et al. (1971)*
		Physicochemical data	Mestecky *et al.* (1975)
Leopard shark macroglobulin	+	Electrophoretic mobility	Klaus *et al.* (1971)
		Physicochemical data	Klaus *et al.* (1971)
Turtle	0	Antigenic cross-reaction	Kobayashi *et al.* (1973)
Paddlefish	0	Electrophoretic mobility	Weinheimer *et al.* (1971)
Gar	0	Electrophoretic mobility	Weinheimer *et al.* (1971)
Nurse shark	0	Electrophoretic mobility	Weinheimer *et al.* (1971)

Schrohenloher (1974a). Convenient fragmentation of the IgA or IgM polymer requisite to this identification was achieved by cyanogen bromide, which cleaves the eight COOH-terminal amino acids of both α and μ, releasing the almost intact J chain and attached H chain fragment(s). A second useful method was the production of the Fc5μ fragment (and attached J chain) by trypsinization at an elevated temperature (Plaut and Tomasi, 1970; Inman and Ricardo, 1974).

The J chain appears to be attached to both IgA subunits in dimeric IgA, requiring two disulfide bonds; for tetrameric IgA, two molecules of J chain are found (Chapuis and Koshland, 1975). Diagonal mapping of the cyanogen-bromide fragments of myeloma IgA and attached J, however, has thus far demonstrated only one J-chain peptide (Ala-Cys-Arg) to which an α-chain fragment was attached (Mendez *et al.*, 1973b). While the J chain could presumably have two such sequences, it has not been proved that it does. In any case, studies on IgA and IgM show that the J chain is bound to at most two H chains—where it may serve as a disulfide "clasp," joining IgM monomeric subunits one and five, while in IgA, the J chain binds the two subunits of IgA (Chapuis and Koshland, 1975).

3.4. J Chain and the Attachment of the Secretory Component

Some evidence has been presented that tends to show that the presence of J chain is necessary for the binding of the SC to IgA. In the IgA myeloma proteins that lacked J chain, SC binding was poor (Brandtzaeg, in press). Such IgA proteins would have to be analyzed for sequence deletions, however, to fully evaluate this. As pointed out above, the SC is likely to bind to the α chain in the C_H1, C_H2, or hinge region. A deletion in one of these, in addition to a deletion in the region of the penultimate cystine, could explain both poor SC and J binding. Other evidence that SC binding may depend on the J chain concerns antisera to the J chain which can block the binding of the SC to IgA or IgM (Brandtzaeg, 1975). Whether this indicates that the SC and the J chain must interact directly, or whether nonspecific steric hinderance of the J-chain antisera produced this result, is uncertain. As pointed out above, the SC and the J chain are not ultimately covalently bonded to each other, since cyanogen bromide cleavage of the C_H3 region and attached J chain does not disturb the SC and α-chain attachment (Cunningham-Rundles, 1974; Mestecky *et al.*, 1974b). At present, Figure 2 appears to be the best structural model of the assembled SIgA molecule.

3.5. Immunoglobulin Assembly

The J chain is attached to IgA or IgM within the immunocyte either before or at the time of Ig secretion (Della Corte and Parkhouse, 1973). Since the J chain is not found in monomeric Ig's, it has been generally assumed that this polypeptide initiates or facilitates the dimerization of IgA and polymerization of IgM, but whether the J chain is essential to the polymerization process is still disputed. In one series of experiments, 7 S IgM could be polymerized if both J chain and an enzyme catalyzing a disulfide exchange were supplied, but if the J chain alone was present, polymerization did not occur (Della Corte and Parkhouse, 1973). Other laboratories reported, however, that IgM polymerization may proceed in the absence of J chain (Eskeland and Harboe, 1973; Kownatzki and Drescher, 1973). Another recent study showed that while a secreted murine IgM had 1 mol J chain/mol 19 S IgM, the intracellular J was present as only 0.5–0.6 mol/mol 19 S IgM. This finding would again indicate that J chain may not be required for polymer assembly (Stott, 1976). In addition, there are scattered reports of naturally occurring polymeric human IgA and human and shark IgM that lack detectable J chain (Eskeland and Brandtzaeg, 1974; Brandtzaeg, in press). Thus, it appears that polymeric IgA or IgM may be formed in the absence of J chain.

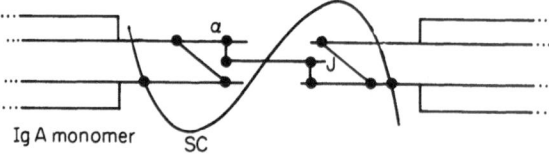

Figure 2. A proposed model of SIgA, particularly using the data of Mestecky (1977), Underdown (1975), and Cunningham-Rundles and Lamm (1975).

Recently, it was observed that the J chain can be detected in cells that secrete IgG, although J chain itself has not been found as a secreted product. The presence of the J chain in such cells may be a residual feature of previously existing IgM synthesis (Kaji and Parkhouse, 1974, 1975). While J chain was not detectable in plasma cells that did not synthesize Ig, it was found in cells that synthesized, but did not secrete. In addition, in one cell line with deficient H chain synthesis, J chain was present in the usual concentrations. This finding would indicate that the control of H-chain and J-chain synthesis is probably not connected (Kaji and Parkhouse, 1974, 1975).

At least in theory, a J-chain myeloma protein could be produced by an abnormal clone of plasma cells, but this occurrence has never been reported. Even in the presence of Bence Jones proteins, finding J chain in the urine is quite rare. As noted in Table 8, a trace of J chain was detected in the urine of only 2 of 100 patients with myeloma (Meinke and Spiegelberg, 1974).

ACKNOWLEDGMENTS

The author is grateful to Drs. E. Lindh, I. Bjork, S. Svensson, and J. Mestecky for preprints of material in press. Support to the author's laboratory is provided by National Cancer Institute grants CA-08748, CA-17404, and CA-05826.

References

Asofsky, R., and Hylton, M. B., 1968, Secretory IgA synthesis in germ-free and conventionally reared mice, *Fed. Proc. Fed. Am. Soc. Exp. Biol.* **27**:617 (abstract).

Barger, B. O., and Inman, F. P., 1976, Physico-chemical characterization of murine J chain, *Immunochemistry* **13**:165–169.

Björk, I., and Lindh, E., 1974, Binding of secretory component to dimers of immunoglobulin A *in vitro*, *Eur. J. Biochem.* **45**:135–145.

Bloth, B., and Svehag, S. E., 1971, Further studies on the ultra-structure of dimeric IgA of human origin, *J. Exp. Med.* **133**:1035–1042.

Bourne, F. J., 1974, Structural features of pig IgA, *Immunol. Commun.* **3**:157–163.

Brandtzaeg, P., 1970, Unfolding of human secretory immunoglobulin A, *Immunochemistry* **7**:127–130.

Brandtzaeg, P., 1974, Mucosal and glandular distribution of immunoglobulin components: Differential localization of free and bound SC in secretory epithelial cells, *J. Immunol.* **112**:1553–1559.

Brandtzaeg, P., 1975, Blocking effect of J chain and J chain antibody on the binding of secretory component to human IgA and IgM, *Scand. J. Immonol.* **4**:837–842.

Butler, J. E., 1971, Physicochemical and immunochemical studies on bovine IgA and glycoprotein-A, *Biochim. Biophys. Acta* **251**:435–449.

Butler, J. E., Groves, M. L., and Coulson, E. J., 1970, The identification of a secretory immunoglobulin in the cow that is antigenetically related to glycoprotein-A, *Fed. Proc. Fed. Am. Soc. Exp. Biol.* **29**:642 (abstract).

Cebra, J. J., and Robbins, J. B., 1966, γ-A Immunoglobulin from rabbit colostrum, *J. Immunol.* **97**:12–24.

Cederblad, G., Johansson, B. G., and Rymo, L., 1966, Reduction and proteolytic degradation of immunoglobulin A from human colostrum, *Acta Chem. Scand.* **20**:2349–2357.

Capuis, R. M., and Koshland, M. E., 1975, Linkage and assembly of polymeric IgA immunoglobulins, *Biochemistry* **14**:1320–1325.

Chuang, C.-Y., Capra, D. J., and Kehoe, J. M., 1973, Evolutionary relationship between carboxyterminal region of a human alpha chain and other immunoglobulin heavy chain constant regions, *Nature (London)* **244**:158–160.

Cunningham-Rundles, C., 1974, The Secretory Component of Exocrine Immunoglobulin A, Ph.D. Thesis, New York University.

Cunningham-Rundles, C., and Lamm, M. E., 1974, Reactive half-cystines of the secretory component, *Fed. Proc. Fed. Am. Soc. Exp. Biol.* **33**:3041 (abstract).

Cunningham-Rundles, C., and Lamm, M. E., 1975, Reactive half-cystine peptides of the secretory component of human exocrine immunoglobulin A, *J. Biol. Chem.* **250**:1987–1991.

Cunningham-Rundles, C., Lamm, M. E., and Franklin, E. C., 1974a, Studies on the primary structure of human secretory component, *Adv. Exp. Med. Biol.* **45**:241–243.

Cunningham-Rundles, C., Lamm, M. E., and Franklin, E. C., 1974b, Human secretory component, *J. Biol. Chem.* **249**:5654–5657.

Della Corte, E., and Parkhouse, R. M. E., 1973, Biosynthesis of immunoglobulin A (IgA) and immunoglobulin M (IgM), *Biochem. J.* **136**:597–606.

Eskeland, T., and Brandtzaeg, P., 1974, Does J chain mediate the combination of 19S IgM and dimeric IgA with the secretory component rather than being necessary for their polymerization?, *Immunochemistry* **11**:161–163.

Eskeland, T., and Harboe, M., 1973, 7 S Immunoglobulin M (IgM) from serum purified by anti μ chain immunoadsorbent: Comparison of the reassociation properties of 7 S IgM and various 19 S IgM subunits, *Scand. J. Immunol.* **2**:511–521.

Ghetie, V., and Mota, G., 1973, The decrease of human colostral immunoglobulin A resistance to papain action after gradual release of the secretory component, *Immunochemistry* **10**:839–840.

Grey, H. M., Abel, C. A., Yount, W. J., and Kunkel, H. G., 1968, A subclass of γA globulins (αA2) which lacks the disulfide bonds linking heavy and light chains, *J. Exp. Med.* **128**:1223–1236.

Halpern, M. S., and Coffman, R. L., 1972, Polymer formation and J chain synthesis in mouse plasmacytomas, *J. Immunol.* **109**:674–680.

Halpern, M. S., and Koshland, M. E., 1970, Novel subunit in secretory IgA, *Nature (London)* **228**:1276–1278.

Heimer, R., Jones, D. W., and Maurer, P. H., 1969, The immunoglobulins of sheep colostrum, *Biochemistry* **8**:3937–3944.

Hong, R., Pollara, B., and Good, R. A., 1966, A model for colostrial IgA, *Proc. Natl. Acad. Sci. U.S.A.* **56**:602–607.

Hurlimann, J., Waldesbühl, M., and Zuber, C., 1969, Human salivary immunoglobulin A: Some immunological and physicochemical characteristics, *Biochim. Biophys. Acta* **181**:393–403.

Hurvitz, A. I., Kehoe, J. M., and Capra, J. D., 1971, Characterization of three homogeneous canine immunoglobulins, *J. Immunol.* **107**:648–654.

Inman, F. P., and Mestecky, J., 1974, The J chain of polymeric immunoglobulins, *Comtemp. Top. Mol. Immunol.* **3**:111–141.

Inman, F. P., and Ricardo, M. J., 1974, The association of J chain with the Fc region of human IgM, *J. Immunol.* **112**:229–233.

Jerry, L. M., Kunkel, H. G., and Adams, L., 1972, Stabilization of dissociable IgA2 proteins by secretory component, *J. Immunol.* **109**:275–283.

Johnstone, A. P., and Mole, L. E., 1975, N-Terminal sequences of secretory piece and α chains of different allotype in rabbit secretory IgA, *Nature (London)* **256**:339–341.

Kaji, H., and Parkhouse, R. M. E., 1974, Intracellular J chain in mouse plasmacytomas secreting IgA, IgM, and IgG, *Nature (London)* **249**:45–47.

Kaji, H., and Parkhouse, R. M. E., 1975, Control of J chain biosynthesis in relation to heavy and light chain synthesis, polymerization and secretion, *J. Immunol.* **114**:1218–1220.

Kang, Y. S., Calvanico, N. J., and Tomasi, T. B., 1974, Human J chain: Isolation and molecular weight studies, *J. Immunol.* **112**:162–167.

Kehoe, J. M., Tomasi, T. B., Jr., Ellouz, F., and Capra, J. D., 1972, Identification of J chain in a homogeneous canine IgA immunoglobulin, *J. Immunol.* **109**:59–64.

Klaus, G. G. B., Halpern, M. S., Koshland, M. E., and Goodman, J. W., 1971, A polypeptide chain from leopard shark 19 S immunoglobulin analogous to mammalian J chain, *J. Immunol.* **107**:1785–1790.

Knight, K. L., Rosenzweig, M., Lichter, E. A., and Hanley, W. C., 1974, Rabbit secretory IgA: Identification and genetic control of two allotypes of secretory components, *J. Immunol.* **112**:877–882.

Kobayashi, K., 1971, Studies on human secretory IgA—Comparative studies of the IgA bound secretory piece and the free secretory piece protein, *Immunochemistry* **8**:785–800.

Kobayashi, K., Vaerman, J.-P., Bazin, H., Labacq-Verheyden, A.-M., and Heremans, J. F., 1973, Identification of J chain in polymeric immunoglobulins from a variety of species by cross-reaction with rabbit antisera to human J chain, *J. Immunol.* **111**:1590–1594.

Koshland, M. E., 1975, Structure and function of the J chain, *Adv. Immunol.* **20**:41–67.

Kownatzki, E., 1971, Studies on a fragment of human IgM macroglobulins related to the "J chain", *Eur. J. Immunol.* **1**:486–491.

Kownatzki, E., and Drescher, M., 1973, Antigen binding and complement fixing activity of IgM molecules reassociated in the presence and absence of J chains, *Clin. Exp. Immunol.* **15**:557–564.

Kunkel, H. G., 1974, Discussion section, *Adv. Exp. Med. Biol.* **45**:263.

Lamm, M. E., and Greenberg, J., 1972, Human secretory component: Comparison of the form occurring in exocrine immunoglobulin A to the free form, *Biochemistry* **11**:2744–2750.

Lawton, A. R., Asofsky, R., and Mage, R. G., 1970, Synthesis of secretory IgA in the rabbit, *J. Immunol.* **104**:388–396.

Lindh, E., 1975, Increased resistance of immunoglobulin A dimers to proteolytic degradation after binding of secretory component, *J. Immunol.* **114**:284–286.

Lindh, E., and Björk, I., 1976a, Binding of secretory component to dimers of immunoglobulin A *in vitro*, *Eur. J. Biochem.* **62**:263–270.

Lindh, E., and Björk, I., 1976b, Binding of secretory component to immunoglobulin IgM, *Eur. J. Biochem.* **62**:271–278.

Mach, J. P., 1970, *In vitro* combination of human and bovine free secretory component with IgA of various species, *Nature (London)* **228**:1278–1282.

Mehta, S. K., Plaut, A. G., Calvanico, N. J., and Tomasi, T. B., Jr., 1973, Human immunoglobulin A: Production of an Fc fragment by an enteric microbial proteolytic enzyme, *J. Immunol.* **111**:1274–1276.

Meinke, G. C., and Spiegelberg, H. L., 1974, Antigenic studies of J chain, *J. Immunol.* **112**:1401–1406.

Mendez, E., Frangione, B., and Franklin, E. C., 1973a, Structure of immunoglobulin A: Amino acid sequence of cysteine-containing peptides from the J chain, *Biochemistry* **12**:1119–1123.

Mendez, E., Prelli, F., Frangione, B., and Franklin, E. C., 1973b, Characterization of a disulfide bridge linking the J chain to the alpha chain of polymeric immunoglobulin A, *Biochem. Biophys. Res. Commun.* **55**:1291–1296.

Mestecky, J., 1977, Structural aspects of human polymeric IgA, *Ric. Clin. Lab.* (in press).

Mestecky, J., and Schrohenloher, R. E., 1974, Site of attachment of J chain to human immunoglobulin M, *Nature (London)* **249**:65 –652.

Mestecky, J., Zikan, J., and Butler, W. T., 1971, Immunoglobulin M and secretory immunoglobulin A: Presence of a common polypeptide chain different from light chains, *Science* **171**:1163–1165.

Mestecky, J., Kulhavy, R., and Kraus, F. W., 1972a, Studies on human secretory immunoglobulin A. II. Subunit structure, *J. Immunol.* **108**:738–747.

Mestecky, J., Zikan, J., Butler, W. T., and Kulhavy, R., 1972b, Studies on human secretory immunoglobulin A. III. J chain, *Immunochemistry* **9**:883–889.

Mestecky, J., Kulhavy, R., Wright, G. P., and Tomana, M., 1974a, Studies on human secretory immunoglobulin A. VI. Cyanogen bromide cleavage, *J. Immunol.* **113**:404–412.

Mestecky, J., Schrohenloher, R. E., Kulhavy, R., Wright, G. P., and Tomana, M., 1974b, Site of J chain attachment to human polymeric IgA, *Proc. Natl. Acad. Sci. U.S.A.* **71**:544–548.

Mestecky, J., Kulhavy, R., Schrohenloher, R. E., Tomana, M., and Wright, G. P., 1975, Identification and properties of J chain isolated from catfish macroglobulin, *J. Immunol.* **115**:993–997.

Morrison, S. L., and Koshland, M. E., 1972, Characterization of the J chain of human polymeric immunoglobulins, *Proc. Natl. Acad. Sci. U.S.A.* **69**:124–128.

Mosmann, T., and Baumal, R., 1975, Synthesis but not secretion of J chain by variant mouse myeloma cells which lose α-chain-synthesizing ability, *J. Immunol.* **115**:955–962.

Newcomb, R. W., Normansell, D., and Stanworth, D. R., 1968, A structural study of human exocrine IgA globulin, *J. Immunol.* **101**:905–914.

Niedermeier, W., Tomana, M., and Mestecky, J., 1972, The carbohydrate composition of J chain from human serum and secretory IgA, *Biochim. Biophys. Acat* **257**:527–530.

O'Daly, J. A., and Cebra, J. J., 1971, Chemical and physiocochemical studies of the component polypeptide chains of rabbit secretory immunoglobulin A, *Biochemistry* **10**:3843–3850.

Pahud, J. J., and Mach, J. P., 1970, Identification of secretory IgA, free secretory piece and serum IgA in the ovine and caprine species, *Immunochemistry* **7**:679–786.

Pahud, J. J., and Mach, J. P., 1972, Equine secretory IgA and secretory component, *Int. Arch. Allergy Appl. Immunol.* **42**:175–186.

Parkhouse, R. M. E., 1972, Biosynthesis of J chain in mouse immunoglobulin A [IgA] and IgM, *Nature (London) New Biol.* **236**:9–11.

Parkhouse, R. M. E., and Della Corte, E., 1973, Biosynthesis of immunoglobulin A (IgA) and immuno-globulin M (IgM), *Biochem. J.* **136**:607–609.

Plaut, A. G., and Tomasi, T. B., 1970, Immunoglobulin M: Pentameric Fcμ fragments released by trypsin at higher temperatures, *Proc. Natl. Acad. Sci. U.S.A.* **65**:318–322.

Poger, M. E., and Lamm, M. E., 1974, Localization of free and bound secretory component in human intestinal epithelial cells, *J. Exp. Med.* **139**:629–635.

Porter, P., and Allen, W. D., 1970, Intestinal IgA in the pig, *Experientia* **26**:90–95.

Rejnek, J., Kostka, J., and Kotynek, O., 1966, Electrophoretic behavior of H and L chains of human serum and colostrum gammaglobulin, *Nature (London)* **209**:926–928.

Reynolds, H. Y., and Johnson, J. S., 1971, Structural units of canine serum and secretory immunoglobu-lin A, *Biochemistry* **10**:2821–2827.

Ricardo, M. J., and Inman, F. P., 1974, The incorporation of J chain into reassembled human immuno-globulin M, *Biochem. J* **137**:79–83.

Ricardo, M. J., Brewer, J. M., and Inman, F. P., 1974, The molecular weight of J chains derived from human immunoglobulin M, *Biochem. J.* **137**:79–83.

Rosenstein, R. W., and Jackson, P., 1973, The binding of a naphthalene dye associated with J chain attachment in an immunoglobulin A mouse immunoglobulin, *Biochemistry* **12**:1659–1664.

Schrohenloher, R. E., Mestecky, J., and Stanton, T. H., 1973, Molecular weight of a human J chain, *Biochim. Biophys. Acta* **295**:576–581.

Sletten, K., Christensen, T. B., and Brandtzaeg, P., 1975, Human secretory component. III. Carbohy-drates, amino acids, and *N*-terminal sequence, *Immunochemistry* **12**:783–785.

South, M. A., Cooper, M. D., Wollheim, F. A., Hong, R., and Good, R. A., 1966, The IgA system. I. Studies of the transport and immunochemistry of IgA in the saliva, *J. Exp. Med.* **123**:615–627.

Stott, D. I., 1976, Biosynthesis and assembly of IgM: Addition of J chain to intracellular pools of 8 S and 19 S IgM, *Immunochemistry* **13**:157–159.

Svehag, S. E., and Bloth, B., 1970, Ultra-structure of secretory and high polymer serum immunoglobulin A of human and rabbit origin, *Science* **168**:847–849.

Svensson, S., Lindh, E., Lindahl, U., and Björk, I., in press.

Thompson, R. E., Reynolds, H. Y., and Waxdal, M. J., 1975, Structural composition of canine secretory component and immunoglobulin A, *Biochemistry* **14**:2853–2859.

Tomasi, T. B., 1965, Studies on the Immunoglobulin A Proteins of Serum and Nonvascular Fluids, Ph.D. thesis, Rockefeller University.

Tomasi, T. B., and Bienenstock, J., 1968, Secretory immunoglobulins, *Adv. Immunol.* **9**:1–96.

Tomasi, T. B., and Calvanico, N., 1968, Human secretory γA, *Fed. Am. Soc. Exp. Biol. Fed. Proc.* **27**:617 (abstract).

Tomasi, T. B., and Capra, J. D., 1974, Discussion section, *Adv. Exp. Med. Biol.* **45**:263.

Tomasi, T. B., and Grey, H. M., 1972, Structure and function of immunoglobulin A, *Prog. Allergy* **16**:81–185.

Tomasi, T. B., and Hauptman, S., 1974, Modulation of the assembly of immunoglobulin subunits by J chain, *Adv. Exp. Med. Biol.* **45**:111–120.

Underdown, B. J., 1975, Is secretory component disulfide-bonded to both monomer subunits in human secretory IgA dimer?, *Biochem. Biophys. Res. Commun.* **62**:54–62.

Vaerman, J. P., Naccache-Corbic, M. C., and Heremans, J. F., 1975, Secretory component of the guinea pig, *Immunology* **29**:933–937.

van Munster, P. J. J., Stoelinga, G. B. A., and Poels-Zanders, S., 1971, Isolation of free secretory component (S.C.) from human milk, determination of its molecular weight, *Immunochemistry* **8**:471–477.

Weicker, J., and Underdown, B. J., 1975, A study of the association of human secretory component with IgA and IgM proteins, *J. Immunol.* **114**:1337–1344.

Weinheimer, P. F., Mestecky, J., and Acton, R. T., 1971, Species distribution of J chain, *J. Immunol.* **107**:1211–1212.

Wilde, C. E., and Koshland, M. E., 1973, Molecular size and shape of the J chain from polymeric immunoglobulins, *Biochemistry* **12**:3218–3224.

Zikan, J., 1973, J chain in pig immunoglobulin, *Immunochemistry* **10**:351–354.

6

The Structural Basis for the Biological Properties of Immunoglobulins

J. MICHAEL KEHOE

1. Introduction

Immunoglobulins (Ig's) are polyfunctional molecules. The most thoroughly studied, and currently best understood, of the numerous functions of this protein family is antigen-binding, a subject that is discussed in detail in several other chapters of this volume. The various other functions are collectively referred to as the *biological properties,* or *effector functions,* of antibodies. These properties are mediated by the constant (C) regions of the heavy (H) chains of the various Ig molecules. In fact, most of the properties recognized at present have been associated with that carboxyterminal subcomponent of the H-chain C region referred to as the Fc (constant) segment, or fragment.

A considerable number of biological properties of Ig's have been recognized and studied to varying degrees up to the present. Such properties are listed in Table 1. There is considerable reason to believe that future research may uncover additional, presently unappreciated, properties that have definite physiological significance. In addition, it seems likely, on the basis of contemporary analyses of previous evolutionary trends, that future evolutionary developments, such as the appearance of additional subclasses of Ig's through H-chain C-region gene duplication and divergence, will be due, at least in part, to favorable selection pressures for still other Ig biological properties, the exact nature of which we can perceive only dimly at present.

2. Nature of Immunoglobulin Biological Properties

In a general sense, the biological properties of Ig's play two major functional roles. They may come into play after the antibody has bound antigen and serve to

J. MICHAEL KEHOE • Department of Microbiology/Immunology, The Northeastern Ohio Universities College of Medicine, Rootstown, Ohio 44272.

TABLE 1. Currently Known Biological Properties (Effector Functions) of Immunoglobulin Molecules

Antigen-dependent properties
1. Complement fixation (classical pathway)
2. Complement fixation (alternate pathway)
3. Opsonic activity (neutrophils and monocytes)

Antigen-independent properties
1. Attachment to mast cells and basophils
2. Macrophage-binding
3. Lymphocyte-binding
4. Placental-passage regulation
5. Intestinal-passage regulation
6. Immunoglobulin-catabolism regulation
7. Passive cutaneous anaphylaxis (PCA)
8. Interaction with protein "A" of *Staphylococcus aureus*
9. Antigenic target for rheumatoid factors

amplify or extend the physiological consequences of antigen-binding (the true *effector function* of Edelman, 1970). A prototypic function of this sort is complement fixation by the classical pathway. Alternatively, the biological property capability of an antibody might assure that the molecule is available in a particular site to provide for a *subsequent* encounter with some antigen with which its variable (V) region is able to interact. Examples of this type of property would be regulated passage across a membrane such as the placenta, or the specific attachment to a cell that is likely to encounter antigen, such as a macrophage. Some other biological properties, such as the interaction of antigenic determinants of the Fc segment with rheumatoid factors, may simply represent pathological, or even incidental, consequences of certain structural attributes of the H-chain C region.

Given the multiplicity of biological properties characteristic of the Ig family, it is not always clear exactly what teleological significance any given function has at a given moment. Certainly the Fc region is subjected to a wide variety of distinct selection pressures that are doubtless mutually contradictory on some occasions. For example, a protein structure ideal for complement fixation may be quite inappropriate for the mediation of the passage of this very molecule across a placental membrane. A unique pressure on the Fc region of many Ig's is thus to provide for the *simultaneous* presence of a number of functional capabilities that may be required on different occasions. All attempts to relate structure to function for this region of the antibody molecule must take this fact into account. It seems clear that this kind of selection pressure has been an important element in the appearance of the numerous classes and subclasses of Ig's that have been observed to date among the various species.

2.1. Antigen-Dependent Properties

2.1.1. Complement Fixation (Classical Pathway)

This is clearly one of the most important biological properties of Ig's. It is a prototypic effector function, as mentioned previously, in that it amplifies the effect of antigen-binding and leads to the capacity for directed cell-membrane destruction and the generation of physiologically active by-products. The subject of the complement cascade itself has been exhaustively reviewed elsewhere (Müller-Eberhard, 1975; Good and Day, 1977) and will not be considered further here. The precise mechanism by which an Ig molecule initiates the classical complement cascade is a relevant and controversial subject, however, and is worthy of additional comment.

The first significant point to emphasize is that not all Ig molecules are capable of interacting with C1q, the subcomponent of the intact first component (C1) of the complement system that is known to provide the linkage between the Ig and complement systems (Schumaker *et al.*, 1976). Table 2 summarizes this information for human Ig's. Clearly, some of the C-region structural differences among these various proteins are responsible for the modulation of their respective capacities to interact with the C1q molecule. As discussed below, there are, as yet, no definitive correlations between the primary structure of localized segments of Ig H-chain C regions and the presence or absence of the complement-binding function. Some recent studies with synthetic peptides do suggest, however, that such correlations may soon be forthcoming (Johnson and Thames, 1976; Prystowsky *et al.*, 1977).

There is no question concerning the dependence of the expression of a latent C1q-binding potentiality of an antibody on the union of this antibody with antigen. One indication of this dependence is the general observation that normal antibodies in serum, or myeloma proteins alone, do not initiate the complement cascade. Such an Ig may be induced to bind C1q with sufficient affinity to stimulate the classical complement cascade, however, if its V region does bind an appropriate antigen, or if the molecule is sufficiently distorted, as by heat denaturation or intramolecular cross-linking by chemical reagents. The latter processes presumably mimic, to some extent at least, alterations in the antibody molecule that occur subsequent to the specific binding of an antigen.

One of the most controversial aspects concerning the mechanisms of activation of the classical complement cascade by Ig is the question whether or not a conformational change in the antibody due to antigen-binding is responsible for the induction of the C1q-binding capacity. Strong views and considerable experimental data have been cited on both sides of the issue. For example, Metzger (1974), in a most thorough analysis of the general question of the effects of antigen-binding on antibody, pointed out that three different kinds of processes could be envisioned to

175

THE STRUCTURAL
BASIS FOR THE
BIOLOGICAL
PROPERTIES OF
IMMUNOGLOBULINS

TABLE 2. Interaction of Human Immunoglobulins with the C1q Subcomponent of the Complement System

Protein	Interaction capacity
IgM	+++
IgG1	+++
IgG2	++
IgG3	++++
IgG4	+
IgA1	−
IgA2	−
IgD	−
IgE	−

account for the induction of latent activities in antibody molecules:

1. An *allosteric* model. As the name suggests, this process would involve an antigen-induced conformational change in the antibody, utilizing the energy of binding in the V region, to reveal appropriate binding sites in other segments of the molecule, such as the Fc region. Such a process obviously assumes some kind of signal passage from the Fab (antigen-binding) to the Fc region, an occurrence numerous investigators have found difficult to establish.
2. A *distortive* model. This process would result from the marked stretching of the antibody molecule that could occur when widely spaced antigenic determinants were bound by a multivalent antibody.
3. An *associative* model. This model sees the role of antigen as merely bringing several or many antibody molecules into close physical approximation to one another. The associated molecules, *as a group,* could possess functional capabilities that individual antibodies would possess only very weakly, or not at all. The capacity to bind C1q could be one such function.

The analysis by Metzger (1974) of all the published experiments then available on the structure of Ig's and their degradation products, the properties of antigen–antibody complexes, and the requirements of antigen participation in complement fixation led him to conclude that there was little evidence to be found for both his allosteric and distortive models and that one was consequently left, by difference, with the associative model, which was consistent with all the known experimental data. This interpretation has not been formally refuted in the intervening period, but, as will be shown below, additional experiments suggesting the occurrence of antigen-induced conformational alterations of antibody have been reported.

Lancet and Pecht (1976) studied the kinetics of hapten-binding to a homogeneous murine IgA myeloma protein by chemical relaxation. The observance of two relaxation times, one bimolecular and the other monomolecular, were interpreted by these authors as kinetic evidence for a conformational change in the Ig induced by the bound ligand. They considered their data consistent with an allosteric model for the effect of antigen or antibody.

Brown and Koshland (1975) analyzed the reaction of an induced IgM antihapten antibody (anti-phenyl-β-lactoside, or Lac) and various hapten conjugates with respect to the complement-binding function. These workers found that the capacity to fix complement was independent of the presence of antigen–antibody aggregates as revealed by analytical ultracentrifugation. Brown and Koshland thus inferred that some intrinsic changes in the IgM molecule itself had occurred. To distinguish whether this intrinsic change was due to extensive cross-linkage by multivalent antigen (distortion) or to a conformational change transmitted to Fc (allosterism), monovalent Lac reagents were prepared. Since these reagents, when reacted with the anti-Lac antibody, resulted in complement fixation levels essentially as high as the multivalent preparations, it was concluded that an allosteric rather than a distortive mechanism was operative, and that the structural changes associated with the binding of an antigenic determinant are not restricted to the Fab segment, but are transmitted across domains to the Fc region. It is conceivable, however, that the mechanisms of C1q-binding that hold for the polymeric IgM molecule may not be valid for IgG.

177

THE STRUCTURAL
BASIS FOR THE
BIOLOGICAL
PROPERTIES OF
IMMUNOGLOBULINS

Some recent evidence from X-ray diffraction analyses of IgG's provided some suggestions as to how alterations in the Fc region could be induced by antigen-binding in Fab. For example, Deisenhofer and Huber and their colleagues (Deisenhofer *et al.*, 1976; Huber *et al.*, 1977) interpreted their crystallographic data of a human IgG1 molecule to indicate a highly flexible molecule in solution when antigen is not bound. These workers suggest, however, that once a specific ligand is bound to the Fab region, a pronounced stiffening of the molecule could occur due to increased *longitudinal* interdomain contact from the Fab region toward Fc. Such structural alterations could unmask previously covered C1q-binding sites or could induce an Fc structural change (in the C_H2 domain see Section 3.1) that increased the affinity of the Ig for C1q. This conception thus also offers support for the allosteric model as described by Metzger (1974).

Another indication of an antigen-induced conformational change in the Fc region was observed by Schlessinger *et al.* (1975). These authors analyzed the conformational changes induced in a number of different antigen–antibody systems by studying the circular polarization of fluorescence due to tryptophan residues. Using this technique, they observed changes in the conformation of intact antibodies that differed from those characteristic of the Fab region alone. They thus inferred that some Fab–Fc interaction and, very likely, an alteration in the conformation of the Fc region had occurred due to antigen-binding. The studies also indicated that the integrity of the inter-H-chain disulfide bonds was essential for the transmission of the conformational alteration to the Fc region.

Thus, in the several years that have elapsed since the analysis by Metzger (1974) of the possible mechanisms for signal transmission from the region of antigen contact in the Fab segment to the Fc region where most biological properties are mediated, several pieces of evidence for allosteric transformation have been obtained. Still, no absolute proof of such transitions has been put forth. The definitive resolution of this question may well require crystallographic data on the *same molecule* in both the native and ligand-bound states. In the meantime, the associative model remains an appealing, if equally difficult to prove, hypothesis.

2.1.2. Complement Fixation (Alternate Pathway)

The existence of this system, now considered the equivalent of the properdin system originally described by Pillemer (Müller-Eberhard, 1975), is no longer in doubt. The system involves the direct activation of the complement cascade at the level of C3, rather than having the C1,4,2 interaction sequence as a preliminary. Among the human Ig's, both IgA and IgE have been reported to participate in the alternate pathway (Gotze and Müller-Eberhard, 1971; Ishizaka, T., *et al.*, 1971). The exact mechanism of activation of this pathway by these two classes is not known, although some kind of interaction with "initiating factor," or IF (Müller-Eberhard, 1974), seems likely to be involved, as it presumably is with other activators of this system.

2.1.3. Opsonic Activity (Neutrophils and Monocytes)

It has been known for some time that IgG's are cytophilic for neutrophils (Messner and Jelinek, 1970; Ishizaka, K., *et al.*, 1970) and macrophages (Huber *et al.,* 1971). This phenomenon can be quite logically, and experimentally, associated with the long-known phenomenon of opsonization, that process whereby phagocytosis is enhanced in the presence of specific antibody. For both macrophages and neutrophils, the binding of the antibody is known to occur through the interaction of some site within the Fc region of the antibody and a specific cell-membrane receptor. The specificity of the membrane receptor for the Fc region was originally shown by inhibition experiments using appropriate purified Fc fragments (Berken and Benacerraf, 1966). As with the complement system, an antigen-induced effect on cells that possess bound antibody specific for that antigen could occur by several mechanisms. An antigen-induced conformational change, or allosteric effect, could clearly play a role here, in principle. One study (Phillips-Quagliata *et al.,* 1971) indicated, however, that the simple aggregation of bound cell receptors by polyvalent antigen (associative model) could lead to improved binding. This question may have to be reexamined in the light of the more recent evidence for conformational changes in complement-binding referred to above.

An important, and unique, feature of biological activities involving the cell-binding of antibody concerns the fact that the Fc-mediated binding usually occurs *before* the binding of antigen to the Fab segment. In the binding of C1q, the preponderance of evidence suggests that no matter what the actual mechanism involved, the antigen-binding step occurs first. In the opsonic process, the Ig is obviously serving as a bifunctional link between the foreign antigen (e.g., *Staphylococcus aureus*) and a cell that is capable of destroying this organism. The physiological advantages of such facilitated ingestion are clear.

Not all Ig's are capable of fixing to the cell-membrane receptors, a situation again analogous to that previously discussed with respect to C1q-binding (see Table 2). Many studies (e.g., Huber *et al.,* 1971) have shown that the human IgG1 and IgG3 subclasses bind with the highest affinity. Other workers (Lawrence *et al.,* 1975) find that IgG4 proteins will also bind to neutrophils and monocytes. These investigators also observed that IgA1 and IgA2 proteins, as well as secretory IgA, would bind to neutrophils but not to monocytes. In this study, native Ig's bound with a higher affinity than did the Fc fragment alone. Also, even though significant inhibition of binding of intact IgG could be obtained with Fc fragments alone, significantly greater inhibition was noted using other intact IgG molecules. This observation may well be related to the increased state of flexibility of the intact IgG molecule as compared with its constituent proteolytic fragments, as observed in the X-ray diffraction studies of Deisenhofer *et al.* (1976). Of considerable interest was the observation of Lawrence *et al.* (1975) that different IgG subclasses were capable of cross-inhibition, indicating that the cell-membrane receptor was not specific for subclass. No reciprocal inhibition was observed for the IgG and IgA proteins, however, suggesting the presence of distinct membrane receptors for these two classes of Ig's.

Lawrence *et al.* (1975) also found that particularly for IgG, mild reduction and alkylation markedly reduced cytophilic activity for monocytes. This implies that the Fc sites involved in this function are very sensitive to the influence of the interchain disulfide bonds on the conformational state of the intact protein.

It is therefore evident that the capacity to interact with specific cell-membrane receptors on monocytes and neutrophils is one of the most important biological properties of antibodies. This function, which is responsible for specific opsoniza-

tion, is not possessed by all antibody proteins, however. We need to know
considerably more about the chemistry of the interaction between the Ig and the cell
receptors and, especially, additional details concerning the effect of antigen-binding
on the relationship of the bound antibody to the cell to which it is bound.

179

THE STRUCTURAL
BASIS FOR THE
BIOLOGICAL
PROPERTIES OF
IMMUNOGLOBULINS

2.2. Antigen-Independent Properties

2.2.1. Attachment to Mast Cells and Basophils

The significance of this Fc function is almost exclusively related to the extraordinary affinity of IgE, the reaginic antibody, for specific receptors on the cell membrane of basophils and mast cells (Ishizaka, T., and Ishizaka, 1975), an occurrence that is responsible for an important amount of clinical disease in the form of immediate hypersensitivity reactions in both man and lower animal species. The other Ig classes show little or no affinity for these cell types, a fact that was important in leading the Ishizakas to reason, before the discovery of IgE, that some then unknown Ig species was responsible for reaginic activity. This conception allowed a reassessment of the idea that a previously known class of Ig, β_{2A}-globulin or IgA, was associable with reaginic activity (Heremans and Vaerman, 1962; Fireman et al., 1963). The careful purification of a reagin-rich fraction from whole human serum led to the recognition of a unique Ig class that was antigenically distinct from any of the known human Ig proteins (Ishizaka, K., et al., 1966). The existence of this separate class, termed IgE, was definitively established when the properties of the isolated reagin were shown to correspond exactly to those of a newly discovered class of myeloma paraproteins (Bennich et al., 1969). Subsequent studies, both fundamental and applied, have amply confirmed the validity of the conclusion that IgE is the Ig responsible for reaginic activity. To date, no subclasses of the IgE class have been identified.

There is no evidence that the antigen-combining function of IgE molecules is mediated in a manner any different from that of other Ig's (see Chapters 1, 4, and 11). This observation is totally consistent with the concept of the two gene–one polypeptide chain hypothesis and the translocation of V-region genes as applied to the Ig system (see Chapter 9). Clearly, the most novel and significant structural feature involving the IgE molecule concerns its Fc component and its affinity for specific receptors on the surface of mast cells and basophils. The interaction is specific in that only mast calls and basophils, and not neutrophils, eosinophils, and monocytes, have the capacity to bind IgE (Ishizaka, K., et al., 1970b; Sullivan et al., 1971). The exact nature of the basophil-membrane IgE Fc receptor is not known at present. Cell-membrane components containing the receptor have been isolated, however, from disrupted basophils (Carson et al., 1975; Isersky et al., 1977), and knowledge about receptor properties is accumulating rapidly.

A number of attempts have been made to estimate the number of IgE molecules specifically bound to basophils. In one study (Ishizaka, T., et al., 1973), 10,000–40,000 IgE molecules per cell were found. Most interestingly, the values were more or less the same for both normal and atopic individuals. The number of IgE molecules on basophils from normal individuals could be increased severalfold, however, by incubation of the cells with pure, exogenous IgE, while the number on the cells of atopic patients could not be so increased. Since a proportion of the bound IgE could be replaced by adding exogenous IgE under appropriate conditions (Ishizaka, T., *et al.*, 1973), the binding is clearly a reversible process. This is obviously an important point relevant to possible attempts to intervene in the binding process.

Kulcyzcki and Metzger (1974) examined quantitative aspects of the binding of rat IgE to rat basophils that grow as cultivable leukemia cells. These studies showed that the rat cells contained an average of 1×10^6 receptor sites for IgE per cell, and that the average equilibrium constant for the Ig–receptor interaction was 9×10^9 M^{-1}. These cells thus had a larger total number of IgE receptor sites than did the human cells alluded to earlier.

Taken together, the various results to date concerning the dynamics of the IgE–cell receptor interaction imply that the sensitivity of a given mast cell to a given allergen is a function of the number of IgE molecules *with V-region specificity for that allergen* that are bound to that cell. The higher the number of such bound antibodies, the greater the sensitivity of that cell for that allergen. Possible mechanisms of cell triggering by the allergen–IgE cell receptor complex are described below.

As with complement fixation and the interaction of antigen–antibody complexes with the receptors of other cell types, it is important to try to understand the exact role of the Ig in effecting the release of pharmacological mediators by a specifically sensitized mast cell or basophil. *A priori,* the allosteric, distortive, or associative model of Metzger (1974) could be applied to the IgE–basophil system. While the data are not as complete as one might wish, the observations that IgE not bound to antigen binds to basophils with a high affinity (10^8–10^9 M^{-1}) and that preformed allergen–IgE complexes also bind to reactive cells (Ishizaka, K., and Ishizaka, 1968) could be taken to mean that an antigen-induced allosteric change does not play a major role in the Fc–receptor interaction.

An explicit proposal for a bridging, or associative, model of IgE triggering was put forth by K. Ishizaka and Ishizaka (1971). This suggestion is based on the following observations: (1) monomeric IgE binds strongly to basophils (e.g. a myeloma protein), but will not, by itself, elicit degranulation; (2) univalent fragments (Fab) of anti-IgE antibodies will not cause degranulation of cells to which intact IgE molecules are affixed; (3) any form of cross-linking of bound IgE including that induced by antigen, or anti-IgE antibodies, or anti-light-chain antibodies, does lead to cell degranulation; (4) the bound Fc fragment of IgE, when cross-linked either by antibody or by chemical means such as bis-diazotized benzidine, will lead to degranulation; and (5) finally, preformed allergen–IgE complexes will induce degranulation, but only when the complexes are not formed in extreme antigen excess where a large number of complexes with the stoichiometric relation ship Ag_2Ab_1 exists. Such complexes would preclude the ready formation of extensive bridging between the various IgE molecules on the cell surface. Thus, although a number of additional details concerning the participation of IgE, and particularly its Fc segment, in cellular stimulation remain to be worked out, the current evidence favors some kind of associative phenomenon as playing a major role. Further understanding will more likely require more information concerning the basophil-cell membrane and the disposition of its Fc receptors than further data concerning the IgE molecule itself.

181

THE STRUCTURAL
BASIS FOR THE
BIOLOGICAL
PROPERTIES OF
IMMUNOGLOBULINS

As indicated above, contrary to earlier reports (Ishizaka, K., and Ishizaka, 1971), the IgE molecule can fix the terminal components of the complement system through the alternate (properdin) pathway. The significance of this capacity for the pathogenesis of allergic disease is not totally clear at the moment.

2.2.2. Macrophage-Binding

There is no evidence so far that this process differs in any significant respects from the binding of Ig to monocytes discussed in Section 2.1.3, a not unexpected observation given the close relationship of these two cell types. It is nonetheless conceivable that additional study will discern some minor differences akin to those that have been observed between other related cell types, as, for example, the difference in binding of IgA by neutrophils (positive) vs. basophils (negative). In this context, it is perhaps noteworthy that Rhodes (1973) observed a receptor for monomeric IgM on guinea pig macrophages, while Lawrence *et al.* (1975) did not detect any significant binding of human IgM to human monocytes when in either the monomeric (8 S) or polymeric (19 S) form. Of course, the possibility of significant species differences cannot be completely ruled out in such cases.

2.2.3. Lymphocyte-Binding

The *passive* binding of exogenous, cytophilic antibody to lymphocytes, as contrasted with the short-term membrane association of a monoclonal protein that has been synthesized in a given cell, has received increased attention recently (Wisloff *et al.*, 1974; Lawrence *et al.*, 1975; Ramasamy *et al.*, 1975). The studies of Lawrence *et al.* (1975) showed that, in the native state, only the IgG1 and IgG3 subclasses bound to human lymphocytes. The IgG2 and IgG4 subclasses, as well as IgM, IgA1, IgA2, IgD, and IgE proteins, were negative. Preaggregation of the proteins showed, however, that the IgG2 and IgG4 subclasses, as well as IgE, but not members of the other classes, could be induced to bind to lymphocytes. As in the case of the neutrophil and monocyte systems, reciprocal inhibition of the binding of *native* IgG1 and IgG3 proteins was observed, indicating the lack of subclass specificity of the membrane receptor.

Basten *et al.* (1972) had earlier presented evidence for the presence of a receptor for antibodies on the surface of murine B lymphocytes. These authors postulated that antibody bound to these receptors might well participate in antibody-mediated cytotoxicity as well as function to concentrate antigen as a prelude to an active immune response. Dickler and Kunkel (1972) demonstrated that aggregated human γ-globulin will bind to a subpopulation of human B cells. The results with unaggregated proteins were less consistent, possibly because of an unfavorable display or concentration of the appropriate Fc binding sites. The region on the B-cell membrane surface involved in binding the preaggregated γ-globulin was distinct from that occupied by the cell's own surface Ig.

A most interesting surface receptor for the Fc region of IgG was observed on a subpopulation of murine T lymphocytes by Stout and Herzenberg (1975). These cells, which were analyzed by the fluorescence-activated cell sorter, were shown to be unrelated to T helper cells. The functional significance of this Ig–cell interaction remains to be elucidated.

It is of considerable interest that both native and aggregated IgM proteins fail to bind to the lymphocyte in view of the established role of nascent IgM as an antigen receptor on the clonally committed lymphocyte. Two distinct mechanisms may well be involved in these two processes. The question merits further study.

2.2.4. Placental-Passage Regulation

A number of species, including man, are known to receive the major part of their passive, maternal, humoral immune protection by the passage of Ig across the placental membrane from mother to fetus. Although passive immunity is indeed the result, the process by which this antibody transfer occurs is by no means passive. In fact, it is now known to involve still another specific interaction between a site, or sites, in the Fc region of the relevant Ig's and a membrane receptor on placental cells. Such a specific Ig–cell receptor interaction was first postulated by Brambell (Brambell *et al.*, 1960; Brambel, 1966) for the passage of rabbit Ig across the yolk sac membrane. These investigators localized the placental-passage function to the Fc region just shortly after the discovery of the Fc region itself. As pointed out by McNabb *et al.* (1976), however, the process by which a mesodermal organ such as the placenta modulates Ig passage might well differ considerably from that characteristic of an entodermal organ such as the yolk sac, or the digestive tract in the case of those species that derive their passive maternal antibody from colostrum after birth. Until recently, the details of neither process (yolk sac or placenta) have been analyzed in much greater detail.

The studies of McNabb *et al.* (1976) established that the human placenta possesses unique receptors that bind Ig's of the IgG class. They further showed that the affinity of the various IgG subclasses varied as follows: IgG1 = IgG3 > IgG4 > IgG2. Neither IgM nor IgA proteins bound to this receptor, a finding that is in accord with the long-standing clinical observation that neither of these classes appears in normal human fetal serum.

An IgG1 Fc fragment bound to these placental receptor molecules just as efficiently as the native molecule, but in contrast to the situation with the intact Ig, the binding capacity of Fc was not affected by mild reduction and alkylation. The binding of the whole IgG1 molecule was totally abolished by such treatment. This observation may also be rationalizable by the observed differences alluded to previously concerning the flexibility of the intact molecule as compared with its subfragments, as inferred from the results of X-ray diffraction studies (Huber *et al.*, 1976).

2.2.5. Intestinal-Passage Regulation

As indicated above, not all species provide for the passage of a significant amount of passive humoral immunity from mother to fetus *in utero* by Ig transport across the placental membrane. Many such species, which include rodents and ruminants (Brambell, 1970), among other animals, obtain the largest proportion of their maternal humoral immune protection through the intake of colostrum and the passage of antibody across the intestinal epithelium into the fetal circulation. The mechanism of this passage has not been thoroughly analyzed from a molecular point of view for any species. Guyer *et al.* (1976), however, recently studied this phenomenon in some detail in the newborn mouse, with special emphasis on the binding of Ig molecules to epithelial-cell receptors in the gut. The experiments showed that while IgG proteins were readily transported across the lining epithelium, IgA and IgM were not. The latter two classes were tested in both their monomeric and polymeric forms. In addition, neither of the polymeric classes was able to compete for epithelial binding sites for the IgG antibodies.

Within the four subclasses of murine IgG, some differences in intestinal transport were observed. The IgG2a and IgG1 subclasses each effectively inhibited the binding of proteins or the other subclasses to the epithelial-cell receptors. Guyer and co-workers proposed, on the basis of their studies, that affinities of the various subclasses for the IgG receptor could be ranked as follows: IgG2a = IgG1 > IgG2b ≃ IgG3. This hierarchy, as determined experimentally, correlates exactly with the levels of these various Ig's that are found in normal mouse milk, and one thus has considerable confidence that it is a physiologically meaningful and significant pattern. The determination of additional characteristics of the receptor itself will require its isolation in pure form. This will permit an investigation of, among other details, whether the relevant receptors bear any significant resemblances to other IgG receptors, such as those associated with neutrophil or macrophage membranes. In addition, the active transport of Ig across the intestinal epithelium should be investigated in more detail in other species, such as ruminants, to define significant interspecies similarities and differences related to this important component of the humoral immune system.

2.2.6. Immunoglobulin-Catabolism Regulation

The period of time a given Ig remains in the circulation is closely regulated. The rate of removal of these proteins, and their rate of synthesis, are the main determinants for the establishment of the serum concentration of the various classes and subclasses. As illustrated for human proteins in Table 3, there is considerable variation among the various members of the Ig family regarding the exact values for degradation and synthesis rates. The synthetic rate is, of course, determined by the usual variables that govern protein synthesis, as well as by the extent of the antigenic stimulation of the lymphoid system. The degradation rate, however, is largely a function of some intrinsic property of the Ig molecule itself. Previous

TABLE 3. Parameters Related to the Serum Concentration of Various Human Immunoglobulins[a]

Parameter	IgG1	IgG2	IgG3	IgG4	IgA1	IgA2	IgM	IgD	IgE
Half-life (days)	23	23	16	23	6	6	5.1	2.8	2.5
Catabolic rate (% turnover per day)	7	7	17	7	25	?	18	37	89
Synthetic rate (mg/kg per day)	25	?	3.4	?	24	?	6.7	0.4	0.016
Serum concentration (mg/ml)	5–12	2–6	0.5–1	0.2–1	0.5–2	0–0.2	0.5–1.5	0–0.4	0–0.002

[a]Comparable patterns undoubtedly exist for Ig's of lower species, but these patterns have not been determined in as great detail. Based on Eisen (1974).

studies (for a review, see Waldmann *et al.*, 1971) have shown the importance of the Fc component in the regulation of Ig catabolism. Such studies have, in the main, shown that the Fc fragment of the various Ig's are cleared from the circulation at a rate that corresponds to that of the intact molecule, while the Fab segment alone is cleared much faster. The most common interpretation of this observation is that the Fc region is responsible for the regulation of the catabolic rate of the intact molecule. The complexity of the situation is pointed up by the observations of Spiegelberg and Fishkin (1972), who showed that the differences in clearance rates for the IgG3 subclass (Table 3) could not be attributed to the Fc region alone, since both isolated Fc regions themselves and H-chain disease proteins are catabolized at the same rate irrespective of the subclass of origin. It is conceivable that the unique hinge region of the human IgG3 subclass (Michaelsen *et al.*, 1977), with its duplicated segments that contribute to the increased length of this γ chain, could modulate the rate of removal of this particular subclass by whatever mechanism is involved. There nonetheless seems to be little question of a primary involvement for the Fc segment in this biological property, since, as discussed in Section 3.1, Dorrington and Painter and their associates showed unequivocally that an isolated domain of the IgG Fc region, not just the intact fragment, shares the clearance rate characteristic of the parent protein. The location and nature of any cell-membrane receptors that interact with the site, or sites, on the Ig molecule to initiate the catabolic process have not yet been defined.

2.2.7. Passive Cutaneous Anaphylaxis

Passive cutaneous anaphylaxis (PCA) is an experimental laboratory technique suitable for demonstrating the binding of certain antibody molecules to cells in the skin of the living animal (Ovary, 1964). The response is due mainly to the release of pharmacologically active mediators from mast cells. While the phenomenon is not a totally natural process in the sense that it could be considered a part of the body's normal physiology, it is nevertheless believed to reflect properties of antibodies that are important to some of their physiological functions. In addition, the PCA reaction provides a highly sensitive assay for antibody quantitation. The results of numerous studies have indicated that the area of the antibody involved in the mediation of this function is the Fc region. As discussed below, the exact segment of the Fc region that is involved is subject to controversy at present. Since a number of different Ig's from a variety of species exhibit PCA reactivity, it is possible that more than one binding mechanism is operative in this biological property of antibodies.

The reaction involves the intradermal injection of the material to be tested into the skin of a test animal, usually a rat or guinea pig. After a suitable interval (4 hr) to allow for the possible cellular fixation of the Ig, a challenge reagent is injected intravenously together with a marker dye, usually Evans blue. This challenge reagent can be an antigen with which the putative test antibody will react, or an antibody with specificity (e.g., anti-Fc) for the test protein. If the test material has bound to the skin sites, a vascular reaction leading to a pronounced circular lesion, accentuated by blue dye, will be apparent in the skin. If the test material has not bound, there will be no such reaction. The dependence of the PCA reaction on the Fc region is illustrated by the negative reaction of $F(ab')_2$ and Fab fragments of known positive Ig's.

2.2.8. Interaction with Protein 'A' of *Staphylococcus aureus*

185

THE STRUCTURAL
BASIS FOR THE
BIOLOGICAL
PROPERTIES OF
IMMUNOGLOBULINS

The presence of an extractable product in *Staph. aureus* that could interact with normal γ-globulin was first observed by Jensen (1958). This interaction was first considered a classic antigen–antibody reaction (i.e., a reaction with what is now known as the antigen-combining site in the Fab region of an antibody), as suggested in the title of Jensen's original article. In 1966, however, Forsgren and Sjoquist (1966) made the surprising observation that protein A did not, in fact, react with the Fab region of the IgG molecule, but rather was bound to the Fc segment. Although IgG isolated from a wide variety of mammalian species will react with protein A (Kronvall *et al.*, 1970), there is still a rather remarkable specificity shown within the members of the human IgG class, since no reaction can be demonstrated with proteins of the IgG3 subclass, even though all three of the other subclasses react strongly (Kronvall and Williams, 1969). The precise structural basis for this distinction has not yet been worked out, although the unique hinge region of the IgG3 protein would have to be considered strongly (Michaelsen *et al.*, 1977).

It was shown that at least two, and possibly more, molecules of IgG are bound per molecule of protein A (Sjoquist *et al.*, 1972). The rationale for this observation was made clearer by the results of amino acid sequence analysis of protein A. Although the complete sequence has not yet been determined, the partial sequence (Sjödahl, 1976) suggests the presence of three highly conserved regions of internal homology, each of which could serve as a binding site for an IgG molecule. The accuracy of this prediction and the detailed stoichiometry involved will have to await additional structural analyses of this protein.

The biological significance of the activity of protein A and its possible effect on the host–parasite relationship, though it has been extensively discussed, remains unclear. Strains of *Staph. aureus* with a high content of protein A are readily agglutinated in normal serum, a process that clearly could have an influence on the pathogenesis of staphylococcal disease. An effect that could be advantageous to the growth and spread of the bacterium was described by Forsgren and Nordström (1974). These workers demonstrated that protein A had a markedly inhibitory effect on the heat-labile opsonins of serum. The antiphagocytic effect could be demonstrated with both *Staph. aureus* and *Escherichia coli,* and was demonstrably independent of any direct effect on the phagocytic cell, the human neutrophil in this case.

It therefore seems that although the exact nature and extent of the effects of the staphylococcus–IgG interaction on this host–parasite relationship are unclear, some consequences favorable to the host (e.g., agglutination of bacteria) and others favorable to the bacterium (e.g., antiphagocytic effect) do occur. The full teleological significance of the interaction obviously requires further definition.

2.2.9. Antigenic Target for Rheumatoid Factors

The serum of patients with a number of chronic diseases, including rheumatoid arthritis, often contains Ig proteins the antibody-combining sites of which are directed toward antigenic determinants of other Ig's. These "rheumatoid factors" thus qualify as bona fide autoantibodies and are, in fact, anti-antibodies. The large majority, but not all, of these anti-antibodies have specificities directed toward antigenic determinants located on the Fc segment of IgG's. A number of rheumatoid factors have been shown to have activities directed against allotypic determinants of IgG molecules. In fact, the observations of Grubb (for a review, see Grubb, 1970) on the specific reactivities of rheumatoid factors led to the original recognition of the existence of the genetic (allotypic) variants of human Ig's.

Some rheumatoid factors react more strongly with denatured than with native Ig's. In these cases, either novel antigenic determinants are exposed by the denaturation process, to yield stronger reactions, or the denaturation process leads to aggregates of Ig with more readily accessible native determinants and an effective increase in determinant valence.

In those usual instances in which IgG is the target for the anti-γ-globulin, differences have been noted in the reactivity with the different IgG subclasses. For example, a frequent observation is that the rheumatoid factors show the strongest reactivities for the IgG1 subclass, somewhat less for IgG2 and IgG4, and none at all for IgG3 (Allen and Kunkel, 1966; Gaarder and Natvig, 1970). In these cases, the antibody activity has been shown to be directed against a particular isotypic antigenic determinant referred to as Ga, which is present on all human IgG proteins except members of the IgG3 subclass.

The specific reactivities of a series of anti-γ-globulin antibodies taken from human patients with hypergammaglobulinemic purpura or mixed cryoglobulinemia were examined as a prelude to the selection of antibodies with known activities for studies of V-region structure–function correlates (Capra et al., 1971). The patterns of reactivity with the various human subclasses were examined and, considered in relation also to the patterns of cross-idiotypic specificity involved (Kunkel et al., 1973), were used as model proteins for V-region amino acid sequence analysis (Capra and Kehoe, 1974) (see also Chapter 11). The anti-Fc specificities of these proteins, although complex, have thus proved of great value in relating the antigen-combining function, idiotypy, and covalent structure of the antibody-combining site.

Some rheumatoid-factor activities have been reported against IgM (Mackenzie et al., 1969), IgA (Strober et al., 1968), and IgE (Williams et al., 1972) proteins. It appears that marked increases in the levels of the target protein can lead to the appearance of rheumatoid-factor activity in serum. Williams et al. (1972) found, for example, that 53% of patients known to suffer from severe allergic disorders had anti-IgE antibodies, while fewer than 10% of patients with other miscellaneous disorders possessed these autoantibodies. It thus appears that intense exposure to the antigen involved markedly increases the probability of producing these kinds of anti-antibodies. The presence of such antibodies in the serum assumes considerable clinical importance because of the potential that is thus generated for severe immediate hypersensitivity reactions due to the immune complex formation that could follow transfusions or other exposure to the relevant antigens.

3. Submolecular Localization of Immunoglobulin Biological Properties

The general localization of the non-antigen-binding, or biological, properties of Ig's to the Fc region was apparent as soon as Porter (1959) showed that whole IgG could be proteolytically cleaved into Fab and Fc segments. Until relatively recently, however, little progress was made toward identifying more limited subsections of the antibody molecule that are responsible for individual biological properties. A major conceptual advance, which considerably circumscribed the issue, was provided by Edelman *et al.* (1969) when they determined the complete primary structure of a human IgG1. The structural features observed led to the enunciation of the "domain" hypothesis for antibody structure, which suggested that the discrete molecular segments, which were apparent from the patterns of amino acid sequence homology, were reflective of the presence of individual functional units (domains) within the Ig molecule. The hypothesis further predicted that each structural domain would be found responsible for the mediation of at least one function characteristic of antibodies. Additional details and implications of this concept were provided by Edelman (1970). A number of studies have now provided experimental data by which the validity of the domain hypothesis, as it relates to biological properties, can be tested.

187

THE STRUCTURAL
BASIS FOR THE
BIOLOGICAL
PROPERTIES OF
IMMUNOGLOBULINS

3.1. Antigen-Dependent Properties

3.1.1. Complement Fixation (Classical Pathway)

This is the first biological property for which an explicit suggestion for a submolecular Fc localization was made. Kehoe *et al.* (1969), in the course of studies on the covalent structure of the H chain of the murine IgG2a protein MOPC 173, showed that a 62-amino-acid fragment localizable to the amino-terminal half of the Fc region was capable of a significant amount of complement-binding. Since no activity could be associated with any of the other constituent fragments of this IgG H chain, Kehoe and co-workers proposed that the C_H2 domain of IgG bore the capacity for complement fixation. This assignment was later verified in several laboratories. Work by Porter and his associates (Connell and Porter, 1971; Colomb and Porter, 1975), for example, showed that it is possible to isolate a large fragment of rabbit antibody that is intact except for the loss of the carboxyterminal H-chain domain, C_H3. Since this enzyme-proteolysis product is able to bind both antigen and complement in quantities one would expect for an intact IgG, the C_H2 domain would clearly seem to be implicated in the complement-binding function. Painter and Dorrington and their colleagues (Ellerson *et al.*, 1972) isolated from a human IgG1 protein an intact C_H2 domain that contained the region corresponding to the murine fragment described by Kehoe *et al.* (1969), and showed that this region was able to bind complement, while an intact C_H3 domain was not. Thus, there is now little question that the activation of the classical complement pathway by IgG involves the C_H2 domain. As discussed in Section 2.1.1, however, the exact mechanism by which this activation of C1q occurs remains to be elucidated.

For IgM, the studies of Hurst *et al.* (1974, 1975) suggested that the C_H4 domain of this Ig class is responsible for the activation of the classical pathway. The approach to this problem was comparable to that used for IgG in that cyanogen bromide fragments isolated from the H chain were tested for their capacity to bind C1, the intact first component of the complement system. The fragments showing activity were localized within the molecule by comparison with the known sequence of human IgM (Watanabe *et al.*, 1973; Putnam *et al.*, 1973). There are as yet no independent verifications by other laboratories of the assignment of the complement-binding function to this domain of the IgM molecule.

There are some perplexing features concerning the exact nature of possible subsites of binding for C1q within the Ig molecule. For example, Kehoe *et al.* (1974) compared the primary structures of the regions of several complement-binding molecules that corresponded to the segment previously shown to be involved in binding C1q in IgG. The absence of common short stretches of sequence led these authors to conclude that there was not some absolutely unique peptide stretch in numerous different Ig's that is responsible for the C1q-binding function, but rather that some common, general conformational feature, very likely modulated by the structure of other sections of the domain involved, could mediate this biological property. Such a conformational feature would not necessarily involve amino acids that are far removed in the linear sequence. This idea is supported by the observation that when one compares the sequence of the strongly binding IgM molecule with the sequences of IgG molecules that also bind C1q tightly, an even lower extent of sequence correspondence is observed, as, for example, between the C_H2 domain of IgG and C_H4 of IgM (Low *et al.*, 1976).

Painter and Dorrington and their associates (Painter *et al.*, 1974; Isenman *et al.*, 1975b) also studied the complement-binding properties of β_2-microglobulin, a protein that has been shown to be the structural equivalent of an Ig domain (Cunningham *et al.*, 1973) as well as an important constituent of histocompatibility antigens (Cresswell *et al.*, 1974). β_2-Microglobulin proved to be a potent participant in the classical complement system (Painter *et al.*, 1974). At first, it seemed surprising that this protein showed classical complement fixation, since sequence analysis indicates that it is slightly more homologous with the non-complement-binding human IgG C_H3 domain than with the C_H2 domain. Moreover, the studies of Isenman *et al.* (1975b) demonstrated that the reduced and alkylated form of β_2-microglobulin, which was believed to be in a random coiled state, also bound C1. One interpretation of this observation is that there is no conformational parameter, even local, involved in the binding of C1q. This interpretation is favored by Isenman *et al.* (1975b). Alternatively, there might be significant, though modest, local conformational features within certain Ig domains that determine the capacity for interaction with C1q. These regions might, in certain cases, be retained in a reduced and alkylated protein. In the native Ig molecule, the disposition of these local regions might well be significantly modulated by other aspects of the protein's structure, as, for example, the relationship of the two C_H2 domains of a given IgG molecule to each other (Deisenhofer *et al.*, 1976), or the integrity of the inter-H-chain disulfide bond. Such functionally significant local conformational features might well be approximated by different primary sequence stretches, as in the C1q-binding regions of IgG and IgM. Conceivably, current studies of chemically synthesized homologues of Ig Fc segments (Johnson and Thames, 1976; Prystowsky *et al.*, 1977) will help clarify some of the details concerning these unresolved paradoxes. Such studies are focusing on tryptophan-containing segments because of the strong indications for the direct involvement of this amino acid in the C1q-binding site (Isenman *et al.*, 1977).

A related question concerning the complement-binding function has to do with the known incapacity of the human IgG4 subclass to interact with C1q (Ishizaka, T., *et al.*, 1967; Schumaker *et al.*, 1976). This fact led at first to a search for primary structure differences in the area of the C_H2 domain known to be involved (Kehoe *et al.*, 1974). No unique covalent feature that could explain the lack of activity of the IgG4 protein was found. Isenman *et al.* (1975a) subsequently showed that the isolated Fc region of an IgG4 protein was able to interact with C1 with the same affinity as that of an Fc fragment from a human IgG1 protein. This finding indicated that there was no intrinsic defect of the IgG4 C_H2 region with respect to the complement-binding function. These authors suggested that steric hindrance from another region of the native IgG4 molecule, most likely the Fab segment, was responsible for its incapacity to interact with C1q.

189

THE STRUCTURAL
BASIS FOR THE
BIOLOGICAL
PROPERTIES OF
IMMUNOGLOBULINS

3.1.2. Complement Fixation (Alternate Pathway)

There is at present no evidence regarding the site of interaction on Ig's that is responsible for activating the alternate pathway.

3.1.3. Opsonic Activity

The site for binding of IgG antibody to monocytes and macrophages was localized to the C_H3 domain in several studies (Yasmeen *et al.*, 1973; Okafor *et al.*, 1974; Ciccimarra *et al.*, 1975). Ovary *et al.* (1976), however, presented evidence, on the basis of a rosetting technique, that C_H2 is involved. These authors suggest that there may be a role for both domains, under different circumstances. The question requires further study.

No data bearing directly on the neutrophil-binding site have yet been presented.

3.2. Antigen-Independent Properties

3.2.1. Attachment to Mast Cells and Basophils

Even though the covalent structure of the C region of the IgE H chain is known (Bennich and von Bahr-Lindstrom, 1974), the precise submolecular location of the site, or sites, that interact with the cell receptor remains unclear. There is no question that the region lies within the Fc fragment (Ishizaka, K., *et al.*, 1970a). The lack of an inhibitory effect on IgE cell sensitization by the Fc' fragment, which comprises approximately the amino-terminal one third of the entire Fc region, suggests that the C_H3 or C_H4 domain might be involved in the cytotropic function. That either site is involved has not been definitively established, however, despite considerable effort.

Dorrington and Bennich (1973) analyzed the conformational changes associated with heating IgE and some of its proteolytic fragments to 56°C, a temperature that is known to destroy the capacity of reagins to bind to basophils and mast cells. The observed changes also strongly implicated the C_H3 and C_H4 domains in the cell-binding function.

Certain disulfide bonds of the IgE molecule are also crucial to the cytophilic property (Takatsu *et al.*, 1975). An intrachain disulfide bond in the Fd region as well as an inter-H-chain bond must be intact for the native molecule to bind firmly to cells. Details of the effects that loss of these bonds have on IgE structure are not yet available.

3.2.2. Macrophage-Binding

Other than the few findings discussed in Sections 2.2.2 and 3.1.3, there are as yet no data on the Ig site responsible for this biological property.

3.2.3. Lymphocyte-Binding

The data in the literature are quite contradictory with respect to this biological property. Ramasamy *et al.* (1975) found evidence for the participation of the IgG C_H3 domain in this function, but Wisloff *et al.* (1974) and Michaelsen *et al.* (1975) believed that their experiments implicated the C_H2 domain, the latter authors at least to the point where some C_H2–C_H3 interaction might be involved. Neither MacLennan *et al.* (1974) nor Ramasamy *et al.* (1975), however, could find any lymphocyte-binding associable with the C_H2 domain. Additional study is clearly required to resolve this issue.

3.2.4. Placental-Passage Regulation

A report by Matre *et al.* (1975) suggested that the C_H3 region of rabbit IgG antibodies is involved in attachment of these molecules to receptors in human placenta. This conclusion was disputed by McNabb *et al.* (1976), who believe the results of Matre and co-workers may be due to the presence of contaminating macrophages. McNabb and co-workers were unable to find any evidence for placental binding by human IgG C_H2 or C_H3 subfragments, in a system in which both intact IgG and Fc fragments isolated from it bound very well. They thus proposed that some form of quaternary interaction between the C_H2 and C_H3 domains in the intact molecule was involved, and that placental passage is, in consequence, an exception to the purest expression of the domain hypothesis, viz., one function equals one domain.

3.2.5. Intestinal-Passage Regulation

Although unequivocally purified IgG domains have not been studied in relation to this biological property, the studies of Guyer *et al.* (1976) suggest that fragments smaller than Fc itself do not participate in this system. Thus, it is possible that some sort of quaternary interaction could be required here also. The phenomenon must be studied further, however, using highly purified, individual domains.

3.2.6. Immunoglobulin-Catabolism Regulation

For IgG, this function was definitively localized to the C_H2 domain by Yasmeen *et al.* (1976). The region involved for other Ig classes is not yet known.

3.2.7. Passive Cutaneous Anaphylaxis

The data for the mediation of this function of IgG are also controversial, since some conflicting observations have been made. Minta and Painter (1972) suggested that the C_H3 domain is active in this phenomenon. This report runs counter to the conclusions of others, including Prahl (1967), Utsumi (1969), Stewart *et al.* (1973), and Ovary *et al.* (1976), none of whom could associate the PCA function with C_H3. No reports of activity for the C_H2 domain alone currently exist. Ovary *et al.* (1976) believe that the *entire* Fc region is required for the expression of this activity. This makes the third biological property for which this form of multidomain activity expression has been formally proposed.

191

THE STRUCTURAL
BASIS FOR THE
BIOLOGICAL
PROPERTIES OF
IMMUNOGLOBULINS

3.2.8. Interaction with Protein 'A' of *Staphylococcus aureus*

The exact site of Fc interaction for this protein is not known at present, although suggestions have been made that the C_H2 domain of IgG may be involved (Kronvall and Frommel, 1970; see also comment in Dorval *et al.*, 1974). Much more evidence is needed to confirm or refute this suggestion.

TABLE 4. Summarized Characteristics of Biological Properties of Human Immunoglobulins[a]

Property	Antigen dependence	Human Ig's involved	Domain localization
Complement fixation			
Classical pathway	+	IgM	C_H4 of IgM
		IgG	C_H2 of IgG
Alternate pathway	−	IgA, IgE	Unknown
Opsonic activity (neutrophils, monocytes)	+	IgG1, IgG3, IgA	Unknown
Mast-cell- and basophil-binding	−	IgE	Unknown
Macrophage-binding	−	IgG1, IgG3	C_H3 of IgG
Lymphocyte-binding	−	IgM, IgG1, IgG3	C_H3 (C_H2?) of IgG
Placental-passage regulation	−	IgG1, IgG2, IgG3, IgG4	Entire Fc required
Intestinal-passage regulation	−	None	Unknown
Immunoglobulin-catabolism regulation	−	All classes and subclasses	C_H2 of IgG
Passive cutaneous anaphylaxis	−	IgG1, IgG3, IgG4	C_H3, or entire Fc
Interaction with protein A of *Staphylococcus aureus*	−	IgG1, IgG2, IgG4	Unknown
Antigenic target for rheumatoid factors	−	IgG1, IgG2, IgG4, IgM, IgA, IgE	Not clear; most likely involves determinants throughout the Fc region

[a]See the text for details and references.

J. MICHAEL KEHOE

3.2.9. Antigenic Target for Rheumatoid Factors

As indicated in Section 2.2.9, various rheumatoid factors have activity against antigenic determinants throughout the Fc region. Additional studies may show whether certain regions are favored because of especially prominent determinant targets.

4. Summary and Conclusions

With the prospect of a complete molecular picture of how antibody molecules bind antigen close at hand, increased attention has been given to the biological properties, or effector functions, mediated by these proteins. Table 4 summarizes what is known of these properties, as presented in this chapter.

Some of these properties, such as complement fixation, have a close functional linkage to the antigen-binding process. The detailed nature of this linkage is not yet fully understood, especially with respect to the manner in which the latency of the complement-binding function is revealed. Other important biological properties of Ig's are designed to assure that these molecules are available at sites where their function may be crucial to survival. An example is the provision of passive maternal humoral immunity to the newborn, be it by placental membrane transport *in utero* or passage across the intestinal epithelium following the ingestion of milk.

Many molecular details of these functions are still unclear, but considerable progress has been made in localizing certain of them to discrete regions of the Fc segment, such as the C_H2 domain of the IgG molecule for classical complement fixation. Much additional information is required, however, especially with respect to the dynamics of the interaction of relevant antibody Fc sites with receptor proteins on cells such as macrophages or basophils. The complex character of the biological properties as a whole is pointed up by the fact that both clearly beneficial effects, such as opsonization, and clearly detrimental effects, such as the sensitization of mast cells or basophils by IgE, are mediated by the Fc region of Ig's.

References

Allen, J. C., and Kunkel, H. G., 1966, Hidden rheumatoid factors with specificity for native γ globulins, *Arthritis Rheum.* 9:758–768.

Basten, A., Miller, J. F. A. P., Sprent, J., and Prize, J., 1972, A receptor for antibody on B lymphocytes. I. Method of detection and functional significance, *J. Exp. Med.* 135:610–626.

Bennich, H., and von Bahr-Lindstrom, H., 1974, Structure of immunoglobulin E (IgE), *Prog. Immunol. II* 1:49–58.

Bennich, H., Ishizaka, K., Ishizaka, T., and Johansson, S. G. O., 1969, Immunoglobulin E: A comparative antigenic study of γE globulin and myeloma IgND, *J. Immunol.* 102:826–831.

Berken, A., and Benacerraf, B., 1966, Properties of antibodies cytophilic for macrophages, *J. Exp. Med.* 123:119–144.

Brambell, F. W. R., 1966, The transmission of immunity from mother to young and the catabolism of immunoglobulins, *Lancet* 2:1087–1088.

Brambell, F. W. R., 1970, in: *The Transmission of Passive Immunity from Mother to Young* (A. Neuberger and E. L. Tatum, eds.), pp. North-Holland, Amsterdam and London.

Brambell, F. W. R., Hemmings, W. A., Oakley, C. L., and Porter, R. R., 1960, Relative transmission of the fractions of papain hydrolyzed homologous γ-globulin from the uterine cavity to the foetal circulation in the rabbit, *Proc. R. Soc. London Ser. B* **151**:478–482.

Brown, J. C., and Koshland, M. E., 1975, Activation of antibody Fc function by antigen-induced conformational changes, *Proc. Natl. Acad. Sci. U.S.A.* **72**:5111–5115.

Capra, J. D., and Kehoe, J. M., 1974, Structure of antibodies with shared idiotypy: The complete sequence of the heavy chain variable regions of two immunoglobulin M anti-gamma globulins, *Proc. Natl. Acad. Sci. U.S.A.* **71**:4032–4036.

Capra, J. D., Kehoe, J. M., Winchester, R. J., and Kunkel, H. G., 1971, Structure–function relationships among anti-gamma globulin antibodies, *Ann. N.Y. Acad. Sci.* **190**:371–381.

Carson, D., Kulczycki, A., Jr., and Metzger, H., 1975, Interaction of IgE with rat basophilic leukemic cells. IV. Release of intact receptors on cell-free particles, *J. Immunol.* **114**:158–160.

Ciccimarra, F., Rosen, F. S., and Merler, E., 1975, Localization of the IgG effector site for monocyte receptors, *Proc. Natl. Acad. Sci. U.S.A.* **72**:2081–2086.

Colomb, M., and Porter, R. R., 1975, Characterization of a plasmin-digest fragment of rabbit immunoglobulin gamma that binds antigen and complement, *Biochem. J.* **145**:177–183.

Connell, G. E., and Porter, R. R., 1971, A new enzymic fragment (Facb) of rabbit immunoglobulin G, *Biochem. J.* **124**:53p.

Cresswell, P., Springer, T., Strominger, J. L., Turner, M. J., Grey, H. M., and Kubo, R. T., 1974, Immunological identity of the small subunit of HLA antigens and beta 2 microglobulin and its turnover on the cell membrane, *Proc. Natl. Acad. Sci. U.S.A.* **71**:2123–2127.

Cunningham, B. A., Wang, J. L., Berggård, I., and Peterson, P. A., 1973, The complete amino acid sequence of β_2 microglobulin, *Biochemistry* **12**:4811–4822.

Deisenhofer, J., Colman, P. M., Epp, O., and Huber, R., 1976, Crystallographic structural studies of a human Fc fragment. II. A complete model based on a Fourier map at 3.5 Å resolution, *Hoppe-Seyler's Z. Physiol. Chem.* **357**:1421–1434.

Dickler, H. B., and Kunkel, H. G., 1972, Interaction of aggregated γ globulin with B lymphocytes, *J. Exp. Med.* **136**:191–196.

Dorrington, K. J., and Bennich, H., 1973, Thermally induced structural changes in immunoglobulin E, *J. Biol. Chem.* **248**:8378–8384.

Dorrington, K. J., and Painter, R. H., 1974, Functional domains of immunoglobulin G, *Prog. Immunol. II* **1**:75–84.

Dorval, G., Welsh, K. I., and Wigzell, H., 1974, Labelled staphylococcal protein A as an immunological probe in the analysis of cell surface markers, *Scand. J. Immunol.* **3**:405–411.

Edelman, G. M., 1970, The covalent structure of a human γG-immunoglobulin. XI. Functional implications, *Biochemistry* **9**:3197–3205.

Edelman, G. M., Cunningham, B. A., Gall, W. E., Gottlieb, P. D., Rutishauser, U., and Waxdal, M. J., 1969, The covalent structure of an entire γG immunoglobulin molecule, *Proc. Natl. Acad. Sci. U.S.A.* **63**:78–85.

Eisen, H. N., 1974, *Immunology,* p. 483, Harper and Row, Hagerstown, Maryland.

Ellerson, J. R., Yasmeen, D., Painter, R. H., and Dorrington, K. J., 1972, A fragment corresponding to the C_H2 region of immunoglobulin G (IgG) with complement fixing activity, *FEBS Lett.* **24**:318–322.

Fireman, P., Vannier, W. E., and Goodman, H. C., 1963, The association of skin-sensitizing antibody with the β_{2a} globulins in sera from ragweed sensitive patients, *J. Exp. Med.* **117**:603–619.

Forsgren, A., and Nordström, K., 1974, Protein A of *Staphylococcus aureus:* The biological significance of its reaction with IgG, *Ann. N.Y. Acad. Sci.* **236**:252–266.

Forsgren, A., and Sjoquist, J., 1966, Protein A from *S. aureus.* I. Pseudo-immune reaction with human γ-globulin, *J. Immunol.* **99**:822–827.

Gaarder, P. I., and Natvig, J. B., 1970, Hidden rheumatoid factors reacting with "Non a" and other antigens of native autologous IgG, *J. Immunol.* **105**:928–937.

Good, R. A., and Day, N. K. (eds.), 1977, *Comprehensive Immunology,* Vol. 2, *Biological Amplification Systems in Immunology,* Plenum Press, New York.

Gotze, O., and Müller-Eberhard, H. J., 1971, The C3-activator system: An alternate pathway of complement activation, *J. Exp. Med.* **134**:90s.

Grubb, R., 1970, *The Genetic Markers of Human Immunoglobulins,* Springer-Verlag, New York.

Guyer, R. L., Koshland, M. E., and Knopf, P. M., 1976, Immunoglobulin binding by mouse intestinal epithelial cell receptors, *J. Immunol.* **117**:587–593.

Heremans, J. F., and Vaerman, J. P., 1962, β_{2a}-Globulin as a possible carrier of allergic reaginic activity, *Nature (London)* **193**:1091–1092.

Huber, H., Douglas, S. D., Nusbacher, J., Kochwa, S., and Rosenfield, R. E., 1971, IgG subclass specificity of human monocyte receptor sites, *Nature (London)* **229**:419–420.

Huber, R., Deisenhofer, J., Colman, P. M., Matsushima, M., and Palm, W., 1976, Crystallographic structure studies of an IgG molecule and an Fc fragment, *Nature (London)* **264**:415–420.

Huber, R., Deisenhofer, J., Colman, P., Matsushima, M., and Palm, W., 1977, X-ray diffraction analysis of immunoglobulin structure, in: *Mosbacher Kolloquium der Gesellschaft für Biologische Chimie: Das Immunsystem* (F. Melchers and K. Rajewsky, eds.), pp. 26–40, Springer-Verlag, Berlin—Heidelberg—New York.

Hurst, M. M., Volanakis, J. E., Hester, R. B., Stroud, R. M., and Bennett, J. C., 1974, The structural basis for binding of complement by immunoglobulin M, *J. Exp. Med.* **140**:1117–1121.

Hurst, M. M., Volanakis, J. E., Stroud, R. M., and Bennett, J. C., 1975, C1̄ fixation and classical complement pathway activation by a fragment of the $C\mu 4$ domain of IgM, *J. Exp. Med.* **142**:1322–1326.

Isenman, D. E., Dorrington, K. J., and Painter, R. H., 1975a, The structure and function of immunoglobulin domains. II. The importance of interchain disulfide bonds and the possible role of molecular flexibility in the interaction between immunoglobulin G and complement, *J. Immunol.* **114**:1726–1729.

Isenman, D. E., Painter, R. H., and Dorrington, K. J., 1975b, The structure and function of immunoglobulin domains: Studies with beta-2-microglobulin on the role of the intrachain disulfide bond, *Proc. Natl. Acad. Sci. U.S.A.* **72**:548–552.

Isenman, D. E., Ellerson, J. R., Painter, R. H., and Dorrington, K. J., 1977, Correlation between the exposure of aromatic chromophores at the surface of the Fc domains of immunoglobulin G and their ability to bind complement, *Biochemistry* **16**:233–240.

Isersky, C., Mendoza, G., and Metzger, H., 1977, Reaction of antibodies with the cell surface receptor for IgE, *Fed. Proc. Fed. Am. Soc. Exp. Biol.* **36**:1217.

Ishizaka, K., and Ishizaka, T., 1968, Induction of erythema-wheal reactions by soluble antigen–γE antibody complexes in humans, *J. Immunol.* **101**:68–78.

Ishizaka, K., and Ishizaka, T., 1971, IgE and reaginic hypersensitivity, *Ann. N. Y. Acad. Sci.* **190**:443–456.

Ishizaka, K., Ishizaka, T., and Hornbrook, M. M., 1966, Physicochemical properties of human reaginic antibody. IV. Presence of a unique immunoglobulin as a carrier of reaginic activity, *J. Immunol.* **97**:75–85.

Ishizaka, K., Ishizaka, T., and Lee, E. H., 1970a, Biologic function of the Fc fragments of E myeloma protein, *Immunochemistry* **7**:687–702.

Ishizaka, K., Tomioka, H., and Ishizaka, T., 1970b, Mechanisms of passive sensitization. I. Presence of IgE and IgG molecules on human leukocytes, *J. Immunol.* **105**:1459–1467.

Ishizaka, T., and Ishizaka, K., 1975, Biology of immunoglobulin E: Molecular basis of reaginic hypersensitivity, *Prog. Allergy* **19**:60–121.

Ishizaka, T., Ishizaka, K., Salmon, S., and Fudenberg, H., 1967, Biologic activities of aggregated immunoglobulins of different classes, *J. Immunol.* **99**:82–91.

Ishizaka, T., Sian, C. M., and Ishizaka, K., 1971, Complement fixation by aggregated IgE through the alternate pathway, *J. Immunol.* **108**:848–851.

Ishizaka, T., Soto, C., and Ishizaka, K., 1973, Mechanisms of passive sensitization. III. Number of IgE molecules and its receptor sites on human basophil granulocytes, *J. Immunol.* **111**:500–511.

Jensen, K., 1958, A noramlly occurring staphylococcus antibody in human serum, *Acta Pathol. Microbiol. Scand.* **44**:421–428.

Johnson, B. J., and Thames, K. E., 1976, Investigations of the complement fixing sites of immunoglobulins, *J. Immunol.* **117**:1491–1494.

Kehoe, J. M., Fougereau, M., and Bourgois, A., 1969, Immunoglobulin peptide with complement fixing activity, *Nature (London)* **224**:1212–1213.

Kehoe, J. M., Bourgois, A., Capra, J. D., and Fougereau, M., 1974, Amino acid sequence of a murine immunoglobulin fragment that possesses complement fixing activity, *Biochemistry* **13**:2499–2504.

Kronvall, G., and Frommel, D., 1970, Definition of staphylococcal protein A reactivity for human immunoglobulin G fragments, *Immunochemistry* **7**:124–126.

195

THE STRUCTURAL
BASIS FOR THE
BIOLOGICAL
PROPERTIES OF
IMMUNOGLOBULINS

Kronvall, G., and Williams, R. C., Jr., 1969, Differences in anti-protein A activity among IgG sub-groups, *J. Immunol.* **103**:828–833.

Kronvall, G., Seal, U. S., Finstad, J., and Williams, R. C., Jr., 1970, Phylogenetic insight into evolution of mammalian Fc fragment of γG globulin using staphylococcal protein A, *J. Immunol.* **104**:140–147.

Kulczycki, A., Jr., and Metzger, H., 1974, The interaction of IgE with rat basophilic leukemia cells. II. Quantitative aspects of the binding reaction, *J. Exp. Med.* **140**:1676–1695.

Kunkel, H. G., Agnello, V., Joslin, F. G., Winchester, R. J., and Capra, J. D., 1973, Cross idiotypic specificity among monoclonal IgM proteins with anti-γ-globulin activity, *J. Exp. Med.* **137**:331–342.

Lancet, D., and Pecht, I., 1976, Kinetic evidence for hapten-induced conformational transition in immunoglobulin MOPC-460, *Proc. Natl. Acad. Sci. U.S.A.* **73**:3549–3553.

Lawrence, D. A., Weigle, W. O., and Spiegelberg, H. L., 1975, Immunoglobulins cytophilic for human lymphocytes, monocytes, and neutrophils, *J. Clin. Invest.* **55**:368–376.

Low, T. L. K., Liu, Y.-S. V., and Putnam, F. W., 1976, Structure, function, and evolutionary relationships of Fc domains of human immunoglobulins A, G, M, and E, *Science* **191**:390–392.

Mackenzie, M. R., Warner, N. L., Linscott, W. D., and Fudenberg, H. H., 1969, Differentiation of human IgM subclasses by the ability to interact with a factor resembling the first component of complement, *J. Immunol.* **103**:607–612.

MacLennan, I. C. M., Connell, G. E., and Gotch, F. M., 1974, Effector activating determinants on IgG. II. Differentiation of the combining sites for Clq from those for cytotoxic K-cells and neutrophils by plasmin digestion of rabbit IgG, *Immunology* **26**:303–310.

Matre, R., Tonder, O., and Endresen, C., 1975, Fc receptors in human placenta, *Scand. J. Immunol.* **4**:741–745.

McNabb, T., Koh, T. Y., Dorrington, K. J., and Painter, R. H., 1976, Structure and function of immunoglobulin domains. V. Binding of immunoglobulin G and fragments to placental membrane preparations, *J. Immunol.* **117**:882–888.

Messner, R. P., and Jelinek, J., 1970, Receptors for human γG globulin on human neutrophils, *J. Clin. Invest.* **49**:2165–2171.

Metzger, H., 1974, Effect of antigen binding on the properties of antibody, *Adv. Immunol.* **18**:169–207.

Michaelsen, T. E., Wisloff, F., and Natvig, J. B., 1975, Structural requirements in the Fc region of rabbit IgG antibodies necessary to induce cytotoxicity by human lymphocytes, *Scand. J. Immunol* **4**:71.

Michaelsen, T. E., Frangione, B., and Franklin, E. C., 1977, Primary structure of the "hinge" region of human IgG3: Probable quadruplication of a 15-amino acid residue basic unit, *J. Biol. Chem.* **252**:883–889.

Minta, J. O., and Painter, R. H., 1972, A re-examination of the ability of pFc′ and Fc′ to participate in passive cutaneous anaphylaxis, *Immunochemistry* **9**:1041–1048.

Müller-Eberhard, H. J., 1974, Patterns of complement activation, *Prog. Immunol. II* **1**:173–182.

Müller-Eberhard, H. J., 1975, Complement, *Annu. Rev. Biochem.* **44**:697–724.

Okafor, G. O., Turner, M. W., and Hay, F. C., 1974, Localization of monocyte binding site of human immunoglobulin G, *Nature (London)* **248**:228–230.

Ovary, Z., 1964, Passive cutaneous anaphylaxis, in: *Immunological Methods* (J. F. Ackroyd, ed.), p. 259, Blackwell, London.

Ovary, Z., Salsuk, P. H., Quijada, L., and Lamm, M. E., 1976, Biologic activities of rabbit immunoglobulin G in relation to domains of the Fc region, *J. Immunol.* **116**:1265–1271.

Painter, R. H., Yasmeen, D., Assimeh, S. N., and Poulik, M. D., 1974, Complement fixing and macrophage opsonizing activities associated with β_2 microglobulin, *Immunol. Commun.* **3**:19–34.

Phillips-Quagliata, J. M., Levine, B. B., Quagliata, F., and Uhr, J. W., 1971, Mechanisms underlying binding of immune complexes to macrophages, *J. Exp. Med.* **133**:589–601.

Porter, R. R., 1959, The hydrolysis of rabbit γ-globulin and antibodies with crystalline papain, *Biochem. J.* **73**:119–126.

Prahl, J. W., 1967, Enzymatic degradation of the Fc fragment of rabbit immunoglobulin IgG, *Biochem. J.* **104**:647–655.

Prystowsky, M. B., Erickson, B. W., and Kehoe, J. M., 1977, Interaction of synthetic peptides from the C_H2 domain of immunoglobulin G with the C1q component of serum complement, *Fed. Proc. Fed. Am. Soc. Exp. Biol.* **36**:1310.

Putnam, F. W., Florent, G. Paul, C., Shinoda, T., and Shimizu, A., 1973, Complete amino acid sequence of the mu heavy chain of a human IgM immunoglobulin, *Science* **182**:287–291.

Ramasamy, R., Secher, D. S., and Adetugbo, K., 1975, C_H3 domain of IgG as binding site to Fc receptor on mouse lymphocytes, *Nature (London)* **253**:656.

Rhodes, J., 1973, Receptor for monomeric IgM on guinea pig splenic macrophages, *Nature (London)* **243**:527–528.

Schlessinger, J., Steinberg, I. Z., Givol, D., Hochman, J., and Pecht, I., 1975, Antigen induced conformational changes in antibodies and their Fab fragments studied by circular polarization of fluorescence, *Proc. Natl. Acad. Sci. U.S.A.* **72**:2775–2779.

Schumaker, V. N., Calcott, M. A., Spiegelberg, H. L., and Müller-Eberhard, H. J., 1976, Ultracentrifuge studies of the binding of IgG of different subclasses to the C1q subunit of the first component of complement, *Biochemistry* **15**:5175–5181.

Sjödahl, J., 1976, Repetitive sequences in protein A from *Staphylococcus aureus:* Three highly homologous Fc-binding regions, *FEBS Lett.* **67**:62–67.

Sjoquist, J., Meloun, B., and Hjelm, H., 1972, Protein A isolated from *Staphylococcus aureus* after digestion with lysostaphin, *Eur. J. Biochem.* **29**:572–578.

Spiegelberg, H. L., and Fishkin, B. C., 1972, The catabolism of human γG immunoglobulins of different heavy chain subclasses. III. The catabolism of heavy chain disease proteins and of Fc fragments of myeloma proteins, *Clin. Exp. Immunol.* **10**:599–607.

Stewart, G. A., Smith, A. K., and Stanworth, D. R., 1973, Biological activities associated with the Facb fragment of rabbit IgG, *Immunochemistry* **10**:755–760.

Stout, R. D., and Herzenberg, L. A., 1975, The Fc receptor on thymus-derived lymphocytes, *J. Exp. Med.* **142**:611–621.

Strober, W., Wochner, R. D., Barlow, M. H., McFarlin, D. E., and Waldman, T. A., 1968, Immunoglobulin metabolism in ataxia telangiectasia, *J. Clin. Invest.* **47**:1905–1915.

Sullivan, A. L., Grimley, P. M., and Metzger, H., 1971, Electron microscopic localization of immunoglobulin E on the surface membrane of human basophils, *J. Exp. Med.* **134**:1403–1416.

Takatsu, K., Ishizaka, T., and Ishizaka, K., 1975, Biological significance of disulfide bonds in human IgE molecules, *J. Immunol.* **114**:1838–1845.

Utsumi, S., 1969, Stepwise cleavage of rabbit immunoglobulin G by papain and isolation of four types of biologically active Fc fragments, *Biochem. J.* **112**:343–355.

Waldmann, T. A., Strober, W., and Blaese, R. M., 1971, Metabolism of immunoglobulins, in: *Progress in Immunology I* (B. Amos, ed.), pp. 891–903, Academic Press, New York.

Watanabe, S., Barnikol, H. U., Horn, J., Bertram, J., and Hilschmann, N., 1973, Die Primärstruktur eines monoklonalen IgM-Immunoglobulins (Makroglobulin Ga1), KK: Die Aminosäuresequenz der H-kette (μTyp, Subgruppe III), Struktur des gesamten IgM-Moleküls, *Hoppe-Seyler's Z. Physiol. Chem.* **354**:1505–1509.

Williams, R. C., Griffiths, R. W., Emmons, J. D., and Field, R. C., 1972, Naturally occurring human antiglobulins with specificity for γE, *J. Clin. Invest.* **51**:955–963.

Wisloff, F., Michaelsen, T. E., and Froland, S. S., 1974, Inhibition of antibody-dependent human lymphocyte mediated cytotoxicity by immunoglobulin classes, IgG subclasses, and IgG fragments, *Scand. J. Immunol.* **3**:29–35.

Yasmeen, D., Ellerson, J. R., Dorrington, K. J., and Painter, R. H., 1973, Evidence for the domain hypothesis: Location of the site of cytophilic activity toward guinea pig macrophages in the C_H3 homology region of human immunoglobulin G, *J. Immunol.* **110**:1706–1709.

Yasmeen, D., Ellerson, J. R., Dorrington, K. J., and Painter, R. H., 1976, The structure and function of immunoglobulin domains. 4. The distribution of some effector functions among the Cγ2 and Cγ3 homology regions of human immunoglobulin G, *J. Immunol.* **116**:518–526.

7

The Significance of Gene Duplication in Immunoglobulin Evolution (Epimethean Natural Selection and Promethean Evolution)

SUSUMU OHNO

1. Introduction

Antibodies produced by B cells of man and other mammals are specified by three autosomally inherited gene clusters that are not linked to each other. The first cluster is for κ-type light (L) chains, while the second is for λ-type L chains. The third specifies various classes of heavy (H) chains (Grubb, 1970; Mage *et al.,* 1973). Each cluster apparently contains a small number (1–10 or so) of constant (C)-region genes and a greater number (up to the order of 10^2) of variable (V)-region genes (Hood *et al.,* 1975). Inasmuch as L and H chains are the components of a single antibody molecule, the observed nonlinkage of relevant genes reveals that verte-brates are perfectly capable of coordinating the activities of nonlinked genes. In fact, the nonlinkage of coordinately regulated genes is a rule rather than an exception; i.e., hemoglobin α- and β-chain genes are not linked. Furthermore, even the observed close linkage between V-region and C-region genes within each cluster may be no functional prerequisite, merely reflecting their evolutionary origin in that they arose as tandem repeats of an ancestral gene. It now appears (see Greaves, 1975) that for their cell-bound antibodies or receptors, T cells also utilize the same

SUSUMU OHNO • Department of Biology, City of Hope National Medical Center, Califor-nia 91010.

set of V-region genes as B cells, but they make use of an entirely different set of C-region genes that may reside within the major histocompatibility locus, i.e., *H-2* of mice and *HLA* of man (Gally and Edelman, 1972). Indeed, the *HLA* gene complex of man, which is carried by chromosome 6, is not linked to any of the three gene clusters for immunoglobulins (Ig's). Furthermore, the β_2-microglobulin locus is on yet another chromosome: chromosome 15 (Goodfellow *et al.*, 1975). Not only does β_2-microglobulin polymerize with HLA antigens on the cell surface, but also there exists a considerable sequence homology between β_2-microglobulin and a particular third of the H-chain C region, thus suggesting common ancestry.

The aforementioned nonlinkage of functionally related genes of the immune system, many of which apparently evolved from a common ancestral gene by a series of gene duplications, is fully compatible with the view that most of the gene-duplication events that generated vertebrate-specific genes occurred at the stage of fish when polyploid evolution was still possible (Ohno, 1970). Indeed, respectable Ig's of the IgM type are already present in elasmobranchian, chondrostean, and holostean fish (Litman *et al.*, 1971). On the other hand, the observation that antibodies generated by lampreys representing the most primitive jawless state bear no resemblance to Ig's of other vertebrates appears to suggest that the most primitive vertebrates had experimented with various approaches to the establishment of immune systems before deciding on the one approach that led to the perfection of the immune system as we understand it today (Litman *et al.*, 1970).

As vertebrates evolved beyond the amphibian stage, polyploid evolution ceased to be a factor in generating new genes from redundant copies of the old. By then, of course, the groundwork had already been laid. Thus, tandem duplication within each gene cluster was sufficient for further refinement of the immune system. For example, an initial H-chain gene cluster apparently contained only a C-region gene for μ-type H chain. To this cluster, clusters for various classes of γ-type H chains as well as those for α-type and ϵ-type H chains have gradually been added. This, then, is the broad picture of evolution by gene duplication of the immune system in vertebrates (Table 1). As such, however, it is no different from that of the hemoglobin system or that of the lactate dehydrogenase isozyme system.

TABLE 1. **Evolution of Genes of the Immune System in Vertebrates**[a]

Nonlinkage	β_2-M, Ig κ-L, Ig λ-L, Ig H, and MHC not linked to each other	Gene duplication occurred at the stage of fish due to polyploidy.
Close linkage	V and C of Ig κ-L, V and C of Ig λ-L, V and C of Ig H, and ubiquitous antigens and *Ir* of MHC closely linked	Gene duplication occurred even at later stages due to tandem repeat.
Functional coordination between unlinked genes	Between Ig κ-L or Ig λ-L and Ig H and between β_2-M and MHC ubiquitous antigens	Polymerization
	Between V of Ig κ-L, Ig λ-L or Ig H, and *Ir* of MHC?	Splicing?
Functional coordination between closely linked genes	Between V and C of Ig κ-L and Ig λ-L, as well as Ig H	Splicing

[a] (β_2-M) β_2-Microglobulin (110 residues); (Ig κ-L) κ-type L chains (110 × 2 residues); (Ig λ-L) λ-type L chains (110 × 2 residues); (Ig H) various classes of H chains (110 × 4 residues); (V, C) variable and constant regions of each Ig chain type; (MHC) major histocompatibility gene complex, i.e., *HLA* of man, *H-2* of the mouse; *(Ir)* immune response genes.

199

THE SIGNIFICANCE
OF GENE
DUPLICATION IN
IMMUNOGLOBULIN
EVOLUTION

As far as I am concerned, the uniqueness of the immune system lies in its ability to cope with all sorts of previously unexperienced contingencies, thus giving an impression of having evolved in anticipation of future needs (Cohn, 1970; Ohno, 1970). The Darwinian concept of evolution by natural selection does not predict the development of a system that can cope with the future. It follows, then, that the immune system must have developed on the basis of a new evolutionary principle. Since antigen-binding sites reside within the V region (110 residues from the amino terminus) of L as well as H chains, further discussion will be confined to evolution of V-region genes.

2. Epimethean Nature of Evolution by Natural Selection

In one version of Greek mythology, the task of creating animals on this earth was assigned to two brother Titans: Prometheus and Epimetheus. Unfortunately, Epimetheus had the first hand at the creation. Having only hindsight, he first gave away all the good attributes to beasts, e.g., strength to lions and tigers and swiftness to horses and gazelles. By the time he came around to creating man, there was nothing left to give; thus, man was made naked and powerless. Fortunately, at this point, Prometheus realized his brother's mistake. Having foresight, he stole fire from heaven and gave it to man. Zeus punished him greatly for this deed. Such is a parable on hindsight and foresight.

Natural selection, as we understand it, also has only hindsight, and is thus Epimethean in character. In this sense, it is no better than a general who always prepares for the future battle solely on the basis of historical precedents. Consequently, like troops under the general's command, a population evolving by natural selection suffers enormous casualties whenever it encounters a drastic change in environment. There is a slim chance of survival by adaptation that depends entirely on a chance presence of appropriate mutants that can cope with the new environment. In this manner, the old species represented by a majority of a previous population dies off, while those few appropriate mutants become the founders of a new species. This new species, in turn, is not at all prepared to cope with the next change in environment that is sure to come. Inasmuch as natural selection always operates after the fact by favoring already existing mutants, genetic polymorphism can confer the ability to cope with future environmental changes only to a population as a whole, but never to every member of a population. Furthermore, at any given moment, the range of environmental changes that a genetically polymorphic population can cope with is quite limited. For example, let us assume that only the presence of an appropriate mutant gene at each of the 10 independent loci can ensure the survival of an individual in a new environment that is very different from the present one. The probability that even a very large population (10^6 members) will by chance contain a pair of such individuals is infinitesimally small, i.e., $2 \times (10^{-5})^{20}$.

All the living organisms of this earth apparently evolved from a common ancestor—witness, for example, the universality of condons—and together they created the biological world dominated by 6 carbon D-sugars and 20 L-amino acids. Needless to say, natural selection made certain that all the metabolic as well as catabolic pathways were specifically tailored to deal with this world. For this very reason, were we to be divorced from our evolutionary kin and placed in another biological world of 7 carbon L-sugars and D-amino acids, our highly refined metabolic as well as catabolic enzyme systems would become totally useless. Despite various problems associated with recent population explosions, it would be very surprising indeed if the entire world population contained a single mutant individual who can metabolize 7 carbon L-sugars and utilize D-amino acids as building blocks of proteins.

This hypothetical example serves to illustrate an inherent limitation of the power of Epimethean natural selection. We can be reasonably certain, however, that our immune system, in sharp contrast to our metabolic and catabolic pathways, would continue to perform well in that alien world, for this system has demonstrated ample capability to deal with all sorts of odd, man-made molecules that are the products of post-World War II chemistry. It is almost certain that this biological world has never experienced many of these man-made molecules until the present. It follows, then, that the immune system has apparently risen above the Epimethean world of evolution by natural selection, for it gives us an impression of having evolved in anticipation of man's eventual success in contaminating this biological world with odd, man-made molecules. This is true of the immune system not only of man, but also of the horse, goat, rabbit, and mouse.

3. Why the Promethean Evolution of the Immune System?

In the Epimethean world of evolution by natural selection, one cannot conceive of the *lac*-operon's becoming the species characteristic of *Escherichia coli* before *Esch. coli*'s first encounter with lactose in the gut of suckling mammalian infants that occurred with the emergence of mammals. Thus, were we to plate a related species of bacteria that had never lived in the mammalian gut on an agar plate containing lactose as a sole carbohydrate source, we would expect to select for a specific mutant clone by killing off the rest. Yet immunologists concoct all sorts of nonbiological haptens and fully expect to raise specific antibodies against them in any randomly chosen rabbit or mouse, and these experimental animals usually do not disappoint them. It follows, then, that in the immune system, the ability to cope with any previously unexperienced contingency is conferred on almost every individual, instead of on a few appropriate mutants in a population. Indeed, the immune system has evolved according to the Promethean principle.

When one realizes that the immune system must have evolved primarily to combat pathogenic parasites (bacteria and viruses), it becomes clear that the development of this system could not have obeyed the Epimethean law of evolution by natural selection. As Charles Darwin already realized (Stauffer, 1975), a peculiar evolutionary relationship exists between parasitic organisms and their hosts. The worst that parasitic organisms (viruses and bacteria) can become is to be too successful, for a too-virulent and too-reproductively proficient strain would exterminate a host population and, in so doing, exterminate itself. Natural selection should thus favor a reasonable benignancy in pathogenic parasitic organisms, so that the reproductive performance of a parasitized host population would not be too severely impaired. The only problem is that the generation time of viruses and bacteria is extraordinarily short by our standard, so that a mutant strain that is either exceptionally virulent or prolific or both can take a very quick, although temporary, advantage and do a great deal of harm to a host population. Such harm is bearable so long as the host's generation time is also reasonably short and its body size reasonably small, so that a limited environment can sustain a large host population. Indeed, insects are quite content to deal with pathogenic parasites without enlisting help from the immune system, their sole defense being based on phagocytic activity of wandering cells, and also possibly of interferons. Vertebrates, on the other hand, tend to be large-bodied, a characteristic that is usually associated with a rather long generation time, and they extract heavy tolls from the environment not only in the amount of food they consume, but also in the amount of wastes they produce. Thus, a given area can sustain only a limited number of individuals. Accordingly, occasional great havoc wrought by particularly virulent mutant strains of parasitic organisms may readily exterminate a vertebrate species. I believe that herein lies the *raison d'être* of the immune system that is unique to vertebrates.

Since there is a difference of several orders of magnitude between the generation time of bacteria and viruses and that of vertebrate hosts, as long as the host's immune system remained under the surveillance of customary Epimethean natural selection, it could never cope with the periodic occurrence of new virulent mutants. Development of the immune system had to depend on a new evolutionary mechanism based on the Promethean principle, so that the system could readily cope with previously unencountered mutant strains of bacteria and viruses.

4. Strategy of Promethean Evolution

Germ-line theorists thought, in their original crude formulation, that the apparent ability of the immune system to cope with all sorts of previously unencountered contingencies is a mere reflection of the fact that the genome of higher vertebrates came to contain an enormous number of V-region genes. Unfortunately, a mere quantitative increase, no matter how great, does not provide an answer. A gene can maintain its integrity only if it comes under strict surveillance by Epimethean natural selection. A V-region gene shelved in the genome in anticipation of a future need does not contribute to the well-being of individuals. While it is ignored by natural selection, there is nothing to prevent it from undergoing random changes due to mutations. Thus, a shelved V-region gene is likely to become a derelict before the need for it arises.

It follows, then, that the V-region genes, to be kept in the genome, must necessarily specify antigen-binding sites directed against common pathogens of the present world. Only then would mutant individuals bearing defective V-region genes become unfit to survive in the present environment, so that natural selection can eliminate them to conserve the functional integrity of each V-region gene. This argument shows that even Promethean evolution has no choice but to ultimately depend on Epimethean natural selection. The ability to cope with the future should somehow be linked to the proved and tested ability of coping with the past and the present. The cross-reactivity by virtue of similarity between an evolutionary familiar antigen and a previously unencountered antigen should play only a minor role in the link between the past and the future. First of all, the power of anticipation based on the similarity to experiences of the past is extremely limited in scope. Furthermore, the ability to discriminate a nonself from a self even if the two differ only by a few amino acid substitutions is a cornerstone of the immune system. Thus, natural selection should have always favored the kinds of antibodies that can single out specific molecules from the group of similars.

What, then, is the nature of the link between the past and the future that enables the immune system to cope with all sorts of previously unencountered contingencies? Somatic mutation theorists have an elegant explanation (Cohn, 1968; Jerne, 1971). During ontogenic development of individuals, somatic mutations affecting stem cells of the immune system randomly modify those heritable V-region genes that have been approved by Epimethean natural selection. A wide variety of antibody-producing clones thus generated are no longer bound to the past; thus, some of them can, by chance, recognize odd, previously unencountered molecules as antigens. Since each clone produces only one specific V-region sequence each of L and H chain, an antigen itself can provide a necessary selective pressure in singling out appropriate clones that are its antagonists and stimulating them to grow in size. Those clones producing antibodies that are either nonsensical or ahead of their time receive no stimuli, thus remaining as insignificant minorities. Accordingly, the immune system is quite content to waste a large number of clones that are never called to action in an individual's lifetime. In this manner, the benefit to be derived from genetic polymorphism generated by randomly sustained mutations is transferred from a population as a whole to every member of a population, and the immune system gains the Promethean character.

In the case of very small mammals with rather short life spans such as mice, however, one wonders whether somatic mutations occur frequently enough to generate sufficiently diverse antibody-producing clones. Yet 6-month-old mice appear to be as immune-competent as 25-year-old men. Fortunately, one can think of two other mechanisms that supplement or even supplant somatic mutations as the means of giving foresight to the immune system. Inasmuch as only those V-region genes that can be placed under strict surveillance by Epimethean natural selection are worth keeping in the genome of germ cells, the total number of V-region genes in the mammalian genome cannot be too great. Indeed, all the mammalian species that have been thoroughly studied have shown that all classes of V-region genes (κ-type L-chain class, λ-type L-chain class, and H-chain class) share in common segments of species-specific sequences. That they do shows at least that at the time of each speciation, the number of V-region genes in the genome must have become quite small (Hood et al., 1975). Indeed, the germ-line theorists are now content with a total number of V-region genes of the order of 10^2 instead of 10^4 or even 10^5 (Hood et al., 1975), which appears to be in keeping with the most recent DNA–RNA hybridization data (Tonegawa et al., 1974). Nevertheless, somatic amplification of the number of V-region genes can compensate for the rarity of somatic mutations. Even if the spontaneous somatic mutation rate per locus per cell generation is 10^{-7}, if the total number of V-region genes in stem cells of the immune system is amplified to 10^4, the overall mutation rate per cell generation now becomes 10^{-3}. Ostensibly, periodic expansions in the number of V-region genes in the germ-line genome can accomplish the same end as somatic amplification (Hood et al., 1975). This mechanism, however, appears to be less efficient and more cumbersome than somatic amplification. Furthermore, a species faces the greatest danger of becoming extinct at its very beginning when it is emerging as an incipient species. Inasmuch as it has done well with a small number of V-region genes in the germ-line genome at this most critical period, I do not see much sense in a species' subsequently expanding the number of V-region genes after it has secured its existence.

The last alternative mechanism, which I personally favor over both somatic mutation and either somatic amplification or periodic germ-line expansion, is the existence of a built-in link between the past and the future within each V-region gene. What if the evolutionary history of V-region genes and the physicochemical property of antigen-binding in combination provide each V-region sequence with two separate binding sites for two very different antigenic determinants? Then, each V-region gene in the genome, which is concerned by natural selection because it provides one binding site directed against common pathogens of the present world, is automatically endowed with the ability to specify an extra binding site with which it can anticipate a future need. In this manner, the link between the past and the future becomes inherent within each V-region gene. Indeed, recent evidence favors the presence of two separate antigen-binding sites within a single V-region sequence (Richards *et al.*, 1975).

It should be noted that the three alternative mechanisms discussed above, which are illustrated in Figure 1, are not necessarily mutually exclusive. It may be that all three mechanisms in combination give unique Promethean character to the immune system.

5. Conclusions

Inasmuch as natural selection has only hindsight, genetic polymorphism as such can confer the ability to cope with previously unencountered environmental changes only on a population as a whole in the form of randomly generated mutant individuals within the population.

203

THE SIGNIFICANCE
OF GENE
DUPLICATION IN
IMMUNOGLOBULIN
EVOLUTION

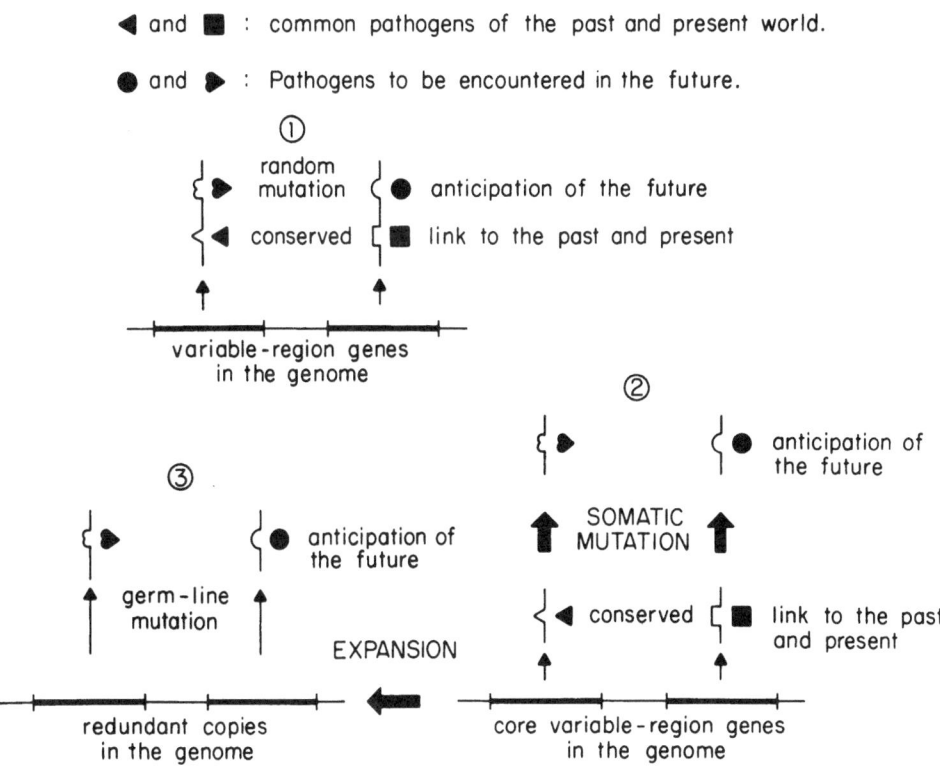

Figure 1. Three alternative mechanisms that confer Promethean character on the immune system.

In the case of the immune system, on the other hand, almost every individual in a mammalian population appears capable of producing antibodies against all sorts of evolutionarily unfamiliar molecules. Mere duplication of V-region genes cannot confer such foresight on the immune system. As far as the V-region genes are concerned, the benefit to be derived from randomly generated mutations has somehow been conferred on almost every member of a population. This chapter has discussed briefly three different but not mutually exclusive mechanisms that may have given Promethean character to the immune system.

References

Cohn, M., 1968 The molecular biology of expectation, in: *Nucleic Acids in Immunology* (O. J. Plescia and W. Braun, eds.), pp. 671–715, Springer-Verlag, New York.

Cohn, M., 1970, Anticipatory mechanisms of individuals, in: *Ciba Found. Symp.: Control Processes in Multicellular Organisms* (G. E. W. Wolstenholme and J. Knight, eds.), pp. 255–297, J. & A. Churchill, London.

Gally, J. A., and Edelman, G. M., 1972, The genetic control of immunoglobulin synthesis, *Annu. Rev. Genet.* **6**:1–46.

Goodfellow, P. N., Jones, E. A., van Heyningen, V., Solomon, E., Bobrow, M., Maggiano, V., and Bodmer, W. F., 1975, The β_2-microglobulin gene is on chromosome 15 and not in the *HL-A* region, *Nature (London)* **254**:267–269.

Greaves, M., 1975, Antigen receptors on T lymphcytes: A solution in sight?, *Nature (London)* **256**:92–93.

Grubb, R., 1970, *The Genetic Markers of Human Immunoglobulins*, Springer-Verlag, New York.

Hood, L., Campbell, J. H., and Elgin, S. C. R., 1975, The organization, expression and evolution of antibodies and other multigen families, *Annu. Rev. Genet.* **9**.

Jerne, N. K., 1971, The somatic generation of immune recognition, *Eur. J. Immunol.* **1**:1–9.

Litman, G. W., Frommel, D., Finstad, J., Howell, J., Pollara, B. W., and Good, R. A., 1970, The evolution of the immune response. VIII. Structural studies of the lamprey immunoglobulin, *J. Immunol.* **105**:1278–1285.

Litman, G. W., Frommel, D., Chartrand, S. L., Finstad, J., and Good, R. A., 1971, Significance of heavy-chain mass and antigenic relationship in immunoglobulin evolution, *Immunochemistry* **8**:345–349.

Mage, R., Lieberman, R., Potter, M., and Terry, W. D., 1973, Immunoglobulin allotypes, in: *The Antigens*, Vol. I (M. Sela, ed.), pp. 300–377, Academic Press, New York.

Ohno, S., 1970, *Evolution by Gene Duplication*, Springer-Verlag, New York.

Richards, F., Konigsberg, W., Rosenstein, R., and Varga, J., 1975, On the specificity of antibodies, *Science* **187**:130–137.

Stauffer, R. C. (ed.), 1975 *Charles Darwin's Natural Selection: Being the Second Part of His Big Species Book Written from 1856 to 1858*, Cambridge University Press, New York.

Tonegawa, S., Steinberg, C., Dube, S., and Bernardini, A., 1974, Evidence for somatic generation of antibody diversity, *Proc. Natl. Acad. Sci. U.S.A.* **71**:4027–4031.

8

The Phylogenetic Origins of Immunoglobulin Structure

GARY W. LITMAN and J. MICHAEL KEHOE

1. Introduction*

Comparative analyses of protein structure in different species can be useful guides to developments in evolutionary history (Arnheim, 1973). This approach is as applicable to the field of immunochemistry as it is to any other biological discipline. Such an analysis involves a search for clues to the origins and developmental processes of a currently extant biological system, e.g., the humoral immune response, by an examination of various aspects of the system as they exist in contemporary representatives of various phylogenetic levels of the animal kingdom. Such an approach assumes that current representatives of older phylogenetic categories are, in fact, reliable indicators of the nature of the particular functions as they existed millions of years ago. The validity of this assumption is perhaps never completely provable, but is nonetheless widely regarded as reasonable. Often, this assumption is the only basis on which certain inferences concerning evolutionary history can be made.

With regard to the evolutionary history of the humoral immune system itself, a number of important questions remain, including: What is the precise extent of the similarities and differences among immune proteins from different species? Can a molecular precursor of vertebrate immunoglobulins (Ig's) be found in any invertebrate species? Do the combining sites of various noninduced ligand-binding mole-

*Abbreviations used in this chapter: (β_2m) β_2-Microglobulin; (CD) circular dichroism; (C region) constant region; (DNP) 2,4-dinitrophenyl; (H chain) heavy chain; (HMW) high-molecular-weight; (Ig) immunoglobulin; (IMW) intermediate-molecular-weight; (J chain) joining chain; (KLH) keyhole limpet hemocyanin; (L chain) light chain; (LMW) low-molecular-weight; (MHC) major histocompatibility complex; (SDS-PAGE) sodium dodecyl sulfate–polyacrylamide gel electrophoresis; (SIg) surface immunoglobulin; (SRBC) sheep erythrocytes; (V region) variable region.

GARY W. LITMAN • Memorial Sloan-Kettering Cancer Center, New York, New York 10021. J. MICHAEL KEHOE • Department of Microbiology/Immunology, The Northeastern Ohio Universities College of Medicine, Rootstown, Ohio 44272.

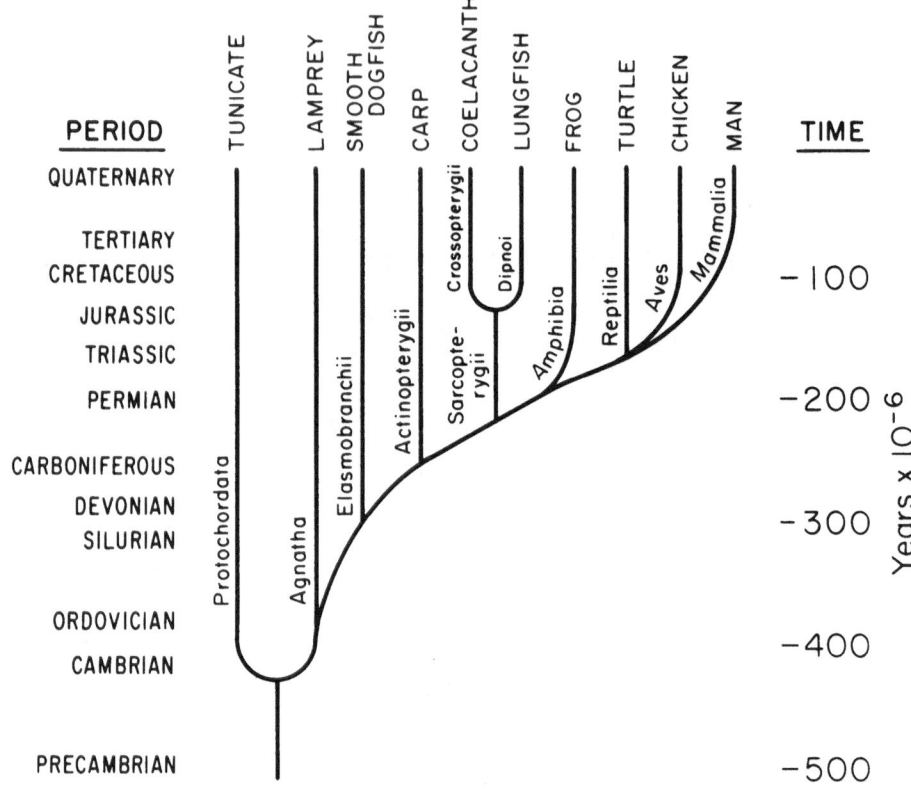

Figure 1. Phylogenetic emergence of vertebrate species. Based on Romer (1970).

cules found in invertebrate species share any structural features with Ig variable (V) regions or parts of other biologically active proteins found in more advanced species?

This chapter covers a number of aspects of these, and related, questions. Emphasis is placed on comparisons of the structure of protein products that either are or may be components of the humoral immune system of various species. A phylogenetic emergence scale is presented in Figure 1 to provide chronological points of reference for the various species discussed.

2. Invertebrate Humoral Immunity—Agglutinins

A number of noninducible glycoproteins reactive with surface structures of bacterial, protozoan, and various mammalian cells are found widely distributed throughout the invertebrate phyla. Considerable speculation has arisen concerning the relationship of these proteins, commonly referred to as agglutinins, to the functionally related Ig's. The physicochemical properties of some of the more thoroughly characterized agglutinins are outlined in Table 1. Although the agglutinins resemble antibody, from the standpoint of structural heterogeneity and function, they are not inducible and can be distinguished from antibody by differences in subunit structure, requirements for divalent cation(s), and thermal stability. While

TABLE 1. Physicochemical Properties of Agglutinins Isolated from Invertebrate Species

Species	Reactivity[a]	Specificity[b]	Temperature stability	Divalent cation[c]	Molecular size	Subunit size	Intersubunit bonding	Heterogeneity[d]	Carbohydrate composition	Ref. No.[e]
Snail (*Helix pomatia*)	HuRBC (Group A)	MeNAcGal, NAc, Gal	Stable: 100°C, 15 min	NR	79,000	26,000 13,000	Noncovalent Covalent	Multiple bands on polyacrylamide gel electrophoresis	Hexose, 7.3% (galactose, 4%; mannose, 3.3%); hexosamine, trace	1
Oyster (*Crassostrea virginica*)	SRBC	NAc Glu, NAcGal, D-Galactose	Stable: 56°C, 30 min Unstable: 70°C, 30 min	Ca²⁺	33.4 S	20,000 Single N-terminal	Noncovalent	ND	Hexose, 6.5%; glucosamine, 6.6%	2
Horseshoe crab (*Limulus polyphemus*)	Ho RBC, HuRBC, PRBC	NANA, NAcGlu	Unstable: 65°C, 30 min	Ca²⁺	399,000	22,500 Single N-terminal	Noncovalent	Multiple bands on electrofocusing	Neutral sugar, 1.8%; glucosamine, 1.8%	3
Lobster (*Homarus americanus*)	MRBC, HRBC (LAg-1)	NANA	Unstable: 56°C, 15 min	Ca²⁺	19 S	55,000	Noncovalent	Two different size classes	Detected, but not quantitated	4
	MRBC (LAg-2)	NAcGal	Unstable: 56°C, 15 min	Ca²⁺	15 S	55,000	Noncovalent	Two different size classes	Detected, but not quantitated	

[a] Reactivity refers only to those cell types commonly employed in analysis of agglutinin activity and is not meant to indicate the complete range of activity of an agglutinin. (Hu-, Ho-, M-, P-, SRBC) Human, horse, mouse, pig, and sheep erythrocytes, respectively.

[b] (MeNAcGal) Methyl α-D-N-acetyl galactosamine; (NAcGal) N-acetyl galactosamine; (NAcGlu) N-acetyl glucosamine; (NANA) N-acetyl neuraminic acid.

[c] Original sources should be consulted for determining divalent cation requirements, since divalent cation removal often leads to loss of one specificity but not another, and in some cases, Ca²⁺ can be substituted for another cation, resulting in only partial loss of activity. (NR) Not required.

[d] (ND) Not determined.

[e] References: (1) Hammarström (1974); (2) Acton et al. (1969); (3) Marchalonis and Edelman (1968a), Finstad et al. (1972, 1974), Roche and Monsigny (1974); (4) Hall and Rowlands (1974a,b).

the minor subunits of some agglutinins are similar in molecular weight to mammalian Ig light (L) chains, amino acid composition and limited sequence analyses have failed to define any significant degree of homology with the subunits of higher or lower vertebrate Ig (Finstad *et al.*, 1974; Kaplan *et al.*, 1977). It was demonstrated that foreign cells coated with lobster agglutinins are engulfed more rapidly by hemocytes than are noncoated cells, suggesting one possible functional role for these proteins (Hall and Rowlands, 1974b). No relationship between the agglutinins and the system of cell-mediated immunorecognition existing in invertebrates such as annelids, echinoderms, and protochordates has been defined (Hildemann, 1974). Work to date has suggested that rather than consider the agglutinins as possible ancestral prototypes of Ig's, it is probably more realistic to consider them as components of invertebrate host recognition that yet may be reflected in non-Ig-mediated immune processes in ostracoderm- and placoderm-derived vertebrates (Sigel, 1974; Litman, 1975).

3. Immunoglobulins of Ostracoderm-Derived Vertebrates

In addition to being capable of rejecting allografts (Hildemann and Thoenes, 1969; Perey *et al.*, 1968), both the Pacific hagfish *(Eptatretus stoutii)* and the sea lamprey *(Petromyzon marinus)* mount an inducible, specific humoral immune response to complex antigens such as human blood group O erythrocytes, sheep erythrocytes (SRBC), *Brucella abortus* bacteria, f-2 bacteriophage, and keyhole limpet hemocyanin (KLH) (Marchalonis and Edelman, 1968b; Pollara *et al.*, 1970). In the Pacific hagfish, antibody to both SRBC and KLH is associated with a heat-stable (56°C, 30 min), $\approx$ 24 S macroglobulin (Linthicum and Hildemann, 1970). The heat stability of the agglutinating activity associated with the macroglobulin fraction is of importance in distinguishing inducible antibody activity from naturally occurring, heat-labile erythrocyte agglutinins also found in these species. Recently, the isolation and purification of the Ig from nonimmune hagfish serum was accomplished using a combination of ultra-centrifugation and both ion-exchange and gel-filtration chromatography techniques (De Ioannes and Hildemann, 1975). The purified Ig gave a single line in double diffusion when reacted with antiserum to whole hagfish serum. When reduced and alkylated Ig was subjected to sodium dodecyl sulfate–polyacrylamide gel electrophoresis (SDS-PAGE), four components varying in molecular weight from 17,000 to 33,000, with a principal component of $\approx$ 22,000 mol. wt., were noted. Higher-molecular-weight material was not noted in the stained gels. When the Ig preparations were subjected to analytical gel filtration in guanidine-HCl, the majority of the material applied eluted in the void volume of a Sephadex G-200 column. The basis for the difference in dissociation behavior of hagfish Ig in SDS vs. guanidine-HCl is not clear. These authors concluded that the 1 $\times$ 10^6 mol. wt. Ig was comprised of L-chain-like subunits and that heavy (H) chains apparently did not evolve until after the emergence of the hagfishes.

The antibody formed in the sea lamprey in response to immunization with bacteriophage f-2 was found to be associated with both $\approx$ 14 S and $\approx$ 7 S serum fractions (Marchalonis and Edelman, 1968b). The purified low-molecular-weight (LMW) Ig exhibited an $S_{20 w} \approx 6.6$ and was apparently comprised of two $\approx$ 70,000 mol. wt. and two $\approx$ 25,000 mol. wt. noncovalently bonded subunits. Complex dissociation of the protein during ultracentrifugation precluded assignment of an absolute molecular weight; however, the estimate of $\approx$ 188,000 mol. wt. (Marchalonis and Cone, 1973) is reasonable. Although the lack of interchain disulfide bonds and lability of antibody activity associated with 6.6 S Ig distinguish this protein from most other lower-vertebrate Ig's, the amino acid composition of the lamprey Ig H chain appears to be related to higher- and lower-vertebrate Ig μ-type H chains (Marchalonis, 1972).

The sea lamprey was shown to respond to immunization with group O human erythrocytes and *Br. abortus* with production of an $\approx$ 9 S Ig (Pollara *et al.*, 1970; Litman *et al.*, 1970). The antibody to the group O erythrocytes is specific for the H surface antigen and coelutes during gel-filtration and ion-exchange procedures with antibody to *Br. abortus*. The antibody molecule is $\approx$ 320,000 mol. wt. and is comprised of $\approx$ 75,000 mol. wt. noncovalently bonded subunits. The secondary structure of the 9 S lamprey Ig is distinct from that of other lower-vertebrate Ig's, and is discussed in detail below. Dissociation of the native molecule with concomitant loss of antibody activity takes place during storage or in the presence of weak denaturing agents. When fully reduced and alkylated Ig was subjected to gel filtration in 6 M guanidine-HCl, a predominant peak representing the native $\approx$ 75,000 mol. wt. subunit and lesser amounts of an $\approx$ 5000 mol. wt. component were noted. No evidence was found for subunits resembling 22,000–25,000 mol. wt. L chains. The reason for the apparent structural differences between the 6.6 S and 9 S lamprey Ig are not clear, although it must be remembered that major differences exist in the antigenic character of f-2 bacteriophage and mammalian erythrocytes. It was suggested previously that the 9 S lamprey Ig may represent an inducible form of the agglutinating glycoproteins found distributed throughout the invertebrates (Litman *et al.*, 1970). It has also been suggested that multimeric, carbohydrate-reactive serum proteins such as the noninducible human blood group O hemagglutinin found in the eel *(Anguilla rostrata)* (Bezkorovainy *et al.*, 1971), nurse shark *(Ginglymostoma cirratum)* fructosan-specific protein (Harisdangkul *et al.*, 1972), and plaice *(Pleuronectes platessa)* inducible C-reactive protein (Baldo and Fletcher, 1973) may represent contemporary expressions of more phylogenetically primitive humoral recognition macromolecules such as the 9 S lamprey Ig (Litman, 1975). More extensive structural characterization of these proteins will be required to resolve some of the ambiguities in the origin and fate of the gene systems involved with production of Ig-like molecules in ostracoderm-derived vertebrates.

4. Immunoglobulins of Placoderm-Derived Vertebrates

4.1. Chondrichthyes

Although no H-chain constant (C)-region primary structure homology or serological partial identity has yet been established between mammalian IgM and the principal Ig class of the Elasmobranchii, it is generally felt that the inducible antibodies of sharks represent prototypic forms of mammalian IgM (Marchalonis and Cone, 1973; Litman, 1975). The most primitive shark species (Frommel *et al.*, 1971b), along with their more recent evolutionary counterparts (Marchalonis and Edelman, 1966b; Clem and Small, 1967), possess both high-molecular-weight (HMW) and LMW Ig's that resemble mammalian IgM in polypeptide chain composition, carbohydrate content, and amino acid composition. Similarities in antigenic character, amino and carbohydrate composition, chain mass, and peptide composition have suggested that the HMW and LMW proteins do not represent distinct Ig classes, but reflect only a difference in polymer composition. The 900,000 mol. wt. HMW Ig consists of five equivalent disulfide-linked, 180,000 mol. wt. subunits, each comprised of two H chains (mol. wt ≈ 70,000) and two L chains (mol. wt. ≈ 23,000) joined through interchain disulfide bonds. A joining (J)-chain-like structure was detected in the HMW but not in the LMW Ig's isolated from several shark species (Klaus *et al.*, 1971b; McCumber and Clem, 1976). The latter are structurally equivalent to the 180,000 mol. wt. subunits of the HMW Ig and have been detected in the serum of all elasmobranch species thus far examined, with the exception of a species of ray that possesses an ≈ 360,000 mol. wt. (dimeric) LMW Ig in addition to a characteristic HMW protein (Marchalonis and Schonfeld, 1970). Measurements of clearance half-lives for isotopically labeled HMW and LMW nurse or lemon shark Ig's suggest that the LMW Ig is neither a precursor nor a catabolic product of HMW Ig (Small *et al.*, 1970).

Both HMW and LMW Ig classes exhibit multivalent (agglutinating) activity for complex bacterial antigens (Schulkind *et al.*, 1971; Frommel *et al.*, 1971b), and the range of combining-site specificities exhibited by elasmobranch antibody includes bacterial, carbohydrate, cell-surface, protein, synthetic hapten, and viral antigens. Observations of electrophoretic heterogeneity in H and L chains subjected to alkaline urea PAGE, production of antiidiotypic antibody in guinea pigs immunized with purified nurse shark antibody to group A variant streptococcal vaccine (Clem *et al.*, 1975), and probable localization of hypervariable regions in horned shark (*Heterodontus franciscii*) (Litman *et al.*, 1976; Kehoe *et al.*, 1977), Ig L chains suggest that diversity in the antigen-binding function is achieved through substitution of contact residues in active-site portions of elasmobranch Ig, very likely in a fashion analogous to that of higher species.

4.2. Osteichthyes

The basic pentamer–monomer arrangement of elasmobranch Ig's is not seen in any of the Actinopterygii. This order, which contains all the bony fishes, is comprised of the chondrosteans, the holosteans, and the teleosts. Definitive characterization has been made of the Ig's of only one chondrostean, the paddlefish (*Polyodon spathula*) (Acton *et al.*, 1971b). The HMW Ig possesses an apparent molecular weight of ≈ 660,000 and is comprised of ≈ 165,000 mol. wt. subunits comprised of disulfide-linked H- and L-chain pairs arranged in a tetrameric configuration. The paddlefish LMW Ig is equivalent to the LMW Ig found in various species of shark (Pollara *et al.*, 1968). A holostean, the bowfin (*Amia calva*), also possesses a ≈ 660,000 mol. wt., presumably tetrameric, HMW Ig along with a LMW Ig (Litman *et al.*, 1971b). Examination of the LMW protein indicated that its H chain has a molecular weight of ≈ 53,000, different from the ≈ 70,000 mol. wt. H chain of the HMW Ig; however, failure to detect major antigenic differences or differences in carbohydrate composition in the H chains of the HMW and LMW Ig's suggested that the LMW Ig was not representative of a distinct class. It was felt, rather, that the H chain of the LMW Ig may lack an ≈ 12,000 mol. wt. segment equivalent to higher-vertebrate Ig C regions or domains.

The other holosteans, two species of gar (*Lepisosteus osseus* and *Lepisosteus platyrhincus*), were characterized as possessing only HMW, tetrameric forms of IgM-like Ig (Acton *et al.*, 1971a; Bradshaw *et al.*, 1971). Affinity chromatography of radiolabeled whole gar serum on agarose columns conjugated with antiserum to gar

Ig L chain failed to reveal even trace amounts of naturally occurring LMW Ig (Litman, unpublished). The restriction of Ig to the HMW class has been noted in several other teleost fish and one amphibian species (see below). Since there is no direct evidence that transient proteolysis accounts for the absence of LMW Ig, it is likely that all H and L chains synthesized are polymerized into a tetrameric configuration. This process may be influenced by the J-chain-like structures associated with the HMW Ig's (Weinheimer *et al.*, 1971).

The most complex pattern of Ig size class distribution in bony fishes is seen in the teleosts. Goldfish *(Carassius auratus)* and carp *(Cyprinus carpio)* appear to synthesize only tetrameric, HMW Ig's equivalent to those found in paddlefish, bowfin, and gar (Marchalonis, 1971). A second pattern of size class distribution is found in a marine teleost, the grouper *(Epinephelus itaira)*, which synthesizes a tetrameric IgM along with a LMW Ig of ≈ 120,000 mol. wt. consisting of two L chains and two H chains (≈ 38,000 mol. wt.) (Clem, 1971). As with the bowfin LMW Ig, similarities in amino acid composition, peptide map characteristics, and carbohydrate composition between HMW and LMW Ig's precluded assignment of the LMW Ig to a distinct class. It was felt that the mass difference between the ≈ 70,000 mol. wt. HMW Ig H chain and the ≈ 38,000 mol. wt. LMW Ig H chain could be accounted for by the deletion of two H-chain C regions. A third pattern of Ig size class distribution was noted in another marine teleost, the margate *(Haemulon album)* (Clem and McLean, 1975). The HMW Ig of this species is comprised of H chains (≈ 70,000 mol. wt.) and L chains (≈ 22,500 mol. wt.), and is most probably tetrameric in configuration. The LMW Ig H and L chains are identical in mass to those of the tetrameric, HMW protein.

Although definitive physicochemical analyses have not been made of the tetrameric Ig's of all the bony fishes mentioned above, the studies that have been reported suggest that both disulfide content and disulfide distribution (intersubunit vs. interchain or intrachain), amino acid composition, and carbohydrate composition are similar to those of mammalian IgM. A detailed compilation of this structural data was reported elsewhere (Litman, 1976). The LMW Ig's found in some of the species resemble, for the most part, the elasmobranch LMW molecules and are composed of equal numbers of L chains (≈ 22,000 mol. wt.) and H chains (≈ 70,000–38,000 mol. wt.). The selective advantage in maintaining a tetrameric configuration in the HMW population may relate to the role of polymer number in expression of effective valence, an important component in the recognition of complex antigenic surfaces such as those of naturally occurring pathogens and parasites. The deviations in H-chain mass noted in the LMW Ig's may relate to the extravascular distribution and expression of the biological (effector) functions of this Ig class.

The first indication for divergence of a second Ig class distinct from the HMW and LMW IgM-like Ig's of the Elasmobranchii and Actinopterygii is found at the phylogenetic level of the Crossopterygii. Both the Australian lungfish *(Neoceratodus forsteri)* (Marchalonis, 1969) and the African lungfish *(Protopterus aethiopicus)* (Litman *et al.*, 1971d) possess a HMW Ig resembling a pentameric form of IgM and an ≈ 120,000 mol. wt. LMW Ig globulin comprised of two H chains (≈ 38,000 mol. wt.) and two L chains (≈ 22,500 mol. wt.). The HMW and LMW Ig's are antigenically distinct and dissimilar in amino acid and carbohydrate composition. The carbohydrate composition of the LMW protein is distinguished from that of other Ig's in that it contains only trace amounts of sialic acid (Frommel *et al.*,

1971a). In addition to HMW and LMW Ig's, lesser amounts of an ≈ 170,000 mol. wt. protein comprised of L chains (≈ 22,500 mol. wt.) and antigenically distinct H chains (≈ 65,000 mol. wt.) were detected in the African lungfish (Litman, 1975). This intermediate-molecular-weight (IMW) protein does not appear to represent the equivalent of 7 S IgM, but appears to be similar to the IMW Ig's found in some amphibian, reptilian, and avian species.

4.3. Amphibia

The Ig's of several amphibian species have been characterized. With the exception of the mud puppy *(Necturus maculosus)*, which synthesizes only HMW Ig (Marchalonis and Cohen, 1973), all amphibians synthesize both HMW and IMW Ig's. The HMW Ig's of most amphibians are ≈ 900,000 mol. wt. and possess typical L chains and ≈ 70,000 mol. wt. H chains. These molecules are probably of a pentameric configuration. The HMW Ig isolated from one amphibian species, the clawed toad *(Xenopus laevis)*, appears, however, to have a hexameric configuration (Parkhouse *et al.,* 1970). Early studies with the IMW Ig of the bullfrog *(Rana catesbiana)* suggested that it may be structurally homologous to mammalian IgG in terms of H-chain mass, amino acid composition, and carbohydrate content (Marchalonis and Edelman, 1966a). Recently, more comprehensive analyses of the IMW Ig's of the bullfrog, clawed toad, and marine toad *(Bufo marinus)* suggested that these Ig's are more homologous with IMW Ig's of dipnoan, reptilian, and avian species than with the IgG-like proteins found in mammalian species (Atwell and Marchalonis, 1975). The IMW Ig's contain equal numbers of H chains (≈ 62,000 mol. wt.) and L chains (≈ 22,000 mol. wt.). It was demonstrated that the IMW Ig of the bullfrog exists in two classes that can be distinguished antigenically and by the tendency of one class to aggregate during gel filtration (Steiner *et al.,* 1975). When the isolated Ig's are subjected to SDS-PAGE, dissociation of the L chains from the H chains occurs in the absence of reducing agent, analogous to the dissociation patterns of human IgA_2 and certain IgG proteins. Comparable analyses of interchain noncovalent bonding with the IMW proteins of other amphibians have not yet been carried out.

4.4. Reptilia

The reptilian Ig's that have been most thoroughly characterized to date were isolated from three different genera of turtle: *Chelydra serpentina* (Chartrand *et al.,* 1971), *Pseudemys scripta* (Leslie and Clem, 1972), and *Chelonia mydas* (Benedict and Pollard, 1972). It appears as though these species synthesize a HMW Ig of a pentameric configuration, an IMW Ig similar to that described in dipnoan and avian species, and a LMW (≈ 120,000 mol. wt.) Ig also found in dipnoan and avian species. The LMW Ig's exhibit bivalent (agglutinating) functions and are comprised of pairs of disulfide-bonded H chains (≈ 38,0000 mol. wt.) and L chains (≈ 23,000 mol. wt.). The carbohydrate content of the LMW Ig is <0.6%, which suggests that the molecule may lack an equivalent of an ≈ 12,000 mol. wt. domain equivalent to the CH_2 (carbohydrate-containing) domain of the γ-type human H chain (Litman *et al.,* 1971a). The IMW Ig detected in two turtle species is ≈ 178,000 mol. wt. and is comprised of two H chains ($\approx$ 64,000 mol. wt.) and two L chains ($\approx$ 22,500 mol. wt.). It is antigenically dissimilar from the HMW Ig, but is partially related to the LMW Ig. Attempts to detect IgA-like Ig in secretions from reptilians were not successful (Vaerman *et al.*, 1975), and it was suggested that IgM-like Ig's are the principal forms of secretory Ig in these species (Portis and Coe, 1975).

4.5. Aves

The Ig's of two avian species, the domestic chicken *(Gallus domesticus)* (Leslie and Clem, 1969) and the Peking duck *(Chordapa aves)* (Zimmerman *et al.*, 1971), have been extensively characterized. The chicken possesses a HMW Ig, most probably of a pentameric configuration, which is serologically cross-reactive with antiserum to mammalian IgM. In addition, an IMW Ig, commonly termed IgY, is found in the serum of these species. The IMW protein contains $\approx$ 6% carbohydrate and is comprised of H chains ($\approx$ 65,000 mol. wt.) and L chains ($\approx$ 22,500 mol. wt.). No evidence has yet been presented for the presence of an $\approx$ 120,000 mol. wt. LMW Ig in this species. An additional class of Ig was detected in bile, saliva, seminal plasma, and lachrymal and intestinal secretions of the chicken. The high concentration of this Ig in these fluids as well as its presence in the plasma cells from the lamina propria of the intestinal mucosa suggest that it may represent a homologue of mammalian secretory IgA (Vaerman *et al.*, 1975). The H chains of the IgA-like Ig isolated from chicken bile and intestinal secretions are noncovalently linked to their respective L chains. The 9–12 S IgA-like Ig isolated from chicken intestinal secretions contains a secretory component, while the 15–16 S IgA-like Ig isolated from bile lacks this structural component (Lebacq-Verheyden *et al.*, 1972). On the basis of these findings as well as certain primary structure considerations (see Section 7), IgA may represent the next homologue of mammalian Ig to appear after IgM during phylogenetic development.

Serum from ducks immunized with bacteria, protein, or hapten-substituted bacteria contains HMW, IMW, and LMW Ig's. The HMW molecule is of $\approx$ 900,000 mol. wt. and cochromatographs with the HMW isolated from turtle (Litman *et al.*, 1973). The IMW Ig resembles the IMW Ig present in dipnoan, amphibian, and reptilian species in terms of H-chain mass ($\approx$ 62,000 mol. wt.) and antigenic relationship to autologous HMW and LMW Ig H chains (Zimmerman *et al.*, 1971). The H chain of the duck IMW Ig cross-reacts with antisera monospecific for chicken IMW Ig H chains. The duck LMW Ig is antigenically deficient in comparison with the IMW Ig, although the H chains of the two Ig classes are similar in amino acid composition. The deficiency of carbohydrate associated with duck LMW Ig is similar to that reported for turtle LMW Ig, and the < 0.6% carbohydrate detectable is apparently L-chain-associated. Unlike the turtle LMW Ig, which fixes both homologous and heterologous complement, duck LMW Ig cannot fix homologous complement (heterologous was not tested) (Zimmerman *et al.*, 1971). It must be noted in interpreting these results, however, that two different methods for analyzing complement fixation were utilized. Studies employing radioactively labeled IMW and LMW Ig's suggest that LMW Ig's are not a breakdown product of IMW Ig (Grey, 1967). It is probable, however, that the H chain of the IMW Ig arose by duplication of a 330-nucleotide segment of a gene coding for the C region of the LMW Ig H chain.

GARY W. LITMAN
AND J. MICHAEL
KEHOE

Although difficulties in obtaining large quantities of homogeneous Ig have restricted conformational analyses of lower-vertebrate Ig, considerable information is available concerning the (1) overall dimensions, (2) secondary structure, (3) interchain noncovalent bonding, (4) susceptibility to limited proteolysis, and (5) segmental flexibility of these proteins. Electron microscopy of negatively stained Ig preparations indicated a hexameric subunit arrangement for clawed toad HMW Ig (Parkhouse *et al.,* 1970) and a tetrameric arrangement for carp (Shelton and Smith, 1970), paddlefish, gar, and catfish *(Ictalurus-punctatus)* (Acton *et al.,* 1971c) HMW Ig's. The tetrameric Ig's of the latter group spanned 300–400 Å across the arms and possessed a central core region of 95–100 Å.

The secondary structure of HMW, IMW, and LMW Ig's from eight species were compared utilizing the technique of circular dichroism (CD) (Litman *et al.,* 1971c). With the exception of the 9 S sea lamprey Ig, all vertebrate Ig's examined displayed a prominent CD band at 217 nm, which suggested the presence of β sheet conformation. The relative intensities of the 217 nm band in the CD spectra of higher- and lower-vertebrate Ig's were equivalent, suggesting similar contents of β structure. As in the CD spectra of human Ig's, the CD spectra of lower-vertebrate Ig was devoid of contributions from the α-helix conformation. A less prominent CD band at 235 nm (which in the case of human IgG and IgM has been shown to reflect conformation in the Fc portion of the H chain) was noted in the CD spectra of several different lower-vertebrate Ig's. In one case (Litman *et al.,* 1971b), this CD band was detected in isolated H chains, suggesting that the Fc regions of higher- and lower-vertebrate Ig's may share some conformational features. Unlike the remarkably similar CD spectra of the Ig's found in species originating from the primitive Placoderms, the CD spectra of the 9 S Ig of the sea lamprey displayed a prominent CD band $[\Theta'] = -17,750$, $\gamma_{min} = 210$ nm, consistent with the presence of significant amounts of α helix, which has not been detected spectroscopically in any other Ig or Ig subunit thus far examined. High-resolution crystal models of Fab fragments and L-chain dimers indicate β-sheet structure to be the predominant form of organized secondary structure in Ig's (see Chapter 1).

A variety of noncovalent forces serve to stabilize the interactions between Ig H and L chains. Since these associations have been shown to be critical in defining the combining site of higher-vertebrate antibody, considerable attention has been given to the nature of these interactions in both solution and crystal states. Information concerning interchain associations in lower-vertebrate Ig's has been gained largely from examination of H- and L-chain dissociation patterns during gel filtration of reduced and alkylated Ig's. In general, reduced and alkylated Ig's isolated from the serum of elasmobranch (Marchalonis and Edelman, 1966b) and chondrostean (Pollara *et al.,* 1968) species require the presence of concentrated guanidine or urea solutions to effect H- and L-chain dissociation, suggesting high levels of interchain noncovalent bonding. Ig's obtained from holostean (Litman *et al.,* 1971b) and teleostean (Clem, 1971) species can be resolved into H and L chains using relatively weak dissociating conditions, suggesting reduced levels of interchain noncovalent bonding. The reduced and alkylated LMW Ig's of dipnoan (Litman *et al.,* 1971d), reptilian (Chartrand *et al.,* 1971), and one avian (Zimmerman *et al.,* 1971) species require strong denaturing conditions for effective chain separation, while the reduced and alkylated IMW Ig of another avian species can be resolved into H and L chains by gel filtration in neutral aqueous buffer (Dreesman and Benedict, 1965). With dipnoan (Litman, 1975), reptilian (Leslie and Clem, 1972), and avian (Zimmerman *et al.,* 1971) LMW Ig's, mild reduction followed by alkylation and gel filtration in neutral aqueous solvents yields a half-molecule consisting of a single L-chain disulfide bonded to a single H chain. Such a finding, taken with the H–L chain dissociation data, would be consistent with strong inter-H–L-chain and diminished inter-H-chain noncovalent bonding. No overall trends in relative degree of noncovalent interchain bonding can be discerned from existing studies; it is reasonable to conclude, however, that interchain noncovalent bonding in lower-vertebrate Ig is equivalent to or greater than that associated with mammalian Ig.

One component of Ig conformation, segmental flexibility, is felt to be particularly important in the expression of antibody-binding function and the possible transmission of conformational change from the antigen-binding site to other regions of the Ig. Segmental flexibility in HMW and IMW Ig's isolated from amphibian, reptilian, and mammalian species was estimated by Richter *et al.* (1972) and Zagyansky (1975). These workers estimated rotational correlation times for dansyl probes attached to the Ig's and concluded that frog (Θ_h = 65–69 nsec), tortoise (Θ_h = 67–70 nsec), and chicken (Θ_h = 43 nsec) IMW Ig's were more rigid than rat or human IgG (Θ_h = 20 nsec). Similarly, carp (Θ_h = 128 nsec), frog (Θ_h = 129–145 nsec), and tortoise (Θ_h = 102–103 nsec) HMW Ig's were found to be more rigid than human IgM (Θ = 27–47 nsec). In interpreting these studies, it should be noted that the location of the fluorescent dansyl probe was not determined, thus complicating analysis of data, More recently, nanosecond decay fluorometry was utilized to examine and compare segmental flexibility in horse IgM, pig IgM, and nurse shark HMW Ig (Holowka and Cathou, 1976). Rather than covalently modify the antibody molecules with the dansyl probes, these workers induced antibody to the dansyl group and immobilized a dansyl-Lys hapten in the antibody active site, thereby defining and restricting the location of the probe. When antibody preparations from the three species bound the dansyl hapten, similar blue shifts and enhanced fluorescence yields of the dansyl group were noted, suggesting similarities of the active sites of the different Ig's. The time-dependent emission anisotropy of dansyl-Lys–shark antidansyl antibody possessed one rapid component (τ = 4.5 nsec) not seen with the horse and pig IgM, suggesting either that the hapten was exposed to solvent or that it was less rigidly bound in the active site of nurse-shark antibody. The major conclusion that can be drawn from this work at present is that shark IgM does display segmental flexibility like mammalian IgM, but to a somewhat lesser degree.

As compared with our understanding of the antigen-combining site of higher-vertebrate antibody, only limited information concerning the combining sites of lower-vertebrate antibody is available. The existing data for combining-site properties of lower-vertebrate Ig reactive with the 2,4-dinitrophenol (DNP) determinant are summarized in Table 2. In terms of relative affinity, hydrophobicity (induced spectral shifts), depth, and reactivity with affinity labels, lower-vertebrate antibody closely resembles mammalian antibody where direct comparisons can be made. Binding-site heterogeneity, reflecting differences in structural composition of active sites within a given species, has also been noted in several lower vertebrate species immunized with DNP-substituted carriers. Other studies have stressed similarities

GARY W. LITMAN
AND J. MICHAEL
KEHOE

TABLE 2. Properties of Lower- and Higher-Vertebrate Antibody to 2,4-Dinitrophenol

Species	Ig class	Immunogen	Test ligand[a]	Association constant, k_0 $(M^{-1})^a$	Combining sites/ molecule[a]	Induced shift in DNP spectrum; difference maxima[a]	Residues modified MNBDF[a,b]	H/L chain labeling ratio[a]	Combining site depth[a]	Ref. No.[c]
Nurse shark (*Ginglymostoma cirratum*)	HMW	DNP-bovine γ-globulin	ε-DNP-L-Lys	10^5–5×10^6	10 (5 high-, 5 low-affinity)	378; 425 nm	ND	ND	ND	1
Rainbow trout (*Salmo gairdneri*)	HMW	DNP-KLH; DNP-human γ-globulin	ND	ND	ND	ND	ND	ND	10–12 Å	2
Snapping turtle (*Chelydra serpentina*)	LMW	DNP-*Br. abortus*	ε-DNP-L-Lys	1.7×10^6	1.7 ± 0.1	390; 468 nm	Tyr/His (5:1)	2.7:1	ND	3
Duck (*Chordapa aves*)	LMW	DNP-*Br. abortus*	ε-DNP-L-Lys	3.8×10^6	1.5 ± 0.1	396; 474 nm	Tyr	1.4:1	ND	3
Rabbit (*Oryctolagus cuniculus*)	IgG	DNP-Bovine serum albumin	ε-DNP-L-Lys	2.5×10^6	2.0 ± 0.1	390 ± 2; 470 ± 3 nm	Tyr	2:1	10–12 Å[d]	4

[a]ND Not determined.
[b](MNBDF) *M*-Nitrobenzenediazonium fluoroborate.
[c]References: (1) Voss *et al.* (1969); (2) Roubal *et al.* (1974); (3) Litman *et al.* (1973); (4) Goodman *et al.* (1967).
[d]The value reported is for rabbit antibody analyzed in parallel with trout antibody (Roubal *et al.*, 1974).

between higher- and lower-vertebrate antibody directed at other simple haptenic and complex antigenic determinants. It is generally accepted that the basic features of the antigen-combining site arose early in evolutionary development and have sustained only moderate degrees of change in response to varying antigenic pressures. This conclusion has been supported by the limited amino acid sequence analyses that have been carried out to date on Ig's from lower species.

6. Proteolytic Cleavage Products of Immunoglobulins from Lower Species

Probably no single technique has contributed more to our ultimate understanding of Ig structure than the use of various proteolytic enzymes to effect cleavage of the proteins into major fragments. Evidence for the organization of Ig into discrete functional units for antigen-binding and mediation of biological properties was first obtained by analysis of the Fab and Fc fragments resulting from treatment of IgG with papain (Porter, 1959). Subsequent studies revealed the susceptibility to proteolysis of polypeptide segments between the C domains of Fc, the V and C regions of human Ig L chains and the H-and L-chain V regions and their respective C regions in the Fab' of a mouse IgA myeloma protein (Edelman and Gall, 1969) (see also Chapter 6). Papain or trypsin proteolysis of lemon shark LMW Ig possessing antibody activity for *Salmonella* results in formation of an $\approx$ 110,000 mol. wt. fragment that retains the agglutinating activity of the parent molecule (Klapper *et al.*, 1971). Partial reduction and alkylation converts the fragment to an $\approx$ 60,000 mol. wt. component that lacks agglutinating activity but binds to the bacteria. Further treatment of the 60,000 mol. wt., 4–5 S fragment with trypsin converts it to a 3.5 S fragment retaining binding activity and reactivity with antibody to lemon shark Ig L chain. The findings with the shark Ig are somewhat similar to cleavage patterns observed with mammalian IgG and IgM. Unlike the case with IgM, however, partial reduction of lemon shark LMW Ig followed by papain digestion results in a breakdown of the molecule to small peptides. Evidence was presented that duck IMW, but not LMW, Ig can be cleaved into Fab and Fc fragments analogous to those formed during limited proteolysis of mammalian IgG (Zimmerman *et al.*, 1971). Chicken IMW (IgY) and turtle IMW Ig's can both be cleaved in a similar fashion into Fab'$_2$-like and Fc-like components (Leslie and Clem, 1972). Since only small amounts of material are required for studies utilizing limited proteolysis as a structural probe, it is anticipated that considerably more information concerning lower-vertebrate Ig structure can be gained employing this approach.

7. Primary Structure

Amino acid sequence analysis provides a most direct probe of evolutionary relationships among proteins. This approach has been especially fruitful for Ig's, both with respect to direct structure–function correlates and in suggesting important phylogenetic relationships. The regional differentiation of Ig's into V and C regions had led to a somewhat separate emphasis on the primary structural attributes of these two regions among various species. Until recently, the V regions have received far greater attention than the C regions, since it has been hoped that they would reveal much about the genetic origins of antibody diversity.

GARY W. LITMAN
AND J. MICHAEL
KEHOE

7.1. Variable-Region Sequences

Specific information concerning the relationship of V-region primary structure to combining-site specificity, idiotype, and other aspects of the ligand-binding function of Ig's is covered in Chapter 11. Consequently, the discussion here will be restricted to some specific comments concerning the comparative phylogenetic patterns of V-region structure, with special reference to lower species. Regrettably, the amount of amino acid sequence data currently available for Ig's from lower species is much less than that for higher species such as the mouse, the rabbit, and man.

Primary structure data presently available for V regions of lower species are displayed in Table 3, together with some representative sequences from proteins of higher animals for comparison. In the absence of myeloma proteins or homogeneous elicited antibodies from most of the lower species, the determination of primary structure for these animals has been performed on pooled Ig preparations. While this method has many technical and conceptual disadvantages, it is advantageous in the single sense of providing some estimate of the extent of heterogeneity present in pools of normal antibodies. The degree of accuracy of such estimates is obviously dependent on the accuracy of the detection systems used (e.g., use of quantitative determinations of amino acid yields at each step of the sequence degradation). When such procedures have been used on selected pools, useful estimates of the extent of variation in pooled antibodies of a number of species have been obtained. Even considering the limited amount of data that is currently available, the primary structure patterns of Ig V regions among the various species have shown a surprising degree of relatedness. This relatedness has held especially true for H chains (Capra *et al.*, 1973; Kehoe and Capra, 1974; Wasserman *et al.*, 1974). This conservation pattern for H chains has extended below mammals to both elasmobranch (Sledge *et al.*, 1974) and hybodont sharks (Litman *et al.*, 1976; Kehoe *et al.*, 1977). As Table 3 illustrates there is more apparent diversity in the L chains from the various species, possibly indicating some important functional attribute of the shorter Ig polypeptide.

As a specific example of the use of the quantitative approach, analyses of the amino-terminal section of the L and H chains of the 7 S Ig produced by the horned shark *(Heterodontus francisci)* suggested that the extent of variation present in this section of the V region of both the L and H chains is less than in corresponding sections of these chains in certain mammalian species (Litman *et al.*, 1976; Kehoe *et al.*, 1977). Such a pattern could be reflective of fewer germ-line V-region genes in the more primitive species. If such a pattern holds up when numerous other lower species have been examined, important questions would be raised concerning the size of the potentiality pool possessed by these more primitive species. Do such species have a more limited repertoire of available combinding specificities, or, at least, of framework sections than do more advanced animals? Combining-site-related, or idiotypic, determinants were demonstrated by Clem in a higher elasmobranch, the nurse shark (Clem *et al.*, 1975). This finding, when considered with the overall conformational features of elasmobranch antibody mentioned previously, indicates that the general features characteristic of mammalian Ig's are also characteristic of at least one other lower vertebrate species.

The studies on the horned shark Ig also revealed a significant homology of the H chains with those of a number of higher species, including man. Partial sequence studies of the L chains, in contrast, showed that these polypeptides were indeed sequenceable, but that the observed sequences were considerably less related to the κ or λ chains of higher species. When the horned shark Ig H- and L-chain sequences were compared with equivalent sequences of nurse shark Ig's, it was noted that these two L chains were only as homologous with each other as either was with human κ and λ chains ($\approx$ 35%). The shark H chains, on the other hand, were much more homologous ($\approx$ 70%). These results suggest a somewhat greater selection pressure on H chains to retain their primary structure and could imply that an appropriate, highly effective H-chain V-region structure had already appeared over 400×10^6 years ago.

A most interesting conserved pentapeptide sequence stretch was found in the V region of L chains from a wide variety of species including the nurse shark, birds, ruminants, the whale, the dog, and man (Stanton *et al.,* 1974). The functional significance of this pentapeptide area is not totally clear but, as suggested by these workers, is most likely a highly significant aspect of L-chain structure in general.

7.2. Constant-Region Sequences

At present, there is much less comparative information available for Ig C regions than for V regions, especially with reference to species lower than mammals, for which hardly any data exist. An interesting comparison of available information for λ L chains from man, the pig, and the mouse was presented, however, by Novotny and Franek (1975). This comparison suggests, in the light of recent X-ray crystallographic data for Ig's that marked differences exist in the extent of sequence variation that occurs among these three species for different segments of the λ C region. Specifically, the surface-loop regions are much less constrained in their variation than are those segments that are intimately involved in the formation of the β-pleated sheet sections through strong, noncovalent interactions. It is to be hoped that additional comparative analyses of the C-region structure of L chains from still other species will demonstrate how universal this pattern may be. Amino acid sequence analysis of the carboxyterminal sections of human IgM and IgA molecules suggested a close evolutionary relationship between these two classes (Chuang *et al.,* 1973) and implied that the IgA class had diverged from IgM relatively recently in evolutionary time. The lack of IgA in reptilian species alluded to earlier is consistent with this conclusion. A definitive answer must also await additional H-chain C-region sequences from a number of lower species. Additional currently available information on H-chain C regions is discussed in Chapter 6, and will not be repeated here.

8. Cell-Surface Immunoglobulin and Immunoglobulin-Related Structure(s)

Ig has been detected by immunofluorescence on the surface of lymphocytes obtained from elasmobranch (Ellis and Parkhouse, 1975), teleost (Emmrich *et al.,* 1975; Warr *et al.,* 1976; Cuchens *et al.,* 1976), and amphibian (DuPasquier *et al.,* 1973) species. Of considerable interest in these studies has been the detection of Ig on thymus lymphocytes in contrast to observations with avian and mammalian T lymphocytes. In the lower vertebrate species, higher percentages of Ig-positive cells

GARY W. LITMAN
AND J. MICHAEL
KEHOE

TABLE 3. Amino-Terminal Variable-Region Sequences of Representative Immunoglobulins from Various Species[a]

Light chains

Species		0	1	2	3	4	5	6	7	8	9	10	11	12	13	14	15	16	17	18	19	20	21	22	23	Ref. No.[b]
Man	V$_\kappa$I prototype		Asp	Ile	Gln	Met	Thr	Gln	Ser	Pro	Ser	Ser	Leu	Ser	Ala	Ser	Val	Gly	Asp	Arg	Val	Thr	Ile	Thr	Cys	1
	V$_\kappa$II prototype		Glu	Ile	Val	Leu	Thr	Gln	Ser	Pro	Gly	Thr	Leu	Ser	Leu	Ser	Pro	Gly	Glu	Arg	Ala	Thr	Leu	Ser	Cys	1
	V$_\kappa$III prototype		Asp	Ile	Val	Met	Thr	Gln	Ser	Pro	Leu	Ser	Leu	Pro	Val	Ser	Pro	Gly	Glu	Pro	Ala	Ser	Ile	Ser	Cys	1
	V$_\lambda$I prototype		PCA	Ser	Val	Leu	Thr	Gln	Pro	Pro	Ser	Val	Ser	Ala	Ala	Thr	Gly	Gln	Lys	Val	Thr	Ser	Ser	Cys	Ser	1
	V$_\lambda$II prototype		His	Ser	Ala	Leu	Thr	Gln	Pro	Ala	Ser	Val	Ser	Gly	Ser	Pro	Gly	Gln	Ser	Ile	Thr	Ile	Ser	Cys	Thr	1
	V$_\lambda$III prototype		Ser	Tyr	Glu	Leu	Thr	Gln	Pro	Pro	Ser	Val	Ser	Val	Ser	Leu	Gly	Gln	Thr	Ala	Val	Ile	Thr	Cys	Ser	1
	V$_\lambda$IV prototype		PCA	Ser	Ala	Leu	Thr	Gln	Pro	Pro	Ser	Ala	Ser	Gly	Ser	Pro	Gly	Gln	Ser	Val	Thr	Ile	Ser	Cys	Thr	1
	V$_\lambda$V prototype		(−)	Ser	Glu	Leu	Thr	Gln	Asp	Pro	Ala	Val	Ser	Gly	Ser	Pro	Gly	Gln	Ser	Val	Thr	Ile	Ser	Cys	Thr	1
Pig	λ prototype		Glu	Thr	Val	Leu	Leu	( )	Gln	Glu	Pro	Ala	Met	Ser	Val	Ala	Leu	Gly	Gln	Thr	Val	Arg	Ile	Thr	Cys	Gln	1
Pig	κ prototype	Ala	( )	Ile	Val*	Leu*	Thr*	Glx	Ser	Pro	Ser*	Leu	Leu*	Ala*	Ser	Pro	Gly	Gly	Thr	Arg	Thr	Leu	Thr	Cys	?	2
Mouse	κ prototype		Asp	Ile	Val	Leu	Thr	Gln	Ser	Pro	Ala	Ser	Leu	Ala	Val	Pro	Leu	Gly	Gln	Arg	Ala	Thr	Ile	Ser	Cys	3
Rat	κ		Asp	Ile	Gln	Met	Thr	Gln	Ser	Pro	Ser	Leu	Leu	Ser	Ala	Ser	Val	Gly	Asx	Arg	Val	Thr	Leu	Ser	Cys	1
Rabbit	κ	Ala	Ala	Val	Val	Met	Thr	Glx	Thr	Pro	Ala	Ser	Val	Ser	Ala	Ser	Val	Gly	Gly	Thr	Val	Thr	Ile	–	Cys	4
Turkey	Pool		( )	( )	( )	Leu	Thr	Gln	Pro	Ala	( )	Ser	Val	Ser	Ala	Ala	Pro	Gly	Gly	Thr	Val	Lys	Ile	Thr	Cys	1
Chicken	Pool		( )	( )	( )	Leu	Thr	Gln	Pro	Ala	( )	Ser	Val		Ala	Asx	Pro	Gly	Gly	Thr	Val	Lys	Ile	Thr	Cys	5
Duck	Pool		( )	( )	( )	Leu	Thr	Gln	Pro	Ala	Ser	Ser		Ala	Asx		Gly		Gly		Val	Lys		Thr		5
Axolotl	Pool (HMW)		Asp	( )	( )	Leu	Thr	Glx		Ala	Ser	Met	–	Val												6
African lungfish	Pool		Asp	( )	( )	Leu	Thr	Glx	Asx	Ala	Ser	Met	–	Val												7
Gar	Pool (HMW)		PCA	Ile*	Val	Ile	Thr	Glx	Pro	Gly*	Ser	Val	Leu													8
Paddlefish	Pool		Asp	Ile*	Val*	Ile	Thr	Glx	Pro	Pro	Pro	Val														9
Leopard shark	Pool		Asp	Ile*	Val*	Leu*	Thr	Glu	Ser	Pro	Pro	Val	Leu											Ser	Cys	10
Nurse shark	Pool		Asp	Thr	Thr	Met*	Thr	Glu	Ser	Pro	Pro	Val	Leu	Ser	Val	Gly	Leu	Gly	Gln	Thr	Ala	Thr	Ile	Thr	Cys	11
Horned shark	Pool		Val	Pro*	Val	Leu	Asp*	Gln*	Thr	Pro	Ile	Pro	Asp*	Pro	Val	Ser	Ala	Gly	Glu	Thr	Ser	Glu*	Leu	Gly	Cys	12

Heavy chains

Species	Sample	Sequence	Ref.
Man	VₕI prototype	PCA Val His Leu Val Glu Ser Gly Ala Gly Val Lys Lys Pro Gly Ala Ser Met Lys Val Ser Cys Ala	1
	VₕII prototype	PCA Val Thr Leu Thr Gly Ser Ser Pro Ala Leu Lys Lys Pro Lys Gln Pro Leu Thr Leu Thr Cys Ala	1
	VₕIII prototype	Glu Val Gln Leu Val Glu Ser Gly Gly Gly Leu Val Gln Pro Gly Gly Ser Leu Arg Leu Ser Cys Ala	1
Pig	IgG pool	Glu Glu Gln Leu Val Glu Ser Gly Gly Gly Leu Val Gln Pro Gly Gly Ser Leu ? Leu Ser Cys Val	14
Dog	IgG pool	Glu Val Gln Leu Val Glu Ser Gly Gly Asp Leu Val Gln* Pro Gly Gly Ser Leu Arg Leu Ser Cys Val	15
Cat	IgG pool	Asp Val Gln Leu Val Glu Ser Gly Gly Asp Leu Val Gln Pro Gly Gly Ser Leu Arg Leu Thr Cys Val	15
Seal	IgG pool	Glu Val Lys Leu Val Glu Ser Gly Gly Asp Leu Val Gln Pro Gly Gly Ser Leu Arg Leu Ser Cys Ala	15
Sea lion	IgG pool	Glu Val Gln Leu Val Glu Ser Gly Gly Asp Leu Val Gln Pro Gly Gly Ser Leu Arg Thr Ser Cys Ala	15
Mink	IgG pool	Glu Val Gln Leu Val Glu Ser Gly Gly Gly Leu Val Gln Pro Gly Gly Ser Leu Arg Leu Ser Cys Ala	15
Guinea pig	IgG pool	Glu* Val Gln Leu Val Glu Ser Gly Gly Gly Leu Val Gln Pro Gly Gly Ser Leu Arg Leu Ser Cys Val	15
Rat	IgG pool	Glu* Val Lys Leu Val Glu Ser Gly Gly Gly Leu Val Gln Pro Gly Gly Ser Leu Arg Leu Ser Cys Ala	15
Mouse	IgG pool	Glu Val Gln Leu Val Glu Ser Gly Gly Asp Leu Val Gln Pro Gly Gly Ser Leu Lys Leu Ser Cys Ala	15
Opossum	IgG pool	Glu Ile Gln Leu Val Glu Ser Gly Gly Gly Leu Val Gln Pro Gly Gly Ser Leu Arg Leu Ser Cys Ala	15
Chicken	IgG pool	Ala Val Thr Leu Asp Glu Ser Gly Gly Gly Leu Gln Thr Pro Gly Gly Ser Ala Arg Leu Val Cys Gly	16
Turkey	IgG pool	Ala Val* Gln Leu* Val Glu Ser Gly Gly Gly Val Gln Gly Pro Gly Val Ser Leu Arg Leu Val Cys Gly	16
Duck	IgG pool	Ala Ala Thr Leu Asp Glu Ser Gly Gly Gly Leu Val Gly Pro Gly Val Gln Leu Arg Leu Val Cys Gly	16
Goose	IgG pool	Ala Ile Gln* Leu Asp Glu Ser Gly Gly Val Leu Val Gly Pro Gly Val Gln Leu Arg Leu Val Cys Gly	16
Pigeon	IgG pool	Ala Ile Ile Leu Val Glu Ser Gly Gly Gly Leu Val Gln Pro Gly Gly ?* Leu Arg Leu Val Cys Gly	16
Marine toad	HMW	( ) Ser Ile Leu — Glu Ser Gly Gly Gly Leu Val Gln Pro Gly Gly ?* Leu Arg Leu Val Cys Gly	17
Axolotl	Pool	Asp — — Val — — — Glx — — — — — — — — — — — — — — —	7
Gar	HMW	Asp Ala* Val* Ile — — Pro Glx Ala Glx — — — — — — — — — — — Cys Gly	18
Paddlefish	pool	Asp Ile Val Val Thr Thr — — — — — — — — — — — — — — — — —	10
Leopard shark	pool	Glu Ile Val Leu Thr Gln Pro Glx Ala Glx — — — — — — — — — — — — —	11
Nurse shark	Homogeneous antibody	Asp Val Thr Leu Thr* Glx Pro Glx Ala Glx Ser Gly Lys Pro Gly Gly Ala Leu Arg Leu Thr Cys Glx	12
Horned shark	Pool	Asp Val Val Leu Thr Gln Pro Glu Ala Glu Gly Gly Pro Gly Gly Ser Leu Arg Leu Thr Cys ?	13

[a] Prototype sequences are taken from Gally (1973), which should be consulted for original references. Positions marked with asterisks showed varying degrees of multiple residues. Parentheses indicate the assumed locations of deletions.

[b] References: (1) Gally (1973); (2) Novotny et al. (1972); (3) Novotny et al. (1970); (4) Wang et al. (1975); (5) Grant et al. (1971); (6) Hood et al. (1970); (7) Hood and Fougereau (1972); (8) Litman et al. (1971d); (9) Acton et al. (1971a); (10) Pollara et al. (1968); (11) Klaus et al. (1971a); (12) Sledge et al. (1974); (13) Kehoe et al. (1977); (14) Franek et al. (1975); (15) Capra et al. (1973); (16) Wasserman et al. (1974); (17) Acton et al. (1972); (18) Acton et al. (1970).

have been detected in lymphocytes of thymic origin (presumably representing T-cell equivalents) than have been detected with lymphocyte populations felt to represent B-cell equivalents. Both patching and capping of surface Ig (SIg) were observed in all the studies. Following modulation by anti-Ig reagents, resynthesis of thymocyte SIg occurs, suggesting that the SIg was not of endogenous origin. Competitive inhibition by purified Ig of the binding of anti-bream *(Lepomis macrochirus)* serum Ig to the surface of bream lymphocytes indicated that these cells contain approximately 0.7×10^{-12} g Ig/cell compared with approximately 1.0×10^{-12} g Ig/cell detected on mouse splenic lymphocytes analyzed in parallel (Cuchens *et al.,* 1976).

Attempts have been made to examine the covalent structure of both bream (Cuchens *et al.,* 1976) and goldfish (Warr *et al.,* 1976) cell-surface Ig using surface-restricted, lactoperoxidase-catalyzed radioiodination, serological precipitation with anti-Ig reagents, and analysis of serological precipitates by SDS-PAGE. The Ig present on goldfish splenocytes appears to consist of a principal component resembling a mammalian μ chain in gel retardation characteristics along with a lower-molecular-weight component similar in relative migration to L chains. Significant quantities of additional components also appear in the precipitates; however, no attempt has been made to characterize them. Goldfish thymocyte Ig consists of a principal component with an apparent molecular weight intermediate between the molecular weights of μ and γ H chains. L-chain-like material and significant amounts of HMW components were also noted. The latter substances reflect a difference in the ability of NP4O to solubilize thymocyte vs. splenocyte SIg.

The Ig found on the surface of bream lymphocytes of different origin consists largely of two components similar in gel retardation characteristics to mammalian μ H and L chains. Substantial amounts of material not solubilized by NP4O have also been observed. Attempts to liberate labeled SIg by pronase digestion were not successful, suggesting a major difference in vectorial disposition of bream lymphocyte SIg vs. mammalian lymphocyte Ig. Biochemical data on lymphocyte Ig from both teleost species are too incomplete to speculate on possible relationships among serum, thymocyte, and other lymphocyte Ig's.

Antisera to human β_2-microglobulin (β_2m), a 12,000 mol. wt. polypeptide that shares substantial homology with certain mammalian Ig C-region domains (Cunningham and Berggård, 1974), were found to be reactive in an indirect immunofluorescence assay with 1–2% of shark (horned shark, nurse shark, dogfish shark) peripheral blood leukocytes (Litman *et al.,* 1976). The reactive cells possessed a lobulated nucleus and granular basophilic cytoplasm and were typical of neither mononuclear lymphocytes nor polymorphonuclear leukocytes. These observations are of particular interest, since studies with mammalian leukocytes have shown β_2m to be associated with the H chain of mouse H-2 and human HLA antigens. A β_2m-like component may also be associated with the corresponding B histocompatibility antigen found in chickens (Ziegler and Pink, 1975). Although antisera to β_2m coprecipitate mammalian leukocyte histocompatibility antigens, attempts to precipitate a β_2m-like (reactive with antiserum to human β_2m) component and any additional surface polypeptides from detergent (NP4O)-solubilized, radioiodinated shark leukocyte preparations were unsuccessful. This negative result may relate, in part, to the difficulties in detergent solubilization of antigens from lower-vertebrate lymphocytes noted by other groups (Warr *et al.,* 1976; Cutchens *et al.,* 1976).

Polypeptides reactive with antiserum to mammalian β_2m were detected in the unfractionated serum of one species of shark, and in two avian species with the use of a heterologous (inhibition of binding of rabbit β_2m with goat antihuman β_2m) radioimmunoassay system (Gordon and Kindt, 1976). An $\approx 12,000$ mol. wt. polypeptide reactive with antiserum to human β_2m was partially purified from nurse shark serum (Litman *et al.*, 1976). The isolated component comigrated with human β_2m in SDS-PAGE and possessed an intrachain disulfide linkage. Further characterization of the half-cystine-containing peptides isolated from the β_2m-like material in lower vertebrate species, along with the known associations between mammalian β_2m and major histocompatibility complex (MHC) products, have profound implications in the interpretation of the evolutionary origins of allogeneic recognition and the relationship between Ig structural genes and the MHC.

9. Summary and Conclusions

All attempts to identify a precursor to mammalian Ig's in invertebrate species have been unsuccessful. These studies include structural analyses of a number of invertebrate agglutinins that possess binding activity for a wide variety of ligands.

IgM-like Ig has been identified in many vertebrates. The evolution of Ig classes distinct from IgM has been observed in the development of most vertebrate species, which includes the Crossopterygii and eventually culminates with the emergence of mammals. These Ig's are comprised of equal numbers of H and L chains and range in molecular weight from $\approx 900,000$ to $180,000$. In most species thus far studied, both LMW and IMW or two classes of IMW Ig have been detected. The relationship, if any, of dipnoan amphibian, reptilian, and avian LMW Ig's to mammalian IgG, IgA, IgD, or IgE has not yet been fully elucidated.* The best evidence for the similarity between lower-vertebrate non-IgM Ig and mammalian Ig is in the case of human and avian secretory IgA. While variation in polymer composition and, to a lesser extent, deviation in H-chain mass characterised the evolution of the HMW and LMW Ig's of the Elasmobranchii and members of the Actinopterygii, Ig evolution along the line of the Crossopterygii involved divergence of multiple, distinct classes of Ig. Physiological distribution, interaction with complement, selective assocations with cell surfaces, and transfer to the developing embryo represent likely non-antigen-dependent selective pressures associated with the functions of specialized segments of the H-chain C regions of all these Ig's.

A most interesting general observation that has arisen from comparative studies of the Ig's of vertebrates concerns the large degree of overall structural similarity possessed by the molecules from the various species. This similarity is reflected in the observation that all bona fide Ig's examined to date possess both H and L chains and share basic conformational features. Also, a high degree of primary structure conservation is apparent in the framework sections of the V

---

*D. Hädge, G. Fiebig, and H. Ambrosius have recently provided convincing physicochemical evidence for the relatedness of IMW Ig isolated from amphibian, reptilian, and avian species. In addition, they further characterized the LMW Ig from these species as being antigenically deficient to the IMW Ig. They were unable, however, to establish a convincing identity between IMW Ig and human IgG and IgD.

regions from widely divergent animal species. There are, in addition, some preliminary indications of similar placements of hypervariable regions in antibodies of phylogenetically distinct species. It is likely that future studies, especially involving amino acid sequence analysis, will define more clearly the exact extent of these common patterns, as well as the details and functional significance of the variations that are seen in different members of the animal kingdom.

ACKNOWLEDGMENTS

Support to the laboratory of G.W.L is provided by NCI CA 08748, AI 14454, and AI 13528, and to J.M.K. by AI 09810.

References

Acton, R. T., Bennett, J. C., Evans, E. E., and Schrohenloher, R. E., 1969, Physical and chemical characterization of an oyster hemagglutinin, *J. Biol. Chem.* **244**:4128–4135.

Acton, R. T., Weinheimer, P. F., Wolcott, M., Evans, E. E., and Bennett, J. C., 1970, *N*-Terminal sequences of immunoglobulin heavy and light chains from three species of lower vertebrates, *Nature (London)* **228**:991–992.

Acton, R. T., Weinheimer, P. F., Dupree, H. K., Evans, E. E., and Bennett, J. C., 1971a, Phylogeny of immunoglobulins: Characterization of a 14S immunoglobulin from the gar, *Lepisosteus osseus, Biochemistry* **10**:2028–2036.

Acton, R. T., Weinheimer, P. F., Durpree, H. K., Russel, T. R., Wolcott, M., Evans, E. E., Schrohenloher, R. E., and Bennett, J. C., 1971b, Isolation and characterization of the immune macroglobulin from the paddlefish, *Polyodon spathula, J. Biol. Chem.* **246**:6760–6769.

Acton, R. T., Weinheimer, P. F., Hall, S. J., Niedermeier, W., Shelton, E., and Bennett, J. C., 1971c, Tetrameric immune macroglobulins in three orders of bony fishes, *Proc. Natl. Acad. Sci. U.S.A.* **68**:107–111.

Acton, R. T., Evans, E. E., Weinheimer, P. F., Niedermeier, W., and Bennett, J. C., 1972, Purification and characterization of two classes of immunoglobulins from the marine toad, *Bufo marinus, Biochemistry* **11**:2751.

Arnheim, N., 1973, Evolution of proteins, in: *The Antigens* (M. Sela, ed.), Vol. I, pp. 377–416, Academic Press, New York.

Atwell, J. L., and Marchalonis, J. J., 1975, Phylogenetic emergence of immunoglobulin classes distinct from IgM, *J. Immunogenet.* **1**:367–391.

Baldo, B. A., and Fletcher, T. C., 1973, C-reactive protein-precipitins in plaice, *Nature (London)* **246**:145–146.

Benedict, A. A., and Pollard, L. W., 1972, Three classes of immunoglobulins found in the sea turtle, *Chelonia mydas, Folia Microbiol. (Prague)* **17**:75–78.

Bezkorovainy, A., Springer, G. F., and Desai, P. R., 1971, Physicochemical properties of the eel anti-human blood-group H (O) antibody, *Biochemistry* **10**:3761–3764.

Bradshaw, C. M., Clem, L. W., and Sigel, M. M., 1971, Immunologic and immunochemical studies on the gar, *Lepisosteus platyrhincus.* II. Purification and characterization of immunoglobulin, *J. Immunol.* **106**:1480–1487.

Capra, J. D., Wasserman, R. L., and Kehoe, J. M., 1973, Phylogentically associated residues within the $V_H III$ subgroup of several mammalian species: Evidence for a "pauci-gene" basis for antibody diversity, *J. Exp. Med.* **138**:410–427.

Chartrand, S. L., Litman, G. W., Lapointe, N., Good, R. A., and Frommel, D., 1971, The evolution of the immune response. XII. The immunoglobulins of the turtle: Molecular requirements for biological activity of the 5.7S immunoglobulin, *J. Immunol.* **107**:1–11.

Chuang, C., Capra, J. D., and Kehoe, J. M., 1973, Immunoglobulin evolution—Relationship between carboxyterminal region of a human α-chain and other immunoglobulin heavy chain constant regions, *Nature (London)* **244**:158–160.

Clem, L. W., 1971, Phylogeny of immunoglobulin structure and function. IV. Immunoglobulins of the giant grouper, *Epinephelus itaira, J. Biol. Chem.* **246**:9–15.

Clem, L. W., and McLean, W. E., 1975, Phylogeny of immunoglobulin structure and function. VII. Monomeric and tetrameric immunoglobulins of the margate: A marine teleost fish, *Immunology* **29**:791–799.

Clem, L. W., and Small, P. A., Jr., 1967, Phylogeny of immunoglobulin structure and function. I. Immunoglobulins of the lemon shark, *J. Exp. Med.* **125**:893–920.

Clem, L. W., McLean, W. E., and Shankey, V., 1975, Quantitative and qualitative aspects of the antibody library of sharks in: *Immunologic Phylogeny* (W. H. Hildemann and A. A. Benedict, eds.), pp. 231–239, Plenum Press, New York.

Cuchens, M., McLean, E., and Clem, L. W., 1976, Lymphocyte heterogeneity in fish and reptiles, in: *Phylogeny of Thymus and Bone Marrow-Bursa Cells* (R. K. Wright and E. L. Cooper, eds.), pp. 205–213, Elsevier/North-Holland, Amsterdam.

Cunningham, B. A., and Berggård, I., 1974, Structure, evolution, and significance of β_2-microglobulin, *Transplant. Rev.* **21**:3–14.

De Ioannes, A. E., and Hildemann, W. H., 1975, Preliminary structural characterization of Pacific hagfish immunoglobin. *Adv. Exp. Med. Biol.* **64**:151–160.

Dreesman, G. R., and Benedict, A. A., 1965, Reductive dissocation of chicken γG immunoglobulins in neutral solvents without a dispersing agent, *Proc. Natl. Acad. Sci. U.S.A.* **54**:822–830.

DuPasquier, L., Weiss, N., and Loor, F., 1973, Direct evidence for immunoglobulins on the surface of thymus lymphocytes of amphibian larvae, *Eur. J. Immunol.* **2**:366–370.

Edelman, G. M., and Gall, W. E., 1969, The antibody problem, *Annu. Rev. Biochem.* **38**:415–466.

Ellis, A. E., and Parkhouse, R. M. E., 1975, Surface immunoglobins on the lymphocytes of the skate, *Rasa naevus, Eur. J. Immunol.* **5**:726–728.

Emmrich, F., Richter, R. F., and Ambrosius, H., 1975, Immunoglobulin determinants on the surface of lymphoid cells of carps, *Eur. J. Immunol.* **5**:76–78.

Finstad, C. L., Litman, G. W., Finstad, J., and Good, R. A., 1972, Evolution of the immune response. XIII. Agglutinators of *Limulus polyphemus* and *Asterias forbesi*: Purification and characterization, *J. Immunol.* **108**:1704–1711.

Finstad, C. L., Good, R. A., and Litman, G. W., 1974, The erythrocyte agglutinin from *Limulus polyphemus* hemolymph: Molecular structure and biological function, *Ann. N. Y. Acad. Sci.* **234**:170–182.

Franek, F., Wasserman, R. L., Novotny, J., and Kehoe, J. M., 1975, The amino-terminal sequence of the V_HIII subgroup of pooled porcine IgG, *Eur. J. Immunol.* **5**:427–429.

Frommel, D., Litman, G. W., Chartrand, S., Seal, U. S., and Good, R. A., 1971a, Significance of carbohydrate composition in immunoglobulin evolution, *Immunochemistry* **8**:573–577.

Frommel, D., Litman, G. W., Finstad, J., and Good, R. A., 1971b, Evolution of the immune response. XI. Immunoglobulins of the horned shark: Purification, characterization and biological properties, *J. Immunol.* **106**:1234–1243.

Gally, J. A., 1973, Structure of immunoglobulins, in: *The Antigens* (M. Sela, ed.), Vol. I, pp. 161–298, Academic Press, New York,

Good, A. H., Traylor, P. S., and Singer, S. J., 1967, Affinity labeling of the active sites of rabbit anti-2,4-dinitrophenyl antibodies with *m*-nitrobenzenediazonium fluoroborate, *Biochemistry* **6**:873–881.

Gordon, S. M., and Kindt, T. J., 1976, Detection of β_2-microglobulin in sera from diverse vertebrate species by the use of a heterologous radioimmunoassay, *Scand. J. Immunol.* **5**:505–511.

Grant, J. A., Sanders, B. G., and Hood, L., 1971, Partial amino acid sequences of chicken and turkey immunoglobulin light chains: Homology with mammalian λ chains, *Biochemistry* **10**:3123–3132.

Grey, H. M., 1967, Duck immunoglobulins. II. Biologic and immunochemical studies, *J. Immunol.* **98**:820–826.

Hall, J. L., and Rowlands, D. T., Jr., 1974a, Heterogeneity of lobster agglutinins. I. Purification and physiochemical characterization, *Biochemistry* **13**:821–827.

Hall, J. L., and Rowlands, D. T., Jr., 1974b, Heterogeneity of lobster agglutinins. II. Specificity of agglutinin–erythrocyte binding. *Biochemistry* **13**:828–832.

Hammarström, S., 1974, Structure, specificity, binding properties and some biological activities of a blood Group A-reactive hemagglutinin from the snail, *Helix pomatia, Ann. N. Y. Acad. Sci.* **234**:183–197.

Harisdangkul, V., Kabat, E. A., McDonough, R. J., and Sigel, M. M., 1972, A protein in normal nurse shark serum which reacts specifically with fructosans. II. Physicochemical studies, *J. Immunol.* **108**:1259–1270.

Hildemann, W. H., 1974, Some new concepts in immunological phylogeny, *Nature (London)* **250**:116–120.

Hildemann, W. H., and Thoenes, G. H., 1969, Immunological responses of Pacific hagfish. I. Skin transplantation immunity. *Transplantation* **7**:506–521.

Holowka, D. A., and Cathou, R. E., 1976, Conformation of immunoglobulin M. 2. Nanosecond fluorescence depolarization analysis of sequential flexibility in anti-ε-1-dimethylamino-5-naphthalenesulfonyl-L-lysine anti-immunoglobulin from horse, pig and shark, *Biochemistry* **15**:3379–3390.

Hood, L., Grant, J. A., and Sox, H. C., Jr., 1970, On the structure of normal light chains from mammals and birds: Evolutionary and genetic implications, in: *Developmental Aspects of Antibody Formation and Structure* (J. Sterzl and I. Riha, eds.), 2nd Ed., Vol. I, pp. 283–309, Academic Press, New York.

Houdayer, M., and Fougereau, M., 1972, Phylogenie des immunoglobulines: La réaction immunitaire de l'axolotl *Ambystoma mexicanum;* Cinétique de la réponse immunitaire et caractérisation des anticorps, *Ann. Inst. Pasteur, Paris* **123**:3–28.

Kaplan, R., Li, S., and Kehoe, J. M., 1977 Molecular characterization of limulin, a sialic acid binding lectin from the hemolymph of the horseshoe crab, *Limulus polyphemus, Biochemistry* **16**:4297–4303.

Kehoe, J. M., and Capra, J. D., 1974, Phylogenetic aspects of immunoglobulin variable region diversity, in *Contemporary Topics in Molecular Immunology,* Vol. 3 (G. L. Ada, ed.), pp. 143–159, Plenum Press, New York.

Kehoe, J. M., Gerber-Jenson, B., Sharon, J., and Litman, G. W., 1977 (submitted).

Klapper, D. G., Clem, L. W., and Small, P. A., 1971, Proteolytic fragmentation of elasmobranch immunoglobulins, *Biochemistry* **10**:645–659.

Klaus, G. G. B., Nitecki, D. E., and Goodman, J. W., 1971a, Amino acid sequences of free and blocked N-termini of leopard shark immunoglobulins. *J. Immunol.* **107**:1250–1258.

Klaus, G. G. B., Halpern, M. S., Koshland, M. E., and Goodman, J. W., 1971b, A polypeptide chain from leopard shark IgG immunoglobulin analogous to the mammalian J chain, *J. Immunol.* **107**:1785–1787.

Lebacq-Verheyden, A. M., Vaerman, J. P., and Heremans, J. F., 1972, A possible homologue of mammalian IgA in chicken serum and secretions, *Immunology* **22**:165–174.

Leslie, G. A., and Clem, L. W., 1969, Phylogeny of immunoglobulin structure and function. III. Immunoglobulins of the chicken, *J. Exp. Med.* **130**:1337–1352.

Leslie, G. A., and Clem, L. W., 1972, Phylogeny of immunoglobulin structure and function. VI. 17S, 7.5S and 5.7S anti-DNP of the turtle, *Pseudemys scripta, J. Immunol.* **108**:1656–1664.

Linthicum, D. S., and Hildemann, W. H., 1970, Immunologic responses of Pacific hagfish. III. Serum antibodies to cellular antigens, *J. Immunol.* **105**:912–917.

Litman, G. W., 1975, Relationship between structure and function of lower vertebrate immunoglobulins, *Adv. Exp. Med. Biol.* **64**:217–228.

Litman, G. W., 1976, Physical properties of immunoglobulins of lower species: A comparison with immunoglobulins of mammals, *Comparative Immunology* (J. J. Marchalonis, ed.), pp. 239–275, Blackwell Scientific Publications, Oxford.

Litman, G. W., Frommel, D., Finstad, J., Howell, J., Pollara, B. W., and Good, R. A., 1970, The evolution of the immune response. VIII. Structural studies of the lamprey immunoglobulin, *J. Immunol.* **105**:1278–1285.

Litman, G. W., Frommel, D., Chartrand, S., Finstad, J., and Good, R. A., 1971a, Significance of heavy chain mass and antigenic relationships in immunoglobulin evolution. *Immunochemistry* **8**:345–349.

Litman, G. W., Frommel, D., Finstad, J., and Good, R. A., 1971b, Evolution of the immune response. IX. Immunoglobulins of the bowfin: Purification and characterization, *J. Immunol.* **106**:747–754.

Litman, G. W., Frommel, D., Rosenberg, A., and Good, R. A., 1971c, Circular dichroic analysis of immunoglobulins in phylogenetic perspective, *Biochim. Biophys. Acta* **36**:647–654.

Litman, G. W., Wang, A. C., Fudenberg, H. H., and Good, R. A., 1971d, N-terminal amino acid sequence of African lungfish immunoglobulin light chains, *Proc. Natl. Acad. Sci. U.S.A.* **68**:2321–2324.

Litman, G. W., Chartrand, S., Finstad, C., and Good, R. A., 1973, Active sites of turtle and duck antibody to 2-4-dinitrophenol, *Immunochemistry* **10**:323–329.

Litman, G. W., Howe, C. W. S., Cunningham-Rundles, C., Oshman, R., Gerber-Jenson, B., and Kehoe, J. M., 1976, Structural diversity of lower vertebrate immunoglobulin and related cell surface structures, in: *Phylogeny of Thymus and Bone Marrow-Bursa Cells* (R. K. Wright and E. L. Cooper, eds.), pp. 99–109, Elsevier/North-Holland, Amsterdam.

Marchalonis, J. J., 1969, Isolation and characterization of immunoglobulin-like proteins of the Australian lungfish (*Neoceratodus forsteri*), *Aust. J. Exp. Biol. Med. Sci.* **47**:405–419.

Marchalonis, J. J., 1971, Isolation and partial characterization of immunoglobulins of goldfish (*Carassius auratus*) and carp (*Cyprinus carpio*), *Immunology* **20**:161–173.

Marchalonis, J. J., 1972, Conservatism in the evolution of immunoglobulin, *Nature (London) New Biol.* **236**:84–86.

Marchalonis, J. J., and Cohen, N., 1973, Isolation and partial characterization of immunoglobulin from a urodele amphibian, *Immunology* **24**:395–407.

Marchalonis, J. J., and Cone, R. E., 1973, The phylogenetic emergence of vertebrate immunity, *Aust. J. Exp. Biol. Med. Sci.* **51**:461–488.

Marchalonis, J. J., and Edelman, G. M., 1966a, Phylogenetic origins of antibody structure. II. Immunoglobulins in the primary immune response of the bullfrog, *Rana catesbiana*, *J. Exp. Med.* **124**:901–913.

Marchalonis, J., and Edelman, G. M., 1966b, Polypeptide chains of immunoglobulins from the smooth dogfish (*Mustelus canis*), *Science* **154**:1567–1568.

Marchalonis, J., and Edelman, G. M., 1968a, Phylogenetic origins of antibody structure. III. Antibodies in the primary immune response of the sea lamprey, *Petromyzon marinus*, *J. Exp. Med.* **127**:891–913.

Marchalonis, J., and Edelman, G. M., 1968b, Isolation and characterization of a hemagglutinin from *Limulus polyphemus*, *J. Mol. Biol.* **32**:453–465.

Marchalonis, J. J., and Schonfeld, S. A., 1970, Polypeptide chain structure of stingray immunoglobulin, *Biochim. Biophys. Acta* **3**:604–611.

McCumber, L. J., and Clem, L. W., 1976, A comparative study of J chain: Structure and stoichiometry in human and nurse shark IgM, *Immunochemistry* **13**:479–484.

Novotny, J., and Franek, F., 1975, Different degrees of interspecies homology in immunoglobulin λ chain constant domain correlated with three-dimensional structure, *Nature (London)* **258**:641–643.

Novotny, J., Franek, F., and Sorm, F., 1970, Large scale isolation, characterization and classification of pig immunoglobulin κ-chains, *Eur. J. Biochem.* **14**:309–316.

Novotny, J., Dolejs, I.., and Franek, F., 1972, Uniformity and species specific features of the *N*-terminal amino-acid sequence of porcine immunoglobulin λ chains, *Eur. J. Biochem.* **31**:277–289.

Parkhouse, R. M. E., Askonas, B. A., and Dourmashkin, R. R., 1970, Electron microscopic studies of mouse immunoglobulin M; Structure and reconstitution following reduction, *Immunology* **18**:575–584.

Perey, D. Y. E., Finstad, J., Pollara, B., and Good, R. A., 1968, Evolution of the immune response. VI. First and second set skin homograft rejections in primitive fishes, *Lab. Invest.* **19**:591–597.

Pollara, B., Suran, A. A., Finstad, J., and Good, R. A., 1968, *N*-terminal amino acid sequences of immunoglobulin chains in *Polyodon spathula*, *Proc. Natl. Acad. Sci. U.S.A.* **59**:1307–1312.

Pollara, B., Litman, G. W., Finstad, J., Howell, J., and Good, R. A., 1970, The evolution of the immune response. VII. Antibody to human "O" cells and properties of the immunoglobulin in lamprey, *J. Immunol.* **105**:738–745.

Porter, R. R., 1959, The hydrolysis of rabbit γ-globulin and antibodies with crystalline papain, *Biochem. J.* **73**:119–126.

Portis, J. L., and Coe, J. E., 1975, IgM: The secretory immunoglobulin of reptiles and amphibians, *Nature (London)* **258**:547–548.

Richter, R., Nuhn, P., Ambrosius, M., Zagyansky, Yu. A., Tumerman, L. A., and Nezlin, R. S., 1972, Restricted flexibility of carp 15 S immunoglobulin molecules as revealed by fluorescence polarisation, *FEBS Lett.* **27**:184–186.

Roche, A.-C., and Monsigny, M., 1974, Purification and properties of limulin: A lectin (agglutinin) from hemolymph of *Limulus polyphemus*, *Biochim. Biophys. Acta* **371**:242–254.

Romer, A. S., 1970, in: *The Vertebrate Body*, 4th Ed., W. B. Saunders Co., Philadelphia.

Roubal, W. T., Etlinger, H. M., and Hodgins, H. O., 1974, Spin-label studies of a hapten-combining site of rainbow trout antibody, *J. Immunol.* **113**:309–315.

Schulkind, M. L., Robbins, J. B., and Clem, L. W., 1971, Reactivities of shark 19S and 7S IgM antibodies to *Salmonella typhimurium*, *Nature (London) New Biol.* **230**:182–183.

Shelton, E., and Smith, M., 1970, The ultrastructure of carp (*Cyprinus carpio*) immunoglobulin: A tetrameric macroglobulin, *J. Mol. Biol.* **54**:615–617.

GARY W. LITMAN
AND J. MICHAEL
KEHOE

Sigel, M. M., 1974, Primitive immunoglobulins and other proteins with binding functions in the shark, *Ann. N. Y. Acad. Sci.* **234**:198–215.

Sledge, C., Clem, L. W., and Hood, L., 1974, Antibody structure: Amino terminal sequences of nurse shark light and heavy chains, *J. Immunol.* **112**:941–948.

Small, P. A., Klapper, D. G., and Clem, L. W., 1970, Half-lives, body distribution and lack of interconversion of serum 19S and 7S IgM of sharks, *J. Immunol.* **105**:29–37.

Stanton, T., Sledge, C., Capra, J. D., Woods, R., Clem, W., and Hood, L., 1974, A sequence restriction in the variable region of immunoglobulin light chains from sharks, birds and mammals, *J. Immunol.* **112**:633–640.

Steiner, L. A., Mikoryak, C. A., Lopes, A. D., and Green, C., 1975, Immunoglobulins in ranid frogs and tadpoles, *Adv. Exp. Med. Biol.* **64**:173–183.

Vaerman, J. P., Picard, J., and Heremans, J. F., 1975, Structural data on chicken IgA and failure to identify the IgA of the tortoise, *Adv. Exp. Med. Biol.* **64**:185–195.

Voss, E. W., Russell, W. J., and Sigel, M. M., 1969, Purification and binding properties of nurse shark antibody, *Biochemistry* **8**:4866–4872.

Wang, A.-C., Fudenberg, H. H., and Bazin, H., 1975, The nature of "species-specific" amino acid residues, *Immunochemistry* **12**:505–509.

Warr, G. W., De Luca, D., and Marchalonis, J. J., 1976, Phylogenetic origins of immune recognition: Lymphocyte surface immunoglobulins in the goldfish, *Carassius auratus, Proc. Natl. Acad. Sci. U.S.A.* **73**:2476–2480.

Wasserman, R. L., Kehoe, J. M., and Capra, J. D., 1974, The V_HIII subgroup of immunoglobulin heavy chains: Phylogenetically associated residues in several avian species, *J. Immunol.* **113**:954–957.

Weinheimer, P. F., Mestecky, J., and Acton, R. T., 1971, Species distribution of J chain, *J. Immunol.* **107**:1211–1212.

Zagyansky, Y. A., 1975, Phylogenesis of the general structure of immunoglobulins, *Arch. Biochem. Biophys.* **166**:371–381.

Ziegler, A., and Pink, J. R. L., 1975, Characterization of major histocompatibility (B) antigens of the chicken, *Transplantation* **20**:523–527.

Zimmerman, B., Shalatin, N., and Grey, H. M., 1971, Structural studies of the duck 5.7 S and 7.8 S immunoglobulins, *Biochemistry* **10**:482–488.

9

Evidence for and the Significance of 'Two Genes, One Polypeptide Chain'

AN-CHUAN WANG

1. Basic Immunoglobulin Units

All immunoglobulins (Ig's) consist of one or more basic units composed of identical pairs of heavy (H) and light (L) polypeptide chains (Figure 1). Each chain folds into several compact globular domains, connected by relatively narrower but more exposed areas. Each domain is approximately 110 amino acids in length and characterized by an intrachain disulfide bond connecting two cysteine residues approximately 60 amino acid residues apart (Figure 1). All Ig polypeptide chains can be divided into an amino-terminal portion, the variable (V) region, and a carboxyl-terminal portion, the constant (C) region. The V regions of both H and L chains are equivalent in size to a domain. The C regions of L chains are of similar size, whereas those of H chains are two to four times longer. Based on the degree of amino acid sequence homology, the V regions have been divided into three main groups, $V\kappa$, $V\lambda$, and V_H. The C regions have been divided into κ and λ types (L chains) as well as γ, α, μ, ϵ, and δ classes (H chains) according to their antigenic and serological properties. Some of the L-chain types and H-chain classes are further divided into subtypes and subclasses, respectively. Details of Ig structure are given in earlier Chapters. A general review on this subject was given by Gally (1973). This chapter is devoted to the genetic aspects of the synthesis of Ig polypeptide chains.

2. History

The genetic control of antibody synthesis is one of the most fascinating biological problems to arise during the past century. It has long been apparent that Ig molecules serve two different kinds of functions: the binding of specific antigens

AN-CHUAN WANG • Department of Basic and Clinical Immunology and Microbiology, Medical University of South Carolina, Charleston, South Carolina 29401.

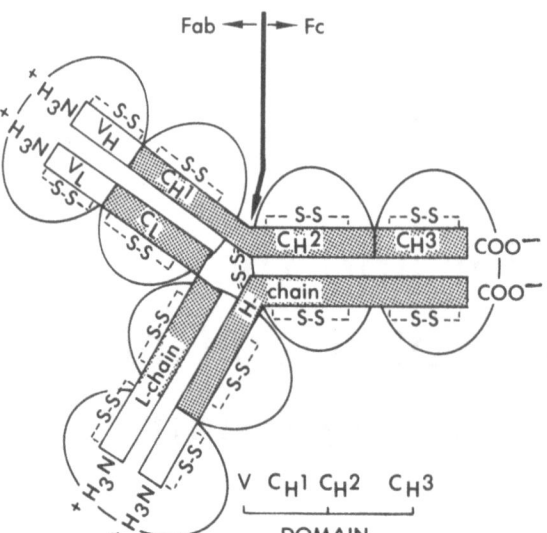

Figure 1. Simplified model of the basic unit of antibodies. Rectangles represent polypeptide chains; dashed lines represent disulfide bonds. Each oval encloses two closely associated domains, termed V_H, V_L, C_L, C_H1, C_H2, and C_H3. (V) Variable region; (C) constant region; (H) heavy chain; (L) light chain.

and a series of biological activities (e.g., complement fixation, placental transfer). Scientists have only recently become aware of the unusual properties of Ig structural genes. In contrast to the classic "one gene, one polypeptide chain" rule (Beadle and Tatum, 1941), which is assumed to govern the synthesis of almost all conventional proteins, each Ig polypeptide chain is apparently synthesized by at least two structural genes.* The "two genes, one polypeptide chain" hypothesis was introduced by Dreyer and Bennett (1965), on the basis of chemical data on κ chains reported by others. At the same time, two laboratories independently showed, by peptide mapping analyses of human Bence Jones κ chains, that all these κ chains appeared to have a variable and an invariable half that are contiguous (Hilschmann and Craig, 1965; Titani and Putnam, 1965). These findings led to the suggestion that two structural genes participate in the synthesis of each κ chain, a hypothesis not generally accepted during the 1960's. Different interpretations of the data on κ-chain amino acid sequences were made, since these data could not distinguish between two alternative explanations: either (1) two genes code for each κ chain, the gene coding for the carboxyl-(C)-terminal half being common to all κ chains, but the gene coding for the amino-(N)-terminal half being unique for each κ-chain V region; or (2) one gene codes for the entire κ chain, genes for different κ chains differing only in the portion coding for the N-terminal half. As will become apparent, the second explanation has not been supported by subsequent studies, while the first is consistent with most of the data. The concept of "two genes for one polypeptide chain" was reviewed previously by Hood (1972).

3. Allotypes of Rabbit Heavy-Chain Variable Regions

Todd (1963) observed that a pair of rabbit allotypic markers was present in both IgG and IgM molecules. These markers, designated a1 and a3, were subsequently

---

*The phenomenon of two genes contributing to the synthesis of a single polypeptide chain is not unique to Ig. The polypeptide chain of another protein, β-galatosidase of *Escherichia coli*, appears to be synthesized by two genes (Apte and Zipser, 1973).

found also in IgA molecules (Feinstein, 1963). Biochemical and serological studies demonstrated that they were associated with the V regions of H chains (Mole *et al.*, 1975), while genetic studies showed that they were linked with the γ-chain C-region allotypic markers (i.e., d11, d12, e14, e15) with documented cases of recombination (Mage *et al.*, 1971; Kindt and Mandy, 1972; Hamers-Casterman and Hamers, 1975).

231

EVIDENCE FOR AND
THE SIGNIFICANCE
OF 'TWO GENES, ONE
POLYPEPTIDE
CHAIN'

The sharing of V-region allotypes by γ, μ, and α chains supported the concept that the V and C regions of each H chain are synthesized by separate genes. It was found, however, that amino acid compositions (Koshland *et al.*, 1969) and partial amino acid sequences (Mole *et al.*, 1975; Jaton *et al.*, 1973) of H chains with different a-group allotypes are very dissimilar, with multiple amino acid differences. Such large-scale amino acid substitutions have never been observed in the allelic forms of any conventional protein system studied thus far, except perhaps in the Cκ allotypes of the rabbit (i.e., b4, b5, b6, b9) (Appella *et al.*, 1969; Goodfleish, 1975) and of the rat (i.e., RL-1a, R1-1b) (Vengerova *et al.*, 1972; Nezlin *et al.*, 1974). It is questionable whether these a-group allotypes really represent allotypes of structural genes coding for the H-chain V regions. It was postulated that the rabbit a-group allotypes may actually be allelic forms of a hypothetical "regulatory gene," and that each allele of this hypothetical "regulatory gene" controls the expression of a set of closely linked V_H genes (Wang, 1975). The differences observed in multiple amino acids between Ig polypeptide chains with such "allotypes" would seem to reflect the differences between sets of functionally related structural genes (their expression is controlled by the hypothetical regulatory gene), rather than between the allelic forms of a single gene. It is likely that the b-group allotypes of the Cκ region in rabbits and the RL-group allotypes of the Cκ region in rats are similar types of genetic systems.

4. Sharing of a Single Constant Region by Variable Regions

To date, more than 100 monoclonal human Ig polypeptide chains have been subjected to peptide mapping analysis, and over 50 have been analyzed for their complete amino acid sequences (Kabat, E. A. *et al.*, 1976; Dayhoff, 1976). The results of these studies demonstrate that the C-terminal half of the L chains is always identical within a given type of chain (κ or λ), with the exception of allotypic or isotypic differences, but that each L chain gives rise to a unique set of peptides in the N-terminal half, distinguishing each chain from all others (Schneider and Hilschmann, 1975).

For example, the C region of all human κ chains has an identical amino acid sequence except for single alternatives at positions 153 and 191. These alternatives are associated with the Km (formerly Inv) allotypic markers: Km(1) κ chains have valine at position 153 and leucine at position 191; Km(3) κ chains have alanine at position 153 and valine at position 191; Km(1,2) κ chains have alanine at position 153 and leucine at position 191 (Steinberg *et al.*, 1974). Both the alanine–valine and the leucine–valine interchanges can result from a single-step point mutation. The biochemical and genetic data are therefore consistent with the concept that the C regions of human κ chains are coded for by a single gene. In contrast, the V regions of human κ chains differ from one another by up to 50% in their amino acid sequences (Dayhoff, 1976; Kabat, E. A., *et al.*, 1976), with the exception of certain rare cases of double myeloma (Wang *et al.*, 1969; Seon *et al.*, 1973a; Wolfenstein-Todel *et al.*, 1974a) in which the V regions of two distinct myeloma proteins are apparently synthesized by the same gene. The degree of difference among the V regions of most κ chains is so striking that practically all immunogeneticists agree that these Vκ regions must be synthesized by many germ-line genes (Cohn *et al.*, 1974). Multiple V-region genes therefore appear to be associated with a single C-region gene for the synthesis of κ chains.

5. Sharing of a Single Variable Region by Constant Regions

Since the genetic control of the V regions of Ig polypeptide chains is still under debate, better experimental support for the "two genes, one polypeptide chain" hypothesis came from the observation that identical V-region amino acid sequences were found to associate with different C regions. Wang *et al.* (1970a) reported chemical and serological studies on monotypic IgG2(κ) and IgM(κ) prepared from a single patient (Til) (Figure 2). These two molecules share idiotypic antigenic determinants not present in any of a large number of monotypic Ig molecules tested (Nisonoff *et al.*, 1972), and the V regions of the μ and γ2 chains have identical amino acid sequences (Wang *et al.*, 1977). In contrast, the C regions of the two chains have less than 30% amino acid sequence homology (Wang *et al.*, 1973). The

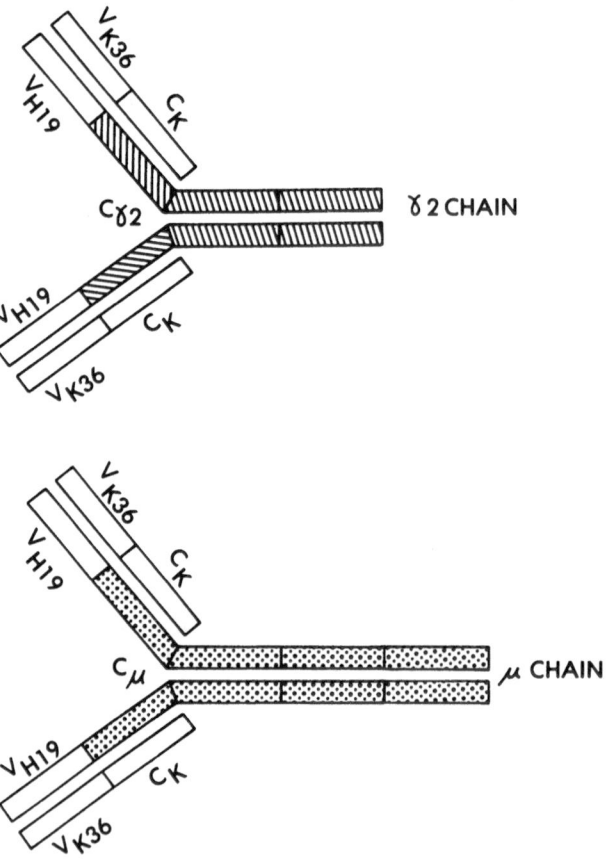

Figure 2. Diagrammatic representation of IgG2(κ) and IgM(κ) from patient Til. White rectangles represent identical portions between the two molecules.

233

EVIDENCE FOR AND
THE SIGNIFICANCE
OF 'TWO GENES, ONE
POLYPEPTIDE
CHAIN'

C region of the μ chain is serologically and biochemically indistinguishable from the C regions of other human μ chains reported by Putnam *et al.* (1973a) and Watanabe *et al.* (1973), whereas the C region of the $\gamma2$ chain is indistinguishable from the C regions of other human $\gamma2$ chains and shows over 90% amino acid sequence homology with human $\gamma1$ chains at the positions compared (Wang and Fudenberg, 1972).

Pedigree studies of large informative families have clearly established that the μ and $\gamma2$ chains are synthesized by different structural genes (Steinberg, 1969; Wells *et al.*, 1973), and that the $C\gamma$ gene diverged from the $C\mu$ gene over 200 million years ago in evolution (Wang and Fudenberg, 1974). The V regions of both Til H chains have 115 amino acid residues, whereas the C regions of human γ and μ chains contain 329 and 452 amino acid residues, respectively (Edelman *et al.*, 1969; Putnam *et al.*, 1973a). There is no known genetic mechanism that would allow two genes to maintain an identical stretch of 345 nucleotides through a period of 200 million years and simultaneously permit the remaining 987 or more nucleotides to diversify to the extent of reflecting 65% difference on polypeptide chains coded by them. The only logical explanation for this observation, therefore, is that the C and V regions of each H chain are synthesized by different structural genes, whereas the same V-region gene codes for the 115 amino acid residues at the N-terminal ends of both H chains.

Subsequently, observations similar to those described above were made on the monotypic proteins of several other patients. The sharing of similar (if not identical) idiotypic antigenic determinants or indistinguishable L chains and V_H regions, or of both, was observed between an IgG and an IgM (Penn *et al.*, 1970), an IgA(κ) and an IgM(κ) (Seon *et al.*, 1973a,b; Yagi and Pressman, 1973), and an IgA1(λ) and an IgG2(λ) (Wolfenstein-Todel *et al.*, 1974a), and an IgA(κ) and an IgG2(κ) (Fair *et al.*, 1975). Although relatively limited data were presented in these studies, they are nevertheless all consistent with the concept that different C regions may share a given V region.

6. Reciprocal Sharing of Variable and Constant Regions in Heavy Chains

Fewer amino acid sequence data are available for the H chains than for the L chains. To date, the complete amino acid sequences of three human $\gamma1$ chains (Edelman *et al.*, 1969; Cunningham *et al.*, 1971; Ponstingl and Hilschmann, 1972), two human μ chains (Putnam *et al.*, 1973a; Watanabe *et al.*, 1973), two human α chains (Kratzin *et al.*, 1975; Liu *et al.*, 1976), and one human ϵ chain (Bennich and von Bahr-Lindstrom, 1974) have been determined. Partial amino acid sequences are available for human $\gamma1$, $\gamma2$, $\gamma3$, and $\gamma4$ chains (Milstein and Pink, 1970; Wang *et al.*, 1971; Florent *et al.*, 1974; Capra and Kehoe, 1975; Wang and Fudenberg, 1975). The known sequences are consistent with the idea that the C regions of different H-chain classes and subclasses are coded for by different genes. Based on the degree of amino acid sequence homology, the V regions of H chains can be divided into at least four non-class-specific subgroups (Kohler *et al.*, 1970a; Wang *et al.*, 1970b; Capra and Kehoe, 1975), each being encoded by at least one (but perhaps many) gene(s). As illustrated in Figure 3, a given V-region subgroup may be found in association with C regions of α, μ, ϵ, and γ chains of various classes and subclasses.

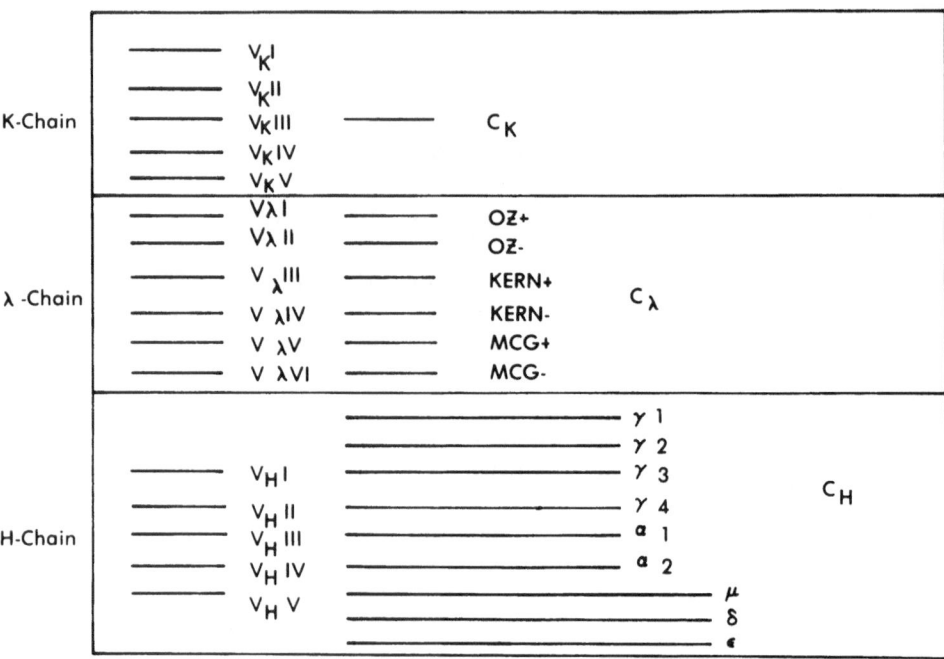

Figure 3. Diagrammatic representation of the association between V regions and C regions of human Ig. Each box encloses products of a family of V-region and a family of C-region genes that are linked. For the C_L (κ- and λ-chain) and C_H regions, each horizontal line represents the product of a single gene; for V regions, each line represents the product(s) of at least one (but more likely many) gene(s). Several $C\lambda$ genes have been identified based on the presence or absence of amino acid substitutions at five C-region positions represented by three myeloma λ chains, Oz, Kern, and Mcg. The combinations clearly established are: Oz+/Kern−/Mcg−, Oz−/Kern+/Mcg−, Oz−/Kern−/Mcg−, Oz−/Kern+/Mcg+. Humans may have a large number of $C\lambda$ genes. [Additional $C\lambda$ variants were described recently by Lieu *et al.* (1977).]

Thus, it is clear that the expression of V_H regions is independent of the expression of C_H regions, supporting the concept that the V region and the C region of each H chain are coded for by two different structural genes.

7. DNA–RNA Hybridization

The most convincing piece of evidence supporting the "two genes, one polypeptide chain" hypothesis was reported recently by Hozumi and Tonegawa (1976). These investigators digested and fractionated mouse DNA with *Bacillus amyloliquefaciens* strain H restriction enzyme. DNA fragments carrying nucleotide sequences coding for the V and C regions of κ chains were detected by hybridization with purified, ^{125}I-labeled κ-chain mRNA and with its 3′-end half. The pattern was entirely different in the genome of mouse embryo cells and of plasmacytoma cells from adult mice. The embryo DNA showed two hybridization components, one of which had a molecular weight of 6 million and contained the $C\kappa$ gene and the

235

EVIDENCE FOR AND
THE SIGNIFICANCE
OF 'TWO GENES, ONE
POLYPEPTIDE
CHAIN'

other of which had a molecular weight of 3.9 million and contained the corresponding Vκ gene as specified by the mRNA (from MOPC 321 plasmacytoma) used in the hybridization. In contrast, the adult tumor DNA had only one hybridization component. This component had a molecular weight of approximately 2.4 million and contained both V-region and C-region gene sequences. These data indicated that the V and the C regions of mouse κ chain are coded for by different genes that are separated from each other on the chromosome in embryonic cells. A somatic rearrangement of Ig genes occurred during differentiation, however, and as a result, the Vκ and Cκ genes were brought to close approximation in adult mice.

8. Fusion of the Variable and Constant Regions

8.1. Hypothetical Models

Theoretically, the V-region and C-region genes or their products may fuse at one of three levels: DNA, mRNA, or protein. The fusion of the two regions of *Esch. coli* β-galactosidase was shown to take place at the protein level (Apte and Zipser, 1973). In the case of Ig, however, fusing at the protein level was ruled out by four lines of evidence: (1) Pulse-labeling with [^{3}H]leucine demonstrated that mouse Ig H chains were synthesized from a single growing point proceeding from *N*-terminus to *C*-terminus (Knopf *et al.*, 1967; Fleischman, 1967). (2) The sizes of polysomes for the synthesis of Ig polypeptide chains are appropriate for those with molecular weights of 55,000 and 23,000, respectively, corresponding to entire H and L chains (Scharff, 1967). (3) mRNA prepared from a mouse myeloma (Stavenger and Huong, 1971) and from normal mouse lymph node (Ralph and Rich, 1971) carried out the *in vitro* synthesis of complete Ig polypeptide chains. (4) Chemical studies on a purified L-chain mRNA from mouse myeloma cells established that the V region and the C region of each L chain were coded for by a single mRNA molecule (Milstein *et al.*, 1974a). The DNA–RNA hybridization experiment described in Section 7 strongly favors a DNA level of fusion. Fusion at the level of mRNA cannot be totally excluded, however, until the DNA/RNA hybridization experiment is confirmed in other species. It is interesting that an RNA ligase from T4-phage-infected *Esch. coli* cells was found to catalyze the covalent joining of two polynucleotide fragments derived from yeast phenylalanine-tRNA (Kaufmann and Littaure, 1974).

Several models have been proposed to explain how the V-region and C-region genes come together. Dreyer and Grey (1968) postulated a "copy–splice" mechanism operating through a special organelle in a programmed manner, systematically expressing all V-region genes in the genome and fusing them with C-region genes by a "breakage-and-reunion" process. D. Kabat (1972) postulated a "looping-out" mechanism, suggesting that a given V-region gene may be joined to a C-region gene by deleting as a circle all the DNA in between. When the same V-region gene is joined to a new C-region gene, once again the DNA in between is lost as a circle. Gally and Edelman (1970) suggested a model (Figure 4) in which one of the tandem array of V-region genes is moved to a C-region gene in another part of the same chromosome by a crossing-over event resembling integration of the λ phage genome into a specific part of the *Esch. coli* genome. The existence of highly specific

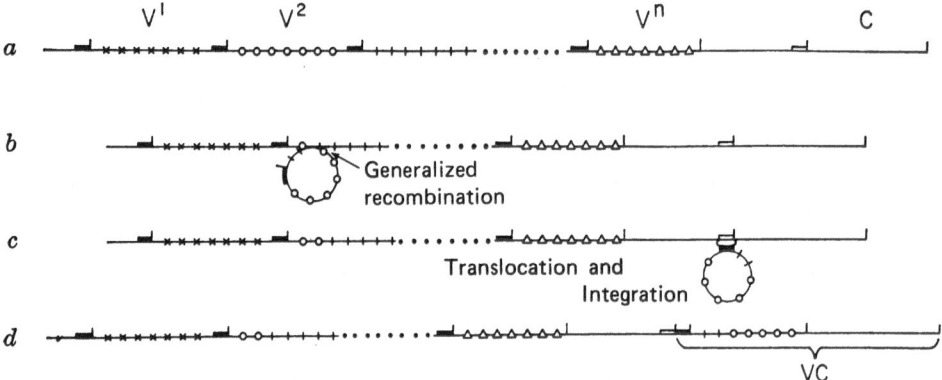

Figure 4. Translocation model for the fusion of V-region and C-region genes. Reproduced from Gally and Edelman (1970) with permission.

enzymes that catalyze the breaking and forming of phosphodiester bonds at particular gene loci was postulated. The central thesis of all these models involves the translocation of a V-region gene to a C-region gene, and this translocation commits a given immunocyte to the production of a specific H or L chain.

A somewhat different model (Figure 5), the "DNA network," was proposed by Smithies (1973). In this hypothesis, genes that encode V regions are arranged in parallel and are connected via a region of one double helix of DNA to parallel C-region genes within each group of linked Ig genes (see Section 9 for a detailed description of linkage groups). Control over the transcriptional pathway through these DNA networks was proposed to account for the expression of only one functional V-region and C-region gene among families of V_H, C_H, V_L, and C_L genes in the genome for the production of one particular kind of Ig molecule in a given plasma cell. The finding that Vκ and Cκ genes are physically separated in mouse embryonic cells (Hozumi and Tonegawa, 1976) is against this model.

8.2. Amino Acid Sequences near the Junction between the Variable and Constant Regions

The C-terminal ends of Ig V-regions are lacking in those amino acid residues characteristic of different kinds of V-region subgroups (Kabat, E. A., *et al.*, 1976).

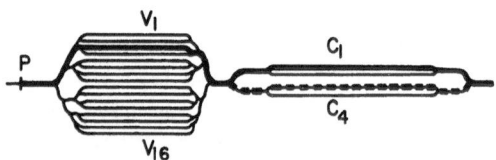

Figure 5. Model of the DNA network, explaining how V-region genes can be connected to the C-region genes at the DNA level. Each line represents a DNA double helix. Commitment to one of the possible polypeptide chains encoded by Ig genes is determined by the random setting of its DNA forks in left (L) or right (R) configurations. The path of an RNA polymerase is indicated by the heavy line starting from an RNA promotor site P; it would transcribe mRNA corresponding to V_3 and C_1. Reproduced from Smithies (1973) with permission.

237

EVIDENCE FOR AND
THE SIGNIFICANCE
OF 'TWO GENES, ONE
POLYPEPTIDE
CHAIN'

Wang and Fudenberg (1975) examined available amino acid sequences near the junction of the V and C regions of monotypic human H chains and found that certain amino acids occurred either invariably or almost invariably at certain positions near the *C*-terminal end of the V regions (Figure 6). For example, counting from the V–C junction toward the *N*-terminal side, position 2 is almost always serine; 3 and 5, valine; 4, threonine; 8, and 10 glycine; and 11, tryptophan.

The unexpected lack of variability of amino acid residues near the *C*-terminal end of the V region is not unique to H chains, being observed also in κ and λ chains. Counting from the V–C junction toward the *N*-terminal side, positions 7, 8, 10, and 11 are relatively invariant in human κ chains (Figure 7) and positions 2–4, 7, 8, 10, and 11 in human λ chains (Figure 8).

The invariant nature of these residues is further emphasized by the fact that the V regions of H, κ, and λ chains differ in length, with an average of 117, 108, and 112 amino acid residues, respectively (Dayhoff, 1976: Kabat, E. A., *et al.*, 1976; Capra

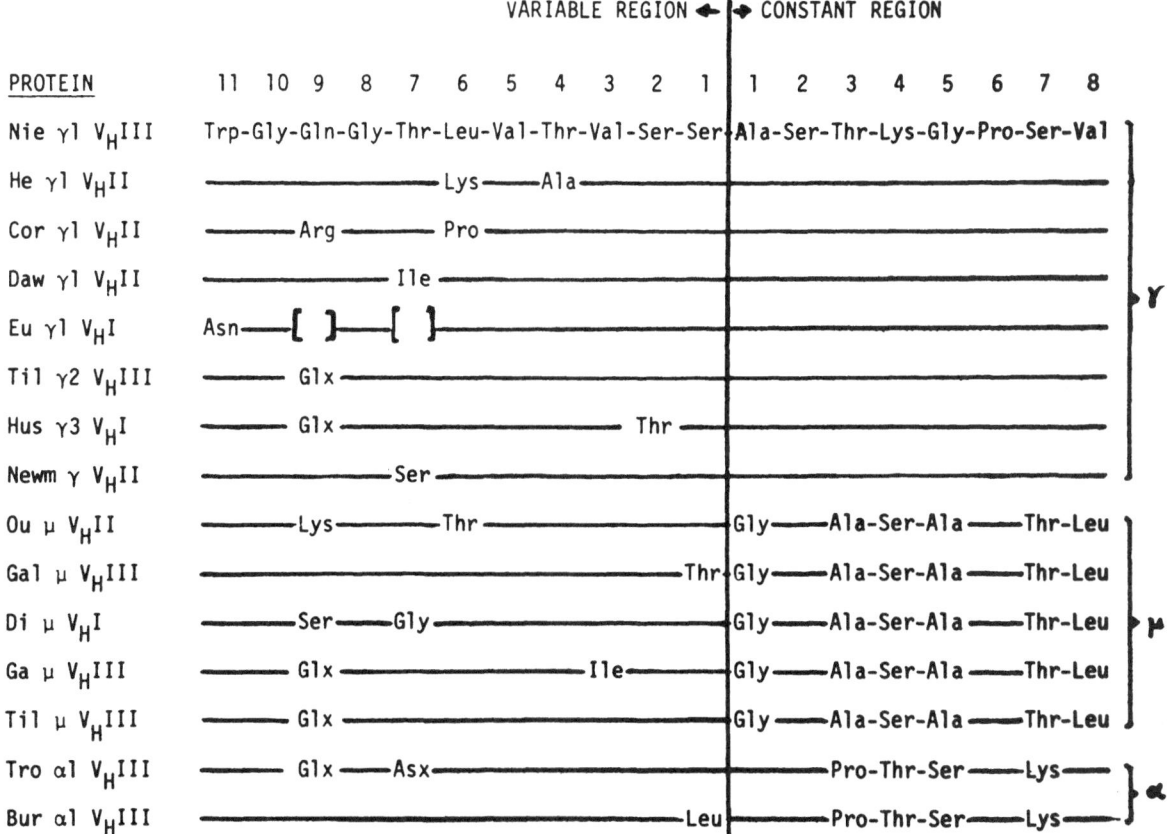

Figure 6. Amino acid sequences near the switch point between the V and C regions of human H chains. Horizontal lines denote identity of amino acid sequences with the sequence at the top. Brackets were introduced in the sequence of the Eu γ1 chain to assure maximum homology with the sequences of other H chains. References: Nie: Ponstingl and Hilschmann (1972); He: Cunningham *et al.* (1971); Cor and Daw: Press and Hogg (1969); Eu: Edelman *et al.* (1969); Til: Wang *et al.* (1977); Hus: Wang and Fudenberg (1975); Newm: Poljak *et al.* (1974); Ou: Putnam *et al.* (1973a); Gal: Watanabe *et al.* (1973); Di and Ga: Florent *et al.* (1974); Tro: Kratzin *et al.* (1975); Bur: Liu *et al.* (1976).

AN-CHUAN WANG

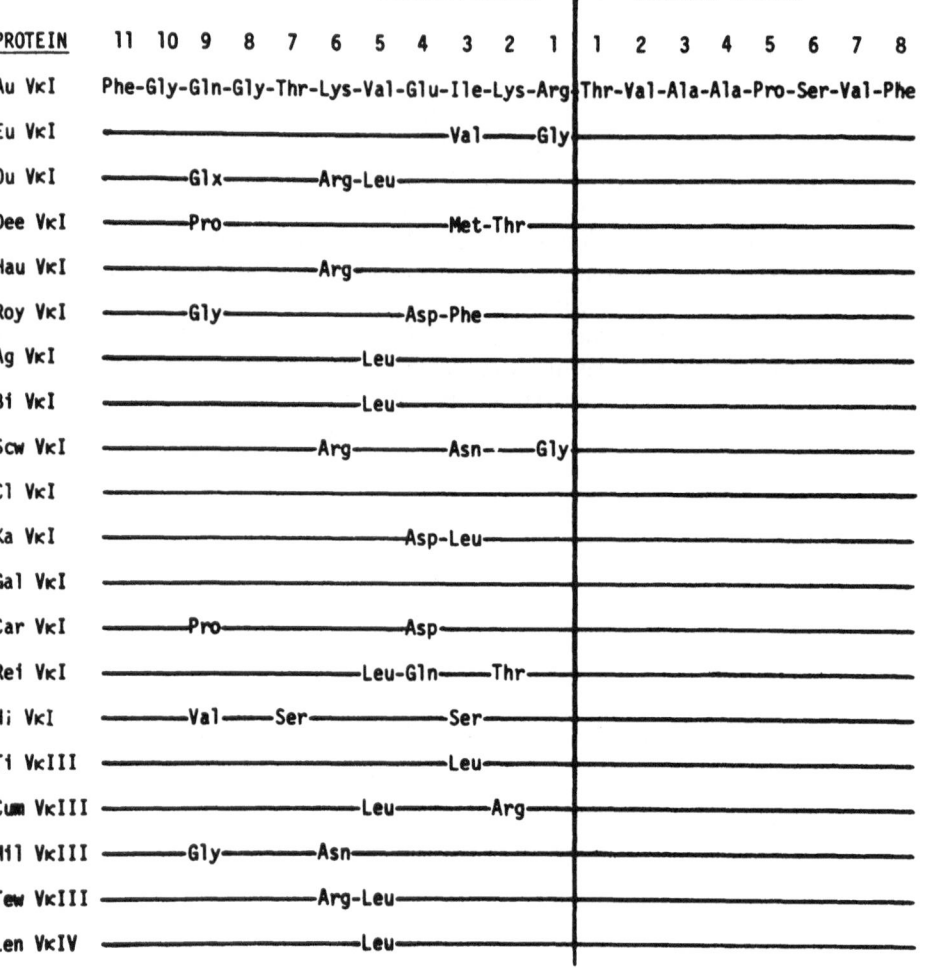

Figure 7. Amino acid sequences near the switch point between the V and C regions of human κ chains. Horizontal lines denote identity of amino acid sequences with the sequence at the top. References: Au: Schiechl and Hilschmann (1971); Eu: Gottlieb *et al* (1970); Ou: Kohler *et al* (1970b); Dee: Milstein and Deverson (1971); Hau: Watanabe and Hilschmann (1970); Roy: Hilschmann (1967); Ag: Titani *et al.* (1969); Bi: Braun *et al.* (1971); Scw: Eulitz *et al.* (1974); Cl: Solomon *et al.* (1975); Ka: Shinoda (1975); Gal: Laure *et al.* (1973); Car: Milstein and Deverson (1974); Rei: Palm and Hilschmann (1975); Ni: Shinoda (1973); Ti: Suter *et al.* (1972); Cum: Hilschmann (1967); Mil: Dreyer *et al.* (1967); Tew: Putnam *et al.* (1973b); Len: Schneider and Hilschmann (1975).

and Kehoe, 1975; Schneider and Hilschmann, 1975). Furthermore, individual polypeptide chains within each of these three V-region groups vary in size at their V regions. For example, the V region of Til H chain has 115 amino acid residues (Wang *et al.*, 1977), whereas that of Ou H chain has 123 residues (Putnam *et al.*, 1973a). Similarly, the V region of Cum κ chain has 116 residues (Hilschmann 1967), while the V regions of Ag κ chain (Titani *et al.*, 1969), Ha λ chain (Shinoda *et al.*, 1970), and X λ chain (Milstein *et al.*, 1968) have 108, 113, and 107 residues, respectively. Yet, counting backward from the V–C junction, many of the positions near that C-terminal end of the V region are surprisingly constant.

239

EVIDENCE FOR AND
THE SIGNIFICANCE
OF 'TWO GENES, ONE
POLYPEPTIDE
CHAIN'

Two glycine residues are of particular interest. They have been found at positions 8 and 10 at the N-terminal side of the V–C junction in all but one (Figure 6: Eu H chain which requires insertion of brackets for obtaining sequence homology) of over 100 Ig polypeptide chains examined (Figures 6–9) (Kabat, E. A., et al., 1976). Another amino acid residue, threonine at position 7 on the N-terminal side of the V–C junction, also showed little variation. It occurred in all but one (Figure 7: Ni) of the L chains and most of the H chains analyzed (Figures 6–9) (Kabat, E. A., et al., 1976). The occurrence of these and other unusually "constant" residues near the C-terminal end of the V regions of all three kinds of Ig polypeptide chains (κ, λ, and H) and in widely separated species (Figure 9: human, mouse, rat, and rabbit) indicates that they may play one or more important roles in antibody synthesis.

The significance of the relatively "constant" residues within the V regions was reviewed from a structural point of view by Poljak (1975). For example, the

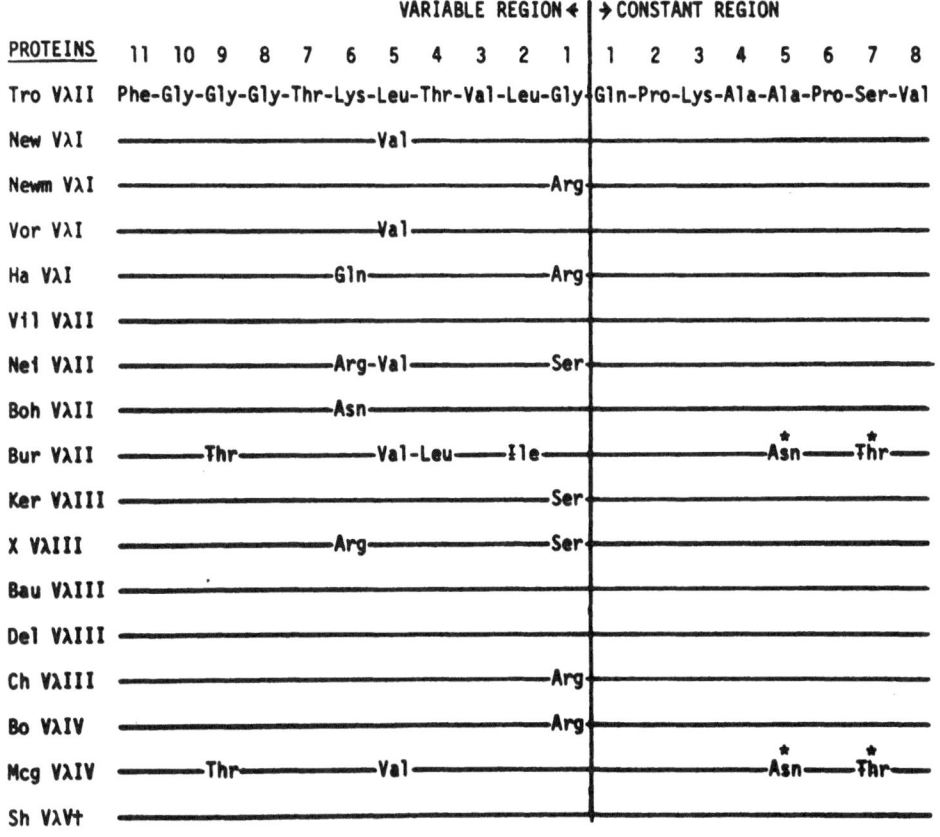

Figure 8. Amino acid sequences near the switch point between the V and C regions of human λ chains. Horizontal lines denote identity of amino acid sequences with the sequence at the top. References: Tro: Scholz and Hilschmann (1975); New: Langer et al. (1968); Newm: B. L. Chen and Poljak (1974): Vor: Engelhard et al. (1974); Ha: Shinoda et al. (1970); Vil: Ponstingl and Hilschmann (1969); Nei: Garver and Hilschmann (1972); Boh: Kohler et al. (1975); Bur: Liu et al. (1976); Ker: Ponstingl et al. (1968); X: Milstein et al. (1968); Bau: Baczko et al. (1974); Del: Eulitz (1974); Ch: Okada et al. (1972); Bo: Wikler and Putnam (1970); Mcg: Fett and Deutsch (1975); Sh: Titani et al. (1970). *Associated with the Mcg isotype (Fett and Deutsch, 1975). †A different classification of VλV was suggested by Sletten et al. (1974).

AN-CHUAN WANG

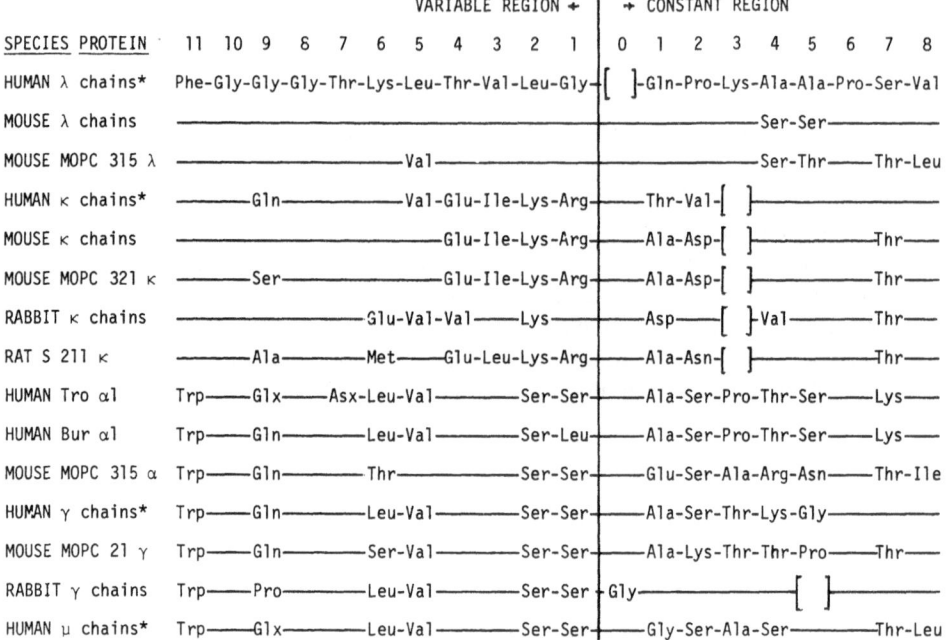

Figure 9. Amino acid sequences near the switch point between the V and C regions of Ig polypeptide chains of various species. Horizontal lines denote identity of amino acid sequences with the sequence at the top. Brackets were introduced to assure maximum homology. References: MOPC 315λ: Dugan *et al.* (1973); MOPC 321κ: McKean *et al.* (1973a); S211κ: Starace and Querinjean (1975); Tro α1: Kratzin *et al.* (1975); Bur α1: Liu *et al.* (1976); MOPC 315 α: Francis *et al.* (1974): MOPC 21γ1: Milstein *et al.* (1974b). References for MOUSE λ chains (at least 17 of which—RPC 20, J558, XS104, SAPC 176, SAPC 178, Y5606, Y5444, HOPC 1, HOPC 2020, J698, H2061, W3159, Y5431, Y5485, Y5830, Y5669, MOPC 511— have the identical amino acid sequence at these positions): Apella (1971); Cesari and Weigert (1973); Cohn *et al.* (1974): References for MOUSE κ chains (at least 4 of which—MOPC 41, MOPC 70, MOPC 63, MOPC 21—have the identical amino acid sequence at these positions): Gray *et al.* (1967); McKean *et al.* (1973b); Milstein *et al.* (1974b): References for RABBIT κ chains (at least 8 of which—4135, BS-1, BS-5, K-25, 2717, 3315, 3374, 120—have the identical amino acid sequence at these positions): K. S. C. Chen *et al.* (1974); Jaton (1974a,b, 1975); Apella *et al.* (1973); Margolies *et al.* (1975): References for RABBIT γ chains (at least 3 preparations of which—BS-1, aa1 pool, aa3 pool—all have the identical amino acid sequences at these positions): Pratt and Mole (1975); Jaton (1976). *Prototype amino acid sequences corresponding to the top sequences in Figure 8 (HUMAN λ chains), Figure 7 (HUMAN κ chains), and Figure 6 (HUMAN γ chains).

phenylalanine residue at position 11 counting from the V–C junction toward the *N*-terminal end of λ chains (Figure 8) has been assumed to be important in the assembling of V_L and V_H domains, whereas the occurrence of the glycine residue at position 8 counting from the V–C junction toward the *N*-terminal end of λ chains (Figure 8) has been attributed to space limitations in terms of a three-dimensional structure. Since a given protein structure need not be limited to performing only one biological function, I would like to suggest another explanation that is not mutually exclusive with the explanations set forth previously by others. I would postulate that the nucleotide sequence coding for the relatively invariant amino acid residues near the *C*-terminal end of the V regions may perform one or both of two additional functions. First, they may serve as markers to be recognized by certain specific

241

EVIDENCE FOR AND
THE SIGNIFICANCE
OF 'TWO GENES, ONE
POLYPEPTIDE
CHAIN'

enzymes (e.g., nucleotidase and ligase) that catalyze the breaking and reforming of phosphodiester bonds at particular gene loci during the translocation of the V- and C-region genes. Second, the pairing of the end of a V-region gene to the stretch of DNA immediately before the beginning of a C-region gene or to the "spacer" DNA between the V- and C-region genes may take place during the translocation. An "invariant" nucleotide sequence near the end of the V-region genes may facilitate this pairing by means of hydrogen bonding between adenine and thymine and between cytosine and guanine, assuming the nucleotide sequence immediately prior to the beginning of a C-region gene (or the corresponding "spacer" DNA sequence) is complementary to that at the end of the V-region genes. It may be possible to examine this assumption by nucleotide sequence determination in future experiments. The stretch of DNA immediately prior to the beginning of the C-region genes might have evolved to perform this function, which indirectly restricted the degree of variability allowed near the end of the V-region genes.

It is speculated that many of the last 11 residues at the C-terminal end of the V region may participate in the fusion in a similar but more restricted manner. For example, counting from the junction between the V and C regions toward the N-terminal end, all human H chains have valine at position 5 (see Figure 6) and all human λ chains have valine at position 3 (see Figure 8), whereas phenylalanine was found at position 11 of all L chains (see Figures 7–9). Perhaps some of these residues may be group-specific, which would be consistent with the fact that only V and C regions belonging to the same linkage group can fuse. Several laboratories observed that human $V_H III$ subgroup is found in higher frequency among α chains (Wang et al., 1971; Capra et al., 1974), and that Vλ chains with a threonine residue at position 9 at the N-terminal side from the V–C junction preferentially associated with a particular C-region isotype (Fett and Deutsch, 1975). Thus, even within a single linkage group, the association of the V and C region may not be entirely at random, and the intragroup amino acid substitutions near the end of the V regions may be responsible for this nonrandom nature of fusion. The exact mechanism for the fusion is not specified. It could be a single crossover within a single DNA molecule, an insertion of a replicated copy of a V-region or a C-region gene, an insertion of an episomal V-region or C-region gene, or fusion of two pieces of mRNA by RNA ligase. As pointed out by Wu and Kabat (1970), there are other relatively invariable positions within the V regions, but not near the C-terminus. These residues seem unlikely to be involved in the pairing process required for the fusion, because in order to align them at the same positions counting from the V–C junction toward the N-terminus, too many gaps must be introduced in most of the H and L chains.

9. Three Linkage Groups

Family analysis of the Ig genetic markers in animals and man demonstrate three linkage groups among antibody structural genes (Milstein and Monro, 1970): κ-chain, λ-chain, and H-chain linkage groups. Each linkage group consists of a family of V-region genes and one or a family of C-region genes (Figure 10). In man, the κ-chain linkage group has one C-region gene, the λ-chain linkage group has at least four C-region genes (Ein, 1968; Hess et al., 1971; Fett and Deutsch, 1975), and the H-chain linkage group has at least nine (Gally and Edelman, 1972). The number of V-region genes in each linkage group is a controversial issue, but most workers

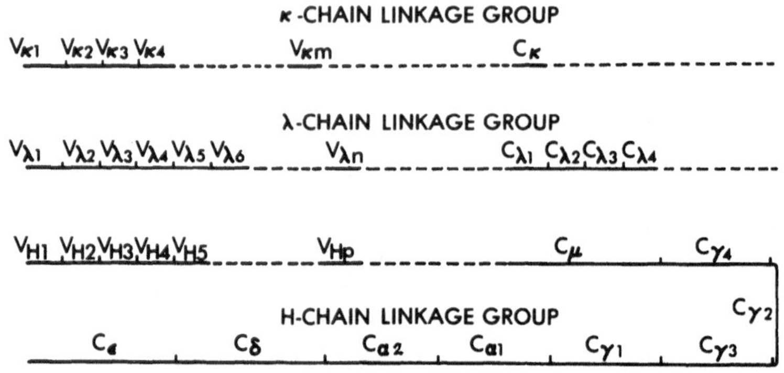

Figure 10. Diagrammatic representation of the three linked antibody gene groups.

agree that it should be much larger than the number of V-region subgroups within each linkage group (Cohn *et al.*, 1974). The evidence for this linkage grouping is as follows: In man (Pink *et al.*, 1971), rabbit (Kelus and Pernis, 1971; Mage *et al.*, 1971; Kindt and Mandy, 1972), mouse (Potter and Lieberman, 1967; Herzenberg *et al.*, 1968), and chicken (Pink and Ivanyi, 1975), all H-chain genes are linked, while in man (Steinberg and Matsumoto, 1964) and rabbit (Kindt, 1975), the C-region genes for κ, λ, and H chain are unlinked. It has been demonstrated that in rabbit, the H-chain V-region allotypes (a1, a2, and a3) are linked to γ-chain C-region allotypes (d11, d12, e14, and e15). Similarly, in mice, idiotypic determinants are linked to H-chain C-region allotypes (Pawlak *et al.*, 1973; Eichman, 1975; Lieberman *et al.*, 1974), and the map distance between a V-region gene (the V_H-DEX) and a C-region gene (Ig-1) was estimated to be approximately 0.4 centimorgan (Riblet *et al.*, 1975). These findings are consistent with the concept that V_H and C_H genes are all linked. Presumably, the same is true of L-chain genes, since *N*-terminal amino acid sequences of rabbit Ig κ chains correlate closely with κ-chain C-region allotypes (Waterfield *et al.*, 1973), whereas the mRNA for a mouse myeloma κ chain contains information coding for both the Vκ and the Cκ regions (Milstein *et al.*, 1974a). This linkage relationship also implies that only V- and C-region genes located in the same chromosome can be fused together to code for a single Ig polypeptide chain.

10. More Than Two Genes for One Polypeptide Chain?

All Ig polypeptide chains consist of repeating homology units (see Figure 1). Each unit is approximately 110 amino acid residues long and has an intrachain disulfide bond bridging two cysteine residues approximately 60 amino acid residues apart. A single L chain is composed of two such units, whereas each H chain is composed of four or five such units. Phylogenetic studies show that genes for Ig polypeptide chains are probably all derived from a common primordial gene that codes for one such unit (Singer and Doolittle, 1966; Hill *et al.*, 1966). Since each L chain is controlled by two genes having the same size as the common ancestor gene, then, by homology, the suggestion that four (or five) genes code for each H chain constitutes an attractive working hypothesis.

243

EVIDENCE FOR AND
THE SIGNIFICANCE
OF 'TWO GENES, ONE
POLYPEPTIDE
CHAIN'

Studies of H-chain-disease (HCD) proteins have provided evidence that the C region of the Fd fragment may be controlled by a separate gene. Amino acid sequence analyses indicated that in three HCD proteins, there are large deleted sections (Frangione and Milstein, 1969; Franklin and Frangione, 1971; Cooper *et al.*, 1972). The deleted sections include almost all the C_H1 domain as well as part of the V region, and the sequences resume at a glutamic acid residue corresponding to position 216 of reference protein Eu. The wholesale deletion of the C_H1 domain led Franklin and Frangione (1971) to suggest that the glutamic acid residue at position 216 may mark the start of a different gene, and that several genes control the synthesis of each H chain. Compelling evidence in support of this concept was obtained from studies of several other HCD proteins, two of which had an internal deletion of 15 amino acids starting at position 216 (Fett *et al.*, 1973; Rivat *et al.*, 1976). A second example, a human $\alpha1$ chain, appeared to have a deletion of the entire C_H3 domain (Despont *et al.*, 1974). The third, also a human $\alpha1$ chain, had an internal deletion comprising the C region of the Fd fragment and a portion of the V region (Wolfenstein-Todel *et al.*, 1974b). Amino acid sequence data on normal and myeloma H chains do not support this hypothesis, however, since within a given subclass of human γ chain, the C_H1 domains of different γ-chain subclasses differ in amino acid sequence (Milstein and Pink, 1970). No reciprocal sharing between the Fc fragment and the C_H1 domain was observed among the four human γ-chain subclasses.

In comparing the V-region amino acid sequences available in the literature, Wu and Kabat (1970) defined three hypervariable regions for human L chains. Subsequently, hypervariable regions were also detected in human H chains and Ig polypeptide chains of other species (Capra and Kehoe, 1975). These hypervariable regions are located within the V region, separated by relatively constant positions called *framework* positions. It was postulated that the genetic information for hypervariable regions is contained in the form of episomes in some extrachromosomal DNA (Wu and Kabat, 1970). The hypervariable-region episomes (or genes) are incorporated into the DNA of structural genes for the framework portion of V regions by translocation. This hypothesis has generated considerable interest among immunogeneticists, and has been supported by the following observations: (1) Two human λ chains of different $V\lambda$ subgroups have an identical amino acid sequence in their first hypervariable regions (Wu *et al.*, 1975). (2) H chains of two anti-gammaglobulins have identical amino acid sequences at two of the four hypervariable regions (Capra and Kehoe, 1974). (3) Two antistreptococcal C carbohydrate antibodies with different V_H allotypes from a single rabbit share identical idiotypic determinants (Kindt *et al.*, 1973). (4) An IgG and an IgM with H chains of different V_H subgroups from one patient shared V_H idiotypic determinants (Hopper *et al.*, 1976).

11. Specific Gene Activation and Differential Gene Expression

Genetic and biochemical studies in higher organisms demonstrate that in a given individual heterozygous for an H-chain genetic marker, a single Ig-producing cell generally synthesizes the H chain of one allele only, not of the other (reviewed by Mage *et al.*, 1973; Fudenberg *et al.*, 1972). The same appears to be true for L chains. This phenomenon, designated *allelic exclusion,* superficially resembles the X-chromosome inactivation described by Lyon (1968), in which it was found that in a given cell, all X chromosomes but one are inactivated early in development. The phenomenon found in Ig is much broader. Structural and genetic studies having demonstrated that multiple genes are involved in the synthesis of both the V and C regions of Ig polypeptide chains (Gally and Edelman, 1972; Wang and Fudenberg, 1974). At least nine C-region genes ($\gamma1$, $\gamma2$, $\gamma3$, $\gamma4$, $\alpha1$, $\alpha2$, μ, δ, and ϵ) for human H chains and six for human λ chains (Figure 3) have been clearly defined. Although the exact number of V-region genes has not been established, it is likely to be much larger than the number of subgroups thus far described (Fudenberg *et al.,* 1972). The genome of each lymphocyte therefore contains multiple genes coding for each of the V_H, C_H, V_L, and C_L regions, and yet under normal conditions, any given lymphocytes synthesized only one specific kind of antibody molecule. Only one member among each family (i.e., V_H, C_H, V_L, and C_L) of genes is expressed, all others being repressed. This phenomenon was termed *specific gene activation* by Steinberg *et al.* (1970). The mechanism for specific gene activation is unknown, but it must be involved, in conjunction with the fusion mechanism of the V- and C-region genes, in the differentiation of lymphocytes that leads to antibody specificity.

Analysis of published amino acid sequence data in the literature shows that the V region of a human λ chain has more sequence homology with the V regions of chicken and turkey L chains than with those of other L chains, including human λ chains (Wang, 1975). This observation has led to the speculation that all vertebrates share large numbers of similar, but not identical, V-region genes. These genes are similar because they evolved from a common primordial gene, but they differ from one another, and differ in different species, because after duplication, each gene has evolved independently. Different sets of these genes are assumed to be expressed in different species. Control at a level equivalent to "regulatory genes" decides which set of genes is to be expressed. The concept of "differential gene expression" offers a logical explanation (Wang, 1975) for the puzzling observation made on rabbit V_H allotypes (a1, a2, and a3), and has been supported by the following observations: (1) The V-region amino acid sequence of a rat κ chain (S211) showed more homology with that of a human κ chain (Roy) than with the sequences of mouse κ chains (Starace and Querinjean, 1975). (2) The rabbit a1 allotypic marker was found in many human sera (Knight *et al.,* 1975). (3) Cultured Ig-producing cells often "mutated" to produce fragments of Ig polypeptide chains (Birshtein *et al.,* 1974). (4) Cultured lymphocytes of homozygous Glm(1−) individuals produced Glm(1) molecules *in vitro* (Rivat *et al.,* 1973). (5) In serial transplantation of human lymphoid tumor lines in hamsters, Glm(1) molecules were detected in one of the lines in which the donor was Glm(1−) (Pothier *et al.,* 1974). (6) A rabbit expressed three allotypes in each of the *a* and *b* loci (Strosberg *et al.,* 1974). (7) Some rabbits (Mudgett *et al.,* 1975), rats (Hunt and Duvall, 1976), and mice (Bosma and Bosma, 1974) can express certain allotypes that could not be inherited via Mendelian segregation. Although a detailed discussion of this subject is beyond the scope of this chapter, the phenomena described here do indicate that the expression of Ig structural genes must be under precise control by the "regulatory genes" in eukaryotic systems, and that they are likely interrelated with the fusion process between V- and C-region genes.

The "genetic switch" hypothesis was proposed by Wang *et al.* (1970a), on the basis of the study of monotypic IgM(κ) and IgG2(κ) from a single patient (see Section 5). According to this hypothesis, during the differentiation of the immune system, a given clone of antibody-producing cells can maintain its V-region specificity while switching from the expression of one class of antibody to another. Such a switch involved the repression of a C-region gene (Cμ) and the simultaneous derepression of another C-region gene (Cγ), whereas the other Ig structural genes (V$_L$, C$_L$, and V$_H$) remain unchanged (Figure 11). In this manner, a single V$_H$ gene (or its copies) may fuse with two or more C$_H$ genes during the differentiation of Ig-producing cells. This hypothesis is supported by many other observations: (1) Several additional cases of double gammopathy (Penn *et al.*, 1970; Seon *et al.*, 1973a,b; Wolfenstein-Todel *et al.*, 1974a; Fair *et al.*, 1975) and a case of triple gammopathy (Grubb and Zettervall, 1975) also demonstrated the sharing of presumably identical L chains and V$_H$ regions. (2) A few days after the immunization of a rabbit, a small fraction of the cells produced both IgM and IgG (Nossal *et al.*, 1971; Pernis *et al.*, 1971; Greaves, 1971); presumably these cells were examined during the switch. (3) Anti-*Salmonella* antibodies of the IgM and IgG classes from an individual rabbit shared idiotypic antigenic determinants (Oudin and Michel, 1969). (4) Clones of cells derived from a single stimulated B lymphocyte produced antibodies of identical idiotype but diverse Ig class (Gearhart *et al.*, 1975). (5) The incidence of multiple myeloma is approximately 1 in 20,000 people, but the frequency of double gammopathy is approximately 1 in 100 patients with multiple myeloma or Waldenström's macroglobulinemia or both (Bihrer *et al.*, 1974), a figure too high to be expected for two independent events.

Experiments done by Kincade *et al.* (1970) provide additional support for the "genetic switch" mechanism. Treatment of 13-day-old chick embryo with purified antibodies to IgM combined with bursectomy at hatching suppressed both IgM and IgG synthesis. Administration of anti-IgM after bursectomy at hatching, however, suppressed only IgM but not IgG synthesis. These result indicate that an IgM-to-

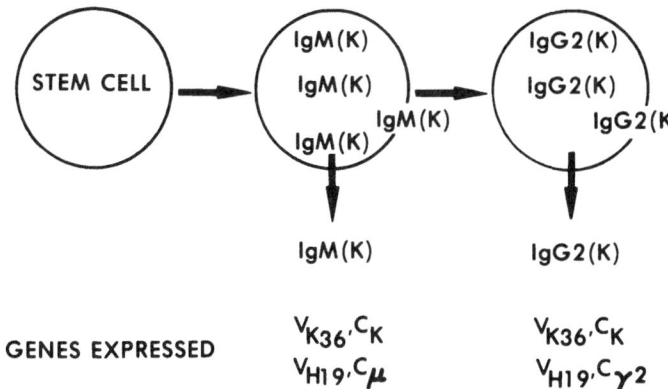

Figure 11. Hypothetical model exemplifying the "genetic switch." It was suggested that only a small fraction of the IgM-producing cells undergo the switching process.

IgG switch takes place inside the bursa of Fabricus in birds. Bursectomy of chick embryos at various stages starting on the 16th day of incubation showed that the birds later may have one of three Ig combinations: IgM only, IgM + IgG, or IgM + IgG + IgA, a situation usually maintained over a long period of time (Kincade and Cooper, 1973) These data support the model for lymphocyte maturation proposed by Cooper *et al.* (1972), who suggested that there is a sequential development from IgM- to IgG- to IgA-forming cells, and that the switch is not driven by antigen. Studies with cultured mouse spleen cells showed, however, that the switch may be driven by antigen (Pierce *et al.,* 1973). Other studies in chickens (Martin and Leslie, 1974; Perez and Bienenstock, 1973) and mice (Manning, 1974) indicate that IgA-producing cells may be derived directly from IgM-producing cells. In addition, a patient with double gammopathy had both monotypic IgM and IgA in his plasma (Yagi and Pressman, 1973). The combined evidence is more compatible with an alternative model (Warner, 1974; Manning, 1974) of lymphocyte maturation, in which a multipotential IgM precursor cell may, by separate pathways, give rise to clones of lymphocytes, each of which produces any one of the other classes of Ig's.

Still other evidence suggests that the switch need not originate from IgM-producing cells (Kishimoto and Ishazaka, 1971) and is not restricted to C_H regions (Wang *et al.,* 1972). Both IgD and IgM were found together on a large proportion of peripheral blood lymphocytes in normal persons (Rowe *et al.,* 1973a) as well as in patients with chronic lymphocytic leukemia (Fu *et al.,* 1974; Kubo *et al.,* 1974). It was noticed that idiotypic antibodies specific for the isolated serum IgM reacted with both the IgM and IgD on the cell membrane (Fu *et al.,* 1975). A parallel finding was made on one patient in whom both IgM and IgD molecules on the same cell had antibody specificity to IgG (Pernis *et al.,* 1974). Rowe *et al.* (1973b) also found that the percentage of lymphocytes positive for IgD is much higher in newborns than in adults, raising the possibility that the gene coding for the C region of the δ chain may participate in the genetic switch and play an important role in the ontogeny of Ig-producing cells.

A slightly different situation is found in mice (Vitetta *et al.,* 1975). Newborn mice have only IgM on the lymphocyte membrane. Beginning 10–15 days after birth, an IgD-like molecule begins to appear on the membrane of the spleen lymphocytes and becomes the predominant cell-surface Ig when the mouse is 3 months old. This is true not only in normal mice but also in germ-free and nude mice. Apparently there is a switch from IgM-producing cells to cells synthesizing IgD-like molecules; this switch is not antigen-driven.

Davie and Paul (1974) studied the proliferation of B lymphocytes in thymus-deprived mice following stimulation with antigen. They failed to find γ-chain-bearing antigen-binding cells in a secondary immune response, but μ-chain-bearing antigen-binding cells persisted. This observation suggests that T lymphocytes may be involved in the "genetic switch" through interaction with B lymphocytes.

13. Summary

DNA–RNA hybridization studies on embryonic and adult mouse lymphocytes and amino acid sequence data on Ig polypeptide chains in man and several other vertebrate species established that each Ig polypeptide chain is coded for by at least two structural genes: a V-region gene and a C-region gene. There is likely a somatic

247

EVIDENCE FOR AND
THE SIGNIFICANCE
OF 'TWO GENES, ONE
POLYPEPTIDE
CHAIN'

rearrangement of the genome, probably by translocation of Ig structural genes, during the differentiation of antibody-producing cells that fuses a V- and C-region gene together either directly or via a stretch of untranscribed "spacer" DNA. This fusion is essential in committing the cell for the synthesis of a particular kind of antibody molecule.

Examination of amino acid sequences near the junction between the V and C regions enabled clear establishment of the V–C switch point in H (see Figure 6), κ (see Figure 7), and λ (see Figure 8) chains. It is noteworthy that many positions near the C-terminal end of the V region are remarkably "invariable." Two glycine residues are particularly obvious. They occur at the 8th and 10th positions from the V–C junction toward the N-terminal end of practically all Ig polypeptide chains sequenced to date, including κ, λ, and H chains of various species (human, rabbit, rat, and mouse). These relatively "invariable" residues may be relevant to the fusion process. It is postulated that the nucleotides on the DNA coding for these residues may have evolved to perform either or both of two functions: (1) to serve as a recognition site for certain enzymes catalyzing the fusion process and (2) to facilitate the pairing between the end of a V-region gene and the DNA immediately prior to the beginning of a C-region gene (or portion of the DNA which served as a "spacer" between the coding nucleotide sequences) by hydrogen bonding between complementary nucleotides.

ACKNOWLEDGMENTS

This work was supported in part by grants from the South Carolina Appropriation for Biomedical Research, the U.S. Public Health Service (AI-13388) and the National Science Foundation (BMS-75-09513). The author is the recipient of an American Cancer Society Faculty Research Award (FRA-125). This is publication No. 11 from the Department of Basic and Clinical Immunology and Microbiology, Medical University of South Carolina.

References

Apella, E., 1971, Amino acid sequences of two mouse immunoglobulin lambda chains, *Proc. Natl. Acad. Sci. U.S.A.* **68**:590–594.

Appella, E., Rejnek, J., and Reisfeld, R. A., 1969, Variations at the carboxyl-terminal amino acid sequence of rabbit light chains with b4, b5 and b6 allotypic specificities, *J. Mol. Biol.* **41**:473–477.

Appella, E., Roholt, O. A., Chersi, A., Radzimski, G., and Pressman, D., 1973, Amino acid sequence of the light chain derived from a rabbit anti-*p*-azobenzoate antibody of restricted heterogeneity, *Biochem. Biophys. Res. Commun.* **53**:1122–1129.

Apte, B. N., and Zipser, D., 1973, *In vivo* splicing of proteins: One continuous polypeptide from two independently functioning operons, *Proc. Natl. Acad. Sci. U.S.A.* **70**:2969–2973.

Baczko, K., Braun, D., and Hilschmann, N., 1974, Die Primärstruktur einer monoklonale Immunoglobulin-L-kette vom λ-Typ Subgruppe IV (Bence Jones protein Bau), *Hoppe-Seyler's Z. Physiol. Chem.* **355**:131–154.

Beadle, G. W., and Tatum, E. L., 1941, Genetic control of biochemical reaction in neurospora, *Proc. Natl. Acad. Sci. U.S.A.* **27**:499–506.

Bennich, H., and von Bahr-Lindstrom, H., 1974, Structure of immunoglobulin E (IgE), *Prog. Immunol.* **2**(1):49–58.

Bihrer, R., Flury, R., and Morell, A., 1974, Biklonale Paraproteinämie, *Schweiz. Med. Wochenschr.* **104**:39–45.

Birshtein, B. K., Preud'homme, J. L., and Scharff, M. D., 1974, Variants of mouse myeloma cells that produce short immunoglobulin heavy chains, *Proc. Natl. Acad. Sci. U.S.A.* **71**:3478–3482.

Bosma, M., and Bosma, G., 1974, Congenic mouse strains: The expression of a hidden immungloblin allotype in a congenic partner strain of BALB/c mice, *J. Exp. Med.* **139**:512–527.

Braun, M., Liebold, W., Barnikol, H. U., and Hilschmann, N., 1971, Die Primärstruktur einer monoklonalen Immunoglobulin-L-kette der Subgruppe I vom K-Typ (Bence–Jones protein Bi): Variabilitätsregel der κ-Ketten, *Hoppe-Seyler's Z. Physiol. Chem.* **352**:647–651.

Capra, J. D., and Kehoe, J. M., 1974, Structure of antibodies with shared idiotypy: The complete sequences of the heavy chain variable regions of two IgM antigamma globulins, *Proc. Natl. Acad. Sci. U.S.A.* **71**:4032–4036.

Capra, J. D., and Kehoe, J. M., 1975, Hypervariable regions, idiotypy and the antibody combining site, *Adv. Immunol.* **20**:1–40.

Capra, J. D., Chuang, C., Kaplan, R. D., and Kehoe, J. M., 1974, Amino acid sequence studies of human IgA myeloma proteins, in: *The Immunoglobulin A System* (J. Mestecky and A. R. Lawton, eds.), pp. 191–199, Plenum Press, New York and London.

Cesari, I. M., and Weigert, M., 1973, Mouse lambda-chain sequences, *Proc. Natl. Acad. Sci. U.S.A.* **70**:2112–2116.

Chen, B. L., and Poljak, R. J., 1974, Amino acid sequence of the (λ) light chain of a human myeloma immunoglobulin (IgG New), *Biochemistry* **13**:1295–1301.

Chen, K. S. C., Kindt, R. J., and Kraus, R. M., 1974, Amino acid sequence of an allotype b4 light chain from a rabbit antibody to streptococcal carbohydrate, *Proc. Natl. Acad. Sci. U.S.A.* **71**:1995–1998.

Cohn, M., Blomberg, G., Geckeler, W., Raschke, W., Riblet, R., and Weigert, M., 1974, First order considerations in analyzing the generator of diversity, in: *The Immune System: Genes, Receptors, Signals* (E. Sercarz and A. Williamson, eds.), pp. 98–117, Academic Press, New York.

Cooper, M. D., Lawton, A. R., and Kincade, P. W., 1972, A two stage model for development of antibody-producing cells, *Clin. Exp. Immunol.* **11**:143–149.

Cunningham, B. A., Gottlieb, P. D., Pflumm, N. M., and Edelman, G. M., 1971, Immunoglobulin structure: Diversity, gene duplication and domains, *Prog. Immunol.* **1**:3–24.

Davie, J. M., and Paul, W. R., 1974, Role of T-lymphocytes in the humoral immune response. I. Proliferation of B-lymphocytes in thymus-deprived mice, *J. Immunol.* **113**:1438–1444.

Dayhoff, M. O. (ed.), 1976, *Atlas of Protein Sequence and Structure*, Vol. 5, Supplement 2, pp. 165–190, National Biomedical Research Foundation, Washington, D.C.

Despont, J. J., Abel, C. A., Grey, H. M., and Penn, G. M., 1974, Structural studies on human IgA1 myeloma protein with a carboxyl-terminal deletion, *J. Immunol.* **112**:1517–1525.

Dreyer, W. J., and Bennett, J. C., 1965, The molecular basis of antibody formation, a paradox, *Proc. Natl. Acad. Sci. U.S.A.* **54**:864–869.

Dreyer, W. J., and Grey, W. R., 1968, On the role of nucleic acid as genes concerning precise chemospecificity to differentiated cell lines, in: *Nucleic Acid in Immunology* (D. J. Prescia and W. Braun, eds.), pp. 614–643, Springer-Verlag, New York.

Dreyer, W. J., Grey, W. R., and Hood, L., 1967, The genetic, molecular and cellular basis of antibody formation: Some facts and a unifying hypothesis, *Cold Spring Harbor Symp. Quant. Biol.* **32**:353–367.

Dugan, E. S., Bradshaw, R. A., Simms, E. S., and Eisen, H., 1973, Amino acid sequence of the light chain of a mouse myeloma protein (MOPC 315), *Biochemistry* **12**:5400–5416.

Edelman, G. M., Cunningham, B. A., Gall, E. W., Gottlieb, P. D., and Waxdal, M., 1969, The covalent structure of an entire γG1 immunoglobulin molecule, *Proc. Natl. Acad. Sci. U.S.A.* **63**:78–85.

Eichmann, K., 1975, Genetic control of antibody specificity in mice, *Immunogenetics* **2**:491–506.

Ein, D., 1968, Nonallelic behavior of the OZ groups in human immunoglobulin λ chains, *Proc. Natl. Acad. Sci. U.S.A.* **60**:982–985.

Engelhard, M., Hess, M., and Hilschmann, N., 1974, Die Primärstruktur einer monoklonalen Immunoglobulin-L-kette der Subgroupe I vom λ-Typ, *Hoppe-Seyler's Z. Physiol. Chem.* **355**:85–88.

Eulitz, M., 1974, A new subgroup of human L-chains of the λ-type, primary structure of Bence Jones protein Del, *Eur. J. Biochem.* **50**:49–69.

Eulitz, M., Gotze, D., and Hilschmann, N., 1974, Die Primärstruktur einer humanen Immunoglobulin-L-kette vom κ-Typ (Bence–Jones Scw). I, *Hoppe-Seyler's Z. Physiol.* **355**:819–841.

Fair, D. S., Kreuger, R. G., Sledge, C., Black, B., and Hood, L., 1975, Studies of IgA and IgG monoclonal proteins derived from a single patient. II. Evidence for identical light chains and variable regions of the heavy chain, Biochemistry **14**:5561–5567.

Feinstein, A., 1963, Character and allotype of an immune globulin in rabbit colostrum, *Nature (London)* **199**:1197–1199.

Fett, J. W., and Deutsch, H. F., 1975, A new λ-chain gene, *Immunochemistry* **12**:643–652.

249

EVIDENCE FOR AND
THE SIGNIFICANCE
OF 'TWO GENES, ONE
POLYPEPTIDE
CHAIN'

Fett, J. W., Smithies, O., and Deutsch, H. F., 1973, Hinge-region deletion localized in the IgG1 globulin Mcg, *Immunochemistry* **10**:115–118.

Fleischman, J. B., 1967, Synthesis of the G heavy chain in rabbit lymph node cells, *Biochemistry* **6**:1311–1320.

Florent, G., Lehman, D., and Putnam, F. W., 1974, The switch point in heavy chains of human IgM immunoglobulins, *Biochemistry* **13**:2482–2498.

Francis, S. H., Leslie, R. G. O., Hood, L., and Eisen, H., 1974, Amino acid sequence of the variable region of the heavy (α) chain of a mouse myeloma protein with antihapten activity, *Proc. Natl. Acad. Sci. U.S.A.* **71**:1123–1127.

Frangione, B., and Milstein, C., 1969, Partial deletion in the heavy chain disease protein Zuc, *Nature (London)* **224**:597–599.

Franklin, E. C., and Frangione, B., 1971, The molecular defect in a protein (CRA) found in γ 1 heavy chain disease, and its genetic implications, *Proc. Natl. Acad. Sci. U.S.A.* **68**:187–191.

Fu, S. M., Winchester, R. J., and Kunkel, H. G., 1974, Occurrence of surface IgM, IgD and free light chains on human lymphocytes, *J. Exp. Med.* **139**:451–456.

Fu, S. M., Winchester, R. J., and Kunkel, H. G., 1975, Similar idiotypic specificity for the membrane IgD and IgM of human B-lymphocytes, *J. Immunol.* **114**:250–252.

Fudenberg, H. H., Pink, J. R. L., Stites, D., and Wang, A. C., 1972, *Basic Immunogenetics*, pp. 1–214, Oxford University Press, New York.

Gally, J. A., 1973, Structure of immunoglobulins, in: *The Antigens* (M. Sela, ed.), pp. 161–298, Academic Press, New York and London.

Gally, J. A., and Edelman, G. M., 1970, Somatic translocation of antibody genes, *Nature (London)* **227**:341–348.

Gally, J. A., and Edelman, G. M., 1972, The genetic control of immunoglobulin synthesis, *Annu. Rev. Genet.* **6**:1–46.

Garver, F. A., and Hilschmann, N., 1972, The primary structure of a monoclonal human λ-type immunoglobulin L-chain of subgroup II (Bence–Jones protein Nei), *Eur. J. Biochem.* **26**:10–32.

Gearhart, P. J., Sigal, N. H., and Klinman, N. R., 1975, Production of antibodies of identical idiotype but diverse immunoglobulin classes by cells derived from a single stimulated B cell, *Proc. Natl. Acad. Sci. U.S.A.* **72**:1707–1711.

Goodfleish, R. M., 1975, Constant region cysteine-containing peptides of b4 and b9 rabbit κ-chains isolated by a new diagonal mapping procedure, *J. Immunol.* **114**:910–912.

Gottlieb, P. D., Cunningham, B. A., Rutishauser, U., and Edelman, G. M., 1970, The covalent structure of a human γG-immunoglobulin. VI. Amino acid sequence of the light chain, *Biochemistry* **9**:3155–3161.

Gray, W. R., Dreyer, W. J., and Hood, L., 1967, Mechanism of antibody synthesis: Size differences between mouse kappa chains, *Science* **155**:465–467.

Greaves, M. F., 1971, The expression of immunoglobulin determinants on the surface of antigen-binding lymphoid cells in mice. I. An analysis of light and heavy chain restrictions on individual cells, *Eur. J. Immunol.* **1**:168–194.

Grubb, A. O., and Zettervall, O. H., 1975, Immunochemical evidence for a common variable region in three immunoglobulin classes in the same individual, *Proc. Natl. Acad. Sci. U.S.A.* **72**:4115–4118.

Hamers-Casterman, C., and Hamers, R., 1975, A second crossing-over between *d* and *a* locus in rabbit immunoglobulin γ chain, *Immunogenetics* **2**:597–603.

Herzenberg, L. A., McDevitt, J. O., and Herzenberg, L. A., 1968, Genetics of antibodies, *Annu. Rev. Genet.* **2**:209–244.

Hess, M., Hilschmann, N., Rivat, L., Rivat, C., and Ropartz, C., 1971, Isotypes in human immunoglobulin λ chains, *Nature (London) New Biol.* **234**:58–60.

Hill, R. L., Delaney, R., Fellow, R. E., and Lebowitz, H. E., 1966, The evolutionary origins of the immunoglobulin, *Proc. Natl. Acad. Sci. U.S.A.* **56**:1762–1769.

Hilschmann, N., 1967, Die chemische Struktur von zwei Bence–Jones Proteins (Roy and Cum) vom κ-Typ, *Hoppe-Seyler's Z. Physiol. Chem.* **348**:1077–1080.

Hilschmann, N., and Craig, J. C., 1965, Amino acid sequence studies with Bence–Jones proteins, *Proc. Natl. Acad. Sci. U.S.A.* **53**:1403–1409.

Hood, L., 1972, Two genes, one polypeptide chain—facts or fiction?, *Fed. Proc. Fed. Am. Soc. Exp. Biol.* **31**:177–187.

Hopper, J. E., Noyes, C., Heinrikson, R., and Kessel, J. W., 1976, Comparative studies on monotypic IgM(λ) and IgG(κ) from an individual patient. II. Amino-terminal sequence analyses, *J. Immunol.* **116**:743–746.

Hozumi, N., and Tonegawa, S., 1976, Evidence for somatic rearrangement of immunoglobulin genes coding for variable and constant regions, *Proc. Natl. Acad. Sci. U.S.A.* **73**:3628–3632.

Hunt, S., and Duvall, E., 1976, Rat immunoglobulin allotypes: Expression by thymus-independent cells, *Biochem. Sc. Trans.* **4**:39–41.

Jaton, J. C., 1974a, Amino acid sequence of the N-terminal 139 residues of light chains derived from a homogeneous rabbit antibody, *Biochem. J.* **141**:1–13.

Jaton, J. C., 1974b, Comparison of the amino acid sequences of the variable regions of light chains derived from two homogeneous rabbit anti-pneumococcal antibodies, *Biochem. J.* **141**:15–25.

Jaton, J. C., 1975, Comparison of amino acid sequences of the variable domains of two homogeneous rabbit antibodies to type III penumococcal polysaccharide, *Biochem. J.* **147**:235–247.

Jaton, J. C., 1976, The V-region sequence of the H chain from a third rabbit anti-pneumococcal antibody, *Biochem. J.* **157**:449–459.

Jaton, J. C., Braun, D. G., Strosberg, A. D., Haber, E., and Morris, J. E., 1973, Restricted rabbit antibodies: Amino acid sequences of rabbit H chains of allotype *a1, a2* and *a3* in the region 80 to 94, *J. Immunol.* **111**:1838–1843.

Kabat, D., 1972, Gene selection in hemoglobulin and antibody-synthesizing cells: A process of intrachromosomal crossing-over selects and activates genes in two different tissues, *Science* **175**:134–140.

Kabat, E. A., Wu, T. T., and Bilofsky, H., 1976, *Variable Regions of Immunoglobulin Chains*, pp. 1–130, Bolt Baranek and Newman, Cambridge, Massachusetts.

Kaufmann, G., and Littauer, U. Z., 1974, Covalent joining of phenylalanine transfer ribonucleic acid half-molecules by T4 RNA ligase, *Proc. Natl. Acad. Sci. U.S.A.* **71**:3741–3745.

Kelus, A. S., and Pernis, B., 1971, Allotypic marker of rabbit IgM, *Eur. J. Immunol.* **1**:123–143.

Kincade, P. W., and Cooper, M. D., 1973, Immunoglobulin A: Site and sequence of expression in developing chicks, *Science* **179**:398–400.

Kincade, P. W., Lawton, A. R., Bockman, D. E., and Cooper, M. D., 1970, Suppression of immunoglobulin G synthesis as a result of antibody-mediated suppression of immunoglobulin M synthesis in chickens, *Proc. Natl. Acad. Sci. U.S.A.* **67**:1918–1925.

Kindt, T. J., 1975, Rabbit immunoglobulin allotypes: Structure, immunology and genetics, *Adv. Immunol.* **21**:35–86.

Kindt, T. J., and Mandy, W. J., 1972, Recombination of genes coding for constant and variable regions of immunoglobulin heavy chains, *J. Immunol.* **108**:1110–1113.

Kindt, T. J., Klapper, D. G., and Waterfield, M. D., 1973, An idiotypic cross-reaction between allotype *a3* and allotype *a* negative antibodies to streptococcal carbohydrate. *J. Exp. Med.* **137**:636–648.

Kishimoto, R., and Ishizaka, K., 1971, Regulation of antibody response *in vitro*. I. Suppression of secondary response by anti-immunoglobulin heavy chains, *J. Immunol.* **107**:1567–1575.

Knight, K. L., Malek, T. R., and Dray, D., 1975, Human immunoglobulins with allotypic determinants of rabbit immunoglobulin heavy chains, *Nature (London)* **253**:216–217.

Knopf, P. M., Parkhouse, R. M. E., and Lennox, E. S., 1967, Biosynthetic units of an immunoglobulin heavy chain, *Proc. Natl. Acad. Sci. U.S.A.* **58**:2288–2295.

Kohler, H., Shimizu, A., Paul, C., Moore, V., and Putnam, F. W., 1970a, Three variable region gene pools common to IgM, IgG and IgA immunoglobulins, *Nature (London)* **227**:1318–1320.

Kohler, H., Shimizu, A., Paul, C., and Putnam, F. W., 1970b, Macroglobulin structure: Variable sequence of light and heavy chains, *Science* **169**:56–59.

Kohler, H., Rudofsky, S., and Kluskens, L., 1975, The primary structure of a human lambda II chain, *J. Immunol.* **114**:415–421.

Koshland, M. E., Davis, J. J., and Fujita, N. J., 1969, Evidence for multiple gene control of a single polypeptide chain: The heavy chain of rabbit immunoglobulin, *Proc. Natl. Acad. Sci. U.S.A.* **63**:1274–1281.

Kratzin, J., Altevogt, P., Ruban, E., Kortt, A., Staroscik, K., and Hilschmann, N., 1975, Die Primärstruktur eines monoklonalen IgA-immunoglobulins (IgA Tro). II. Die Aminosäuresequenz der H-kette, α-Typ, Subgruppe III Struktur des gesamten IgA-molekuls, *Hoppe-Seyler's Z. Physiol. Chem.* **356**:1337–1342.

Kubo, R. T., Grey, H. M., and Pirofsky, B., 1974, IgD: A major immunoglobulin on the surface of lymphocytes from patients with chronic lymphatic leukemia, *J. Immunol.* **112**:1952–1954.

Langer, B., Steinmetz-Kayne, N., and Hilschmann, N., 1968, The primary structure of a monoclonal human λ-type immunoglobulin L-chain of subgroup I (New), *Hoppe-Seyler's Z. Physiol. Chem.* **349**:945–951.

251

EVIDENCE FOR AND
THE SIGNIFICANCE
OF 'TWO GENES, ONE
POLYPEPTIDE
CHAIN'

Laure, C. J., Watanabe, S., and Hilschmann, N., 1973, Die Primärstruktur eines monoklonalen IgM-Immunoglobulins (Makro-globulin Ga1). I. Die Aminosäesequenz der L-kette K-Typ, Subgruppe I, *Hoppe-Seyler's Z. Physiol. Chem.* **354**:1503–1504.

Lieberman, R., Potter, M., Mushinski, E. B., Humphrey, W., Jr., and Rudikoff, S., 1974, Genetics of a new IgV$_H$ (T15) idiotype marker in the mouse regulating natural antibody to phosphorylcholine, *J. Exp. Med.* **139**:983–1001.

Lieu, T. S., Deutsch, H. F., and Tischendorf, F. W., 1977, Human λ chain sequence variations and serologic associations, *Immunochemistry* **14**:429–433.

Liu, Y. S. V., Low, T. L. K., Infante, A., and Putnam, F. W., 1976, Complete covalent structure of a human IgA1 immunoglobulin, *Science* **193**:1017–1020.

Lyon, M. F., 1968, Chromosomal and subchromosomal inactivation, *Annu. Rev. Genet.* **2**:31–52.

Mage, R., Young-Cooper, G. O., and Alexander, C. B., 1971, Genetic control of variable and constant regions of immunoglobulin heavy chains, *Nature (London) New Biol.* **230**:63–64.

Mage, R., Lieberman, R., Potter, M., and Terry, W. D., 1973, Immunoglobulin allotype, in: *The Antigens* (M. Sela, ed.), pp. 299–376, Academic Press, New York and London.

McKean, D., Potter, M., and Hood, L., 1973a, Mouse immunoglobulin chains: Partial amino acid sequence of a κ chain, *Biochemistry* **12**:749–759.

McKean, D., Potter, M., and Hood, L., 1973b, Mouse immunoglobulin chains: Pattern of sequence variation among κ chains with limited sequence differences, *Biochemistry* **12**:760–771.

Manning, D. D., 1974, Recovery from anti-Ig induced immunosuppression: Implications for a model of Ig-secreting cell development, *J. Immunol.* **113**:455–463.

Margolies, M. N., Cannon, L. E., Strosberg, A. D., and Haber, E., 1975, Diversity of light chain variable region sequences among rabbit antibodies elicited by the same antigen, *Proc. Natl. Acad. Sci. U.S.A.* **72**:2180–2184.

Martin, L. N., and Leslie, G. A., 1974, IgM-forming cells as the immediate precursor of IgA-producing cells during ontogeny of the immunoglobulin-producing system of the chicken, *J. Immunol.* **113**:120–126.

Milstein, C. P., and Deverson, E. V., 1971, The amino acid sequence of a human κ-light chain, *Biochem. J.* **123**:945–958.

Milstein, C. P., and Deverson, E. V., 1974, Primary structure of κ-light chain from a human myeloma protein, *Eur. J. Biochem.* **49**:377–391.

Milstein, C., and Munro, A. J., 1970, The genetic basis of antibody specificity, *Annu. Rev. Microbiol.* **24**:335–358.

Milstein, C., and Pink, J. R. L., 1970, Structure and evolution of immunoglobulins, *Prog. Biophys. Mol. Biol.* **21**:211–263.

Milstein, C., Clegg, J. B., and Jarvis, J. M., 1968, Immunoglobulin λ-chains: The complete amino acid sequence of a Bence–Jones protein, *Biochem. J.* **110**:631–652.

Milstein, C., Brownlee, G. C., Cartwright, E. M., Jarvis, J. M., and Proudfoot, N. J., 1974a, Sequence analysis of immunoglobulin light chain messenger RNA, *Nature (London)* **252**:354–359.

Milstein, C., Adetugbo, K., Cowan, J., and Secher, D. A., 1974b, Clonal variants of myeloma cells, *Prog. Immunol.* **2**(1):157–168.

Mole, L. E., Geier, M. D., and Koshland, M. E., 1975, The isolation and characterization of the V$_H$ domain from rabbit heavy chains of different *a* locus allotype, *J. Immunol.* **114**:1442–1448.

Mudgett, J. B., Kunkel, H. G., and Gedde-Dahl, R., Jr., 1975, Genetic studies of the heavy chain subgroups of γ G globulin: Recombination between the closely linked cistrons, in: *Gamma Globulins* (J. Killander, ed.), pp. 313–328, Almavist and Wiksell, Stockholm.

Nezlin, R. S., Vengerova, T. I., Rokhlin, O. V., and Muchulla, H. K. G., 1974, Allotypic marker of kappa light chains of rat immunoglobulins localized in the constant region of the chain, *Immunochemistry* **11**:517–518.

Nisonoff, A., Fudenberg, H. H., Wilson, S. K., Hopper, J. E., and Wang, A. C., 1972, Individual antigenic specificity in immunoglobulins: Relationship to biosynthesis. *Fed. Proc. Fed. Am. Soc. Exp. Biol.* **31**:206–209.

Nossal, G. J. V., Warner, N. L., and Lewis, H., 1971, Incidence of cells simultaneously secreting IgM and IgG antibody to sheep erythrocytes, *Cell. Immunol.* **2**:41–53.

Okada, Y., Nozu, Y., Titani, K., Watanabe, S., Hara, H., and Kitagawa, N., 1972, Amino acid sequences of λ chain of human immunoglobulin A, *Immunochemistry* **9**:207–210.

Oudin, J., and Michel, M., 1969, Idiotype of rabbit antibodies, *J. Exp. Med.* **130**:619–642.

Palm, W., and Hilschmann, N., 1975, The primary structure of a crystalline monoclonal immunoglobulin κ-type light chain, subgroup I (Bence–Jones protein Res); isolation and characterization of tryptic peptide; the complete amino acid sequence; a contribution to the elucidation of three dimensional structure of antibodies, in particular their combining site, *Hoppe-Seyler's Z. Physiol. Chem.* **356**:167–191.

Pawlak, L. L., Mushinski, E. B., Nisonoff, A., and Potter, M., 1973, Evidence for the linkage of the IgCH locus to a gene controlling the idiotypic specificity of anti-*p*-azophenylarsonate antibodies in strain A mice, *J. Exp. Med.* **137**:22–31.

Penn, G. M., Kunkel, G. H., and Grey, H. M., 1970, Sharing of individual antigenic determinants between a γG and a γM protein in the same serum, *Proc. Soc. Exp. Biol. Med.* **135**:660–665.

Perez, D. Y. E., and Bienenstock, J., 1973, Effects of bursectomy and thymectomy on ontogeny of fowl IgA, IgG and IgM, *J. Immunol.* **111**:633–637.

Pernis, B., Forni, L., and Amante, L., 1971, Immunoglobulins as cell receptors, *Ann. N.Y. Acad. Sci.* **190**:420–431.

Pernis, B., Brovet, J. C., and Seligmann, M., 1974, IgD and IgM on the membrane of lymphoid cells in macroglobulinemia: Evidence for identity of membrane IgD and IgM antibody activity in a case with anti-IgG receptors, *Eur. J. Immunol.* **4**:776–778.

Pierce, C. E., Asofsky, R., and Solliday, S. M., 1973, Immunoglobulin receptors on B-lymphocytes: Shifts in immunoglobulin class during immune responses, *Fed. Proc. Fed. Am. Soc. Exp. Biol.* **32**:41–43.

Pink, J. R. L., and Ivanyi, J., 1975, Close linkage between genes coding for allotypic markers on chicken IgG and IgM, *Eur. J. Immunol.* **5**:506–507.

Pink, J. R. L., Wang, A. C., and Fudenberg, H. H., 1971, Antibody variability, *Annu. Rev. Med.* **22**:145–170.

Poljak, R. J., 1975, X-ray diffraction studies of immunoglobulins, *Adv. Immunol.* **21**:1–33.

Poljak, R. J., Amzel, L. M., Chen, B. L., Phizackerley, R. P., and Saul, F., 1974, Three-dimensional structure of the Fab fragment of a human myeloma immunoglobulin at 2.0-Å resolution, *Proc. Natl. Acad. Sci. U.S.A.* **71**:3440–3444.

Ponstingl, H., and Hilschmann, N., 1969, Vollständige Aminosäuresequenz einer λ-Kette der Subgruppe II (Bence–Jones Protein Vil): Die Evolution als Ursache der Antikörper-spezifizität, *Hoppe-Seyler's Z. Physiol. Chem.* **350**:1148–1152.

Ponstingl, H., and Hilschmann, N., 1972, Die Primärstruktur eines monoklonalen IgG1-Immunoglobulin (Myeloprotein Nie). II. Aminosäuresequenz des konstanten Teils der H-kette, Zuordnung genetischer Faktoren, *Hoppe-Seyler's Z. Physiol. Chem.* **353**:1369–1372.

Ponstingl, H., Hess, M., and Hilschmann, N., 1968, Die vollständige Aminosäuresequenz des Bence–Jones-Protein Ker: Eine neue Untergruppe der Immunoglobulin-L-kette von λ-Typ, *Hoppe-Seyler's Z. Physiol. Chem.* **349**:867–871.

Pothier, L., Borel, H., and Adams, R. A., 1974, Expression of IgG allotypes in human lymphoid tumor lines serially transplantable in neonatal Syrian hamsters, *J. Immunol.* **113**:1984–1991.

Potter, M., and Lieberman, R., 1967, Genetic studies of immunoglobulins in mice, *Cold Spring Harbor Symp. Quant. Biol.* **32**:187–202.

Pratt, D., and Mole, L. E., 1975, Sequence studies on the constant region of the Fd-section of rabbit immunoglobulin G of different allotype, *Biochem. J.* **151**:337–349.

Press, E. M., and Hogg, N. M., 1969, Comparative study of two immunoglobulin G Fd-fragments, *Nature (London)* **223**:807–810.

Putnam, F. W., Florent, G., Paul, C., Shinoda, T., and Shimizu, A., 1973a, Complete amino acid sequence of the mu heavy chain of human IgM immunoglobulin, *Science* **182**:287–291.

Putnam, F. W., Whitley, E. J., Paul, O., and Davidson, J. N., 1973b, Amino acid sequence of a Bence–Jones protein from a case of primary amyloidosis, *Biochemistry* **12**:3763–3780.

Ralph, P., and Rich, A., 1971, Immunoglobulin synthesis in a cell-free system, *Biochemistry* **10**:4717–4725.

Riblet, R., Weigert, M., and Mäkelä, O., 1975, Genetics of mouse antibodies. II. Recombination between V_H genes and allotypes, *Eur. J. Immunol.* **5**:778–781.

Rivat, L., Gilbert, D., and Ropartz, C., 1973, Immunoglobulin allotypic specificities in mixed leukocyte cultures, *Immunology* **24**:1041–1049.

Rivat, C., Schiff, C., Rivat, L., Rofartz, C., and Fougereau, M., 1976, Deletion of hinge region of human

253

EVIDENCE FOR AND
THE SIGNIFICANCE
OF 'TWO GENES, ONE
POLYPEPTIDE
CHAIN'

myeloma IgG1 molecule (protein LEC) associated with nonexpression of Glm(3) and Km (1,2) allotypes. A possible genetic explanation at the DNA level, *Eur. J. Immunol.* **6**:545–551.

Rowe, D. S., Hug, K., Forni, L., and Pernis, B., 1973a, Immunoglobulin D as a lymphocyte receptor, *J. Exp. Med.* **138**:965–972.

Rowe, D. S., Hug, K., Faulk, W. P., McCormick, J. N., and Gerber, H., 1973b, IgD on the surface of peripheral blood lymphocytes of the human newborn, *Nature (London) New Biol.* **252**:155–157.

Scharff, M. D., 1967, The assembly of gamma globulin in relation to its synthesis and secretion in: *Nobel Symp.: Gammaglobulins: Structure and Control of Biosynthesis* (J. Killander, ed.), pp. 385–399, Interscience, New York.

Schiechl, H., and Hilschmann, N., 1971, Die Primärstruktur einer monoklonalen Immunglobulin-L-kette vom κ-Typ, Subgruppe I (Bence–Jones protein-Au), *Hoppe-Seyler's Z. Physiol. Chem.* **353**:345–370.

Schneider, M., and Hilschmann, N., 1975, The primary structure of a monoclonal immunoglobulin L-chain of the κ-type, subgroup IV, *Hoppe-Seyler's Z. Physiol. Chem.* **356**:507–557.

Scholz, R., and Hilschmann, N., 1975, Die Primärstruktur eines monoklonalen IgA Immunoglobulins (IgA Tro). I. Die Aminosäuresequenz der L-kette, λ-Typ, Subgruppe II, *Hoppe-Seyler's Z. Physiol. Chem.* **356**:1333–1335.

Seon, B. K., Yagi, Y., and Pressman, D., 1973a, Monoclonal IgA and IgM in the serum of a single patient (SC). II. Identity of light chains from IgA(κ) and IgM(κ), *J. Immunol.* **110**:345–349.

Seon, B. K., Yagi, Y., and Pressman, D., 1973b, Comparative chemical study of α and μ chains from a single patient (SC), *J. Immunol.* **111**:1285–1287.

Shinoda, T., 1973, Amino acid sequence of a human kappa type Bence–Jones protein II: Chymotryptic peptides and sequence of protein Ni, *J. Biochem.* **73**:433–446.

Shinoda, T., 1975, Comparative structure studies on the light chains of human immunoglobulins I: Protein Ka with Inv (3) allotypic markers, *J. Biochem.* **77**:1277–1296.

Shinoda, T., Titani, K., and Putnam, F. W., 1970, Amino acid sequence of human λ-chains II: Chymotryptic peptides and sequence of protein Ha, *J. Biol. Chem.* **245**:4475–4487.

Singer, S. J., and Doolittle, R. F., 1966, Antibody active site and immunoglobulin molecule, *Science* **153**:13–24.

Sletten, K., Husby, G., and Natvig, J. B., 1974, N-terminal amino acid sequence of amyloid fibril protein AR, prototype of a new λ-variable subgroup VλV, *Scand. J. Immunol.* **3**:833–836.

Smithies, O., 1973, Immunoglobulin genes: Arranged in tandem or in parallel?, *Cold Spring Harbor Symp. Quant. Biol.* **38**:725–737.

Solomon, A., McLaughlin, C. L., and Capra, J. D., 1975, Bence–Jones protein and light chains of immunoglobulins XI: A transient Bence–Jones-related protein associated with corticosteroid therapy, *J. Clin. Invest.* **55**:579–586.

Starace, V., and Querinjean, P., 1975, The primary structure of a rat kappa Bence–Jones protein: Phylogenetic relationships of V- and C-region genes, *J. Immunol.* **115**:59–62.

Stavenger, J., and Huong, R. C. C., 1971, Synthesis of a mouse immunoglobulin light chain in a rabbit reticulocyte cell-free system, *Nature (London) New Biol.* **230**:172–176.

Steinberg, A. G., 1969, Globulin polymorphism in man, *Annu. Rev. Genet.* **3**:25–51.

Steinberg, A. G., and Matsumoto, M., 1964, Studies on the Gm, Inv, Hp and Tf serum factors of Japanese population and families, *Hum. Biol.* **36**:77–85.

Steinberg, A. G., Terry, W. D., and Morrell, A. R., 1970, Human allotype and genetic dogma, *Protides Biol. Fluids Proc. Colloq.* **17**:111–116.

Steinberg, A. G., Milstein, C. P., McLaughlin, C. L., and Solomon, A., 1974, Structure studies on Inv (1,2) kappa chain, *Immunogenetics* **1**:108–117.

Strosberg, A. D., Hamer-Casterman, C., Van der Loo, W., and Hamers, R. A., 1974, A rabbit with the allotypic phenotype a1, a2, a3, b4, b4, b6, *J. Immunol.* **113**:1313–1318.

Suter, L., Barnikol, H. U., Watanabe, S., and Hilschmann, N., 1972, Die Primärstruktur einer monoklonalen Immunoglobulin-L-kette von κ-Typ, Subgruppe III (Bence–Jones-Protein Ti). IV. Die vollständige Aminosäuresequenz und ihre Bedeutung für den Mechanismus der Antikörperbildung, *Hoppe-Seyler's Z. Physiol. Chem.* **353**:189–208.

Titani, K., and Putnam, F. W., 1965, Immunoglobulin structure: Amino-terminal and carboxyl-terminal peptides of type I Bence–Jones proteins, *Science* **147**:1304–1305.

Titani, K., Shinoda, T., and Putnam, F. W., 1969, The amino acid sequence of a kappa type Bence–Jones protein III: The complete sequence and the location of the disulfide bridges, *J. Biol. Chem.* **244**:3550–3560.

Titani, K., Wikler, M., Shinoda, T., and Putnam, F. W., 1970, The amino acid sequence of a λ Bence–Jones protein III: The amino acid sequence and the location of the disulfide bridges, *J. Biol. Chem.* **245**:2171–2176.

Todd, C. W., 1963, Allotype in rabbit 19S protein, *Biochem. Biophys. Res. Commun.* **11**:170–175.

Vengerova, T. I., Rokhlin, O. V., and Nezlin, R. S., 1972, Chemical differences between two allotypic variants of light chains of rat immunoglobulins: Peptide mapping and cyanogen bromide cleavage, *Immunochemistry* **9**:1239–1245.

Vitetta, E. S., Melcher, U., McWilliams, M., Lamm, M. E., Phillips-Quagliata, J. M., and Uhr, J., 1975, Cell surface immunoglobulins. XI. The appearance of IgD-like molecules on murine lymphoid cells during ontogeny, *J. Exp. Med.* **141**:206–215.

Wang, A. C., 1975, Gene expansion and evolution: Evidence for differential expression of immunoglobulin variable region genes in different species, in: *Antibody Structure and Molecular Immunology* (J. Gergely and G. A. Medgyesi, eds.), pp. 19–31, Akademiai Kiado, Budapest, and North-Holland, Amsterdam and London.

Wang, A. C., and Fudenberg, H. H., 1972, Chemical analysis of Fc and Fab fragments derived from papain digestion of human IgG2 myeloma proteins, *Nature (London) New Biol.* **240**:24–25.

Wang, A. C., and Fudenberg, H. H., 1974, IgA and evolution of immunoglobulins, *J. Immunogenet.* **1**:3–31.

Wang, A. C., and Fudenberg, H. H., 1975, Amino acid sequences near the "switch point" of heavy chains of human immunoglobulins: Genetic hypothesis, *Arch. Biochem. Biophys.* **168**:657–664.

Wang, A. C., Wang, I. Y. F., McCormick, J. N., and Fudenberg, H. H., 1969, The identity of light chains of monoclonal IgG and monoclonal IgM in one patient, *Immunochemistry* **6**:451–459.

Wang, A. C., Wilson, S. K., Hopper, J. E., Fudenberg, H. H., and Nisonoff, A., 1970a, Evidence for control of synthesis of the variable regions of the heavy chains of IgG and IgM by the same gene, *Proc. Natl. Acad. Sci. U.S.A.* **66**:337–343.

Wang, A. C., Pink, J. R. L., Fudenberg, H. H., and Ohms, J., 1970b, A variable region subgroup of heavy chains common to immunoglobulins G, A and M and characterized by an unblocked amino-terminal residue, *Proc. Natl. Acad. Sci. U.S.A.* **66**:657–663.

Wang, A. C., Fudenberg, H. H., and Pink, J. R. L., 1971, Heavy chain variable regions in normal and pathological immunoglobulins, *Proc. Natl. Acad. Sci. U.S.A.* **68**:1143–1146.

Wang, A. C., Fudenberg, H. H., Goldrosen, M. H., and Freedman, M. H., 1972, Chemical studies of heavy chains of two IgG1(λ) myeloma proteins from a single patient, *Immunochemistry* **9**:473–479.

Wang, A. C., Gergely, J., and Fudenberg, H. H., 1973, Amino acid sequences at constant and variable regions of heavy chains of monotypic immunoglobulins G and M of a single patient, *Biochemistry* **12**:528–539.

Wang, A. C., Wang, I. Y. F., and Fudenberg, H. H., 1977, Immunoglobulin structure and genetics: Identity between variable regions of a μ and a γ2 chain, *J. Biol. Chem.* **252**:7129–7199.

Warner, N. L., 1974, Membrane immunoglobulins and antigen receptors on B and T lymphocytes, *Adv. Immunol.* **19**:67–216.

Watanabe, S., and Hilschmann, N., 1970, Die Primärstruktur einer monoklonalen Immunoglobulin-L-kette der Subgruppe I vom κ-Typ (Bence–Jones Protein Hau): Untergruppen innerhalb der Subgruppe, *Hoppe-Seyler's Z. Physiol. Chem.* **351**:1291–1295.

Watanabe, S., Barnikol, H. V., Horn, J., Bertram, J., and Hilschmann, N., 1973, Die Primärstruktur einer monoklonalen IgM-Immunoglobulins (Makroglobulin Gal). II. Die Aminosäuresequenz der H-kette (μ-Typ, Subgruppe HIII), Struktur des gesamten IgM-moleküls, *Hoppe-Seyler's Z. Physiol. Chem.* **354**:1505–1509.

Waterfield, M. D., Morris, J. E., Hood, L. E., and Todd, C. W., 1973, Rabbit immunoglobulin light chains: Correlation of variable region sequences with allotypic markers, *J. Immunol.* **110**:227–232.

Wells, J. V., Bleumer, J. F., and Fudenberg, H. H., 1973, Human anti-IgM isoantibodies; detection of IgM allotypic markers, *Proc. Natl. Acad. Sci. U.S.A.* **70**:827–829.

Wikler, M., and Putnam, F. W., 1970, Amino acid sequence of human λ chains. III. Tryptic peptides, and sequence of protein Bo, *J. Biol. Chem.* **245**:4488–4507.

Wolfenstein-Todel, C., Franklin, E. C., and Rudders, R. A., 1974a, Similarities of the light chains and the variable regions of the heavy chains of the IgG2(λ) and IgA1(λ) myeloma proteins from a single patient, *J. Immunol.* **112**:871–876.

255

EVIDENCE FOR AND
THE SIGNIFICANCE
OF 'TWO GENES, ONE
POLYPEPTIDE
CHAIN'

Wolfenstein-Todel, C., Mihaesco, E., and Frangione, B., 1974b, "Alpha chain disease" protein Def: Internal delection of a human immunoglobulin A1 heavy chain, *Proc. Natl. Acad. Sci. U.S.A.* **71**:974–978.

Wu, T. T., and Kabat, E. A., 1970, An analysis of the sequences of the variable regions of Bence–Jones proteins and myeloma light chains and their implications for antibody complementarity, *J. Exp. Med.* **132**:211–250.

Wu, T. T., Kabat, E. A., and Bilofsky, H., 1975, Similarities among hypervariable segments of immunoglobulin chains, *Proc. Natl. Acad. Sci. U.S.A.* **72**:5107–5110.

Yagi, Y., and Pressman, D., 1973, Monoclonal IgA and IgM in the serum of a single patient (SC). I. Sharing of individually specific determinants between IgA and IgM, *J. Immunol.* **110**:335–344.

10

Structure of Atypical Immunoglobulins— Relationship to Genetic Control Mechanisms

BLAS FRANGIONE

1. Introduction

Much of the knowledge of antibody function and structure has been obtained from studies of the homogeneous proteins produced by patients with neoplasms of plasma cells and lymphocytes. There is now little doubt that most of the homogeneous proteins in these patients are structurally normal antibodies or immunoglobulin (Ig) molecules. This conclusion has received further support from the discovery of myeloma proteins and macroglobulins possessing antibody activity. Under normal conditions the synthesis of heavy (H) and light (L) chains is approximately balanced, and plasma cells secrete primarily complete Ig molecules. In certain disease states, however, unbalanced synthesis most commonly manifested by the production of free L chains [Bence Jones proteins (BJP's)] can occur. Only since the discovery of defective H chains in humans [heavy-chain-disease (HCD) proteins (Franklin *et al.,* 1964; Osserman and Takatsuki, 1964)] and of half-molecule IgA proteins in mice (Potter and Kuff, 1964) has the existence of structurally altered molecules in association with plasma-cell and lymphocytic neoplasms been recognized. Since that time, an increasing number of studies have attempted to use mutant proteins and the tumors producing them to obtain structural and genetic information that could not be derived from studies of intact molecules. Since progress in this area has been dependent on the chance occurrence and recognition of structurally altered proteins, attempts have recently been made to induce such mutations in clones of plasma-cell tumors and to study the products of such mutated

---

BLAS FRANGIONE • Department of Pathology, Irvington House Institute, New York University Medical Center, New York, New York 10016.

cells (Baumal *et al.*, 1973; Milstein *et al.*, 1974; Scharff, 1974). The most commonly observed changes are the loss of H- or of both H- and L-chain production. Recent studies, however, have also demonstrated several H-chain variants that resemble quite strikingly some of those previously noted to arise spontaneously in human plasma-cell tumors (Frangione and Franklin, 1973).

In this discussion of structurally altered molecules, we will concentrate on HCD proteins in man, since they remain the most interesting and striking abnormality, and will briefly mention a series of more subtly altered molecules in man and mouse. Finally, some theoretical implications derived from studies of such atypical Ig's in regard to the possible unique genetic mechanisms involved in the control of Ig chains will be discussed.

2. Heavy-Chain Variants: Heavy-Chain-Disease Proteins

HCD proteins will be defined as molecules consisting of part of or the entire H chain and devoid of L chains. The L chains are either not produced, not assembled, or degraded. Of the five potentially recognizable types of HCD in man, those corresponding to γ, α, and μ chains have been described, and the expected frequency of the other two (ϵ- and δ-HCD) is such that their detection may be difficult. To date, there are about 35 cases of γHCD, 80 of αHCD, and 10 of μHCD. The results of physicochemical and immunochemical studies of these molecules are summarized in Table 1.

2.1. γ-Heavy-Chain Disease

γHCD was the first type of HCD to be described (Franklin *et al.*, 1964). It resembles a lymphoma more than multiple myeloma, since bone lesions are extremely rare. Two unusual features that have been described in more than half these subjects are the waxing and waning of the lymphadenopathy and the involvement of nodes in Waldeyer's ring that gives rise to the almost pathognomonic finding of uvular swelling and palatal edema. The disease generally has a fatal outcome in 6 months to 5 years. As in other forms of lymphoid malignancies, fever and infections are often the direct cause of death. Routine examination of bone marrow and peripheral blood cells shows the existence of atypical lymphocytes and sometimes plasma cells in the blood and a malignant lymphoid or plasmacytic infiltrate of marrow or nodes or both. These findings are not sufficient to allow their differentiation from multiple myeloma or other related neoplasms. The diagnosis is

TABLE 1. Properties of γ-, α-, and μ-Heavy-Chain-Disease Proteins

Property	γHCD	αHCD	μHCD
Mobility	Fast γ–β	β	$\alpha 1$
Sedimentation rate	2.8–4 S	4–11 S	10.8–11 S
Molecular weight (monomer)	25,000–58,000	35,000–42,000	35,000–55,000
L-chain production	No	No	Often
J chain	No	Often	In some
Present in the urine	Usually	Sometimes	No
Subclass	$\gamma 1$	Only $\alpha 1$	—
	$\gamma 2$		
	$\gamma 3$		
	$\gamma 4$		

259

STRUCTURE OF
ATYPICAL
IMMUNO-
GLOBULINS—
RELATIONSHIP
TO GENETIC
CONTROL
MECHANISMS

dependent on the demonstration in serum and usually in the urine of an Ig, usually with a fast β mobility and a rather heterogeneous pattern that reacts with antisera to γ chains but not to L chains. The amount of protein in the urine is often sufficiently large to make its detection easy. It should be emphasized that unlike the case in patients with a myeloma protein and a concurrent urinary BJP, in patients with HCD, the serum and urine protein have identical mobilities and BJP's have not been detected in γHCD to date. In general, the sedimentation coefficient of these proteins lies between 3.5 and 4 S and the molecular weight ranges from 45,000 to 120,000 for the dimer. They tend to be rich in carbohydrates. Among the γHCD proteins studied so far, there is an unexpectedly high incidence of molecules belonging to the γ3 subclass. None of these proteins has been shown to possess antibody activity. It is now recognized that γHCD proteins represent a heterogeneous group of molecules ranging from an intact H chain to protein having various types of terminal or internal deletions, and that some are probably the result of proteolytic digestion of a larger precursor molecule.

The proteins with internal deletions have been studied most carefully to date (Figure 1). Three proteins—CRA, GIF, and ZUC—resemble each other in having

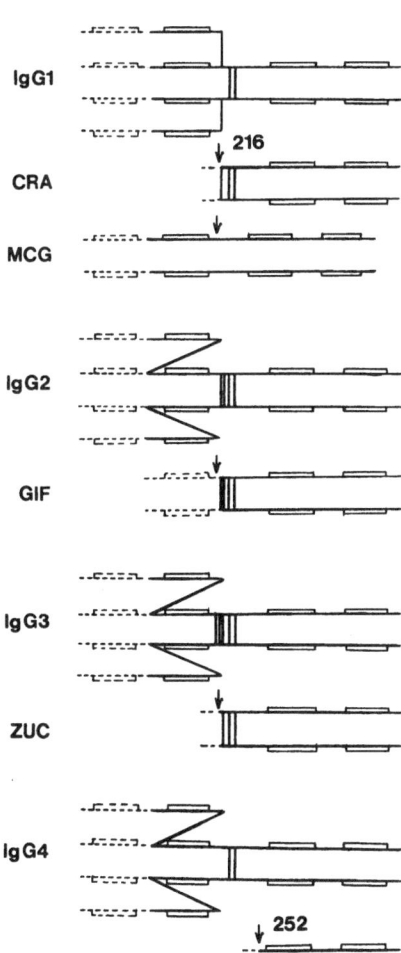

Figure 1. Schematic diagram of variants of human Ig H (γ) chains with internal deletions compared with normal IgG molecules of different subclasses (----) V region; ($\downarrow$) position at which deletions end or start (see the text). The numbering is taken from the γ1 sequence (Edelman *et al.*, 1969). (CRA) A γ1 HCD protein; (MCG) an IgG1 myeloma protein; (GIF) a γ2 HCD protein; (ZUC) a γ3 HCD protein—the hinge region of the γ3 H chain appears to have a series of similar or identical duplications (not shown) (Adlersberg *et al.*, 1975); (HAL) a γ4 HCD protein. For their amino acid sequences, see Frangione and Franklin (1973).

an internal deletion with resumption of the normal sequence at a homologous position: glutamic acid at residue 216 (Figure 1). One of these proteins, ZUC (Frangione and Milstein, 1969), is a γ3 protein containing a gap of about 200 residues starting at 17 or 18 residues after the *N*-terminus of the variable (V) region and including the two intrachain loops of the Fd fragment, the inter-H–L and a major part of the extended hinge normally present in γ3 H chains (Adlersberg *et al.*, 1975). The protein becomes identical to the invariant sequence of γ3 from a glutamic acid residue corresponding to 216, which is the middle of the H chain [γ1 numbering (Edelman *et al.*, 1969)]. CRA (Franklin and Frangione, 1971) is a γ1 protein that lacks almost the entire Fd fragment. The amino terminal is heterogeneous, and after 10 or 11 residues from the V region, normal synthesis resumes at the same position as above. It contains three inter-H–H disulfide bridges instead of the usual two found in γ1 H chains, since in the absence of L chains, the cysteine residue ordinarily involved in forming the H–L disulfide bonds appears to have joined the homologous residue of the other H chain to yield an additional inter-H–H disulfide bond. GIF (Cooper *et al.*, 1972) is a γ2 protein that has a blocked *N*-terminus and contains much of the Fd V region. It has a gap of about 100 residues corresponding to the Fd constant (C) region and involving one intrachain loop and the H–L disulfide bridge. Normal sequence resumes at a glutamic acid residue in a homologous position of the H chain.

Four other proteins seem to be closely related to this group in having an internal deletion of part of the V region, and the C_H1 domain. Since they also lack the whole hinge, however, these molecules dissociate into monomers in the absence of reducing agents, a fact that readily suggests this type of a structural defect. Careful studies of one protein in this group (HAL), a γ4 HCD protein (Figure 1), permitted a precise definition of the nature of the internal deletion (Frangione *et al.*, 1973), and demonstrated clearly that the normal sequence resumes at a methionine residue at 252. Three other proteins with internal deletions have not been studied as carefully in terms of reinitiation of synthesis, but probably resemble HAL in having a deletion that includes the hinge. HI (Terry and Ohms, 1970; Woods *et al.*, 1970) probably lacks the C_H1 domain and the hinge. The other two, PAR (Calvanico *et al.*, 1972) and BAZ (Smith, L. L., *et al.*, 1973) have not been studied sufficiently to map the deletion precisely.

Very often, HCD proteins begin at the hinge region. While such molecules most probably represent examples of proteolytic digestion of a larger precursor molecule, the possibility that they too are synthetic products has not been excluded. Two examples of this type have been published (Terry and Ein, 1972), and we observed two others (Franklin and Frangione, 1975). In these proteins, the larger precursor was never found, nor was it possible to discover an increase in proteolytic activity in the serum. Serious consideration must be given, however, to the possibility that some of these patients synthesize an intact H chain that is then degraded, in view of the recent findings on the origin of the HCD proteins from patient OMM, who has two γ3 HCD proteins in the serum (Adlersberg *et al.*, 1975). One is a polypeptide with a molecular weight of 59,000 daltons after reduction that appears to consist of virtually the entire H chain. In addition, the serum contains a second protein with a molecular weight of 40,000 daltons after reduction, which starts with glycine and consists of the entire hinge region and the remainder of the Fc region. While it is tempting to postulate that the smaller molecule is derived from the larger one by proteolysis, and that this is the first instance in which the precursor has been

261

STRUCTURE OF
ATYPICAL
IMMUNO-
GLOBULINS—
RELATIONSHIP
TO GENETIC
CONTROL
MECHANISMS

found, the possibility of a two-step mutation, one of which originally gave rise to the intact H-chain protein while the second one resulted in the smaller fragment, is given support by the production of only the smaller piece in a clone of cells established from this patient's peripheral lymphocytes with no evidence of intra- or extracellular degradation.

The significance of the γHCD proteins in terms of a normal counterpart remains uncertain. While it seems likely these apparently functionless deleted molecules, no two of which so far appear to be identical, are abnormal, a recent as yet unconfirmed report by Lam and Stevenson (1973) of the isolation from a large pool of normal serum of a small amount of a 35,000 molecular weight H chain with a normal amino-terminal sequence PCA-Val-Gln and presumably an internal deletion has raised the distinct possibility that these molecules are present in trace amounts normally.

2.2. α-Heavy-Chain Disease

For reasons that remain obscure, αHCD appears to be more common than γHCD. Since this disorder was initially and is still most commonly encountered in the Mediterranean area (North Africa, Middle East, and southern Europe), the intestinal form is often referred to as "Mediterranean lymphoma" (Seligman et al., 1969). In more than 90% of the 80 reported cases, a plasmacytic infiltrate of the intestinal tract gave rise to diarrhea, steatorrhea, and severe malabsorption. The disease has now also been encountered in northern Europe and America, although with lower frequency. Other organs that are normally a part of the IgA-producing secretory immune system are on occasion the sites of involvement. At least 4 cases, with a rather benign form of the disease, have had diffuse lymphocyte and plasma-cell infiltrates of the respiratory tract. αHCD occurs often in younger people, and can undergo remissions with a variety of antibiotics and chemotherapeutic agents. This finding, together with the epidemiological characteristics, has suggested an infectious etiology. The diagnosis of αHCD, as is the case with γHCD, is dependent on the immunochemical demonstration of an α-chain-related serum and sometimes urine protein lacking L chains. Because of the not infrequent presence of hidden L chain in IgA myeloma proteins, it is imperative to exclude the existence of L chains by chemical methods. As was the case with γHCD, L-chain excretion in the form of BJP has not been observed in this variant. All αHCD proteins studied to date belong to the α1 subclass. Their molecular weights range between 35,000 and 42,000 for the monomer, and their carbohydrate content is also very high. Antigenic and chemical analysis (Seligman et al., 1971) provided evidence for an intact Fc fragment. Since the amino-terminus in most of these proteins was shown to be heterogeneous, the question arose whether αHCD proteins are normal α chains that undergo postsynthetic intra- or extracellular degradation or whether they contain a primary defect followed by secondary proteolysis. Detailed structural studies have been published for two proteins: DEF and AIT (Wolfenstein-Todel et al., 1974, 1975) (Figure 2). Both molecules contained a short heterogeneous segment corresponding to the V region, and after a gap that encompasses the rest of the V and C_H1 regions, normal synthesis resumed at a valine residue that may be the α-chain counterpart to glutamic acid, position 216 of the γ1 chain. It was postulated, therefore, that αHCD proteins DEF and AIT are synthesized as internally deleted H chains, followed by postsynthetic proteolysis.

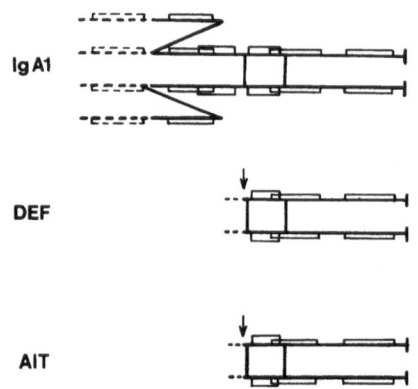

Figure 2. Comparison of deletions detected in variants of human α chains. Top: Schematic diagram of an IgA1 molecule. (----) V region. The arrangement of disulfide bridges is tentative. Note two extra intrachain bridges in association with the hinge region. The last half-cysteinyl residue of the α chain can be linked to the J chain or another α chain. (DEF, AIT) α1 HCD proteins. (↓) Position within the hinge region at which normal sequence starts after internal deletions. The position is homologous with some γHCD proteins (Wolfenstein-Todel *et al.*, 1975).

2.3. μ-Heavy-Chain Disease

μHCD generally accompanies chronic lymphocytic leukemia. Several features are worth mentioning, foremost among which are the existence in the bone marrow of vacuolated plasma cells, which have been seen in most of the patients, and frequently the presence of BJP in the urine in significant amounts (Franklin, 1975). The production of unassembled L chains distinguishes these molecules from those encountered in γ- and αHCD. In one instance, immunofluorescent studies indicated that the L chain was found in the same cell as the μ chain (Zucker-Franklin and Franklin, 1971). In the majority of these patients, routine electrophoresis was normal, except for marked hypogammaglobulinemia, and the diagnosis could be suspected only on the basis of the presence, on immunoelectrophoresis, of a rapidly migrating protein reactive with antisera to μ chain and not with those to L chains. In the case of μHCD, too, it is usually necessary to prove the absence of L chains chemically, since nonreactive L chains have been noted in macroglobulins.

The information on the structure of μHCD proteins is more limited. Most exist in the serum as pentamers similar to the (Fc)μ5 fragment, with molecular weights between 180,000 and 300,000, which explains the failure to find them in the urine. The mechanism for polymer formation remains to be explained, since joining (J) chain is not always present (Dammacco *et al.*, 1974; Bonhomme *et al.*, 1974). The limited chemical studies of three proteins are consistent with immunological findings that most, if not all, of the Fc region is present (Forte *et al.*, 1970; Dammacco *et al.*, 1974; Lebreton *et al.*, 1975). For reasons that are not understood, alanine was found at the N-terminus in each. Although their molecular weights differ, BUR is a μHCD protein that differs from the others in being smaller (35,000 daltons) (Figure 3). Its amino-terminal sequence (Lebreton *et al.*, 1975) appeared to correspond to that of μ-chain OU (Putnam *et al.*, 1973) starting with residue 338, except for the presence of Ala instead of Val. Protein GLI (Forte *et al.*, 1970) has a molecular weight of 50,000–55,000, and its amino-terminal sequence indicates that it starts at alanine position 131 (Frangione *et al.*, 1976). Studies of the cysteine-containing peptides show that all the labile S–S bonds are present including the intersubunit and inter-H–L disulfide bridges. Since unassembled L chains were present in the same cell on the μ chains, it would appear either that the L chain is abnormal or that the V_H region plays a role in modulating the conformation of the H chain to permit the formation of a disulfide bridge.

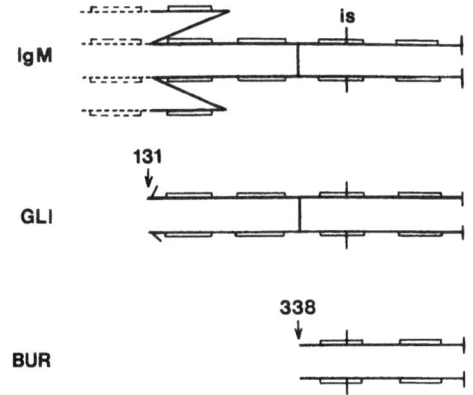

Figure 3. Comparison of deletions detected in variants of human μ chains. Top: Monomer of an IgM molecule. (----) V region. Note the extra C domain present in the H chain. (is) Intersubunit bonds linking the pentamer. The last half-cysteinyl residue of the μ chain is joined to the J chain or another μ chain. (BUR) A μHCD protein with an amino-terminal deletion comprising the first three domains (Lebreton et al., 1975); it starts at residue 338 with an alanine residue [valine is at the same position in a normal μ chain (Putnam et al., 1973]; (GLI) a μ HCD protein with an amino-terminal deletion (V region only), which starts with an alanine residue, but at position 131 (Frangione et al., 1976).

263

STRUCTURE OF
ATYPICAL
IMMUNO-
GLOBULINS—
RELATIONSHIP
TO GENETIC
CONTROL
MECHANISMS

3. Myelomas with Altered Heavy Chains

In recent years, different types of abnormalities have been discovered, either through routine screening of many human proteins or through studies of spontaneous and induced mutations of murine plasma-cell tumors. The alterations in H chains discussed below have been noted.

3.1. Internal Deletion Similar to γ-Heavy-Chain-Disease Proteins

A clone of plasma-cell tumor originally derived from MOPC 21, an IgG1-producing plasmacytoma (Secher et al., 1973), was found to produce a myeloma protein (IF-2) with an internal deletion comprising only the C_H1 region of the H chain (Figure 4). The gap starts at position 121 and ends with Val 215, which is homologous with Glu 216, the site of resumption of normal synthesis in most human γHCD proteins (Milstein et al., 1974).

3.2. Deletion of the Hinge Region Only

There are reports of two crystalline myeloma proteins of the γ1 type with a small deletion involving only the hinge (Deutsch and Suzuki, 1971; Lopes and

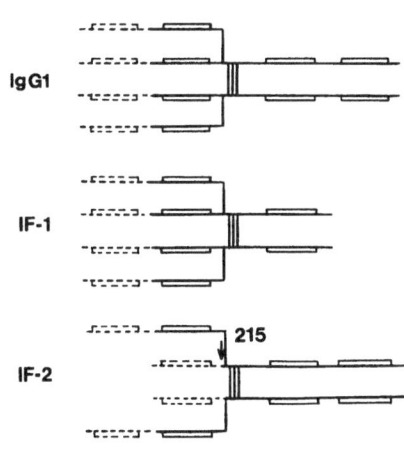

Figure 4. Schematic diagram of normal mouse IgG1 myeloma protein (top) and mutants IF-1 and IF-2 with deletion of C_H3 and C_H1, respectively (Milstein et al., 1974). (↓) Position at which normal synthesis starts after an internal deletion. Note that the site is similar to the sites described in human γ- and α-HCD proteins with internal gaps (see Figures 1 and 2).

Steiner, 1973). Both proteins appear to have a molecular weight (145,000) similar to that of normal IgG molecules in nondissociating solvents. When subjected to urea or acid, however, they yield an L-chain dimer and two free H chains. Dissociation without reduction is due to the absence of all the cysteine residues involved in inter-H chain bridges. In the first protein, MCG, the deletion was clearly mapped and shown to involve residues 216–230 (Fett *et al.*, 1973) (see Figure 1). The second protein, BOB, behaved similarly in dissociating conditions (Lopes and Steiner, 1973). The exact nature of the deletion, however, has not been defined yet.

3.3. Deletion of the Carboxy-Terminal and of the Heavy Chain

Loss of the last domain of the H chain has been detected as a stable variant grown in tissue culture (IF-1) from MOPC 21 tumor in the mouse (Secher *et al.*, 1973), in several mutants of the murine MPC 11 cell line (Scharff, 1974; Morrison *et al.*, 1974), in one human IgA myeloma (Despont and Abel, 1974; Despont *et al.*, 1974), and in several 3.9 S half-molecule IgA tumors of murine origin (Lieberman *et al.*, 1968; Seki *et al.*, 1968; Mushinski, 1971; Robinson *et al.*, 1974). IF-1 variant contains an L chain of normal size and a shorter H chain that contains sialic acid not present in the parent molecule (Secher *et al.*, 1973). The deletion involves the C_H3 region, starting with residue 358 (Milstein *et al.*, 1974) (Figure 4). Studies showing the same size protein intracellularly, and the synthesis of a shorter than normal protein when 18 S in RNA was used in a heterologous reticulocyte, lysate cell-free system, clearly support the view that this is a synthetic product, probably due to point mutation, not the result of proteolysis.

Probably similar in the nature of the defect are some of the mutants induced by IRC 191 treatment of the IgG2b-producing MPC 11 cell line (Baumal *et al.*, 1973; Birshtein *et al.*, 1974; Scharff, 1974). While chemical analyses have not mapped the deletion precisely, fingerprints and preliminary analysis of cyanogen bromide fragments have shown part of the Fc fragment, possibly the carboxyl-terminal end, to be missing. An analogous type of deletion appears to be present in an IgA1 myeloma protein VO, which was antigenically deficient and seemed to lack more than 100 residues, probably the entire C_H3 domain (Despont and Abel, 1974; Despont *et al.*, 1974). VO protein existed purely as a monomeric molecule, perhaps due to the absence of the carboxyl-terminal cysteine residue, which has been shown to be linked to the J chain (Mendez *et al.*, 1973; Mestecky *et al.*, 1974).

A larger deletion encompassing the C_H3 and C_H4 domains of the μ chain appears to have occurred in protein KLO, a (Fab)$_2$ μ fragment disease (DeCoteau et al, 1973). The molecule gave a reaction of partial identity with IgM and nonidentity with Fcμ, had a molecular weight of 130,000, and was composed of two normal-sized L chains and two H chains having molecular weights of 42,000 instead of the usual 60,000–65,000. The molecule lacked the *C*-terminal of normal μ chain and concurrently lacked the J chain. The authors postulated that a nonsense mutation may have led to failure of synthesis of the last two domains (i.e., the Fc fragment). Additional biosynthetic studies are necessary to exclude proteolysis.

Closely related to these deleted H chains, but possibly differing from them in representing a hitherto unrecognized subclass of IgA, are the 3.9 S, two-chain IgA-related molecules initially described by Potter and Kuff (1964). Chemical studies of one (47A) allow the conclusion that the H chain has a molecular weight of 40,000 instead of the 50,000–55,000 usually found for α chains and lacks approximately 100 residues (Robinson *et al.*, 1974), which make up essentially the whole C_H3 domain. This deletion by itself cannot account for the unexpected S–S bond linking the L to the H chain. Because the human IgA subclasses differ in H–L disulfide bridges, they have raised the possibility that the as yet undefined differences in the H–L bond may be related to subclass differences. Biosynthetic studies with the 47A-producing tumor demonstrated the presence of HL as the primary intracellular species and larger amounts of free H chains, while in the secreted material, HL is the predominant (Bevan, 1971). Unfortunately, these studies have failed to provide a definitive mechanism for the failure of obtaining H_2L_2 molecules. A similar example of human IgG molecule was reported (Spiegelberg *et al.*, 1975) in which the H chain is shorter and appears to have a deletion of the C_H3 domain.

265

STRUCTURE OF
ATYPICAL
IMMUNO-
GLOBULINS—
RELATIONSHIP
TO GENETIC
CONTROL
MECHANISMS

4. Myelomas with Altered Light Chains

4.1. Internal Deletion

A large number of amino acid variable sequences of L chain are now available, many of which have small groups of 1–6 residues. Since these sequences occur mainly in the hypervariable region, are small in size, and are as yet of unknown significance (Chen and Poljak, 1974), we will not describe them further.

An unusual situation exists in IgG, κ myeloma protein SAC, which has an internal deletion of the L chains encompassing residues 19–99 (Lewis *et al.*, 1968; Smithies *et al.*, 1971; Parr *et al.*, 1972). This molecule was unusual in having a sedimentation coefficient of 5.4 instead of the normal 6.6 S and a molecular weight of 125,000, with both H and L chains having less than the expected molecular weight. It is believed that the internal deletion of the L chain is the prime and perhaps the sole genetic defect, and that the loss of the V_H region may have been the result of proteolytic digestion (Parr *et al.*, 1972).

Similar in nature is an IgG, λ myeloma protein (SM), recently described by Isobe and Osserman (1974). The protein had a molecular weight of 110,000, L chains with an estimated 15,000 daltons, and H chains of approximately 45,000 daltons. The L-chain C region is intact, whereas the V region has only 30 residues. The V-region segment represents residues 1–30 of normal λ chain, and after a gap of 81 residues, normal synthesis resumes at a glutamyl residue at position 110, the initiation point of the C region (Garver *et al.*, 1975). The reason for the smaller H chain is less well defined and may well be, as has been suggested in the case of SAC, the result of proteolytic digestion. The finding of the Fc fragment in the serum and urine and the progressive change in the molecule during storage support this view.

Of great interest is the recent report by Kuehl and Scharff (1974) demonstrating that the MOPC 11 mouse myeloma cell line, which produces not only H and L chains but also an 11,600-dalton fragment that, on the basis of radiochemical peptide analysis, consists of almost all the C region and lacks all the V-region peptides. This C_L fragment comprises about 1% of the newly synthesized protein, compared with 8% for the complete L chain; less than 20% of the fragment is secreted, whereas the remainder is degraded intracellularly with a half-life of 30 min. On the basis of chemical and biosynthetic data (Kuehl and Scharff, 1974), it is suggested that this is a synthetic, not a degradative, product.

4.2. Elongation

To date, there is only a single example of an elongated L chain, which was found in a κ chain secreted by MPC 11. This κ chain has 12 extra residues at the amino-terminus (Smith, G. P., 1973). The amino acid sequence of these 12 additional residues of the intact MPC 11 L chain shows that the first 6 residues of the extra piece are similar to residues 13–18 of the MPC 11 κ chain or the first 6 residues of other κ chains. Thus, it is postulated that this may be the result of recent breakage and reunion of two κ V-region genes. The origin of residues 7–12 is most difficult to explain and must await the amino acid sequence of the precursor region, which has been identified intracellularly in several mouse L-chain-producing cell lines (Swan *et al.*, 1972; Milstein *et al.*, 1972; Mach *et al.*, 1973; Schecter, 1973).

Another instance of a larger L chain is of that reported to be present on the surface 8 S IgM from a continuous culture of human lymphocytes (Daudi), originally derived from a patient with Burkitt's lymphoma (Kennel, 1974). Since only sodium dodecyl sulfate gels were used to determine molecular weight (33,000 instead of 23,000), additional studies are necessary to document this observation and to delineate precisely the nature of the alteration.

5. Hybrid Molecules

To date, hybrid molecules have been defined mainly by antigenic or genetic analysis. The first was described by Warner *et al.* (1966) in a mouse IgG2b myeloma, GPC 5, produced in an (NZB × BALB/c) F_1 hybrid. On the basis of inhibition studies, at least 95% of the molecules carried specificities of both the IgG2a and IgG2b subclasses. A closely related event seems to have occurred in some of the drug-induced mutants of MPC 11 (IgG2b-producing tumor) that produce normal or larger H chains in addition to normal-sized L chains (Morrison *et al.*, 1974; Scharff, 1974). Five such mutants have been found. The chains have lost almost half the parental H-chain peptides and acquired instead a number of IgG2a peptides. A relationship to IgG2a was further supported by antigenic and biosynthetic studies. The latter studies revealed assembly by the $H_2 \rightarrow H_2L \rightarrow H_2L_2$ pathway characteristic of the IgG2a subclass, rather than the $H_L \rightarrow H_2L \rightarrow H_2L_2$ pathway typical of IgG2b molecules. Thus, on the basis of these preliminary studies, these molecules appear to be hybrids possibly resulting from crossing-over between closely related C-region genes.

Studies of the genetic Gm markers of human IgG proteins have uncovered several examples of hybrid molecules that, on the basis of a similar crossing-over occurring in hemoglobins, might well be referred to as "Lepore" type of hybrid γ-globulins (Kunkel *et al.*, 1969). The first such protein was discovered in 1969, when a patient was found with undetectable levels of γ3 subclass when antisera to γ3 Fc fragment was used, whereas the concentration was markedly elevated with antisera recognizing γ3 determinants on the Fab. When similar studies were carried out with antisera to γ1 determinants, the converse was found. The presence of hybrid molecules having a γ3 Fab and a γ1 Fc fragment was confirmed by precipitation studies. Failure to detect any γ1 or γ3 genetic markers, including the Gm z and f markers (Natvig and Kunkel, 1974) that are characteristics of the γ1 subclass and reflect a change at residue 214, makes it likely that the γ3 part extends up to and possibly beyond the hinge. An even more subtle hybrid was described in members of a Swedish family who had a phenotype Gm (z a⁻x⁻f g b) that had not been observed previously, since in Caucasian individuals, the gene complex of $\gamma 1$ chain is either $Gm^{a,z}$ or Gm^{non-af} (Natvig *et al.*, 1974). The finding of IgG1 molecules, which are $Gm\ (^{non-a,z})$, is likely to be the result of intragenic recombination between $Gm^{a,z}$ and Gm^{non-af} to yield the gene complex $Gm^{non-a,z}$.

Two myeloma proteins that may be the result of similar process have been observed. One, LA (Natvig and Kunkel, 1974), appears, on the basis of antigenic and genetic marker analysis, to be a hybrid of the C_H1 and C_H2 portion of IgG4, and the C_H3 region of IgG2. A subsequent search of 150 normal Negro sera detected 4 that appeared to have similar molecules, thus indicating that it is the product of a rare normal gene in the Negro population. The other, GOE, has the Fd fragment and the hinge region of $\gamma 3$ and the carboxyl end of $\gamma 1$ chain (Prelli *et al.*, 1975).

6. Nonsecretors

Several examples of human and murine plasma-cell tumors unassociated with a serum of urine protein abnormality have been identified. Most represent a failure of Ig synthesis (Gach *et al.*, 1971), and some were shown by immunofluorescence to contain in their cytoplasm L chains that either are not secreted or are degraded intra- and extracellularly (Hurez *et al.*, 1970, 1972). While a defect in the addition of carbohydrate seems possible, in view of the postulated role in the attachment of carbohydrate moieties as a prerequisite for secretion (Schenkein and Uhr, 1970), direct evidence has not been obtained yet in instances in which Ig is not secreted. Studies of several nonsecretory mutants of the MOPC 21 tumor line showed that some of these tumors produce free L chains, which appeared to be degraded intracellularly. Several clones that contained no L chain were shown to have defective H chain. Biosynthetic studies demonstrated that the failure of some of the variants to synthesize L chains was not due to misallocation of mRNA to the free polyribosomes (Ig-chain synthesis is confined to membrane-derived polyribosomes). In fact, fingerprint analysis of the corresponding mRNA showed the presence of an inactive form of this molecule (Cowan *et al.*, 1974).

7. Discussion

The discovery of tumor cells that synthesize and secrete defective Ig chains offered an opportunity to determine whether plasma-cell and lymphocyte mutants would provide the same valuable information as had been obtained from mutants in prokaryotes. It is assumed that in the majority of these mutated cells, transcription and translation of Ig mRNA have occurred faithfully so that the aberrant polypeptide chain can be considered as a gene product. In considering these questions, two points deserve emphasis. First, meaningful information can be obtained only from molecules that are the products of synthesis, not from those for which the possibility of proteolytic degradation of a precursor exists; second, the available methods are very selective and can detect only gross defects. Thus, the possibility exists that subtle changes are much more frequent than one might expect. Even though conclusions regarding the defects in these mutants clearly require more chemical studies, it is obvious, even at this early stage, that the types of structural variants do not appear to be random, and that the mutation rate, at least in the mouse, is surprisingly high [the spontaneous mutation rate in Ig production is about 1×10^{-3} per cell generation, (Baumal *et al.,* 1973)]. This may well be related in some unknown fashion to the generation of antibody diversity, since the genetic instability of these cell lines appears to be specific to Ig production and does not reflect a general genetic instability.

Prominent among these mutants are those leading to deletions of the products of the genes coding for H chains and less frequently for L chains. Deletions can be internal or terminal. In the event that proteolytic digestion of an intact H chain can be excluded the mechanism of deletions starting at the amino-terminus and comprising one third to one half of the H chain as described in some cases of γ- and μHCD proteins (see Sections 2.1.1 and 2.1.3) must await the characterization of the mRNA by studying the specific translated products.

At this time, the simplest molecules to discuss are those that are shorter than normal and lack the carboxyl-terminal segment. These molecules are most likely the result of a mutational event giving rise to a chain termination. The best studied of these molecules is the IF-1 mutant in the mouse, in which the termination occurs at the serine at position 358 (Milstein *et al.,* 1974). The triplet coding for the residue can be changed to a chain-termination codon (UCG to UAG) by a single base change.

The genetic events responsible for extensive, internal gaps are more difficult to define. Sequence analysis of Ig's, the inheritance of their genetic polymorphisms, and evolutionary arguments indicate that the V and C regions of L and H chains are encoded in the germ line by separate structural genes, and evidence favors joining of VC at the DNA level. Two current models have been formulated to account for a possible mechanism of joining V and C genes. The translocation model (Dreyer and Bennett, 1965; Gally and Edelman, 1972) proposes that one of many closely associated V genes becomes excised and transported to and joined with the C genes to form a complete VC cistron. The other model (Smithies, 1973) advocates the occurrence of V genes arranged in parallel, forming a branched network connected to a less extensive network of parallel C genes. Internal deletions in Ig's could conceivably be explained by assuming a translocation error originating either during or after intrachromosomal recombination or by breaks in DNA at nonhomologous positions and strand reunion involving a branch point.

The results of structural studies of human γ- and αHCD proteins indicate that all these molecules have internal deletion of variable size involving part of the V and C regions, and that the hinge region rather than the beginning of the C segment plays an important role as the site at which the gap frequently ends and on occasion begins. The positions involved in human γ and α chains (Edelman *et al.,* 1969; Wolfenstein-Todel *et al.,* 1974) and in the mouse mutant IF-2 (Milstein *et al.,* 1974) appear to be homologous. Position 216 marks the beginning of the hinge region, a section of the H chain between the C_H1 and C_H2 domains that contains the inter-H chain disulfide bonds and that is not homologous with any Ig domains and is highly variable for each class or subclass (Frangione and Franklin, 1972). Moreover, the hinge region can be found as a series of identical or similar repetitive sequences of small fragments (Frangione and Wolfenstein-Todel, 1972; Adlersberg *et al.,* 1975). Although the genetic origin of the hinge region is not known, it seems likely from these studies that the DNA segment coding for the hinge or part of it contains a

269

STRUCTURE OF
ATYPICAL
IMMUNO-
GLOBULINS—
RELATIONSHIP
TO GENETIC
CONTROL
MECHANISMS

special site for recombination that can at times join with a fragment of the V gene to give a viable molecule. If, as postulated by Lam and Stevenson (1973) for human deleted γ chain proteins, these fragments are always produced in small amounts, they may be considered to be perhaps remnants of more primitive types of normal Ig components. The possibility exists that they are specified by structural genes discrete from those determining the intact H or L chains, possibly analogous to the β_2-microglobulins. β_2-Microglobulin present in normal persons is related to the Fc fragment of IgG and is part of HLA molecules (Smithies and Poulik, 1972; Peterson *et al.*, 1974). An important point, which must not be lost sight of, is that with the exception of μHCD, all patients with γ and αHCD proteins fail to synthesize L chains. Since L and H chains are controlled by unlinked genes, the failure of L-chain synthesis is difficult to explain and requires either a second mutation or the existence of some regulatory mechanisms affecting both H- and L-chain synthesis.

The not infrequent occurrence of hybrids of the type described is not unexpected due to the structural homologies among different subclasses and their close genetic linkage. They can be the result of a malalignment at meiosis, with unequal homologous crossing over, or, alternatively, of a deletion of the *C*-terminal end of the first C gene to the *N*-terminal part of the adjacent C region with read-through into the second gene. Detailed chemical studies will be necessary to determine whether each of these crossovers is a random process or involves a complete domain. Studies of such molecules may ultimately prove to be the best way of mapping Ig chain loci and their expression.

References

Aldersberg, J. B., Franklin, E. C., and Frangione, B., 1975, Repetitive hinge region sequences in human IgG3: Isolation of an 11,000-dalton fragment, *Proc. Natl. Acad. Sci. U.S.A.* **72**:723–727.

Baumal, R., Birshtein, B., Coffino, P., and Scharff, M. D., 1973, Mutations in immunoglobulin-producing mouse myeloma cells, *Science* **182**:164–166.

Bevan, M. J., 1971, Interchain disulfide bond formation studied in two mouse myelomas which secrete immunoglobulin A, *Eur. J. Immunol.* **1**:133–138.

Birshtein, B. K., Preud'homme, J. L., and Scharff, M. D., 1974, Variants of mouse myeloma cells that produce short immunoglobulin heavy chains, *Proc. Natl. Acad. Sci. U.S.A.* **71**:3478–3482.

Bonhomme, T., Seligmann, M., Mihaesco, C., Clauvel, J., Danon, F., Brouet, J., Bouvry, P., Martine, J., and Clerc, M., 1974, Mu-chain disease in an African patient, *Blood* **43**:485–492.

Calvanico, N. J., Rabin, B., Plaut, A., and Tomasi, T. B., Jr., 1972, Studies on a new gamma heavy chain disease protein, *Fed. Proc. Abstr.* **13**:771.

Chen, B. L., and Poljak, R. J., 1974, Amino acid sequence of the (lambda) light chain of a human myeloma immunoglobulin (IgG New), *Biochemistry* **13**:1295–1302.

Cooper, S., Franklin, E. C., and Frangione, B., 1972, Molecular defect in a gamma-2 (γ-2) heavy chain, *Science* **176**:187–189.

Cowan, N. J., Secher, D. S., and Milstein, C., 1974, Intracellular immunoglobulin chain synthesis in non-secreting variants of a mouse myeloma: Detection of inactive light-chain messenger RNA, *J. Mol. Biol.* **90**:691–701.

Dammacco, F., Bonomo, L., and Franklin, E. C., 1974, A new case of mu heavy chain disease: Clinical and immunochemical studies, *Blood* **43**:713–719.

DeCoteau, W. E., Calvanico, N. J., and Tomasi, T. B., 1973, Malignant lymphoma with a monoclonal F(ab)mu fragment, *Clin. Immunol. Immunopathol.* **1**:190–202.

Despont, J. P. J., and Abel, C. A., 1974, Glycopeptides of heavy chains from human IgA myeloma proteins, *J. Immunol.* **112**:1623–1627.

Despont, J. P. J., Abel, C. A., Grey, H. M., and Penn, G. M., 1974, Structural studies on a human IgA1 myeloma protein with a carboxy-terminal deletion, *J. Immunol.* **112**:1517–1525.

Deutsch, H. F., and Suzuki, T., 1971, A crystalline Gl human monoclonal protein with an excessive H chain deletion, *Ann. N.Y. Acad. Sci.* **190**:472–486.

Dreyer, W. J., and Bennett, J. C., 1965, The molecular basis of antibody formation: A paradox, *Proc. Natl. Acad. Sci. U.S.A.* **54**:864–869.

Edelman, G. M., Cunningham, B. A., Gall, W. E., Gottlieb, P. D., Rutishauser, V., and Waxdal, M. J., 1969, The covalent structure of an entire gamma G immunoglobulin molecule, *Proc. Natl. Acad. Sci. U.S.A.* **63**:78–85.

Fett, J. W., Deutsch, H. F., and Smithies, O., 1973, Hinge-region deletion localized in the IgG-globulin Mcg, *Immunochemistry* **10**:115–118.

Forte, F., Prelli, F., Yount, F., Jerry, L., Kochwa, S., Franklin, E. C., and Kunkel, H. G., 1970, Heavy chain disease of the gamma (gamma M) type: Report of the first case, *Blood* **36**:137–144.

Frangione, B., and Franklin, E. C., 1972, Chemical typing of the immunoglobulins IgM, IgA1 and IgA2, *FEBS Lett.* **20**:321–323.

Frangione, B., and Franklin, E. C., 1973, Heavy chain diseases: Clinical features and molecular significance of the disordered immunoglobulin structure, *Semin. Hematol.* **10**:53–64.

Frangione, B., Lee, L., Haber, E., and Bloch, K., 1973, Protein Hal: Partial deletion of a "γ" immunoglobulin gene(s) and apparent reinitiation at an internal AUG codon, *Proc. Natl. Acad. Sci. U.S.A.* **70**:1073–1077.

Frangione, B., and Milstein, C., 1969, Partial delection in the heavy chain disease protein ZUC, *Nature (London)* **224**:597–599.

Frangione, B., and Wolfenstein-Todel, C., 1972, Partial duplication in the "hinge" region of IgA1 myeloma proteins, *Proc. Natl. Acad. Sci. U.S.A.* **12**:3673–3676.

Frangione, B., Franklin, E. C., and Prelli, F., 1976, μ Heavy-chain disease—A defect in immunoglobulin assembly, *Scand. J. Immunol.* **5**:623–627.

Franklin, E. C., 1975, Mu-chain disease, *Arch. Intern. Med.* **135**:71–72.

Franklin, E. C., and Frangione, B., 1971, The molecular defect in a protein (CRA) found in gamma-1 heavy chain disease and its genetic implications, *Proc. Natl. Acad. Sci. U.S.A.* **68**:187–191.

Franklin, E. C., and Frangione, B., 1975, Structural variants of human and murine immunoglobulins, in: *Contemporary Topics in Molecular Immunology* (F. P. Inman, ed.), pp. 89–126. Plenum Press, New York.

Franklin, E. C., Lowenstein, J., Bigelow, B., and Meltzer, M., 1964, Heavy chain disease—a new disorder of serum gamma-globulin: Report of the first case, *Am. J. Med.* **37**:332–350.

Gach, J., Simar, L., and Salmon, J., 1971, Multiple myeloma without M-type proteinemia: Report of a case with immunologic and ultrastructure studies, *Am. J. Med.* **50**:835–844.

Gally, J. A., and Edelman, G. M., 1972, The genetic control of immunoglobulin synthesis, *Annu. Rev. Genet.* **6**:1–46.

Garver, F. A., Chang, L., Mendicino, J., Isobe, T., and Osserman, E. F., 1975, Primary structure of a deleted human lambda type immunoglobulin light chain containing carbohydrate: Protein Sm λ, *Proc. Natl. Acad. Sci. U.S.A.* **72**:4559–4563.

Hurez, D., Preud'homme, J. L., and Seligmann, M., 1970, Intracellular "monoclonal" immunoglobulin in non-secretory human myeloma, *J. Immunol.* **104**:263–264.

Hurez, D., Flandren, G., Preud'homme, J. L., and Seligmann, M., 1972, Unreleased intracellular monoclonal macroglobulin in chronic lymphocytic leukaemia, *Clin. Exp. Immunol.* **10**:223–234.

Isobe, T., and Osserman, E. F., 1974, Plasma cell dyscrasia associated with the production of incomplete (?deleted) IgGλ molecules, gamma heavy chains, and free lambda chains containing carbohydrate: Description of the first case, *Blood* **43**:505–526.

Kennel, S. J., 1974, The κ chains of immunoglobulins from a continuous culture of human lymphocytes (Daudi) have an unusual molecular size, *J. Exp. Med.* **139**:1031–1036.

Kuehl, W. M., and Scharff, M. D., 1974, Synthesis of a carboxyl-terminal (constant region) fragment of the immunoglobulin light chain by a mouse myeloma cell line, *J. Mol. Biol.* **89**:409–421.

Kunkel, H. G., Natvig, J. B., and Joslin, F. G., 1969, "Lepore" type of hybrid gammaglobulin, *Proc. Natl. Acad. Sci. U.S.A.* **62**:144–149.

Lam, C. W., and Stevenson, G. T., 1973, Detection in normal plasma of immunoglobulin resembling the protein of gamma-chain disease, *Nature (London)* **246**:419–421.

Lebreton, J., Ropartz, C., Rousseaux, J., Roussel, P., Dautrevaux, M., and Biserte, G., 1975, Immuno-chemical and biochemical study of a human Fc μ-like fragment (μ-chain disease), *Eur. J. Immunol.* **5**:179–184.

271

STRUCTURE OF
ATYPICAL
IMMUNO-
GLOBULINS—
RELATIONSHIP
TO GENETIC
CONTROL
MECHANISMS

Lewis, A. F., Bergsagel, D. E., Bruce-Robertson, A., Schachter, R. K., and Connell, G. E., 1968, An atypical immunoglobulin, *Blood* **32**:189–204.

Lieberman, R., Mushinski, J. F., and Potter, M., 1968, 2-Chain immunoglobulin A molecules: Abnormal or normal intermediates in synthesis, *Science* **159**:1355–1357.

Lopes, A. D., and Steiner, L. A., 1973, A structural defect in a crystallizable myeloma protein, *Fed. Proc. Abstr.* **32**:1003.

Mach, B., Faust, C., and Vasalli, P., 1973, Purification of 14S messenger RNA of immunoglobulin light chain that codes for a possible light-chain precursor, *Proc. Natl. Acad. Sci. U.S.A.* **70**:451–455.

Mendez, E., Prelli, F., Frangione, B., and Franklin, E. C., 1973, Characterization of a disulfide bridge linking the J chain to the alpha chain of polymeric immunoglobulin A, *Biochem. Biophys. Res. Commun.* **55**:1291–1297.

Mestecky, J., Schrohenloher, R. E., Kulhavy, R., Wright, G. P., and Tomane, M., 1974, Site of J chain attachments to human polyermic IgA, *Proc. Natl. Acad. Sci. U.S.A.* **71**:544–548.

Millstein, C., Brownlee, G. G., Harrison, T. M., and Mathews, B., 1972, A possible precursor of immunoglobulin light chains, *Nature (London) New Biol.* **239**:117–120.

Milstein, C., Adetugbo, K., Cowan, N. J., and Secher, D. S., 1974, Clonal variants of myeloma cells, in: *Progress in Immunology II*, Vol. 1 (L. Brend and J. Holporow, eds.), pp. 157–168, American Elsevier, New York.

Morrison, S. L., Baumal, R., Birshtein, B. K., Kuehl, W. M., Preud'homme, J. L., Frank, L., Jasek, T., and Scharff, M. D., 1974, The identification of mouse myeloma cells which have undergone mutation in immunoglobulin production, in: *Cellular Selection and Regulation in the Immune Response* (G. M. Edelman, ed), p. 233, Raven Press, New York.

Mushinski, J. F., 1971, Gamma-A half molecules: Defective heavy chain mutants in mouse myeloma proteins, *J. Immunol.* **106**:41–50.

Natvig, J. B., and Kunkel, H. G., 1974, A hybrid IgG4–IgG2 immunoglobulin, *J. Immunol.* **112**:1277–1284.

Natvig, J. B., Michaelsen, T. E., Gedde-Dahl, T., Jr., and Fischer, T., 1974, IgG1 subclass protein with the genetic Gm markers (Gm) (2 plus non-a plus): Another example of intragenic hybridization among IgG subclass genes, *Immunogenetics* **1**:33–41.

Osserman, E. F., and Takatsuki, K., 1964, Clinical and immunochemical studies of four cases of heavy (Hγ) chain disease, *Am. J. Med.* **37**:351–373.

Parr, D. M., Percy, M. E., and Connell, G. E., 1972, A human immunoglobulin G with deletions in both heavy and light polypeptide chains, *Immunochemistry* **9**:51–63.

Peterson, P. A., Rask, L., and Lindblom, J. B., 1974, Highly purified papain-solubilized HL-A antigens contain β_2-microglobulin, *Proc. Natl. Acad Sci. U.S.A.* **71**:35–39.

Potter, M., and Kuff, E. L., 1964, Disorders in the differentiation of protein secretion in neoplastic plasma cells, *J. Mol. Biol.* **9**:537–544.

Prelli, F., Frangione, B., Franklin, E. C., Abel, C. A., and Van Loghem, E., 1975, An unusual γ3 human immunoglobulin heavy chain, *Fed. Proc. Abst.* **34**:970.

Putnam, F. W., Florent, G., Paul, C., Shinoda, T., and Schimuzu, A., 1973, Complete amino acid sequence of the Mu heavy chain of a human IgM immunoglobulin, *Science* **182**:287–291.

Robinson, E. A., Smith, D. F., and Apella, E., 1974, Chemical characterization of a mouse immunoglobulin A heavy chain with a 100-residue deletion: Amino acid and carbohydrate compositions and NH$_2$- and COOH-terminal sequences, *J. Biol. Chem.* **249**:6605–6610.

Scharff, M. E., 1974, The synthesis, assembly and secretion of immunoglobulin: A biochemical and genetic approach, *Harvey Lecture*, Series 69, p. 125.

Schechter, I., 1973, Biologically and chemically pure mRNA for a mouse immunoglobulin L-chain prepared with the aid of antibodies and immobilized oligothymidine, *Proc. Natl. Acad. Sci. U.S.A.* **70**;2256–2260.

Schenkein, I., and Uhr, J., 1970, Immunoglobulin synthesis and secretion. I. Biosynthetic studies of the addition of the carbohydrate moieties, *J. Cell Biol.* **46**:42–51.

Secher, D. S., Cotton, R., and Milstein, C., 1973, Spontaneous mutation in tissue culture—Chemical nature of variant immunoglobulin from mutant clones of MOPC 21, *FEBS Lett.* **37**:311–316.

Seki, T., Apella, E. and Itano, H. A., 1968, Chain models of 6.6S and 3.9S mouse myeloma gamma A immunoglobulin molecules, *Proc. Natl. Acad. Sci. U.S.A.* **61**:1071–1078.

Seligmann, M., Mihaesco, E., and Frangione, B., 1971, Studies on alpha chain disease, *Ann. N. Y. Acad. Sci.* **190**:487–500.

Seligmann, M., Mihaesco, E., Hurez, D., Mihaesco, C., Preud'homme, J. L., and Rambaud, J. C., 1969, Immunochemical studies in four cases of alpha chain disease, *J. Clin. Invest.* **48**:2374–2389.

Smith, G. P., 1973, Mouse immunoglobulin kappa chain MPC11: Extra amino-terminal residues, *Science* **181**:941–943.

Smith, L. L., Barton, B. P., Garver, F. A., Lutcher, C. L., and Faguet, G. B., 1973, Physiochemical and immunochemical characterization of a new IgG1 (γ1) heavy chain disease protein, *Fed. Proc. Fed. Am. Soc. Exp. Biol.* **32**:840 (Abstract).

Smithies, O., 1973, Immunoglobulin genes: Arranged in tandem or in parallel?, *Cold Spring Harbor Symp. Quant. Biol.* **38**:725–737.

Smithies, O., and Poulik, M. D., 1972, Initiation of protein synthesis at an unusual position in an immunoglobulin gene, *Science* **175**:187–189.

Smithies, O., Gibson, D., Fanning, E. B., Percy, M. E., Parr, D. M., and Connell, G. E., 1971, Deletions in immunoglobulin polypeptide chains as evidence for breakage and repair in DNA, *Science* **172**:574–577.

Spiegelberg, H. L., Heath, V., and Lang, J. E., 1975, Human myeloma IgG half molecules: Structural and antigenic analysis, *Biochemistry* **14**:2157–2163.

Swan, D., Aviv, H., and Leder, P., 1972, Purification and properties of biologically active messenger RNA for a myeloma light chain, *Proc. Natl. Acad. Sci. U.S.A.* **69**:1967–1971.

Terry, W., and Ein, D., 1972, Structural studies of gamma heavy chain disease proteins, *Ann. N.Y. Acad. Sci.* **190**:467–471.

Terry, W., and Ohms, J., 1970, Implications of heavy chain disease protein sequence for multiple gene theories of immunoglobulin synthesis, *Proc. Natl. Acad. Sci. U.S.A.* **66**:558–563.

Warner, N., Herzenberg, L. A., and Goldstein, G., 1966, Immunoglobulin isoantigens (allotypes) in the mouse. II. Allotypic analysis of three γG$_2$-myeloma proteins from (NZB × BALB/c)F$_1$ hybrids and of normal γG$_2$-globulins, *J. Exp. Med.* **123**:707.

Wolfenstein-Todel, C., Mihaesco, E., and Frangione, B., 1974, "Alpha chain disease": Protein Def: Internal deletion of a human immunoglobulin A$_1$ heavy chain, *Proc. Natl. Acad. Sci U.S.A.* **71**:974–978.

Wolfenstein-Todel, C., Mihaesco, E., and Frangione, B., 1975, Variant of a human immunoglobulin: "Alpha chain disease" protein AIT, *Biochem. Biophys. Res. Commun.* **65**:47–53.

Woods, R., Blumenschein, G., and Terry, W., 1970, A new type of human gamma heavy chain disease protein: Immunochemical and physical characteristics, *Immunochemistry* **7**:373–381.

Zucker-Franklin, D., and Franklin, E. C., 1971, Ultrastructural and immunofluorescence studies of the cells associated with mu-chain disease, *Blood* **37**:257–271.

11

Patterns of Sequence Variability in Immunoglobulin Variable Regions: Functional, Evolutionary, and Genetic Implications

J. MICHAEL KEHOE and J. DONALD CAPRA

1. Introduction

It is now clear that the humoral immune response is the result of the production of large amounts of immunoglobulin (Ig) by descendants of individual clones of lymphoid cells. These cells also bear that same Ig on their surface as a specific antigen receptor, a fundamental requirement of the clonal selection hypothesis (Jerne, 1955; Burnet, 1959). These receptors, when released from the cell, maintain their capacity to interact with that same antigen. This chapter will concern itself with how that antigen–antibody interaction is mediated from a structural point of view, and will focus especially on the nature of the antibody variability required to cope with the myriads of antigens encountered by vertebrates. The phenomenon of idiotypy and some possible mechanisms for the generation of the required Ig diversity will be included in the discussion, as will some phylogenetic distinctions in Ig structure that are discernible among a number of higher species.

J. MICHAEL KEHOE • Department of Microbiology/Immunology, The Northeastern Ohio Universities College of Medicine, Rootstown, Ohio 44272. J. DONALD CAPRA • Department of Microbiology, University of Texas Health Science Center at Dallas, Southwestern Medical School, Dallas, Texas 75235.

2. Variable Regions Defined: Molecular Limits and Phylogenetic Occurrence

It has been widely assumed since the demonstration of variable (V) regions and constant (C) regions by Hilschmann and Craig (1965) that the V region of the antibody molecule would be responsible for the antigen-binding function. This idea was, in fact, explicitly proposed by Edelman *et al.* (1969) in 1969 as a fundamental tenet of the domain hypothesis. Nonetheless, direct proof that the V regions alone were not only necessary, but sufficient, to fulfill the antigen-binding function came when Inbar *et al.* (1972) showed that the combined V regions of the light (L)-chain and heavy (H)-chain (Fv fragment) of a hapten-binding murine myeloma protein was capable of binding this hapten (dinitrophenol) (DNP) in precisely the same fashion as the intact Ig molecule. These findings, combined with other related studies, led to the formal conclusion that the molecular basis for the antigen-binding function would be found by a structural analysis of V regions alone. Significant insights into the overall structure of antibody V regions have now been obtained by the sequence analysis of the V regions of a number of different Ig's from man and other mammals. This information on the primary structure of Ig V regions, especially when placed in juxtaposition with complementary information on the tertiary structure of Ig's derived from X-ray diffraction studies (discussed in Chapter 1), has now provided a relatively clear picture of how V regions carry out the antigen-binding function.

Figure 1 displays the published complete V-region sequences of several human Ig H chains. These sequences will serve to illustrate a number of the principles that will be individually described. The data indicate the following general points, which will be stated and then discussed in more detail:

1. The precise carboxy-terminal limit of the V region of H chains is not yet fully defined. It may well be position 124 of the H chain using the numbering system shown in Figure 1, but it seems unlikely that even many additional protein sequences can absolutely define the V–C junction point. This problem is discussed in more detail below.

2. Ig's from all species examined to date contain V regions (in both L and H chains).

3. The sequence variability of the V region is not random, but is organized on a surprisingly precise basis. Most notably, as first pointed out for L chains (Wu and Kabat, 1970; Milstein, 1967; Franêk, 1969) and later for H chains (Capra, 1971; Kehoe and Capra, 1971; Capra and Kehoe, 1974a,b), Ig V regions all contain *hypervariable* regions in which the sequence variation from protein to protein is especially marked. In human H chains, four segments can be termed hypervariable, including positions 31–37, 51–68, 84–91, and 101–110. Among these, the first, second, and fourth hypervariable regions have been termed *complementarity-determining* (Wu *et al.*, 1975) because the X-ray diffraction studies of Ig's have shown that these segments do indeed line the antibody-combining site. The function or significance of the H-chain hypervariable region at positions 84–91 is not yet clear. It is conceivable that this segment reflects some important V-region genetic polymorphism that has not yet been elucidated. Any possible genetic significance has been difficult to assess, since all the hypervariable regions in man have been defined using myeloma proteins, a system obviously poorly suited to parent–

275

PATTERNS OF
SEQUENCE
VARIABILITY IN
IMMUNOGLOBULIN
VARIABLE REGIONS

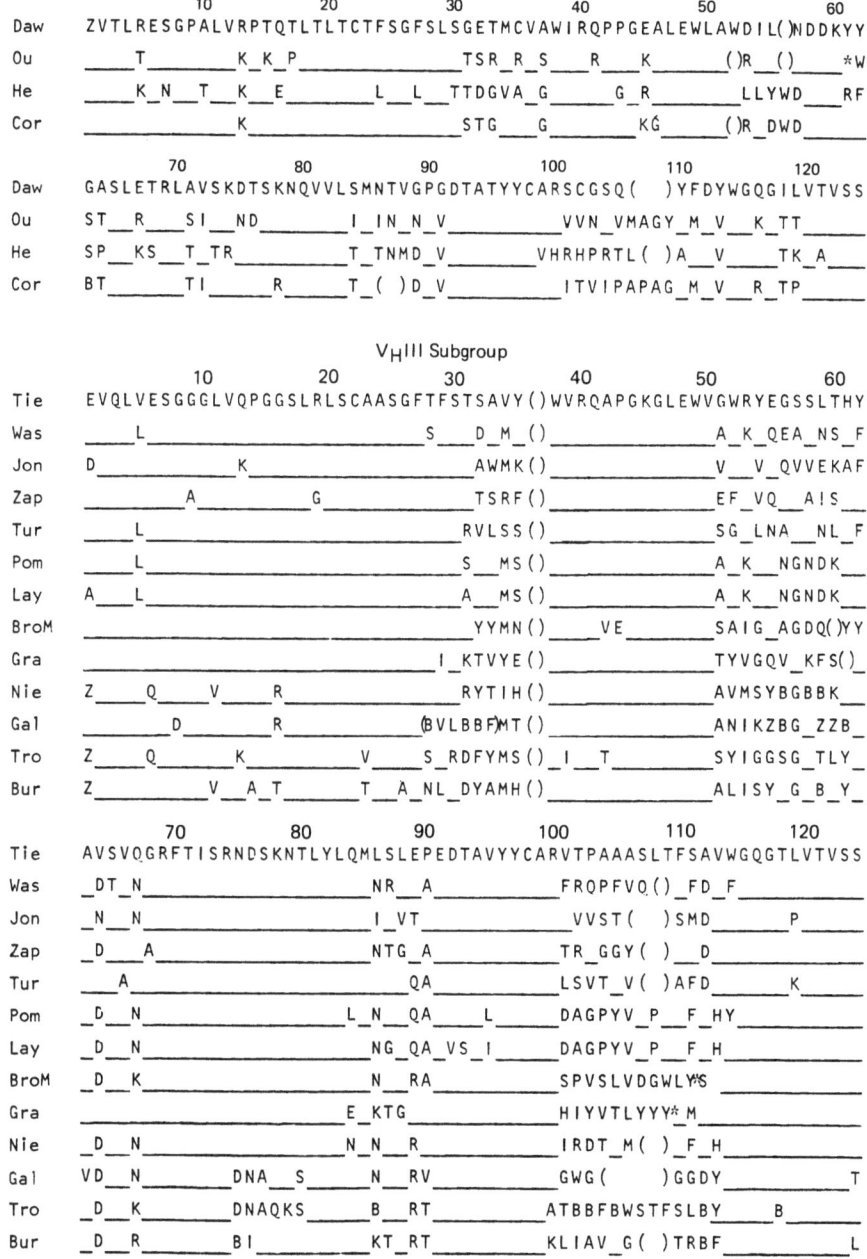

Figure 1. Amino acid sequence of the published complete V regions of human myeloma proteins of the V$_H$II and V$_H$III subgroups. Protein Eu of the V$_H$I subgroup has not been included, since no other similar protein has been completely sequenced (Edelman *et al.*, 1969). The original references for these sequences are: Subgroup V$_H$II—Daw, Cor: Press and Hogg (1970); Ou: Winkler *et al.* (1969); He: Cunningham *et al.* (1969). Subgroup V$_H$III—Tie, Was, Jon, Zap, Tur: Capra and Kehoe (1974a); Pom, Lay: Capra and Kehoe (1974b); BroM: Capra and Hopper (1976); Gra: Capra, (1975); Nie: (Ponstingl *et al.* (1970); Gal: Watanabe *et al.* (1973); Tro: F. W. Putnam (1976, personal communication); Bur: Kratzin *et al.* (1975).

J. MICHAEL KEHOE
AND J. DONALD
CAPRA

offspring tracing of particular hypervariable region structures. Consequently, the reason for the existence of this hypervariable region remains unclear. A more thorough discussion of this point is included in Querinjean *et al.* (1975).

The position of the three complementarity-determining hypervariable regions is the same in a number of different species that have been examined to date. A possible exception is to be found in certain rabbit anticarbohydrate antibodies (Haber *et al.*, 1976). This common location for hypervariable regions across a variety of animal species clearly indicates the selective advantage of this particular mechanism of generating antibody diversity in a wide variety of species existing in quite distinct environments.

Segments of the V region that are not included in the hypervariable segments (comprising 75–80% of the total H-chain V region, for example) can be termed the relatively invariant, or *framework,* regions. As shown by X-ray diffraction analysis, these segments provide a superstructure for positioning the complementarity-determining residues in an appropriate position to make contact with antigen. Especially within a given V region subgroup, the variation between any two proteins in the framework segment is very modest (on the order of 5–10% for H chains, as illustrated in Figure 1). There is now no doubt that the relatively invariant segments of the V regions are responsible for the generally similar three-dimensional structure of the combining region of all antibodies. As with the hypervariable regions, the relatively invariant segments have very comparable dimensions in all Ig's from the various higher animal species that have been studied to date, again indicative of the general biological unity reflected in this component of the humoral immune response.

3. Variable Region–Constant Region Transition

As indicated in Section 2, the exact division between the V region and the C region is not yet known for any Ig chain. There is much reason to believe that the junction in a human κ L chain is at positions 107–108, but no formal proof is yet available. As indicated by Figure 2, the situation with H chains seems even less clear. The problem stems from the now nearly universal belief that separate genes exist for the V region and the C region of a given Ig polypeptide (Cohn, 1971). It has not been possible to identify any recognition sequence of amino acids in the completed polypeptides that would suggest a process by which the V region–C region integration could take place. It may well be that recognition, excision, and integration processes sufficient to provide for V–C joining at the nucleic acid level leave no visible remnant of the process in the proteins eventually synthesized. It would seem that only further information on the specific DNA chemistry involved in the association of V regions with C regions will be able to confirm the actual transition point between these two components of the Ig polypeptide chain.

Figure 2 indicates one possible interpretation of the amino acid sequence data that are available at present on the V–C junction in human Ig H chains. The variation seen in position 124 clearly cannot be correlated with a specific Ig class. Position 125 contains an alanine in all sequenced human IgA and IgA myeloma proteins, but a glycine in the four human IgM proteins sequenced to date. Although it is true that all sequenced proteins have serine in position 126 and that 127 represents the first position in which a unique amino acid has been documented for

277

PATTERNS OF
SEQUENCE
VARIABILITY IN
IMMUNOGLOBULIN
VARIABLE REGIONS

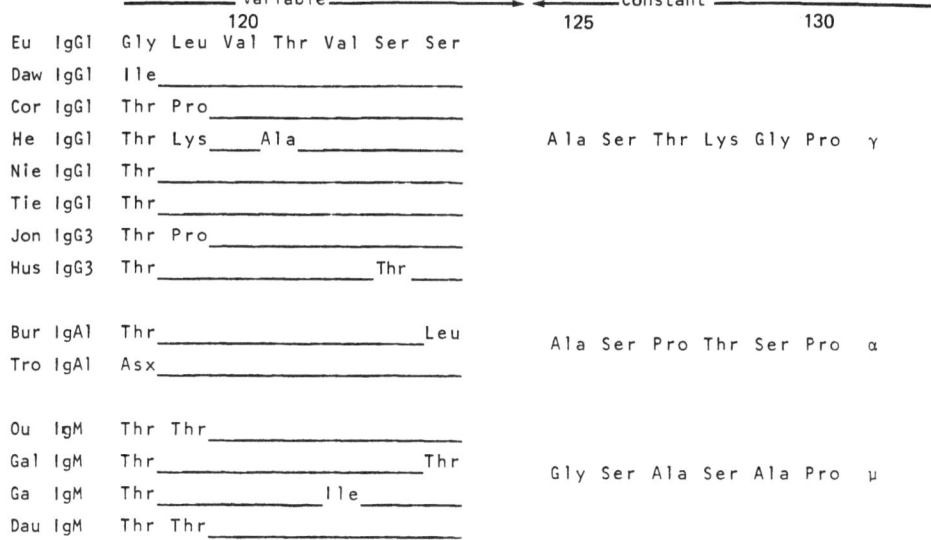

Figure 2. The V–C bridge. The original references for the proteins not given in Figure 1 are: Hus: A. Wang (1976, personal communication); Ga, Dau: Florent *et al.* (1974).

each of the classes, to place the V–C junction at position 126–127, one would have to assume that the glycine in 125 in all IgM proteins was fortuitous and still a portion of the V region. It seems more likely that the junction is between 124 and 125, and that the α and γ chains share the same amino acid in positions 125 and 126. Obviously, additional amino acid sequence data on human IgE and IgD myeloma proteins will be helpful in defining more precisely this important demarcation zone.

4. Subgroups Defined and Their Distribution in Phylogeny

One of the most important contributions of the amino acid sequence analysis of numerous Ig V regions was the revelation of *subgroups* of variability (Niall and Edman, 1967; Köhler *et al.*, 1970), that pattern of sequence variation wherein certain sets of V regions bear a closer sequence relationship to each other than to other V regions assignable to a different subgroup (the principle is illustrated for H chains by the sequences shown in Figure 1). The direct application of sequencing methodology has been crucial here, since the distinction of subgroups serologically by specific antisera has been applicable to Ig H-chain regions only recently, although it was very successfully utilized in the analysis of human κ chains (Solomon and McLaughlin, 1971). In the case of H chains, the identification of the subgroup has often been especially difficult because of the presence of pyrrolidone-carboxylic acid as the amino-terminal amino acid in all proteins except most members of the $V_H III$ subgroup, thus precluding an easy designation by amino-terminal sequence analysis. Consequently, the $V_H III$ subgroup of H chains has received the most study to date in terms of its distribution among the Ig's from different higher-animal species (Kehoe and Capra, 1972; Capra *et al.*, 1973; Wasserman *et al.*, 1974).

J. MICHAEL KEHOE
AND J. DONALD
CAPRA

An early impetus for analysis of the distribution of the $V_H III$ subgroup among several mammalian species was the observation that all of a series of myeloma H chains from dogs and cats could be assigned to this V_H subgroup (Kehoe and Capra, 1972). Two possible explanations for this were either a preferential selection of $V_H III$-like proteins by the neoplastic conversion or the presence of all, or nearly all, $V_H III$ proteins in the normal total pool of the Ig's produced by these species. As reported previously (Capra *et al.*, 1973), the validity of the latter hypothesis was approachable by the application of automated sequencing methodology to normal antibodies isolated from the serum pools of normal animals. The initial results showed that for both dogs and cats, the H chains of the normal IgG antibodies were assignable to the $V_H III$ subgroup in a proportion greater than 90%. Thus, the great preponderance, if not absolutely all, of the H chains expressed by these species are identifiable as $V_H III$ proteins, and it therefore seems most reasonable to assume that this is the explanation for the exclusive classification of myeloma proteins from these species as $V_H III$ H chains.

A comparable analysis of human IgG showed that 20–25% of the proteins contained $V_H III$ H chains (Capra *et al.*, 1973). Subsequently, a series of normal IgG preparations from a wide variety of animal species were similarly examined for their proportional content of $V_H III$ H chains. As shown in Table 1, considerable variation among the different species was noted for this parameter. Most important, however, the proportional distribution of H chains of this subgroup maintained absolute fidelity to the phylogenetic status of the animals concerned; i.e., related animals (man/monkey, cow/sheep, rat/mouse) shared the same proportion of the $V_H III$ subgroups in their IgG pools. It has been of particular interest to see proteins clearly homologous with the human $V_H III$ subgroup represented in animals of much older lineage, such as the leopard shark (*Ginglymostoma cirratum*) (Sledge *et al.*, 1974) and the much older still horned shark (*Heterodontus francisci*) (Kehoe *et al.*, 1977). Clearly, whether or not they represent H-chain V-region progenitor genes, $V_H III$-related genes have served the humoral immune response very effectively over a long period of evolutionary time.

TABLE 1. Proportional Content of $V_H III$ H Chains in IgG Pool for Various Species

Animal	Genus and species	$V_H III$ subgroup (%) in IgG pool
Man	*Homo sapiens*	20–25
Monkey		
Rhesus	*Macaca mulatta*	25–30
African green	*Cercopithecus aethiops*	20–25
Mouse	*Mus musculus*	20–25
Rat	*Rattus rattus*	20–25
Guinea pig	*Cavis cobaya*	20–25
Cow	*Bos taurus*	0
Sheep	*Ovis aries*	0
Moose	*Alces malchis*	0
Dog	*Canis familiaris*	90–95
Cat	*Felis domesticus*	90–95
Mink	*Putorius vison*	95–100

Capra and Kehoe (1975) also examined the association of the $V_H III$ subgroup with human IgA proteins, both from myelomas and from pools of normal serum IgA. The study showed a marked skewing of the association of $V_H III$ V regions with both kinds of IgA (60%) as compared with human IgG (20–25%, as shown in Table 1). More recently, the V_H distribution among human IgM proteins was examined and found to be similar to that in IgG (Capra and Klapper, 1976a,b).

The precise phylogenetic origin of the subgroups has not been clear, but recent evidence suggests that all three of the subgroups defined by the H-chain sequence data have very early phylogenetic origins. It is clear from the preceding discussion that the $V_H III$ subgroup preceded mammalian speciation, since it was found in all avian species studied and is very likely present in sharks. The question remains, however, whether each of the subgroups of other mammals have derived independently within each species from the $V_H III$ subgroup as progenitor, or whether the present human V_H subgroups originated prior to mammalian speciation. Recent amino acid sequence data suggest that the $V_H I$ and $V_H II$ subgroups also exist in other orders of the class Mammalia. For example, the MOPC 315 H-chain sequence is more closely related to the human $V_H II$ subgroup than to any other V_H sequence, and a rat Ig H chain sequenced by Querinjean *et al.* (1975) had marked similarities to the MOPC 315 sequence [see Figure 3 (Section 7.2)]. In the framework of the H chain from positions 1 to 30, rat protein S-216 differs very significantly from other rat myeloma proteins that have been sequenced, but possesses a striking homology with the MOPC 315 mouse α chain. These two proteins have 26 identical positions up to position 31 (see Figure 3). Both have more positions characteristic of the human $V_H II$ subgroup than the human $V_H III$ subgroup. Furthermore, they share seven residues that have yet to be found in H chains from other species. The sequence similarities of these two proteins from different rodents imply that the responsible genes derived from a common precursor that diverged prior to rat–mouse divergence. The similarity of this structure to the human $V_H II$ subgroup further suggests that the origin of the $V_H II$ subgroup, like the origin of the $V_H III$ subgroup, occurred very early in mammalian evolution.

Structural counterparts of the $V_H I$ subgroup have been difficult to discern in nonhuman species. Despite the many mouse myeloma H-chain sequences, few resemble the prototype human $V_H I$ protein Eu. However, induced A/J mouse antiphenylarsonate antibodies that bear a cross-reacting idiotype were recently subjected to extensive amino acid sequence analysis, which showed that these proteins clearly resemble the human $V_H I$ subgroup (Capra *et al.*, 1975). Unpublished data indicate that the region around methionine 83 is remarkably similar to the human $V_H I$ protein Eu, particularly with respect to the position of the methionine residue (83 vs. 85 in $V_H II$ and $V_H III$ proteins) and in the segment between the third and fourth hypervariable region (86–100). Heretofore, no other Ig's have been shown to have the sequence characteristics of Eu in this segment (Capra and Nisonoff, 1977). This remarkable similarity of the induced antiphenylarsonate antibody H chains and the human $V_H I$ protein Eu can most easily be interpreted as indicating that the $V_H I$ subgroup also had its origin prior to mouse–human divergence, and very likely is also of early phylogenetic origin.

Structural studies on the V regions of rabbit Ig H chains have also been revealing in terms of the phylogenetic origin of the V_H subgroups. Until recently, the only amino acid sequence data derived from either pooled Ig from rabbits homozygous at the *a* locus or from homogeneous antibodies bearing one of the *a*

279

PATTERNS OF
SEQUENCE
VARIABILITY IN
IMMUNOGLOBULIN
VARIABLE REGIONS

markers. These studies revealed that while there were 6–8 amino acid differences in the framework region of rabbit antibodies that differed in group *a* allotypic specificities, the general framework of rabbit Ig's was remarkably similar to the human $V_H II$ subgroup (Mole *et al.*, 1971; Pratt and Mole, 1975; Jaton, 1974; Kindt, 1975). Previous studies from our laboratory had indicated that rabbit serum contained little, if any, "unblocked" IgG H chains, and with the exception of a single report (Wang *et al.*, 1975), there was little indication that the rabbit contained structural genes for a human $V_H III$ type protein. Recently, however, Johnstone and Mole (Mole, 1976, personal communication) as well as Fraser *et al.* (1977) demonstrated that both pooled A_0 and a homogeneous antibody bearing no group A markers (presumably A_0) bore a striking resemblance to the human $V_H III$ prototype sequence, with the exception of a blocked *N*-terminal residue and a glutamic acid in position 2, rather than the more customary valine. These studies, along with many previous indications (Kehoe and Capra, 1972; Ponstingl *et al.*, 1970; Cebra *et al.*, 1975; Watanabe *et al.*, 1973; Kratzin *et al.*, 1975; Hood *et al.*, 1971), further point up the difficulties involved in making subgroup assignments on the basis of *N*-terminal amino acid residues alone. Nonetheless, when taken as a whole, the studies indicate that all three Ig H-chain subgroups as defined in man have their counterparts in other mammals, and imply that subgroups probably arose very early in vertebrate evolution.

Similar studies of the phylogenetic distribution patterns of L-chain types had previously been carried out by Hood and co-workers (Hood and Prahl, 1971). Although this is obviously a very different parameter than the H-chain subgroup designation, the principle of similar chain representation in closely related species was observed. The distribution patterns for L-chain type and content of $V_H III$ H chains do not parallel each other, however, since there are species (e.g., cow) with all, or nearly all, λ chains and essentially no unblocked $V_H III$ H chains, while other species (e.g., dog) with predominantly λ L chains have close to 100% $V_H III$ proteins (Table 1). This is, of course, consistent with the observations established by numerous analyses of genetic markers showing that H and L chains are completely unlinked.

The origin of the L-chain V-region subgroups is less clear. Although κ chains closely similar to the human $V_K I$ subgroups have been sequenced in the mouse, rat, and rabbit, and while subgroups clearly exist in each of these species, there appears to be no clear relationship between the subgroups of these various species. Thus, a homologue to the $V_K II$ and $V_K III$ subgroups has not been found to date in either the mouse, rat, or rabbit, for which extensive sequence data on Ig κ chains is available. Recently, however, Wasserman *et al.* (1978) described the amino acid sequence of a canine κ chain that has remarkable similarities to the human $V_K II$ prototypic sequence, even though more than 95% of canine L chains are of the λ type. This single canine κ-chain V region, excluding the hypervariable positions, is more than 85% homologous with the human $V_K II$ subgroup, while less than 50% homologous with the human $V_K I$ or $V_K III$ subgroups. Thus, like the situation in the H chains, the available evidence would suggest that L-chain V-region subgroups also existed prior to mammalian speciation.

5. Phylogenetically Associated Residues

Several analyses of the amino acid sequence of antibody proteins, including myeloma proteins of man and the mouse (Hood and Talmage, 1970) homogeneous antistreptococcal antibodies in the rabbit (Hood *et al.*, 1970), and myeloma proteins of dogs and cats (Kehoe and Capra, 1972), indicated that the amino acids at certain positions in either the L or H chains seem characteristic of proteins from a given animal. As an example, Hood *et al.* (1970) showed that position 11 of the κ L chain of a homogeneous rabbit antibody was valine, whereas it is consistently leucine in both human and mouse κ chains. Correspondingly, Kehoe and Capra (1972) showed, in a study of the H chains of dog and cat myeloma proteins, that certain positions could be correlated with the species of origin. For example, position 21 of the H chain of the dog unfailingly showed a serine residue, while this position was uniformly threonine in the cat. Later studies on normal pooled Ig from these species as well as others (Wasserman *et al.*, 1974) established that the unique residues originally found in the myeloma proteins could also be identified in the pools. There is reason to disfavor the original designation of such residues as "species-specific," since they are not usually absolutely specific for a particular species, but tend to occur within more broadly defined phylogenetic categories. In consequence, the term *phylogenetically associated* was proposed for such residues (Kehoe and Capra, 1972) to emphasize more accurately their precise nature. As will be discussed below, such residues have important implications for the various proposals having to do with the explanation of the origin of antibody diversity.

281

PATTERNS OF
SEQUENCE
VARIABILITY IN
IMMUNOGLOBULIN
VARIABLE REGIONS

6. Nature of Idiotypy and Its Relationship to Hypervariable Regions and the Antibody Combining Site

It has been more than 20 years since the description of individual antigenic specificity of an Ig (Slater *et al.*, 1955). This phenomenon, which has since been renamed *idiotypy*, has become one of the most widely used immunological probes. Examples in which the idiotypic determinants of Ig's have been used span the entire field of immunology, and include their use in mapping of murine V-region genes (Eichmann, 1975) and their elegant application for the elimination or stimulation of specific clones of B cells (Kluskens and Köhler, 1974; Rowley *et al.*, 1973). The recent descriptions of idiotypes on T cells (Binz and Wigzell, 1975; Eichmann and Rajewsky, 1975) have caused widespread interest, and raise the possibility that V-gene products may be present in molecules other than Ig's, or at least in molecules indistinguishable from prototypic B-cell-produced Ig.

6.1. Molecular Localization of the Idiotypic Determinants

In 1955, Slater, Ward, and Kunkel immunized rabbits with human myeloma proteins and observed that when rabbit antisera were absorbed with normal human serum or a series of myeloma proteins of similar class and L-chain type, the antisera continued to react with the immunogens. They further showed that with the exception of the immunizing agent, the antisera would not react with any other myeloma proteins tested, and they reasoned that each myeloma protein contained within its structure unique determinants. These they termed the *individual antigenic specificities* of myeloma proteins.

Some years later, Oudin (1966) and Williams and Kunkel (1963) extended these observations to include induced antibodies. Oudin showed that rabbit anti-*Salmonella* antibodies contained what he termed *idiotypic determinants*, and Williams and Kunkel demonstrated that human antibodies to certain red cell antigens contained unique determinants. Soon, there was substantial agreement that two phenomena, namely, *individual antigenic specificity* and *idiotypy,* were measuring much the same parameter, and the term *idiotypy* is now used to describe this general phenomenon.

About the time these experiments were being done, the four-chain model of γ-globulin was proposed and the important cleavage techniques for separating H and L chains and Fab and Fc became available. The idiotypic determinants were soon localized to the Fab region of Ig molecules (Grey *et al.,* 1965), but localization to either the H or L polypeptide chain proved more difficult. The prevalent interpretation at present is that the expression of the idiotype *usually* requires the interaction of both the H and L polypeptide chains, and is only occasionally restricted to a single chain.

The formal proof that the idiotypic determinants resided in the V regions of the H and L polypeptide chains was provided by Wells *et al.* (1973), who showed that the Fv fragment derived from myeloma protein MOPC 315, which comprised the V region of the H and L polypeptide chain of this mouse myeloma with anti-DNP activity, contained the idiotypic determinants. It seemed unlikely, however, that the entire V region was involved in the formation of the idiotypic determinants. Since amino acid sequence studies have revealed the presence of hypervariable regions within Ig H- and L-chain V regions, and these areas of the V region are extremely heterogeneous in pooled Ig, they were naturally thought to be involved in antibody complementarity. Affinity labeling of the active site has shown that all three hypervariable regions of the L chain and three of the four hypervariable regions of the H chain were near the antibody active site. Thus, the picture has emerged that the antibody-combining site consists of the hypervariable portions of both V regions, clustered in three-dimensional space to form a pocket or groove into which antigen is bound. In recent years, the interrelationships among the hypervariable regions, idiotypy, and the antibody-combining site have become increasingly clear.

6.2. Relationship between Idiotypic Determinants and the Antibody-Combining Site

An investigation of IgM cold agglutinins by Williams *et al.* (1968) provided the first evidence that the idiotypic determinants might relate to the antibody-combining site. This study demonstrated that Ig's with similar specificities shared antigenic determinants (termed *cross-idiotypic specificity* or *shared idiotypy*), and these workers postulated that the structures shared by the cold agglutinins included the antibody-combining site. The inhibition of the reactivity of idiotypic determinants when the cold agglutinins were bound to their red cell antigens provided further evidence for this relationship. Later, the studies were extended to the IgM anti-γ-globulins, and it was demonstrated that these proteins could be classified into two cross-idiotypic groups (Kunkel *et al.,* 1973). Again, evidence was presented that suggested that the antibody-combining site was involved in the idiotypic cross-reactions. The elegant studies of Brient and Nisonoff (1970) demonstrated that the reaction between antiidiotypic antibodies could be inhibited as much as 69% by homologous haptens. Similar results were obtained by Sher and Cohn (1972), who showed that phosphorylcholine inhibited the reaction between a mouse antiphosphorylcholine myeloma protein and its antiidiotypic serum. Weigert *et al.* (1974) studied the relationship between the idiotypes and the combining sites of mouse myeloma proteins with anti-α(1→6)-dextran, anti-α(1→3)-dextran, and anti-levan specificities. They introduced the term *ligand-modifiable idiotype* to denote the ability of a ligand to inhibit an idiotypic reaction. They stressed, however, that although proteins demonstrating idiotypic cross-reactions generally have similar combining specificities, the converse is not true; i.e., all antibodies that bind a specific ligand need not show cross-idiotypic specificity.

283

PATTERNS OF
SEQUENCE
VARIABILITY IN
IMMUNOGLOBULIN
VARIABLE REGIONS

Thus, while it is clear that most idiotypic determinants are somehow related to the antibody-combining site, not all idiotypes can be modified by ligand. Idiotypic determinants not modifiable by ligand may represent portions of the combining site not occupied by hapten, since the X-ray crystallographic studies suggest that the combining site may accommodate molecules larger than simple haptens (Poljak *et al.*, 1974; Segal *et al.*, 1974; Shiffer *et al.*, 1973).

6.3. Relationship between Hypervariable Regions and Idiotypic Determinants

Our laboratory selected two anti-γ-globulin antibodies with cross-idiotypic specificity for complete amino acid sequence analysis of the V regions of the H and L polypeptide chains. These two proteins (Lay and Pom) have only eight amino acid differences in their entire H-chain V regions (Capra and Kehoe, 1974b). Three of the interchanges occur within hypervariable regions and five in the framework residues. Two of the three hypervariable-region interchanges are now known to be in a non-complementarity-determining hypervariable region. As is evident in Figure 1, most V_HIII proteins differ from each other in approximately five residues in their framework—a very similar number to the differences between the Pom and Lay proteins. Randomly chosen Ig's, however, are dramatically different in their hypervariable regions, while Lay and Pom are virtually identical. These data strongly imply that major idiotypic determinants on Ig molecules are related to complementarity-determining hypervariable regions.

More recent studies demonstrating the relationship between the idiotype and the hypervariable regions come from deliberately induced antibodies to the azophenylarsonate group (Capra *et al.*, 1975; Nisonoff *et al.*, 1974). Anti-*p*-azophenylarsonate antibodies have been isolated from individual mice, and separated into two subpopulations—those bearing a cross-reacting idiotype and those devoid of this cross-reacting idiotype. Amino acid sequence analysis of the H chains of the idiotypically related proteins has demonstrated that the first and second hypervariable regions are homogeneous, while those anti-*p*-azophenylarsonate antibodies not bearing the cross-reacting idiotype have a heterogeneous amino acid sequence in the first and second hypervariable regions. One must reserve judgment on the homogeneity of the entire V_H region, since these sequences are not complete, especially since Cebra *et al.* (1975) noted heterogeneity in the fourth hypervariable region of guinea pig antibodies despite homogeneity in the first, second, and third hypervariable regions. Nonetheless, these studies suggest that antibodies selected on the basis of idiotypic specificity demonstrate a homogeneous sequence in at least some of their hypervariable regions and provide additional evidence relating idiotype and hypervariable regions. The L chains of the same murine anti-*p*-azophenylarsonate antibodies were recently sequenced and are homogeneous in their hypervariable positions, but significantly different in their framework (Capra *et al.*, 1976). These findings have important implications for theories of antibody diversity (see Section 7).

6.4. Relationship between Hypervariable Regions and the Antibody-Combining Site

Three lines of evidence link the hypervariable regions to the combining site—affinity labeling, sequence studies, and X-ray crystallographic experiments. In L chains, affinity labels have been localized within hypervariable regions by several authors, and most of the recent work on H chains supports this general view. Ray and Cebra (1972) localized affinity labels to the first and fourth hypervariable regions of guinea pig antibodies, and Koo and Cebra (1974) similarly labeled the second hypervariable region. Haimovich *et al.* (1972) had previously affinity-labeled the second hypervariable region of mouse myeloma protein 315. Thus, the generalization has emerged that the very regions of the molecule that show the highest degree of sequence variation are near or part of those exact regions of the H chains where affinity labels have been localized.

Cebra *et al.* (1975) elegantly demonstrated that guinea pigs immunized with defined haptens produce antibodies in which the first three hypervariable regions are restricted in their sequence and differ in primary structure among the antibodies of differing specificities. This clearly relates the specificity of antibodies to the sequence in their hypervariable regions. Much of the work done on the mouse myeloma proteins, particularly those with antiphosphorylcholine specificity, supports this view.

Finally, the X-ray crystallographic evidence clearly indicates that there is a clustering of hypervariable regions on the surface of the Fv component of the antibody molecule. Here they form a cavity, the depth of which varies as insertions or deletions are made in hypervariable regions (see Chapter 1). The third H-chain hypervariable region plays no role in the combining site, and the second hypervariable region of the L chain may not (Poljak *et al.*, 1974; Segal *et al.*, 1974, Shiffer *et al.*, 1973).

7. Genetic Origin of Variable-Region Sequence Diversity

The genetic origin of antibody diversity remains one of the most interesting unsolved problems of contemporary biology. The reason the question is still open is that the available experimental approaches have been unequal to the task of sufficiently eliminating the ambiguities and *ad hoc* requirements of the proposed alternative explanations. Amino acid sequencing unquestionably sharpened the issues by demonstrating the existence of V regions themselves, subgroups, phylogenetically associated residues, and hypervariable regions, but it now seems clear that this approach alone will not be capable of providing a definitive answer to the question whether each Ig V region has its own gene present in the zygote genome. One important point not always emphasized in discussions on the matter of the number of genes associated with antibody V regions is that *all* the various proposals have a significant germ-line component and acknowledge the existence of a set of germ-line genes that are subject to the various selective pressures over evolutionary time like other sets of mammalian genes. The difference of viewpoint concerns how many such genes each individual possesses at the zygote stage. From an experimental point of view, any absolute demonstration that the number of V-region genes present in a given somatic cell is *any number* less than the total number of V regions expressed by that individual will formally exlude the pure germ-line hypothesis as an explanation of the observed diversity.

All the currently tenable hypotheses for the explanation of diversity assume the correctness of the clonal selection concept originally stated by Jerne and Burnet, as indicated previously. The instructive, or direct template, hypothesis (Breinl and Haurowitz, 1930; Mudd, 1932), which postulates direct intervention by antigen, no longer receives serious consideration by contemporary immunologists, principally because of the demonstration by Haber (1964) that an antibody Fab fragment could be completely denatured and then refolded to regain antigen-binding activity (thus explicitly demonstrating that necessary and sufficient information for antigen-binding is available in the sequence alone), and because amino acid sequencing of numerous Ig V regions has indicated that a sufficiently wide variety of primary structures exist in the general Ig population.

With this as a background, four of the currently favored hypotheses designed to explain the origin of antibody V-region diversity will be discussed.

7.1. The Pure Germ-Line, or Multigene, Theory

This proposal is, in a certain sense, the most traditional of the concepts, since it does not suppose any marked variance with classic genetic mechanisms for the immune system. Simply stated, the theory postulates that for each and every Ig V region, there exists in the germ line a discrete gene that codes for that V region. For however many antibody V regions an individual can express, exactly that many genes, no more and no fewer, exist in the zygote and each and every resulting somatic cell of that individual. In this conception, which was outlined some years ago by Dreyer and Bennett (1965), and has more recently been championed by Hood and his associates (Hood, 1972; Hood et al., 1974), and by Hilschmann and his colleagues (Garver and Hilschmann, 1971), the genetic system for the generation of antibody diversity is just a special adaptation of the same genetic processes that operate for other proteins such as the cytochromes or hemoglobin. No special mechanisms affect the genes responsible for V-region structure, and such genes are subjected only to variations of the same general kinds of selection pressure that affect other genetic systems. As with many of these other systems, gene duplication with subsequent mutation and selection in an *evolutionary* time frame are assumed to be cardinal features of the system. The merits of this concept are quite obvious, especially the consistency with other mammalian genetic systems. Indeed, analogies among the proposed antibody system and other presumably multigene systems have been one of the most important arguments for the proponents of the pure germ-line theory (Smith, 1973).

Nonetheless, there have been some experimental observations that argue strongly against the validity of the pure germ-line idea. Two such findings are the H-chain V-region allotypes of the rabbit (Kunkel and Kindt, 1975; Kindt, 1975) and the phylogenetically associated residues of Ig V regions (Kehoe and Capra, 1974) alluded to earlier. The presence of such residues is difficult to explain under a germ-line basis for the origin of the relatively invariant areas of the V region without invoking some special mechanism for their appearance. To specifically counter the problem of gene-number constraint that is suggested by the presence of phylogenetically associated residues, processes of gene coevolution or expansion have been

285

PATTERNS OF
SEQUENCE
VARIABILITY IN
IMMUNOGLOBULIN
VARIABLE REGIONS

J. MICHAEL KEHOE
AND J. DONALD
CAPRA

advanced (Hood *et al.*, 1974; Smith, 1973), again on the basis of finding some precedent for these processes in biological systems other than the humoral immune response. The gene expansion–contraction model postulates that at some time in the evolutionary development of the species, a given mutation occurs in one of the V-region genes. This altered gene then acts as a seed to repopulate the entire V-region-gene pool, most or all of the other genes are deleted by the contraction process, and the resulting multigene pool will now show the mutation in question as a phylogenetically associated residue.

The presence of the H-chain V-region allotypic markers in the rabbit also argues against a germ-line hypothesis in the same fashion, but the force of this particular argument may be lessened by the increasing indications that these markers may be controlled by a series of regulatory genes (Strosberg *et al.*, 1974).

The strongest objection to the pure germ-line origin of antibody diversity has come from the nucleic acid hybridization studies that actually provide a numerical estimate of the number of genes consecrated to a particular function. As such studies of Ig systems have been more highly refined technically over the last few years, the numerical estimate of the number of V-region genes has decreased. Two recent reports state unequivocally that the number of V-region genes detectable by hybridization procedures is significantly less than would be required by a pure germ-line hypothesis (Tonegawa, 1976; Leder *et al.*, 1976).

7.2. The Insertional, or Episomal, Theory

When hypervariable regions were first detected in Ig L chains by Wu and Kabat (1970), they postulated that special mechanisms might generate the diversity within this portion of Ig molecules and suggested that episomelike genes might be inserted into a basic V-region gene, thus creating a significant amount of antibody diversity. Five years later, faced with the continued contradictions of the germ-line and somatic theories, Capra and Kindt (1975) proposed a reexamination of the insertion idea. They argued that in the ensuing ten years since the original descriptions of the two major theories of antibody diversity, the data had become increasingly irreconcilable. In the view of Capra and Kindt, the full elucidation and appreciation of the extent of phylogenetically associated residues, the clearer definition and structural localization of the rabbit allotypic markers, and the impact of the nucleic acid hybridization data made multigene theories increasingly untenable. On the other hand, the clear evidence for idiotypic inheritance, and more particularly, the documentation of the structural basis of the idiotype, dictated a new germ-line gene for each heritable idiotypic marker. With the number of inheritable idiotypes surpassing 20 (and the upper limits apparently not yet within reach), multigene theories became more attractive. In addition, some specific experimental findings could be readily explained by the genetic insertional model. These findings included: (1) the observation of identical idiotypes in rabbit antibodies of differing allotypes (Kindt *et al.*, 1973); (2) the finding of identical hypervariable regions in human antibodies in which the framework segments were modestly different (Capra and Kehoe, 1974b); (3) the RNA transfer experiments of Bell and Dray (1971); (4) the lymphoid transfer studies of Urbain *et al.* (1975); (5) the description by Hopper and his associates (Hopper, 1975; Hopper *et al.*, 1976; Capra and Hopper, 1976) of two myeloma proteins of identical idiotype but different V_H

287

PATTERNS OF
SEQUENCE
VARIABILITY IN
IMMUNOGLOBULIN
VARIABLE REGIONS

subgroup that arose from a single clone of malignant plasma cells; (6) the demonstration by Braun *et al.* (1976) of different framework residues with identical hypervariable regions in L chains isolated from different rabbit anti-*Streptococcal* antibodies; and (7) the realization that rabbits of different *a* locus allotype can contain identical idiotypes (Kindt *et al.*, 1974).

The fundamental tenet of the gene-interaction model is that the evidence arguing for few V-region genes applies directly to the framework segment of the V region, while the evidence raising the number of presumed V-region genes is directed toward the hypervariable regions (idiotype–antibody combining site component). By assuming the separation of these two entities in the genome, many conflicting data can be reconciled. One is then left with the requirement for some joining mechanism between the framework and hypervariable region gene segments. Such a process, however, would require very complex biochemical control mechanisms.

One prediction of gene interaction involves the issue of the "linkage" between the framework and the hypervariable region–idiotype–antibody combining site. The evidence in favor of this linkage is overwhelming (reviewed in Capra, 1975). Despite this, the exceptions to linkage between framework and hypervariable region–idiotype–combining site are noteworthy and are difficult to reconcile under either major theory of antibody diversity. Clearly, a gene-interaction model accommodates this lack of linkage, since the theory predicts that while linkage is likely, it need not be absolute. For a further discussion of these matters, the original reference (Capra and Kindt, 1975) should be consulted.

In a series of experiments from the laboratory of one of the authors (J.D.C.), hypervariable region identity in proteins of differing V-region subgroups was explored. The induced antiphenylarsonate antibodies in A/J mice were known to contain a single H chain, but two or three L chains (Nisonoff *et al.*, 1974; Capra *et al.*, 1975). The complete amino acid sequence of the L chains of these antibodies has now been reported (Capra *et al.*, 1976), and they have been found to contain homogeneous sequences in the three L-chain hypervariable regions but dramatically different frameworks, probably reflecting their origins in three to four distinct mouse V_K subgroups (Figure 3).

Klapper and Capra (1976) reported the sequence of the L chains of two anti-γ-globulin antibodies that share cross-reacting idiotypic determinants. As noted in Section 6.3, the H chains from these antibodies contain two identical complementarity-determining hypervariable regions, and the V regions of the H chains of these antibodies belong to the same V-region subgroup, although there are eight sequence differences in their framework segments. It was known that the L chains of proteins Lay and Pom belong to different human V_K subgroups, and it was also previously reported that their first H-chain hypervariable regions were significantly different (Capra *et al.*, 1971). The complete amino acid sequence of these L chains has now been reported (Capra and Klapper, 1976b), and despite their belonging to a different V_K subgroup, they contain identical second and third hypervariable regions (Figure 4).

The finding of these identical hypervariable regions in proteins of different V-region subgroups is unprecedented with the exception of the results of a computer search by Wu *et al.* (1975), in which a comparable hypervariable region identity was found. Classic theories of antibody diversity would predict a very low probability

J. MICHAEL KEHOE
AND J. DONALD
CAPRA

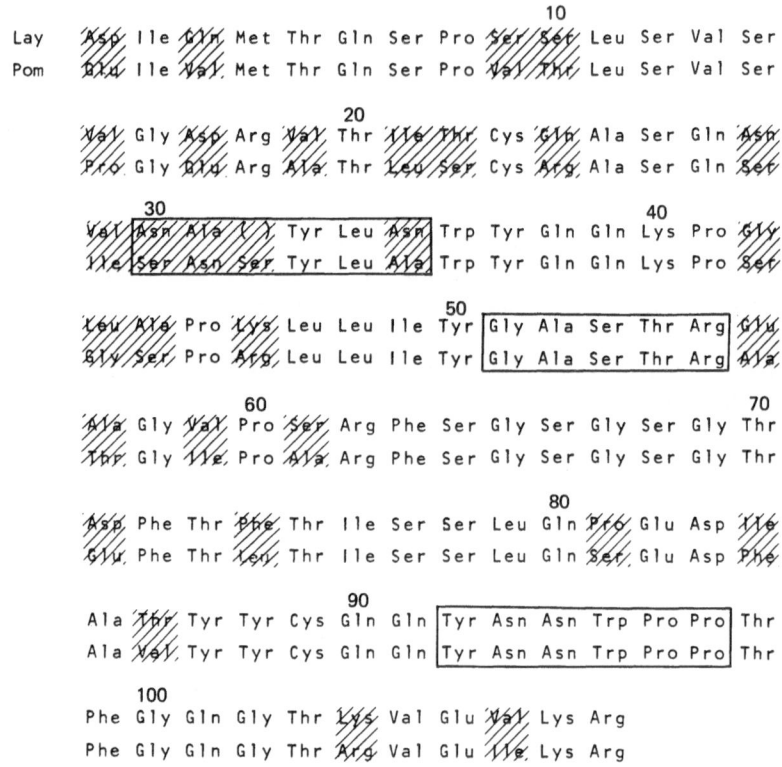

Figure 3. Amino acid sequence of the V regions of the L chains of two IgM anti-γ globulins with shared idiotype. The differences between the sequences are cross-hatched, and the hypervariable regions are boxed. Note that the second and third hypervariable regions have an identical sequence, while there are significant differences in the first hypervariable region (Capra *et al,* 1976; Capra and Klapper, 1976a,b; Klapper and Capra, 1976).

for this occurrence, and the findings seem most easily reconciled by a hypervariable-insertion model. It must be said, of course, that alternative explanations of this data are possible, and adherents of alternative hypotheses for the origin of antibody diversification (including one of the authors, J.M.K.) can offer reasonable interpretations of the data mentioned above within the context of their alternative theories.

The hypervariable-insertion model might be extended to the T cell and easily accommodate much of the data bearing on this sytem available at present. In the rat, the mouse, and the rabbit, it is now evident that the T cell contains a molecule of molecular weight approximately 70,000 that is antigen-specific but contains no known Ig-class-specific markers (Binz and Wigzell, 1976; Krawinkel *et al.,* 1976; Mole, 1976, personal communication). In addition to having a precisely defined antibody specificity, however, the relevant molecule contains idiotypic determinants. Recent studies from two laboratories indicate that in the rabbit, this molecule

Figure 4. Amino acid sequence of the L chains of antiphenylarsonate antibodies bearing the cross-reacting idiotype. Arrows above the sequence pointing right indicate determinations performed on the amino acid sequencer. Below are noted the various citraconylated tryptic (CT) peptides isolated from the mixture, and the yield of each peptide. All three hypervariable regions appear to have a homogeneous sequence despite numerous substitutions in the framework segment (Capra *et al.,* 1976).

289

PATTERNS OF
SEQUENCE
VARIABILITY IN
IMMUNOGLOBULIN
VARIABLE REGIONS

```
                                    10
 Asp Ile Gln Met Thr Gln Thr Pro Ser Ser Leu Ser Ala Ser Leu Gly
         Val                           Ile     Leu

 Asp Ile Gln Met Thr Gln Thr Pro Ser Ser Leu Ser Ala Ser Leu Gly
 ◄─────────────────────────────CT-3-1────────────────────────────
                               (20)
 Asp Ile Val Met Thr Gln Thr Pro Ser Ile Leu Leu Ala Ser Leu Gly
 ◄─────────────────────────────CT-2-1────────────────────────────
                               (24)


           20                                       30
 Asp Arg Val Ser Ile Ser Cys Arg Ala Ser Gln Asp Leu Ser Gln Tyr
             Leu

 Asp Arg Val Ser Ile Ser Cys Arg Ala Ser Gln Asp Leu Ser Gln Tyr
 ──────► ◄─────────CT-5-1─────────► ◄─────              ─CT-1-T-1
                   (32)                                   (20)
 Asp Arg Val Ser Ile Leu Cys Arg Ala Ser Gln Asp Leu Ser Gln Tyr
 ──────► ◄─────────CT-5-2─────────► ◄─────
                   (14)


                              40
 Leu Phe Trp Tyr Gln Gln Lys Pro Gly Gln Pro Pro Lys Leu Leu Ile
         Phe                    Glu     Ala

 Leu Phe Trp Tyr Gln Gln Lys Pro Gly Gln Pro Pro Lys Leu Leu Ile
 ───────────────────────────► ◄──CT-1-T-1──► ◄──CT-1-T5
                                    (20)           (50)
 Leu Phe Trp Phe Gln Gln Lys Pro Glu Gln Ala Pro Lys
 ◄────────────────CT-1-T-3────────────────────►
                  (52)


      50                                60
 Tyr Arg Val Ser Arg Leu Thr Asn Gly Val Pro Asp Arg Phe Ser Gly
 ─────CT-6─────► ◄────────CT-4-1────────► ◄──
      (48)                (57)

                                         Phe Ser Gly
                                         ◄──

                                         Phe Thr Gly
                                         ◄────CT-5-4
                                             (12)

                          70                             80
 Ser Gly Ser Gly Thr Asp Phe Thr Leu Thr Ile Asp Pro Met Glu Glu
 ──────────────────────────────CT-2-2─────────────────────────────
                               (30)
 Ser Gly Ser Arg Thr Asp Phe Thr Leu Thr Ile Ser Ser Val Glu Ala
 CT-5-5─────────► ◄────────────────────────────CT-3-4─────────────
  (24)                                            (26)
 Ser Gly Ser Arg
 ──────────────►

                                    90
 Asp Asp Thr Ala Thr Tyr Phe Cys Gln Gln Ser Arg Leu Ile Pro Arg
 ─────────────────────────────────────────► ◄──CT-4-2──────►
                                                  (63)


 Asp Asp Thr Ala Asp Tyr Phe Cys Gln Gln Ser Arg
 ──────────────────────────────────────────────►

           100
 Thr Phe Gly Gly Gly Thr Lys Leu Glu Ile Lys Arg
 ◄─────────CT-3-3───────────────────────────►
            (28)
 Thr Phe Gly Gln Gly Thr Lys Leu Glu Ile Arg
 ◄───────────CT-3-5──────────────────────►
              (53)
```

J. MICHAEL KEHOE
AND J. DONALD
CAPRA

contains no *a* locus determinants (Cazenave, 1976, personal communication; Jensenius *et al.*, 1976). A possible explanation for these provocative findings would involve the insertion of the very same hypervariable regions that can be expressed on B cells into a "T-cell protein" that was not an Ig in the traditional sense. Histocompatibility molecules or other related or nonrelated membrane proteins might serve as the putative acceptor molecule. This would reationalize the identity of idiotype and combining specificity without involving a separately evolved specificity-determining region of the genome that had the same specificities as the Ig but was in fact not a classic Ig molecule.

7.3. The Somatic Recombination Theory

Specific proposals suggesting somatic recombination as a means of generating V-region diversity were made originally by Smithies (1963) and later in a more complete form by Gally and Edelman (1970). As the name suggests, the postulated process would involve recombination in somatic cells (and in a somatic as well as evolutionary time frame) between closely arrayed genes coding for a specific subgroup, which genes have arisen by duplication. Unequal crossing-over between tandemly arranged duplicated genes would lead to the somatic generation of many variants from an initial number that is lower than the total number of V regions a given animal is actually capable of expressing. As discussed by Gally and Edelman (1970), such a proposal can readily account for subgroup-specific, phylogenetically associated, and allotype-specific residues.

The major difficulty this theory has encountered is that in all the V-region protein sequences that have been obtained to date, little or no indication of recombination has been obtained. If somatic recombination were the only, or even a prominent, mechanism for diversity generation, one might expect to see at least some clear indication of it by this time. It is certainly still conceivable that evidence for such recombinational processes will yet be forthcoming. An excellent general discussion of the elements of this theory and some of the other proposals is to be found in the general review of Ig's by Gally (1973).

7.4. The Somatic Mutation Theory

This hypothesis, like the somatic recombination theory, also places the necessary amplification of V-region gene number mainly in somatic time (the life of the individual), but proposes a different mechanism, mutation, for the generation of the required variant genes. One version of this idea was described by Lederberg (1959) some time ago, but more recently, detailed theoretical and experimental bases for the proposal were provided by Cohn (1971) and by Jerne (1971). As presently formulated, this hypothesis suggests that low-frequency spontaneous variation (especially involving "missense" mutations) of a relatively few germ-line genes is responsible for generating the diversity provided in the mature immune response. Because of the antigen selection for combining specificity, the observed variation in the hypervariable segments of the V regions (both L and H) is much higher than that seen in the relatively invariant segments (Cohn, 1971). Antigen thus does intervene in the humoral immune response, not by acting as a direct template, but by favoring through selection the most suitable combining variants. Since variation by mutation continues throughout the lifetime of the individual, new combining specificities will continually appear and may, or may not, be selected for by antigen. When specific

291

PATTERNS OF
SEQUENCE
VARIABILITY IN
IMMUNOGLOBULIN
VARIABLE REGIONS

clones of lymphocytes are appropriately selected for in this manner, clonal division results with concomitant increased probability of additional mutational variants, some of which will have improved antigen-combining capacities leading to additional preferential selection and the production of higher-affinity antibody, consistent with the pattern that has been seen in a wide variety of experimental systems. Massive doses of antigen, such as would be encountered when anti-self specificities arise, would lead to death of that clone and the loss of that particular combining specificity, i.e., tolerance.

The main objections to this proposal are based on two different considerations. One view argues on the basis of time considerations, indicating that there cannot be enough time available, on a somatic scale, to generate all the potential specificities the selective immune response is known to contain. Another argument against the idea states that it would be enormously, and excessively, wasteful of cells because of the large numbers of unneeded or nonfunctional variants that would be expected to arise. Adherents of the somatic mutation concept, like the adherents of the alternative proposals, simply find the counterarguments unpersuasive. Obviously, both the somatic mutation and somatic recombination hypotheses are readily compatible with the presence of phylogenetically associated residues and the detection of relatively low numbers of V-region genes by nucleic acid hybridization techniques (Tonegawa, 1976; Leder *et al.*, 1976). Admittedly, both the mutation and recombination explanations may have to assume the existence of additional germ-line genes as the number of demonstrated inherited idiotypes increases. But even if several hundred basic genes do exist, this is still far below the total required by the mature immune response, and some amplification mechanism must be invoked. Somatic mutation would seem to be a suitable process to provide for the unique biological demands of the immune system within the context of natural selection.

8. Conclusions

The amino acid sequence analysis of Ig V regions has given, and continues to give, important insights into the function, evolutionary origin, and genetic basis of the humoral immune response. It has become increasingly clear how these data must be integrated with other experimental approaches including genetic analysis through allotypic markers, X-ray diffraction studies of three-dimensional structure, and immunochemical studies to fully exploit the information that sequence analysis provides. Among the most significant findings that sequence studies have helped reveal are the existence of V regions themselves, the occurrence of subgroups, the presence of alternating hypervariable and relatively invariant sections of the V region, the presence of phylogenetically associated residues, and the impressive unity of the mechanism of the antigen-binding function, at least among the more highly evolved species, including man.

References

Bell, C., and Dray, S., 1971, Expression of allelic immunoglobulin in homozygous rabbits injected with RNA extract, *Science* **171**:199–201.

Binz, J., and Wigzell, H., 1975, Shared idiotypic determinants on B and T lymphocytes reactive against the same antigenic determinants. I. Demonstration of similar or identical idiotypes on IgG molecules and T cell receptors with specificity for the same alloantigens, *J. Exp. Med.* **142**:197–211.

Binz, H., and Wigzell, H., 1976, Shared idiotypic determinants on B and T lymphocytes reactive against the same antigenic determinants. V. Biochemical and serological characteristics of naturally occurring, soluble antigen-binding T lymphocyte-derived molecules, *Scand. J. Immunol.* **5**:559–571.

Braun, D. G., Huser, H., and Riesen. W. F., 1976, Rabbit antibody light chains: selective breeding narrows variability in framework and complementarity-determining residues, *Eur. J. Immunol.* **6**(8):570–578.

Breinl, F., and Haurowitz, F., 1930, Die chemische Untersuchung des Präzipitäts auf Hämoglobin und Anti-hämoglobin-serum und Bemerkungen über die Natur der Antikörper, *Z. Physiol. Chem.* **192**:45–57.

Brient, B. W., and Nisonoff, A., 1970, Quantitative investigations of idiotypic antibodies. IV. Inhibition by specific haptens of the reaction of anti-hapten antibody with its anti-idiotypic antibody, *J. Exp. Med.* **132**:951–962.

Burnet, F. M., 1959, *The Clonal Selection Theory of Acquired Immunity*, Vanderbilt University Press, Nashville.

Capra, J. D., 1971, Hypervariable regions of human immunoglobulin heavy chains, *Nature (London) New Biol.* **230**:61–63.

Capra, J. D., 1977, Patterns of variability in variable regions of immunoglobulin heavy chains, in: *Antibodies in Human Diagnosis and Therapy* (E. Haber and R. Krause, eds.), pp. 87–102, Raven Press, New York.

Capra, J. D., and Hopper, J. E., 1976, Comparative studies on monotypic IgM lambda and IgG kappa from an individual patient. III. The complete amino acid sequence of the V_H region of the IgM paraprotein, *Immunochemistry* **13**:995–999.

Capra, J. D., and Kehoe, J. M., 1974a, Variable region sequences of five human immunoglobulin heavy chains of the V_HIII subgroup: Definitive identification of four heavy chain hypervariable regions, *Proc. Natl. Acad. Sci. U.S.A.* **71**:845–848.

Capra, J. D., and Kehoe, J. M., 1974b, Structure of antibodies with shared idiotypy: The complete sequence of the heavy chain variable regions of the two immunoglobulin M anti-gamma globulins, *Proc. Natl. Acad. Sci. U.S.A.* **71**:4032–4036.

Capra, J. D., and Kehoe, J. M., 1975, Distribution and association of heavy and light chain variable region subgroups among human IgA immunoglobulins, *J. Immunol.* **114**:678–682.

Capra, J. D., and Kindt, T. J., 1975, Antibody diversity: Can more than one gene encode each variable region?, *Immunogenetics* **1**:417–427.

Capra, J. D., and Klapper, D. G., 1976a, Distribution and association of heavy and light chain variable region subgroups among human IgM immunoglobulins, *La Riceria Clin. Lab.* **6**(Suppl. 3):34–44.

Capra, J. D., and Klapper, D. G., 1976b, Complete amino acid sequence of the variable domains of two human IgM anti-gamma globulins (Lay/Pom) with shared idiotypic specificities, *Scand. J. Immunol.* **5**:677–684.

Capra, J. D., and Nisonoff, A., 1977, Structural studies of induced antibodies with defined idiotypic specificities. V. The complete amino acid sequence of the light chain variable regions of anti-*p*-azophenylarsonate antibodies from A/J mice bearing a cross-reactive idiotype *J. Immunol.* **119**:993–999.

Capra, J. D., Kehoe, J. M., Winchester, R. W., and Kunkel, H. G., 1971, Structure–function relationships among anti-gamma globulin antibodies, *Ann. N.Y. Acad. Sci.* **190**:371–381.

Capra, J. D., Wasserman, R. L., and Kehoe, J. M., 1973, Phylogenetically associated residues within the V_HIII subgroup of several mammalian species, *J. Exp. Med.* **138**:410–427.

Capra, J. D., Tung, A., and Nisonoff, A., 1975, Structural studies on induced antibodies with defined idiotypic specificities, *J. Immunol.* **115**:414–418.

Capra, J. D., Klapper, D. G., Tung, A. S., and Nisonoff, A., 1976, Identical hypervariable regions in light chains of differing V_K subgroups, *Cold Spring Harbor Symp. Quant. Biol.* **41**:847–853.

Cebra, J. J., Koo, P. H., and Ray, A., 1975, Specificity of antibodies: Primary structural basis of hapten binding, *Science* **186**:263–265.

Cohn, M., 1971, The take-home lesson, *Ann. N.Y. Acad. Sci.* **190**:529–584.

Cunningham, B. A., Pflumm, M. N., Rutishauser, U., and Edelman, G. M., 1969, Subgroups of amino acid sequences in the variable regions of immunoglobulin heavy chains, *Proc. Natl. Acad. Sci. U.S.A.* **64**:997–1003.

Dreyer, W. J., and Bennett, J. C., 1965, The molecular basis of antibody formation: A Paradox, *Proc. Natl. Acad. Sci. U.S.A.* **54**:864–869.

Edelman, G. M., Cunningham, B. A., Gall, W. E., Gottieb, P. D., Rutishauser, U., and Waxdal, M., 1969, The covalent structure of an entire γG immunoglobulin molecule, *Proc. Natl. Acad. Sci. U.S.A.* **63**:78–85.

293

PATTERNS OF
SEQUENCE
VARIABILITY IN
IMMUNOGLOBULIN
VARIABLE REGIONS

Eichmann, K., 1975, Genetic control of antibody specificity in the mouse, *Immunogenetics* **2**:491–506.

Eichmann, K., and Rajewsky, K., 1975, Induction of T and B cell immunity by anti-idiotypic antibody, *Eur. J. Immunol.* **5**:661–666.

Florent, G., Lehman, D., and Putnam, F. W., 1974, The switch point in μ heavy chains of human IgM immunoglobulins, *Biochemistry* **13**:2482–2498.

Franék, F., 1970, The character of variable sequences in immunoglobulins and its evolutionary origin, in: *Symposium on Developmental Aspects of Antibody Formation and Structure*, (J. Sterzl and I. Riha, eds.), pp. 311–313, Czech. Acad. Sci., Prague.

Fraser, B. A., Johnston, A. P., Gordon, S. M., and Kindt, T. J., 1977, The response of rabbits to streptococcal hyperimmunization, *Cold Spring Harbor Symp. Quant. Biol.* **41**:689–698.

Gally, J. A., 1973, Structure of immunoglobulins, in: *The Antigens* (M. Sela, ed.), pp. 161–298, Academic Press, New York.

Gally, J., and Edelman, G. M., 1970, Somatic translocation of antibody genes, *Nature (London)* **227**:341–348.

Garver, F. A., and Hilschmann, N., 1971, The primary structure of a monoclonal λ-type immunoglobulin L-chain of subgroup II (Bence–Jones protein Nei): Evolutionary origin of antibody variability, *FEBS Lett.* **16**:128–132.

Grey, H. M., Mannik, M., and Kunkel, H. G., 1965, Individual antigenic specificity of myeloma proteins, *J. Exp. Med.* **121**:561–575.

Haber, E., 1964, Recovery of antigenic specificity after denaturation and complete reduction of disulfides in a papain fragment of antibody, *Proc. Natl. Acad. Sci. U.S.A.* **52**:1099–1106.

Haber, E., Margolies, M. N., and Cannon, L. E., 1976, Origin of antibody diversity: Insights gained from amino acid sequence studies of elicited antibodies, *Cold Spring Harbor Symp. Quant. Biol.* **41**:647–649.

Haimovich, J., Eisen, H. N., Hurvitz, E., and Givol, D., 1972, Localization of affinity-labeled residues on the heavy and light chain of two myeloma proteins with anti-hapten activity, *Biochemistry* **11**:2389–2398.

Hilschmann, N., and Craig, L. C., 1965, Amino acid sequence studies of Bence–Jones proteins, *Proc. Natl. Acad. Sci. U.S.A.* **53**:1403–1409.

Hood, L. E., 1972, Two genes, one polypeptide chain: Fact or fiction?, *Fed. Proc. Fed. Am. Soc. Exp. Biol.* **31**:177–187.

Hood, L., and Prahl, J., 1971, The immune system: A model for differentiation in higher organisms, *Adv. Immunol.* **14**:291–351.

Hood, L., and Talmage, D. W., 1970, Mechanism of antibody diversity: Germ line basis for variability, *Science* **168**:325–334.

Hood, L., Eichmann, K., Lackland, H., Krause, R. M., and Ohms, J., 1970, Rabbit antibody light chains and gene evolution, *Nature (London)* **228**:1040–1044.

Hood, L., Grant, J. A., and Sox, H. C., Jr., 1971, in: *Developmental Aspects of Antibody Formation and Structure* (J. Sterzl and I. Riha, eds.), Vol. 1, pp. 283–309, Academia, Prague.

Hood, L., Barstad, P., Loh, E., and Nottenberg, C., 1974, Antibody diversity: An assessment, in: *The Immune System: Genes, Receptors, Signals,* (E. E. Sercarz, A. R. Williamson, and C. F. Fox, eds.), pp. 119–139, Academic Press, New York.

Hopper, J. E., 1975, Comparative studies on monotypic IgM lambda and IgG kappa from an individual patient. I. Evidence for shared V_H idiotypic determinants, *J. Immunol.* **115**:1101–1107.

Hopper, J. E., Noyes, C., Heinrikson, R., and Kessel, J. W., 1976, Comparative studies on monotypic IgM λ and IgG κ from an individual patient. II. Amino-terminal sequence analyses, *J. Immunol.* **116**:743–746.

Inbar, D., Hochman, J., and Givol, D., 1972, Localization of antibody-combining sites within the variable portions of heavy and light chains, *Proc. Natl. Acad. Sci. U.S.A.* **69**:2659–2662.

Jaton, J. C., 1974, Completion of the analysis of the primary structure of the variable domain of a homogeneous rabbit antibody to Type III pneumococcal polysaccharide, *Biochem. J.* **143**:723–732.

Jensenius, J. C., Williams, A. F., and Mole, L. E., 1976, Abstracts, Third European Immunology Meetings, p. 68.

Jerne, N. K., 1971, The somatic generation of immune recognition, *Eur. J. Immunol.* **1**:1–9.

Jerne, N. K., 1955, The natural-selection theory of antibody formation, *Proc. Natl. Acad. Sci. U.S.A.* **41**:849–857.

Kehoe, J. M., and Capra, J. D., 1971, Localization of two additional hypervariable regions in immunoglobulin heavy chain, *Proc. Natl. Acad. Sci. U.S.A.* **68**:2019–2021.

J. MICHAEL KEHOE
AND J. DONALD
CAPRA

Kehoe, J. M., and Capra, J. D., 1972, Sequence relationships among the variable regions of immunoglobulin heavy chains from various mammalian species, *Proc. Natl. Acad. Sci. U.S.A.* **69**:2052–2055.

Kehoe, J. M., and Capra, J. D., 1974, Phylogenetic aspects of immunoglobulin variable region diversity, in: *Contemporary Topics in Molecular Immunology*, Vol. 3 (G. L. Ada, ed.), pp. 143–159, Plenum Press, New York.

Kehoe, J. M., Sharon, J., Gerber-Jensen, B., and Litman, G. W., 1978 (submitted).

Kindt, T. J., 1975, Rabbit immunoglobulin allotypes: Structure, immunology and genetics, *Adv. Immunol.* **21**:35–86.

Kindt, T. J., Klapper, D. G., and Waterfield, M. D., 1973, An idiotypic cross-reaction between allotype a3 and allotype a negative rabbit antibodies to streptococcal carbohydrates, *J. Exp. Med.* **137**:636–648.

Kindt, T. J., Thunberg, A. L., Mudgett, M., and Klapper, D. G., 1974, A study of V region genes using allotypic and idiotypic markers, in: *The Immune System: Genes, Receptors, Signals* (E. E. Sercarz, A. R. Williamson, and C. F. Fox, Eds.), pp. 69–88, Academic Press, New York.

Klapper, D. G., and Capra, J. D., 1976, The amino acid sequence of the variable regions of the light chains from two idiotypically cross-reactive IgM anti-gamma globulins, *Ann. Immunol. (Inst. Pasteur)* **127**:261–271.

Kluskens, L., and Köhler, H., 1974, Regulation of immune response by autogenous antibody against receptor, *Proc. Natl. Acad. Sci. U.S.A.* **71**:5083–5087.

Köhler, H., Shimizu, A., Paul, C., Moore, V., and Putnam, F. W., 1970, Three variable-gene pools common to IgM, IgG, and IgA, *Nature (London)* **227**:1318–1320.

Koo, P. H., and Cebra, J., 1974, Affinity labeling of a distinctive lysyl residue within the second hypervariable region of γ_2 chain of guinea pig anti-*p*-azobenzenearsonate antibody, *Biochemistry* **13**:184–195.

Kratzin, J., Altevogt, P., Ruban, E., Kortt, A., Atarogcik, K., and Hilschmann, N., 1975, Die Primärstruktur eines monoklonalen IgA-Immunoglobulins (IgA Tro). II. Die Aminosäuresequenf der H-Kette, Alpha Typ, Subgruppe III, Struktur des Gesamten IgA Moleküls, *Hoppe-Seyler's Z. Physiol. Chem.* **356**:1337–1342.

Krawinkel, U., Cramer, M., and Rajewsky, K., 1976, Abstracts, Third European Immunology Meetings, p. 77.

Kunkel, H. G., and Kindt, T., 1975, *Allotypes and Idiotypes in Immunogenetics and Immunodeficiency* (B. Benacerraf, ed.), pp. 56–80, University Park Press, Baltimore.

Kunkel, H. G., Agnello, V., Joslin, F. G., Winchester, R. J., and Capra, J. D., 1973, Cross-idiotypic specificity among monoclonal IgM proteins with anti-γ-globulin activity, *J. Exp. Med.* **137**:331–342.

Leder, P., Swan, D., Honjo, T., and Seidman, J., 1976, Origin of immunoglobulin gene diversity: The evidence and a restriction–modification model, *Cold Spring Harbor Symp. Quant. Biol.* **41**:855–862.

Lederberg, J., 1959, Genes and antibodies, *Science* **129**:1649–1653.

Milstein, C., 1967, Linked groups of residues in immunoglobulin κ chains, *FEBS Lett.* **2**:301–304.

Mole, L. E., Jackson, S. A., Porter, R. R., and Wilkinson, J. M., 1971, Allotypically related sequences in the Fd fragment of rabbit, *Biochem. J.* **124**:301–318.

Mudd, S., 1932, A hypothetical mechanism of antibody formation, *J. Immunol.* **23**:423–427.

Niall, H. D., and Edman, P., 1967, Two structurally distinct classes of kappa-chains in human immunoglobulins, *Nature (London)* **216**:262–263.

Nisonoff, A., Tung, A., and Capra, J. D., 1974, Factors determining immune responsiveness at the level of B-cells, *Prog. Immunol.* **2**:17–25.

Oudin, J., 1966, The genetic control of immunoglobulin synthesis, *Proc. R. Soc. Ser. B* **166**:207.

Poljak, R. J., Amzel, L. M., Chen, B. L., Phizackerley, R. P., and Saul, F., 1974, The three-dimensional structure of the Fab fragment of a human myeloma immunoglobulin at 2.0 Å resolution, *Proc. Natl. Acad. Sci. U.S.A.* **71**:3440–3444.

Ponstingl, H., Schwartz, J., Reichel, W., and Hilschmann, N., 1970, Die Primärstruktur eines monoklonalen γ1-Immunoglobulins (Myelomprotein Nie). I. Aminosäuresequenz des variablen Teils der H-kette, Subgruppen variabler Teile, *Hoppe-Seyler's Z. Physiol. Chem.* **351**:1591–1594.

Pratt, D., and Mole, L. E., 1975, Sequence studies on the constant region of the Fd sections of rabbit immunoglobulin G of different allotype, *Biochem. J.* **151**:337–349.

Press, E. M., and Hogg, N. M., 1970, The amino acid sequences of the Fd fragments of two human γ-1 heavy chains, *Biochem. J.* **117**:641–660.

295

PATTERNS OF
SEQUENCE
VARIABILITY IN
IMMUNOGLOBULIN
VARIABLE REGIONS

Querinjean, P., Bazin, H., Kehoe, J. M., and Capra, J. D., 1975, Transplantable immunoglobulin-secreting tumors in rats, *J. Immunol.* **114**:1375–1378.

Ray, A., and Cebra, J. J., 1972, Localization of affinity-labelled residues in the primary structures of anti-dinitrophenyl antibody raised in strain 13 guinea pigs, *Biochemistry* **11**:3647–3657.

Rowley, D. A., Fitch, F. W., Stuart, F. P., Köhler, H., and Cozenza, H., 1973, Specific suppression of immune responses, *Science* **181**:1133–1141.

Segal, D. M., Padlan, E. A., Cohen, G. H., Rudikoff, S., Potter, M., and Davies, D. R., 1974, The three-dimensional structure of a phosphorylcholine-binding mouse immunoglobulin Fab and the nature of the antigen binding site, *Proc. Natl. Acad. Sci. U.S.A.* **71**:4298–4302.

Sher, A., and Cohn, M., 1972, Effect of haptens on the reaction of anti-idiotype antibody with a mouse antiphosphorylcholine plasmacytoma protein, *J. Immunol.* **109**:176–178.

Shiffer, M., Girling, R. L., Ely, K. R., and Edmundson, A. B., 1973, Structure of a λ-type Bence–Jones protein at 3.5-Å resolution, *Biochemistry* **12**:4620–4631.

Slater, R. J., Ward, S. M., and Kunkel, H. G., 1955, Immunological relationships among the myeloma proteins, *J. Exp. Med.* **101**:85–108.

Sledge, C., Clem, L. W., and Hood, L. E., 1974, Antibody structure: Amino terminal sequences of nurse shark heavy and light chains, *J. Immunol.* **112**:941–948.

Smith, G. P., 1973, *The Variation and Adaptive Expression of Antibodies,* Harvard University Press, Cambridge, Massachusetts.

Smithies, O., 1963, Gamma-globulin variability: A genetic hypothesis, *Nature (London)* **199**:1231–1236.

Solomon, A., and McLaughlin, C. L., 1971, Bence–Jones proteins and light chains of immunoglobulins. IV. Immunochemical differentiation among proteins within each of the three established κ-chain classes, *J. Immunol.* **106**:120–127.

Strosberg, A. D., Hammers-Casterman, C., van der Loo, W., and Hamers, R., 1974, A rabbit with the allotypic phenotype *a1a2a3 b4b5b6, J. Immunol.* **113**:1313–1318.

Tonegawa, S., 1976, Reiteration frequency of immunoglobulin light chain genes: Further evidence for somatic generation of antibody diversity, *Proc. Natl. Acad. Sci. U.S.A.* **73**:203–207.

Urbain, J., Tasiaux, N., Leuwen Kroon, R., Van Acker, A., and Mariame, B., 1975, Sharing of idiotypic specificities between different antibody populations from an individual rabbit, *Eur. J. Immunol.* **5**:570–575.

Wang, L. S., Hora, J., and Friedenson, B., 1975, Existence of the V_HIII subgroup in rabbit antibody heavy chains, *J. Immunol.* **115**:889–890.

Wasserman, R., Kehoe, J. M., and Capra, J. D., 1974, The V_HIII subgroup of immunoglobulin heavy chains: Phylogenetically associated residues in several avian species, *J. Immunol.* **113**:954–957.

Wasserman, R. W., and Capra, J. D., 1978 (submitted).

Watanabe, S., Barnikol, H. U., Hor, J., Bertram, J., and Hilschmann, N., 1973, Die Primästruktur eines monoklonalen IgM-Immunoglobulins (Makroglobulin Gal). II. Die Aminosäuresequenz der H-Kette (μ-Typ, Subgruppe HIII), Struktur des gesamten IgM-Moleküls, *Hoppe-Seyler's Z. Physiol. Chem.* **354**:1505–1509.

Weigert, M., Raschke, W. C., Carson, D., and Cohn, M., 1974, Immunochamical analysis of the idiotypes of mouse myeloma proteins with specificity for levan or dextran, *J. Exp. Med.* **139**:137–147.

Wells, J. V., Fudenberg, H. H., and Givol, D., 1973, Localization of idiotypic antigenic determinants in the Fv region of murine myeloma protein MOPC-315, *Proc. Natl. Acad. Sci. U.S.A.* **70**:1585–1587.

Williams, R. C., and Kunkel, H. G., 1963, Separation of rheumatoid factors of different specificities using columns conjugated with gamma-globulin, *Arthritis Rheum.* **6**:665–675.

Williams, R. C., Kunkel, H. G., and Capra, J. D., 1968, Antigenic specificities related to the cold agglutinin activity of gamma M globulins, *Science* **161**:379–380.

Winkler, M., Köhler, H., Shinoda, T., and Putnam, F. W., 1969, Macroglobulin structure: Homology of mu and gamma heavy chains of human immunoglobulins, *Science* **163**:75–78.

Wu, T. T., and Kabat, E. A., 1970, An analysis of the sequences of the variable regions of Bence–Jones proteins and myeloma light chains and their implications in antibody complementarity, *J. Exp. Med.* **132**:211–250.

Wu, T. T., Kabat, E. A., and Bilofsky, H., 1975, Similarities among hypervariable segments of immunoglobulin chains, *Proc. Natl. Acad. Sci. U.S.A.* **72**:5107–5110.

12

Genetic Control of Immunoglobulin Synthesis in Man

ANDREAS MORELL and SILVIO BARANDUN

1. Introduction

Most of our current understanding of the immune response is based on (1) investigation of the nature of antigens as the inducing stimulus; (2) investigation of the products of the immune response: sensitized lymphocytes and humoral antibodies; and (3) studies of the kinetics of these products. With growing knowledge on these topics, it became evident that hereditary factors exert an important influence both on the capability of an organism to recognize certain antigens and on the magnitude of the response. About twelve years ago, systematic experimental research on genetic control of immune responsiveness was taken up, and has yielded a great number of important discoveries that have placed this field of immunology in the spotlight of interest.

There is substantial evidence for various types of genetic control of the immune response. Most of the interest today is focused on immune response genes associated with genes coding for the major histocompatibility specificities. Another genetic control mechanism is linked to genes coding for immunoglobulin (Ig) allotypes or other structural traits of Ig molecules. Furthermore, genetic influences on Ig synthesis that are sex-linked or that show no connections with other genetic factors have been demonstrated.

In this chapter, the emphasis will be on the genetic control of Ig and antibody synthesis in man. Animal models will be mentioned only as far as required for a general understanding, since this topic has already been covered by a number of reviews.

ANDREAS MORELL and SILVIO BARANDUN • Institute for Clinical and Experimental Cancer Research, University of Berne, Tiefenau-Hospital, Berne, Switzerland.

ANDREAS MORELL
AND SILVIO
BARANDUN

2. Evidence for Genetic Control of Antibody Synthesis in Experimental Animals

Intensive research on the genetic basis of the immune response during recent years has established that the ability of an animal to recognize certain antigens as immunogens can be controlled by autosomal dominant genes, called *immune response (Ir) genes* (McDevitt and Benacerraf, 1969; Benacerraf, 1974; Green, 1974). So far, such antigen-specific *Ir* genes have been identified in mice, guinea pigs, rats, and rhesus monkeys. Animals that possess the relevant *Ir* gene are able to form an immune response including both cellular immunity and humoral antibodies against the corresponding antigen. Animals lacking the specific *Ir* gene do not develop cellular immunity and synthesize either little or no antibody at all against that antigen.

Three types of antigens have been used for the identification of *Ir* genes:

1. Synthetic polypeptides with a restricted range of L-amino acids, and their hapten conjugates, forming molecules of limited structural diversity
2. Weak native antigens, i.e., alloantigens, differing only slightly from the autologous molecules in the immunized host
3. Native foreign protein molecules with many antigenic determinants, administered in limiting doses allowing the recognition of the strongest immunogenic determinants only

Most investigations were carried out with synthetic polypeptides in inbred strains of mice and in guinea pigs. Several *Ir* genes, each specific for the recognition of a defined synthetic polypeptide, could be identified and were shown to be closely associated with genes controlling major histocompatibility specificities (McDevitt and Chinitz, 1969; Benacerraf and McDevitt, 1972; McDevitt and Bodmer, 1974). In the mouse, most *Ir* genes are located on chromosome 17 in the center of the major histocompatibility complex (MHC) (the *H-2* region) between the *H-2 K* locus, which is the gene for one of the two major serological transplantation antigens, and the Ss locus, a marker near the center of the *H-2* complex controlling the synthesis of a serum β-globulin. Studies with recombinant mice that have portions of the MHC of two different inbred strains allowed a detailed mapping of this chromosomal region, called the *I region* (Shreffler and David, 1975). The number of *Ir* genes in this region is thought to be considerable: many *Ir* genes have been detected in a relatively short time. It is, however, certainly less than the number of genes coding for the different antibody specificities of Ig molecules, since the immune response controlled by a given *Ir* gene always results in a highly heterogeneous population of antibodies.

It is assumed that these histocompatibility-linked *Ir* genes are expressed on immunocompetent cells, predominantly on T lymphocytes. One finding in favor of this hypothesis is that the presence of an *Ir* gene is a prerequisite for the development of cellular immunity, a characteristic T-cell function (Green *et al.*, 1966). Furthermore, no antibody response to an antigen recognized by a given *Ir* gene can be seen in thymectomized animals (Mitchell *et al.*, 1972). Of key importance for the understanding of the immune response mechanism is that the products of the *Ir* genes on T cells are responsible for the recognition of and the immune response to the carrier molecules of hapten–carrier conjugates (Levine *et al.*, 1963). They do not recognize the haptens, which are recognized by receptors on B lymphocytes (Green *et al.*, 1966; Dunham *et al.*, 1972). Thus, an effective immune response to the hapten requires a cooperation between helper T cells specific for the carrier portion and B cells binding the haptenic group of the immunogen (Kindred and Shreffler, 1972; Katz and Benacerraf, 1975). There is evidence that this T-cell–B-cell interaction too is mediated by products of the *Ir* genes that are expressed on the helper T cells and, as receptors of the activated helper T cells or their products, also on B cells (Katz and Benacerraf, 1975).

Thus, the immune response to simple synthetic polypeptides is under the control of single autosomal dominant genes acting at the level of antigen recognition. Similar examples of monogenic control of the antibody response were found with alloantigens and with limiting amounts of complex native protein antigens (Benacerraf and McDevitt, 1972; Green, 1974).

As already mentioned, there are examples in which genetic control of the immune response is associated, not with histocompatibility-linked genes, but with genes coding for Ig allotypes and thus for structural Ig genes. This type of genetic control seems to work at the level of B lymphocytes. One example of such an allotype-linked *Ir* gene was described by Blomberg *et al.* (1972). It concerns the ability of inbred mice to produce either high or low amounts of antibodies of restricted heterogeneity against α-1,3-dextran. This restricted antibody response is an autosomal dominant trait linked to the gene coding for the heavy-(H)-chain allotype. Other systems (Eichmann, 1973; Cramer, 1974) of immune responses resulting in the production of antibodies of highly restricted heterogeneity are dealt with extensively elsewhere in this volume. In this context, the investigations of Biozzi *et al.* (1970) must be mentioned. They studied the genetic regulation of the antibody response by selective breeding of random-bred Swiss mice for the production of either low or high amounts of antibodies against sheep and pigeon erythrocytes. After 16 generations, two lines of mice had developed that differed sharply in the hemagglutinin titers produced after immunization with these multideterminant antigens. Of particular interest was the observation that the two lines of mice showed similar differences in their antibody response to other non-cross-reacting complex antigens such as O and H antigens of *Salmonella typhi* and hen ovalbumin. In addition, quantitative analyses revealed significantly lower serum levels of all Ig classes in the low-responder line than in the high responders, which had concentrations within the normal range for Swiss mice. This difference was more pronounced for IgM and the subclasses of IgG than for IgA, and was even more marked after than before immunization. The two lines also differed in the allotypic markers of their H chains: Three phenotypes were observed in high-responder mice. These animals were either homozygous or heterozygous for the allotypes found in BALB/c and in C57BL inbred strains. All low responders, on the other hand, were homozygous for the same H-chain linkage group that is never seen in commonly used inbred strains of mice but has been observed in wild mice.

It is concluded that these selective breeding experiments probably have resulted in a segregation of genes concerned with the regulation of Ig synthesis irrespective of antibody specificity. In contrast to the monogenic control of the specific responsiveness to simple antigens, the response to multideterminant strong immunogens such as heterologous erythrocytes is controlled by a number of genes that probably act cumulatively.

ANDREAS MORELL
AND SILVIO
BARANDUN

3. Evidence for Genetic Control of Immunoglobulin Synthesis in Man

Thus, there is convincing evidence that genetic control mechanisms act on Ig synthesis under experimental conditions in which both the immunogenic agent and the genetic make up of the recipient are well defined. But are such mechanisms also effective in natural immunological responses in man? There is reason to assume that they in fact are. Many examples of genetic influences on Ig synthesis and antibody production in man have been reported. As in the animal systems, they may be histocompatibility-linked, or associated with Ig allotypes. Moreover, serum levels of certain Ig classes may be sex-linked or under the influence of genes without any known correlation with other genetic traits.

3.1. Genetic Control of the Synthesis of Reaginic Antibodies

During the last few years, associations between antigens of the MHC and susceptibility to specific diseases have been found in mice and—to a surprising extent—also in man (McDevitt and Bodmer, 1974; Dausset *et al.*, 1974). Most of these diseases are correlated with certain serologically detectable antigens controlled by the second locus of the *HLA* complex or with lymphocyte-dependent antigens of the closely linked *MLC* locus on chromosome 6, or with both.* Many if not most of these diseases, such as rheumatoid disorders and autoimmune and allergic diseases, are known to have an immunological background. As a corollary, hypothetical *Ir* genes situated in this chromosomal region have been postulated and are thought to be directly or indirectly responsible for susceptibility to these diseases. Today, evidence for the existence of *Ir* genes in man has been obtained in the case of ragweed hay fever, in which the required three factors (McDevitt and Bodmer, 1974)—i.e., association with a distinct *HLA* type, specific immune response, and relevant clinical symptoms (Svejgaard *et al.*, 1975)—could be demonstrated.

Levine *et al.* (1972) found that in seven families, ragweed hay fever and IgE antibody production to antigen E, the major protein antigen of ragweed pollen, correlated with distinct *HLA* haplotypes in successive generations. This IgE antibody response was detected by anaphylactic-type hypersensitivity reactions after intradermal injection of dilute solutions of antigen E. In one of these families, 4 of 6 members with the *HLA 1,8* haplotype had intensive anaphylactic-type skin reactions to antigen E and severe hay fever. On the other hand, none of 7 relatives who lacked the *HLA 1,8* haplotype had hay fever, and only 1 of them showed some skin reactivity. Data in the other families were similar, although skin reactivity and clinical hay fever were associated with a different *HLA* haplotype in each family. Of the family members who had the hay-fever-associated haplotypes, 77% had IgE-anti-ragweed antibodies and clinical disease. Of the 11 members who lacked these haplotypes, 10 had no skin reactivity, 1 had weak skin reactivity, and none suffered from hay fever. In addition to IgE antibodies, the authors were able to demonstrate IgG serum antibodies to antigen E in selected subjects who had the hay-fever-associated haplotype and showed an intense IgE antibody response. The authors concluded that IgE and IgG responsiveness to antigen E in man is controlled by a

---

*According to the new nomenclature for the MHC, the first locus is designated *HLA-A*, the second *HLA-B*, and the *MLC* locus is now *HLA-D*. (Bach and van Rood, 1976).

genetic locus that is closely linked to the *HLA* system and is inherited as a Mendelian dominant trait.

Blumenthal *et al.* (1974) tried to localize or map this postulated *Ir* locus for antigen E, called *Ir E,* with respect to the *HLA* complex. Their data are based on a study of one large family with 57 members spanning three generations. In this family, IgE antibody production against antigen E, as detected in anaphylactic-type skin hypersensitivity, was associated with the *HLA 2,12* haplotype. In the third generation of this family, they found a recombinant who as a result of a crossing-over between the first and second *HLA* locus, between *HLA 2,12* and *HLA 9,W15,* had a *HLA 9,12* haplotype. She also had the postulated *Ir E* gene. Since no linkage between antibody production to ragweed antigen E and *HLA 2* or other *HLA* antigens could be demonstrated, the authors feel that their data can best be explained with a linkage between the gene for *HLA 12* and the *Ir E* locus or loci controlling hypersensitivity to ragweed antigen E. From this observation and from the number of possible recombinants between the *HLA* loci and the postulated *Ir E* locus, they concluded that the probable map order is: *HLA* first locus–*HLA* second locus–*Ir E* locus. This would place *Ir E* somewhere in the vicinity of the *HLA-D* locus.

The interpretation of the data presented by Levine *et al.* (1972) and by Blumenthal *et al.* (1974) was recently challenged by Bias and Marsh (1975), who questioned the way the data were analyzed and think that there is not enough evidence for linkage between *HLA* and *Ir* genes controlling IgE or IgE and IgG responses to ragweed antigen E. These authors could not find any association between sensitivity to ragweed antigen E and a specific *HLA* type. In their studies, however, they detected a highly significant association between the presence of an antigen of the *HLA 7* cross-reacting group and both IgE and IgG antibody responses to the ragweed pollen antigen Ra 5 (Marsh *et al.,* 1973a,b). This allergen has a low molecular weight of only 5200 with a known primary structure of 45 amino acids, and seems to be a much better tool for studying the immune response than the far more complex antigen E (mol. wt. 38,000).

Even with the aforementioned strong reservations, however, correlations between HLA antigens and sensitivity to ragweed allergens were found by all three groups of investigators. The data both of Blumenthal *et al.* (1974) and of Marsh *et al.* (1973a) are compatible with an association with HLA antigens of the second locus. In contrast to Levine *et al.* (1972) and Blumenthal *et al.* (1974), Bias and Marsh (1975) saw no evidence in family studies for concordant transmission of a familial *HLA* haplotype and IgE or IgG response to any of several pollen allergens, including antigen E. Thus, the situation seems to be more complex than suggested by the first two groups of authors. One reason the effect of *HLA*-linked *Ir* genes may be difficult to visualize is probably related to the observation of Bazaral *et al.* (1971), who found that basal IgE levels, i.e., regulation of biosynthesis and metabolism of all IgE molecules, are genetically controlled. This observation was supported by the results of Hamburger *et al.* (1973) in twin pairs. Further elucidation was obtained in sophisticated family studies by Marsh *et al.* (1974), who were able to pin down the influence of an autosomal recessive gene for high IgE levels (> 95 U/ml) and, accordingly, an autosomal dominant allele for low (< 95 U/ml) IgE serum concentrations. This IgE-regulating locus was shown to have a profound modulating effect on the specific IgE antibody response to allergens. It could easily mask the effect of *HLA*-associated *Ir* genes.

3.2. Other Examples of HLA-Linked Immune Responses in Man

ANDREAS MORELL
AND SILVIO
BARANDUN

Several promising attempts have been undertaken to demonstrate linkage between HLA groups and immune responses to various other antigens. Dausset and Hors (1975) studied the antibody response against Rh(D) erythrocytes in 93 Rh-negative hyperimmunized subjects and could not find any association between the magnitude of the immune response and HLA antigens. Results of studies of the anti-D response in women after multiple Rh-incompatible pregnancies also failed to show such a connection (Petranyi et al., 1974). It is assumed that under these conditions, possible effects of Ir genes are obscured by the multideterminant composition of most naturally occurring antigens, on one hand, and the complexity of the immune response in normal subjects, on the other. In hay fever with hypersensitivity against pollen allergens, the situation is to some extent simplified on the side of the antigens: in this case, we are dealing with relatively small antigens that yet can be subdivided into even smaller components, which are inhaled in minute amounts and have a very potent and easily demonstrable effect in suscepti-ble subjects. This type of immunization is certainly not comparable with most others. The question is whether the problem can also be tackled from the side of the antigen recipient. There are a few observations that point in this direction:

Several groups of investigators have found increased antibody titers against measles and rubella viruses in sera of patients with autoimmune diseases such as rheumatoid arthritis, chronic hepatitis, and multiple sclerosis (Lucas et al., 1972; Triger et al., 1972; Laitinen and Vesikari 1972; Brody et al., 1971). Susceptibility to these diseases is known to be strongly associated with the presence of certain HLA antigens. It has been hypothesized that cell-mediated immune responses to para-myxoviruses and rubella virus may be impaired in these conditions (Jersild et al., 1973), and that the increased humoral response against measles and rubella viruses in multiple sclerosis and other autoimmune diseases might reflect a deviation of the humoral immune response as a result of a deficient cellular immune response. It is still not clear to what extent cellular immunodeficiency is involved in these diseases (Jersild et al., 1975). Okumura and Tada (1971) did show, however, an increased production of anaphylactic antibodies in rats with impaired T-cell function, and C. E. Buckley et al. (1973) suggested an inverse relationship between immediate and delayed-type cutaneous hypersensitivity in man. It might therefore be advanta-geous to study genetic control of antibody responses in partially immunodeficient subjects. In fact, C. E. Buckley et al. (1973) found strong evidence for HLA-linked control of the immune response in three families that were selected on the basis of their delayed-type unresponsiveness to a battery of bacterial, viral, fungal, and plant antigens. In each of these three families, highly significant associations were detected between HLA haplotypes and the magnitude of immediate-type cutaneous hypersensitivity reactions to a number of test antigens. The data are consistent with the assumption of a linkage between HLA haplotypes and genes determining the immune response to various naturally occurring antigens.

Selection of families with a partial defect of the T-cell system has proved to be one promising approach. Preliminary results of another interesting investigation of immune response genes were recently reported by Haverkorn et al. (1975). They studied the antibody response against poliomyelitis viruses, diphtheria toxoid, and rubella, measles, and influenza viruses in 71 monozygotic and 72 dizygotic twin pairs. Comparison of the ratios of antibody titers in mono- and dizygotic twin pairs regardless of HLA haplotypes revealed a significantly greater similarity in monozygotic twins, but only for antibodies against measles, poliomyelitis I virus, and diphtheria toxoid. When the dizygotic twin pairs were divided into HLA-identical and HLA-nonidentical groups and analyzed for antibody titer ratios, significantly greater similarity was found in the HLA-identical group for measles antibodies only, but not for the immune responses against the other antigens. This finding indicates a possible linkage between *HLA* loci and some locus or loci involved in the immune response against measles. The data also underline how difficult it is to grasp hard evidence on this topic even with human "material" considered to be ideal for genetic investigations.

3.3. Correlations between Gm Allotypes and Serum Immunoglobulin Concentrations

In normal human sera, IgG molecules are present in four isotypic variations: subclasses IgG1, IgG2, IgG3, and IgG4. Examples of normal serum concentrations in adults are (in mg/ml): IgG1, 6.63 ± 1.70; IgG2, 3.22 ± 1.08; IgG3, 0.58 ± 0.30; IgG4, 0.46 ± 0.40 (Morell *et al.,* 1972, 1975). Molecules of all four subclasses carry genetically determined structural variations, called Gm factors or Gm allotypes, which are located to different positions in the constant (C) region of the γ chains. Most Gm factors are found on molecules of only one of the four subclasses and allow genetic analyses of the IgG molecules (Grubb, 1970). These allotypic specificities coded for by the structural genes for the IgG subclasses are inherited as codominant Mendelian traits. Each subclass exists in at least two genetic variations. Population studies have shown close linkage between genes coding for allotypes of different subclasses. As a consequence, the chromosomal region with this linked group of genes has been referred to as the *Gm gene complex.* The subclass-specific Gm factors in normal sera constitute a Gm phenotype, and a subject can be described as being homozygous or heterozygous for the various factors (Natvig and Kunkel, 1973). Some relevant Gm factors are listed in Table 1 (for detailed information, see Grubb, 1970, and Natvig and Kunkel, 1973). Gm(a) and Gm(f) are the two antithetical markers of IgG1, Gm(g) and Gm(b) of IgG3 molecules. For IgG2, only one Gm factor has been characterized; thus, IgG2 molecules are either positive or negative for Gm(n). For IgG4 molecules, two allotypic markers, 4a and 4b, have been described that are also expressed on molecules of other subclasses, 4a on IgG1 and IgG3, 4b on IgG2.

TABLE 1. Relationship of Gm Factors to IgG Subclasses[a]

Gm factors		
Original nomenclature	WHO nomenclature	IgG subclasses
Gm(a)	Gm(1)	IgG1
Gm(f)	Gm(4)	IgG1
Gm(g)	Gm(21)	IgG3
Gm(b)	Gm(5)	IgG3
Gm(n)	Gm(23)	IgG2
4a	—	IgG1, IgG3, IgG4
4b	—	IgG2, IgG4

[a]The original Gm nomenclature is used in the text.

ANDREAS MORELL
AND SILVIO
BARANDUN

3.3.1. Correlations between IgG Subclass Serum Levels and Gm Allotypes

During the last few years, correlations between Gm phenotypes and IgG subclass serum concentrations have been established. This is documented best for IgG3: Serum levels of this subclass in subjects homozygous for the IgG3 marker Gm(b) are twice as high as in subjects homozygous for the antithetical marker Gm(g). In heterozygotes, the IgG3 levels were found to be intermediate (Yount *et al.*, 1967). These findings suggest a "gene-dosage effect" of Gm genes on the IgG3 concentration. In our experience, IgG3 levels in heterozygotes tend to be rather high (Morell *et al.*, 1972), which is compatible with a dominant effect of Gm(b) on IgG3 concentrations.

IgG2 serum levels in general are higher in subjects who carry the IgG2 marker Gm(n) than in those who are Gm(n−) (Morell *et al.*, 1972; van der Giessen *et al.*, 1973). Family studies with homozygous and heterozygous members, however, failed to demonstrate a clear-cut influence of this marker on the IgG2 serum level (Steinberg *et al.*, 1973). An interesting observation is the relationship among Gm(n), the IgG2 marker, and the IgG4 levels: Serum concentrations of IgG4 are highest in sera of subjects homozygous for this factor having the genotype Gm^{n+}/Gm^{n+}. In heterozygous Gm^{n+}/Gm^{n-} subjects, IgG4 levels are intermediate, and in the Gm^{n-}/Gm^{n-} subjects who lack this Gm factor, they are lowest (Steinberg *et al.*, 1973). This correlation suggests that the genes coding for IgG4 and IgG2 may be very close to each other or even adjacent, an assumption that has obtained strong support from the recent detection of a hybrid IgG molecule consisting of parts of the subclasses IgG2 and IgG4 (Natvig and Kunkel, 1974).

Examples of such correlations are given in Table 2. In all these investigations, serum concentrations of the IgG subclasses were determined directly either by radial immunodiffusion or by radioimmunoassay using subclass-specific antisera. Litwin and Balaban (1972) were able to measure the Gm concentrations by an automated inhibition of hemagglutination assay. They found striking differences in the serum concentrations of the antithetical IgG3 allotypes, Gm(b) and Gm(g), confirming the results obtained by direct determination of IgG3. In heterozygous sera, Gm(b) constituted 70% of the total IgG3, Gm(g) only 30%. Thus, the gene product of the Gm(b) IgG3 allele is more than twice that of the Gm(g) allele. For IgG1, the differences between the gene products of Gm(f) and Gm(a) were smaller, Gm(f) constituting 54% and Gm(a) 46% of the total IgG1. Taken together, the data show that serum levels of IgG3, IgG4, and, to some extent, also IgG2 and IgG1, are under a genetic control.

TABLE 2. Correlations Between IgG Subclass Serum Levels (Mean Values) and Gm Phenotypes[a]

Gm phenotype	Number of sera	IgG2 (mg/ml)	IgG3 (mg/ml)	IgG4 (mg/ml)
Gm(a+g+)	12	—	0.27	—
Gm(a+f+g+b+)	49	—	0.59	—
Gm(f+b+)	39	—	0.64	—
Gm(n+)	66	3.40	—	0.56
Gm(n−)	38	2.93	—	0.27

[a] From Morell *et al.* (1972).

3.3.2. Correlation of Serum IgD concentration with Gm Allotypes

305

GENETIC
CONTROL OF
IMMUNOGLOBULIN
SYNTHESIS IN MAN

In a recent study, Walzer and Kunkel (1974) reported that IgD serum concentrations are under genetic control similar to that for the IgG subclass levels. Since there are no allotypic markers on IgD molecules, the authors correlated IgD levels with Gm markers of IgG subclasses. The results indicate that subjects who are homozygous for the markers Gm(f) and Gm(b) have significantly lower serum IgD levels than subjects homozygous for the Gm(a), Gm(g) linkage group. It therefore seems that serum concentrations of one Ig class can be directly correlated with allotypic markers of another Ig class. In analogy to the relationships between the IgG2 marker Gm(n) and IgG4 levels, this would suggest a close linkage between the structural genes coding for the C regions of IgD and IgG H chains. Similar relationships do not exist for IgA and IgM, since serum levels of these Ig classes did not differ significantly among the two groups of homozygotes.

3.3.3. Gm Allotypes and the Human Antibody Response to Flagellin

In all the previous studies, Gm allotypes were correlated with Ig class or subclass serum levels representing the sum of the humoral immune responses to the antigenicity of the environment. There is no doubt that allotype-linked genetic influences have an effect on Ig levels, and similarities to the results of Biozzi *et al.* (1970) are striking. Even more detailed information on genetic effects, however, could probably be obtained by comparing Gm allotypes with the humoral response to well-chosen, defined antigens. Unfortunately, today there are still few human data.

Wells *et al.* (1971) studied the humoral response to monomeric flagellin *(Salmonella adelaide)* in relation to Gm factors in 113 Caucasians. The probands were divided into two groups: "Low responders" had low titers (< 100) of natural antibodies to flagellin and a low immune response on injection of flagellin (< 100). "High responders" had high titers (> 600) of natural antibodies or a high response after antigen injection (> 10'000), or both. In the high-responder group, the number of subjects with the markers Gm(a) and Gm(g) was significantly higher than in the low-responder group, in which subjects prevailed who were homozygous for Gm(f) and Gm(b) and thus lacked the other two markers. Thus, it seems that there is an association between the magnitude of the antibody response and the presence of genes coding for IgG1 molecules of the Gm(a) allotype and IgG3 molecules of the Gm(g) allotype. No difference was observed between subjects homozygous and heterozygous for Gm(a) and Gm(g).

Six years after this study was undertaken, the same authors (MacKay *et al.,* 1975) reported mortality data for the two groups: there were significantly more survivors in the high-responder group (82%) than in the low-responder group (56%). One might hypothesize that the low responders who are negative for Gm(a) and Gm(g) have either a lower immune responsiveness to certain bacterial antigens or a greater predisposition to certain illnesses, both of which lower their life expectancy.

3.4. Other Genetic Influences on Immunoglobulin Levels

Titers of isoantibodies to the blood group antigens A and B as well as total IgM serum levels are known to be higher in girls than in boys (Grundbacher, 1972a;

Allansmith *et al.*, 1968). This sex difference becomes manifest at the age of 9–10 years, reaches a maximum at 15–20 years, and tends to decrease later in life. Grundbacher (1972a) found in family studies a much closer correlation between the IgM levels of boys and their mothers than between those of boys and their fathers. He suggested that the X chromosome carries a gene or genes for IgM concentrations. Between daughters and their fathers, on the other hand, the correlation coefficient of serum IgM levels was about twice as high as between daughters and mothers, which is in agreement with the same assumption: the X chromosome transmitted from fathers to daughter is always the same and is the only one that is effective in the father, whereas the mother can transmit either of two or a possible recombination between the two X chromosomes. Thus, both higher mean IgM values in females and higher correlation coefficients between parents and offspring support the hypothesis that the X chromosome carries genes influencing the IgM serum concentrations. It furthermore seems that there is some additive or "gene-dosage" effect: Rhodes *et al.* (1969) noticed that IgM values were highest in females with three X chromosomes, intermediate in normal girls, and clearly lower in XO subjects, in whom IgM levels similar to those in normal males were observed.

Finally, investigations of Ig levels in homozygous and heterozygous twins by Allansmith *et al.* (1969) must be mentioned in this context. They detected a hereditary influence on the levels of IgG, IgD, and IgA. This influence was not associated with other factors.

3.5. Genetic Aspects of Immunoglobulin Synthesis in Immunodeficiency States

It has been suggested that the study of immunodeficiency states might offer some clues for a more thorough understanding of the genetics of immune response (Biozzi *et al.*, 1970; Buckley, C. E., *et al.*, 1973). Some of the immunodeficiency diseases are known to have a more or less well-defined sex-linked recessive, others an autosomal recessive, mode of inheritance. In most instances, however, no clear inheritance patterns can be seen. Can such diseases be assigned to a deficiency of structural Ig genes or of genes with a regulatory function, or to both, or are genes involved that act on the level of antigen recognition or of cell proliferation and differentiation? A great deal of work has been done to clarify these questions. Its contribution to our understanding of the immune response, however, has been modest so far. One of the main problems involved in such investigations may be the enormous variability even of defined immunodeficiency syndromes.

In this chapter, a selection of papers on genetics of Ig synthesis in immunodeficient patients and their relatives is reviewed. Dausset and Hors (1975) determined HLA antigens in 36 children suffering from various immunodeficiencies and observed a significantly increased frequency of HLA 1, an antigen at the first *HLA* locus. This finding is rather exceptional, since most HLA-associated diseases as well as the postulated human *Ir E* genes are correlated with antigens of the second *HLA* locus. The observation is still preliminary and, before conclusions can be drawn, needs confirmation in a larger number of patients with well-defined immunodeficiency syndromes and in their relatives.

Studies of hypogammaglobulinemic patients and their relatives have in rare cases provided some evidence for structural abnormalities in the region of the Gm

heterozygous for abnormal Gm gene complexes with deletions of genes coding for
the genetic markers of IgG3 and IgG1 molecules. The mother lacked the expected
IgG1 marker Gm(f), and the father had no IgG3 marker Gm(g), in their abnormal
haplotypes. The propositus inherited both abnormal gene complexes and was
hypogammaglobulinemic. His hypogammaglobulinemia could not be satisfactorily
explained, however, with the abnormalities of the IgG1 and IgG3 genes alone: He
had a low total IgG and a low IgG1 serum concentration, as expected from the
abnormal IgG1 gene. His IgG (1.03 mg/ml) consisted to about 50% of IgG3. The
IgG3 level, therefore, is not depressed or is only slightly depressed. IgG2 and IgG4
concentrations, however, were below the limit of detectability, and he also had
severely depressed levels of the other Ig classes. Thus, a regulator-gene abnormality seems to be involved as well. Both parents and the patient's sister, who inherited
one abnormal gene complex from her father, had normal IgG levels with a normal
subclass distribution and were in good health.

Quantitative determinations of the IgG1 and IgG3 genetic markers were performed by Litwin and Fudenberg (1972) on the sera of three pedigrees of immunodeficient patients. The authors tried to detect quantitative allotype aberrations that
might be present in carriers of defective structural IgG genes. In fact, they found
deficient concentrations of one Gm allotype or an imbalance between the gene
products of Gm(f) and Gm(a) in the sera of 7 of 27 heterozygous relatives in three
successive generations. They concluded that this number of abnormal sera was not
sufficient for the assumption of recessive genes responsible for defective synthesis
of Gm allotypes, and interpreted their findings as an inherited regulatory-gene
defect in these families.

Isolated absence of the Ig classes IgG and IgM is known, although rare, and
occasionally shows familial clustering (Gitlin, 1966; Stiehm and Fudenberg, 1966).
Isolated absence of IgA has been found by many investigators, and seems to occur
with a frequency of about 1 in 700 subjects (Bachmann, 1965). It thus represents the
most common form of human immunodeficiency (Buckley, R., 1975). Most cases
occur sporadically, but in several instances, familial accumulations have been
observed. Many well-documented studies on the genetic basis of IgA deficiency
with conflicting results can be found in the literature (reviewed by Grundbacher,
1972b). On the basis of his own studies in two families and on the accumulated
evidence in the literature, Grundbacher assumes that a predisposition to IgA
deficiency is inherited by polygenic factors. It may be noteworthy that the incidence
of IgA deficiency is increased in individuals with abnormalities of chromosome 18.

Note Added in Proof: Since this manuscript was submitted, a number of
publications relevant to this topic have appeared. In particular, the authors wish to
mention the articles in *HLA and Allergy* (A. L. de Weck and M. N. Blumenthal,
eds.), 1977, Volume II of *Monographs in Allergy*, S. Karger, Basel.

ACKNOWLEDGMENTS

The authors wish to thank Dr. W. Riesen for helpful discussion and Mrs.
Margreth Blum for secretarial aid.

This work was supported by the Swiss National Foundation for Scientific
Research.

ANDREAS MORELL
AND SILVIO
BARANDUN

Allansmith, M., McClellan, B. H., Butterworth, M., and Maloney, J. R., 1968, The development of immunoglobulin levels in man, *J. Pediatr.* **72**:276–290.

Allansmith, M., McClellan, B., and Butterworth, M., 1969, The influence of heredity and environment on human immunoglobulin levels, *J. Immunol.* **102**:1504–1510.

Bach, F. H., and van Rood, J. J., 1976, The major histocompatibility complex—Genetics and biology, *New Engl. J. Med.* **295**:806–813.

Bachmann, R., 1965, Studies of the serum IgA level. III. The frequency of A-γA-globulinemia, *Scand. J. Clin. Lab. Invest.* **17**:316–320.

Bazaral, M., Orgel, H. A., and Hamburger, R. N., 1971, IgE levels in normal infants and mothers and an inheritance hypothesis, *J. Immunol.* **107**:794–801.

Benacerraf, B., 1974, Immune response genes, *Scand. J. Immunol.* **3**:381–386.

Benacerraf, B., and McDevitt, H. O., 1972, Histocompatibility linked immune genes, *Science* **175**:273–279.

Bias, W. B., and Marsh, D. G., 1975, *HL-A* linked antigen E immune response genes: An unproved hypothesis, *Science* **188**:375–377.

Biozzi, G., Asofsky, R., Lieberman, R., Stiffel, C., Mouton, D., and Benacerraf, B., 1970, Serum concentrations and allotypes of immunoglobulins in two lines of mice genetically selected for "high" or "low" antibody synthesis, *J. Exp. Med.* **132**:752–764.

Blomberg, B., Geckeler, W. R., and Wiegert, M., 1972, Genetics of the antibody response to dextrans in mice, *Science* **177**:178–180.

Blumenthal, M. N., Amos, D. B., Noreen, H., Mendell, N. R., and Yunis, E. J., 1974, Genetic mapping of *Ir* locus in man: Linkage to second locus of *HL-A*, *Science* **184**:1301–1303.

Brody, J. A., Sever, J. L., and Henson, T. E., 1971, Virus antibody titers in multiple sclerosis patients, siblings and controls, *J. Am. Med. Assoc.* **216**:1441–1446.

Buckley, C. E., III, Dorsey, F. C., Corley, R. B., Ralph, W. B., Woodbury, M. A., and Amos, D. B., 1973, *HL-A* linked human immune-response genes, *Proc. Natl. Acad. Sci. U.S.A.* **70**:2157–2161.

Buckley, R., 1975, Clinical and immunologic features of selective IgA deficiency, in: *Birth Defects: Orig. Artic. Ser. 11: Immunodeficiency in Man and Animals* (D. Bergsma, ed.), pp. 134–142, The National Foundation–March of Dimes. Sinauer Associates, Sunderland, Massachusetts.

Cramer, M., 1974, *Zur Genetik der monklonalen Immunantwort von Inzuchtmäusen gegen Streptokokken-Zellwand-polysaccharide*, Inaugural-Dissertation, Walter Kleikamp, Cologne, Germany.

Dausset, J., and Hors, J., 1975, Some contributions of the *HL-A* complex to the genetics of human diseases, *Transplant. Rev.* **22**:44–74.

Dausset, J., Degos, L., and Hors, J., 1974, The association of the HL-A antigens with diseases, *Clin. Immunol. Immunopathol.* **3**:127–149.

Dunham, E. K., Unanue, E. R., and Benacerraf, B., 1972, Antigen binding and capping by lymphocytes of genetic nonresponder mice, *J. Exp. Med.* **136**:403–408.

Eichmann, K., 1973, Idiotype expression and the inheritance of mouse antibody clones, *J. Exp. Med.* **137**:603–621.

Gitlin, D., 1966, Current aspects of the structure, function and genetics of the immunoglobulins, *Annu. Rev. Med.* **17**:1–22.

Green, I., 1974, Genetic control of immune response, *Immunogenetics* **1**:4–21.

Green, I., Paul, W. E., and Benacerraf, B., 1966, The behaviour of hapten-poly-L-lysine conjugates as complete antigens in genetic responder and as haptens in nonresponder guinea pigs, *J. Exp. Med.* **123**:859–879.

Grubb, R., 1970, *The Genetic Markers of Human Immunoglobulins* (A. Kleinzeller, G. F. Springer, and H. G. Wittman, eds.), Springer-Verlag, Berlin—Heidelberg—New York.

Grundbacher, F. J., 1972a, Human X chromosome carries quantitative genes for immunoglobulin M, *Science* **176**:311–312.

Grundbacher, F. J., 1972b, Genetic aspects of selective immunoglobulin A deficiency, *J. Med. Genet.* **9**:344–347.

Hamburger, R. N., Orgel, H. A., and Bazaral, M., 1973, Genetics of human serum IgE levels, in: *Mechanisms in Allergy: Reagin-Mediated Hypersensitivity* (L. Goodfriend, A. H. Sehon, and R. P. Orange, eds.), pp. 131–139, Marcel Dekker, New York.

Haverkorn, M. J., Hofman, B., Masurel, N., and van Rood, J. J., 1975, *HL-A* linked genetic control of immune response in man, *Transplant. Rev.* **22**:120–124.

Jersild, C., Fog, T., Hansen, G. S., Thomsen, M., Svejgaard, A., and Dupont, B., 1973, Histocompatibility determinants in multiple sclerosis, with special reference to clinical course, *Lancet* **2**:1221–1225.

Jersild, C., Dupont, B., Fog, T., Platz, P., and Svejgaard, A., 1975, Histocompatibility determinants in multiple sclerosis, *Transplant. Rev.* **22**:148–163.

Katz, D. H., and Benacerraf, B., 1975, The function and interrelationships of T-cell receptors, *Ir* genes and other histocompatibility gene products, *Transplant. Rev.* **22**:175–195.

Kindred, B., and Shreffler, D. C., 1972, *H-2* dependence of cooperation between T and B cells *in vivo*, *J. Immunol.* **109**:940–943.

Laitinen, O., and Vesikari, T., 1972, Chronic hepatitis with very high rubella and measles virus antibody titers, *Lancet* **2**:1141.

Levine, B. B., Ojeda, A., and Benacerraf, B., 1963, Basis for the antigenicity of hapten-poly-L-lysine conjugates in random bred guinea pigs, *Nature (London)* **200**:544.

Levine, B. B., Stember, R. H., and Fotino, M., 1972, Ragweed hay fever: Genetic control and linkage to *HL-A* haplotypes, *Science* **178**:1201–1203.

Litwin, S. D., and Balaban, S., 1972, A quantitative method for determining human γG allotype antigens (Gm). II. Differences in Gm gene expression for γG1 and γG3 H chains in sera, *J. Immunol.* **108**:991–999.

Litwin, S. D., and Fudenberg, H. H., 1972, Quantitative abnormalities of allotypic genes in families with primary immune deficiencies, *Proc. Natl. Acad. Sci. U.S.A.* **69**:1739–1743.

Lucas, C. J., Brouwer, R., Feltkamp, T. E. W., ten Veen, J. H., and van Loghem, J. J., 1972, Measles antibodies in sera from patients with autoimmune diseases, *Lancet* **1**:115–116.

MacKay, I. R., Wells, J. V., and Fudenberg, H. H., 1975, Correlation of Gm allotype, antibody response, and mortality, *Clin. Immunol. Immunopathol.* **3**:408–411.

Marsh, D. G., Bias, W. B., Hsu, S. H., and Goodfriend, L., 1973a, Association of the *HL-A* 7 cross-reacting group with a specific reaginic antibody response in allergic man, *Science* **179**:691–693.

Marsh, D. G., Bias, W. B., Hsu, S. H., and Goodfriend, L., 1973b, Associations between major histocompatibility antigens (HL-A) and specific reaginic antibody responses in allergic man, in: *Mechanisms in Allergy: Reagin-Mediated Hypersensitivity* (L. Goodfriend, A. H. Sehon, and R. P. Orange, eds.), pp. 113–129, Marcel Dekker, New York.

Marsh, D. G., Bias, W. B., and Ishizaka, K., 1974, Genetic control of basal serum immunoglobulin E levels and its effect on specific reaginic sensitivity, *Proc. Natl. Acad. Sci. U.S.A.* **71**:3588–3592.

McDevitt, H. O., and Benacerraf, B., 1969, Genetic control of specific immune responses, *Adv. Immunol.* **11**:31–74.

McDevitt, H. O., and Bodmer, W. F., 1974, HL-A, immune response genes and disease. *Lancet* **1**:1269–1275.

McDevitt, H. O., and Chinitz, A., 1969, Genetic control of the antibody response: Relationship between immune response and histocompatibility *(H-2)* type, *Science* **163**:1207–1208.

Mitchell, G. F., Grumet, F. C., and McDevitt, H. O., 1972, Genetic control of the immune response: The effect of thymectomy on the primary and secondary antibody response of mice to poly-L-(Tyr-Glu)-poly-D,L-Ala-poly-L-Lys, *J. Exp. Med.* **135**:126–135.

Morell, A., Skvaril, F., van Loghem, E., and Terry, W. D., 1972, Correlation between the four subclasses of IgG and Gm allotypes in normal human sera, *J. Immunol.* **108**:195–206.

Morell, A., Skvaril, F., and Barandun, S., 1975, Quantitative Aspekte der IgG-Subklassen, in: *IgG-Subklassen der menschlichen Immunglobuline: Immunochemische, genetische, biologische und klinische Aspekte*, pp. 29–59, S. Karger, Basel.

Natvig, J. B., and Kunkel, H. G., 1973, Human immunoglobulins: Classes, subclasses, genetic variants and idiotypes, *Adv. Immunol.* **16**:1–59.

Natvig, J. B., and Kunkel, H. G., 1974, A hybrid IgG4–IgG2 immunoglobulin, *J. Immunol.* **112**:1277–1284.

Okumura, K., and Tada, T., 1971, Regulation of homocytotropic antibody formation in the rat. VI. Inhibitory effect of thymocytes on the homocytotropic antibody response, *J. Immunol.* **107**:1682–1689.

Petranyi, G., Ivanyi, R., and Hollan, S., 1974, Relation of HL-A and Rh systems to immune reactivity: A joint report of the results of the HL-A and Immune Response Workshop, Budapest, 1972, *Vox Sang.* **26**:470–482.

Rhodes, K., Markham, R. L., Maxwell, P. M., and Monk-Jones, M. E., 1969, Immunoglobulins and the X-chromosome. *Br. Med. J.* **3**:439–441.

Shreffler, D. C., and David, C. S., 1975, The *H-2* major histocompatibility complex and the *I* immune response region: Genetic variation, function and organisation, *Adv. Immunol.* **20**:125–195.

Steinberg, A. G., Morell, A., Skvaril, F., and van Loghem, E., 1973, The effect of Gm(23) on the concentration of IgG2 and IgG4 in normal human serum, *J. Immunol.* **110**:1642–1645.

Stiehm, E. R., and Fudenberg, H. H., 1966, Clinical and immunologic features of dysgammaglobulinemia type 1, *Am. J. Med.* **40**:805–815.

Svejgaard, A., Platz, R., Ryder, L. P., Staub-Nielsen, L., and Thomsen, M., 1975, HL-A and disease associations: A survey, *Transplant. Rev.* **22**:3–43.

Triger, D. R., Kurtz, J. B., MacCallum, F. O., and Wright, R., 1972, Raised antibody titers to measles and rubella viruses in chronic active hepatitis, *Lancet* **2**:665–667.

van der Giessen, M., Freyee, W., Rossouw, E., and van Loghem, E., 1973, Qualitative and quantitative studies on IgG2 globulins in individual human sera with an antiserum capable of differentiating between Gm(n+) and Gm(n−) proteins, *Clin. Exp. Immunol.* **14**:127–139.

Walzer, P. D., and Kunkel, H. G., 1974, The correlation of serum IgD concentration with Gm allotype, *J. Immunol.* **113**:274–278.

Wells, J. V., Fudenberg, H. H., and MacKay, I. R., 1971, Relation of the human antibody response to flagellin to Gm genotype, *J. Immunol.* **107**:1505–1511.

Yount, W. J., Kunkel, H. G., and Litwin, S. D., 1967, Studies of the Vi (γ2c) subgroup of γ-globulin: A relationship between concentration and genetic type among normal individuals, *J. Exp. Med.* **125**:177–190.

Yount, W. J., Hong, R., Seligmann, M., Good, R., and Kunkel, H. G., 1970, Imbalances of gammaglobulin subgroups and gene defects in patients with primary hypogammaglobulinemia, *J. Clin. Invest.* **49**:1957–1966.

13

Heavy-Chain Variable (V$_H$) Subgroups among Myeloma Proteins, Antibodies, and Membrane Immunoglobulins of Lymphocytes

J. B. NATVIG, Ø. FØRRE, and T. E. MICHAELSEN

1. Introduction

One of the new developments in studying human immunoglobulins (Ig's) is the determination of variable (V) subgroups of heavy (H) and light (L) chains by serological methods using specific anti-V-subgroup antibodies (Førre *et al.*, 1976a; Natvig *et al.*, 1976b; Tischendorf *et al.*, 1970; McLaughlin and Solomon, 1974). Since the early description of V$_H$ subgroups, only a very few proteins have been sequenced. These few include particularly proteins that have been accessible in large amounts, such as myeloma proteins, and a few antibodies, such as monoclonal cold agglutinins and monoclonal rheumatoid factors (Capra and Kehoe, 1975a,b; Kunkel *et al.*, 1974; Köhler *et al.*, 1970; Nisonoff *et al.*, 1975; Gergely *et al.*, 1973).

More studies have been performed on L chains because they have been more readily accessible to sequence analysis and subsequent determination of Vκ or Vλ subgroups (McLaughlin and Solomon, 1974; Nisonoff *et al.*, 1975; Engelhard and Hilschmann, 1976; Smith *et al.*, 1971).

J. B. NATVIG, Ø. FØRRE, and T. E. MICHAELSEN • Institute of Immunology and Rheumatology, Rikshospitalet University Hospital, Oslo, Norway.

With the development of serological typing systems, however, new fields of investigation have been opened up in studying the subgroups of V_H chains. With such tools, V_H subgroups in normal Ig, in myeloma proteins, and in immune antibodies and other antibodies that are present in serum in low concentrations, as well as in membrane Ig on lymphocytes, could be characterized. In this chapter, we will particularly mention some of the new developments in the field of V_H subgroups as markers of Ig's.

2. Anti-V_H-Subgroup Antisera

A most important aspect of this development has been the raising of specific antisera to each of the three main V_H subgroups (Førre *et al.*, 1976a; Natvig *et al.*, 1976b). These antisera were raised primarily in rabbits but also in some cases in monkeys or other primates by immunization with myeloma proteins of known V_H subgroup according to amino acid sequence analysis. Hyperimmune antisera to such proteins were absorbed extensively to make them V_H-subgroup-specific and to eliminate all the antibodies against the constant (C) regions of the H chains and the antibodies against the L chains. For example, anti-V_HI was absorbed with V_HII and V_HIII proteins, approximately 2–3 mg/ml, to remove all contaminating antibody activity to V_HII and V_HIII proteins. In addition, absorption was made with 1–2 mg/ml pooled L chains and with a myeloma protein that was selected to have the same Ig C-region class and subclass as the myeloma protein used for immunization. In this way, all the antibody activity except the one directed against the V_H subgroup antigens and the idiotypes (Kunkel *et al.*, 1963; Natvig and Kunkel, 1973) was eliminated. No elimination of idiotype specific antibodies was possible because absorption with the homologous protein used for immunization to remove the idiotype antibodies would also remove the V_H-subgroup-specific antibodies. For this reason, it was important to avoid idiotype-specific antibodies in the reaction. This could be done by utilizing a myeloma protein for coating of red cells (see below) different from the one used for immunization. Thus, a different myeloma protein with the same V_H subgroup as the one used for immunization was employed for red cell coating. For each V_H subgroup, at least two different antisera were available, one made against a κ and one against a λ protein. In working with the anti-V_H-subgroup sera in the hemagglutination inhibition tests, the myeloma proteins used for the coating of red cells were also selected to be different in κ or λ types from those used for immunization.

The hemagglutination inhibition tests were carried out by red cells coupled by the chromic chloride method to isolated myeloma proteins of known V_H subgroup (Gold and Fudenberg, 1967). The coated red cells were washed four times in sterile 0.9% saline. From a stock solution of 50 mg chromic chloride ($\times$ 6H_2O) in 5 ml 0.9% NaCl, 0.05 ml was diluted in 0.45 ml 0.9% NaCl. Then, 0.05 ml of the last mixture was added to an equal amount of packed red cells, the tube was shaken for 1 min, and 0.1 ml myeloma proteins (2 mg/ml) was added. The mixture was left at room temperature for 4–5 min, and the coated cells were washed four times with 20–40 volumes excess of saline, and used as a 1% suspension within 24 hr in hemagglutination and inhibition tests as described in detail before (Natvig, 1965; Natvig and Kunkel, 1968).

3. Comparison of V_H Subgroups of the Same Proteins Determined Serologically and by Amino Acid Sequence Analysis

The absorbed V_H-subgroup-specific antisera were utilized in hemagglutination inhibition tests specific for each of the three main V_H subgroups. By comparing the V_H subgroup as originally determined by amino acid sequence analysis with the serological V_H-subgroup determination, we always got the same results for any single myeloma protein. Thus, myeloma proteins with a V_H subgroup defined by amino acid sequence analysis inhibited only in systems with the same V_H-subgroup specificity (Table 1). Since both κ and λ proteins belonging to a given V_H subgroup inhibited equally well, there was clearly no relation to κ- or λ L-chain type. Similarly, no relation was seen to constant H-chain determinants such as Ig classes and subclasses. Furthermore, isolated H chains but not L chains inhibited, and as expected, pooled IgG's or their F(ab')$_2$ fragments showed inhibition in all the V_H-subgroup systems. There was only one possible exception in the system—protein Dau, which was thought from previous amino acid sequence analysis to be either the V_HIII or the V_HIV subgroup (Köhler *et al.*, 1970), but gave a strong inhibition in the V_HIII system, and therefore appeared serologically to be subgroup V_HIII. The V_HIV system is not clearly defined, however, and remains to be further character-

TABLE 1. Inhibition of Serological V_H Subgroup Systems by Myeloma Proteins of Chemically Determined V_H Subgroups, Immunoglobulin Chains, and Fragments

Inhibitor		Test systems[a]		
		V_HI	V_HII	V_HIII
V_HI myeloma proteins				
ND	IgE λ	0.002	–	–
Stu	IgG1κ	0.001	–	–
V_HII myeloma proteins				
Lan	IgA2κ	–	0.002	–
Lev	IgG3λ	–	0.008	–
V_HIII myeloma proteins				
Jon	IgG3λ	–	–	0.002
Falk	IgG1κ	–	–	0.002
Dau	IgHκ	–	–	0.002
Ig chains and fragments				
Pool IgG		0.03	0.008	0.002
Pool H chain		0.03	0.004	0.002
Pool L chain		–	–	–
Pool F(ab')$_2$		0.06	0.008	0.002

[a]Test systems using red cells coated by myeloma proteins (V_HI Stu, V_HII Ou, and V_HIII Tei, respectively), and specifically absorbed anti-V_HI, anti-V_HII, and anti-V_HIII antisera. Concentrations (mg/ml) are the lowest that gave inhibition. (–) No inhibition at a starting dilution of 0.5 mg/ml.

ized (Putnam, personal communication). Determination of V_H subgroups has also recently been attempted with types of chemical analysis other than amino acid sequencing. One technique is to determine whether the proteins have blocked (usually V_HI and V_HII proteins) or unblocked (usually V_HIII proteins) *N*-terminal (Capra and Kehoe, 1975b). The other technique uses typing of tryptic or chymotryptic peptides (Moulin *et al.*, 1975). There was also an overall good correlation between serological V_H typing and these two chemical V_H-typing techniques, there being, with only one exception, complete agreement between the serological system and the two chemical systems (Table 2). Whether this one exception could be due to technical difficulties or to other reasons is not known.

4. Serologically Determined V_H Subgroups in Myeloma Proteins with Previously Unknown V_H Subgroups

Altogether, 131 myeloma proteins with previously unknown V_H subgroups were typed serologically in addition to the 36 proteins that had previously been typed by some of the chemical techniques mentioned above. The results are shown in Table 3. All the proteins except two were typable in only one of the three serological subgroups. These two proteins, which were not V_HI, V_HII, or V_HIII by the present test systems, might represent other V_H subgroups or, alternatively, rare genetic variants of these subgroups (Førre *et al.*, 1976a).

The percentage distribution of V_H subgroups in the total material of 167 myeloma proteins was almost the same as in the previously unclassified group. It showed V_HIII to be the predominant subgroup, representing 50% of the total Ig, while V_HII comprised 33% and V_HI about 16% of the total. Thus, there was an overall ratio of approximately 1 : 2 : 3 for V_HI/V_HII/V_HIII. The relative distribution of the V_H subgroups within the different Ig classes and subclasses was also studied. For the IgG class, the distribution was nearly the same as for total Ig, but slightly more V_HII and slightly less V_HIII. Particularly, IgG3 had a rather high percentage for V_HII, and IgG2 was rather high for V_HI. Further analysis of the IgG subclasses is required, however, to establish a significant relationship. In the case of IgA, about 70% belonged to the V_HIII, while the V_HI was low. For the IgM proteins, V_HII was lower and V_HI higher than the average for Ig. Although the IgD and IgE myeloma proteins were rare, the study showed that these proteins also utilized the same V_H pool.

TABLE 2. Comparison of V_H-Subgroup Typing by Serological and Two Chemical Methods

	Serological typing		
Chemical typing	V_HI	V_HII	V_HIII
Peptide analysis			
V_HI	1		
V_HII		2	
V_HIII		1	5
N-terminal amino acid			
Blocked		3	
Unblocked			4

TABLE 3. Relationship among Immunoglobulin Classes, Subclasses, and V_H Subgroups in 167 Myeloma Proteins[a]

Class	V_HI			V_HII			V_HIII			Unclassified		
	U	T	%	U	T	%	U	T	%	U	T	%
IgG1	7	12	(18)	22	25	(37)	23	31	(45)	—	—	—
IgG2	4	4	(27)	4	4	(27)	7	7	(46)	—	—	—
IgG3	0	1	(5)	7	9	(47)	7	8	(42)	1	1	(5)
IgG4	1	1	(11)	1	3	(33)	3	4	(44)	1	1	(11)
Total IgG	12	18	(16)	34	41	(37)	40	50	(45)	2	2	(2)
IgA1	1	1	(5)	3	5	(28)	12	12	(67)	—	—	—
IgA2	—	—	—	1	1	(20)	1	4	(80)	—	—	—
Total IgA	1	1	(4)	4	6	(26)	13	16	(70)	—	—	—
IgM	6	7	(24)	7	8	(28)	9	14	(48)	—	—	—
IgD	—	—	—	—	—	—	2	2	(100)	—	—	—
IgE	0	1	(50)	—	—	—	1	1	(50)	—	—	—
Total Ig	19	27	(16)	45	55	(33)	65	83	(50)	2	2	(1)

[a] (U) Myeloma proteins with unknown V_H subgroups; (T) total of myeloma proteins with chemically defined V_H subgroups and myeloma proteins with unknown V_H subgroups; (%) percentage of classes, subclasses, and total Ig.

5. Relative Amounts of the V_H Subgroups in Different Human Sera

A total of 13 normal Caucasian sera including sera from 3 homozygous $Gm(a+g+)$ and 3 homozygous $Gm(f+b+)$ subjects as well as Japanese and Negro sera were also tested. Semiquantitative hemagglutination inhibition experiments were performed with the V_H-subgroup systems that had similar sensitivity and were inhibited by positive myeloma proteins down to a concentration of 0.002–0.008 mg/ml. In all cases, there was less inhibition in the V_HI system than in the other test systems. The normal sera inhibited in a maximum dilution of 256–512 in the V_HI system, while inhibition was seen in dilutions from 1024 to 4096 in the V_HII and V_HIII systems, again with somewhat stronger inhibition in the V_HIII system. No obvious relationship was observed between the inhibitory capacity in the V_H subgroup systems and the population groups with different Gm types.

6. Restriction of Immune and Natural Human Antibodies for V_H Subgroups

Anti-D, which is the most common anti-Rh antibody specificity, was first tested. ORh(D)-positive erythrocytes were sensitized with each of 45 different anti-D-antisera (Førre *et al.*, 1976b) and subsequently tested with an anti-Ig-antiserum and with anti-V_HI-, anti-V_HII-, and anti-V_HIII-subgroup-specific antisera. Surprisingly, 40 of 45 anti-D antibodies reacted only with anti-V_HII, and not with anti-V_HI or anti-V_HIII (Table 4). Some other antibody preparations showed different patterns, but on the whole, there was a striking restriction to the V_HII subgroup, as discussed in further detail by Natvig *et al.* (1976b).

For some other incomplete IgG antibodies, there was a similar restriction; anti-C was particularly restricted to the V_HIII subgroup, as was anti-Kell. Some other incomplete red cell antibodies, however, showed less restriction. The specificity of the reactions was investigated in a series of experiments, and antibodies that gave a specific reaction with a certain anti-V_H-antiserum could, for example, be used in hemagglutination and inhibition studies to detect the corresponding V_H subgroup (Natvig *et al.*, 1976b).

Also, restrictions of other red cell antibodies were studied, particularly anti-A and anti-B of the IgG class. This was done by coating red cells with subagglutinating doses of the IgG antibody and performing similar tests as described above for anti-Rh antibodies using the same anti-V_H antisera (Table 5). These studies showed that anti-A was primarily restricted to V_HI, while anti-B was mostly V_HIII. Some absorption experiments were also performed that indicated that the IgM anti-A

TABLE 4. Subgroup of IgG Anti-D Antibodies

Total	Anti-Ig (R : 115)	Anti-V_HI (R : 483)	Anti-V_HII (R : 161)	Anti-V_HIII (R : 349)
21	256–2048	< 2	256–512	< 2
16	256–1024	< 2	64–128	< 2
3	256–512	< 2	16–32	< 2
2	512–1024	8	128	< 2
1	2048	32	512	64
2	512	< 2	< 2	16–64

TABLE 5. Distribution of Serological V$_H$ Subgroups Among Anti-A, Anti-B, and Anti-Duffy IgG Antibodies

Cells sensitized with:	N^a	Titers obtained with various antisera			
		Anti-Ig (R : 115)	Anti-V$_H$I (R : 483)	Anti-V$_H$II (R : 161)	Anti-V$_H$III (R : 349)
IgG anti-A	6	128–1024	16–64	< 2	< 2
	2	128–512	16	4	< 2
	3	128–1024	32–64	4–8	2–4
	2	64–1024	< 2	< 2	16–32
IgG anti-B	21	64–1024	< 2	< 2	8–64
	1	512	4	< 2	32
	4	1024	4	4	64
IgG anti-Fy(a)	3	128–256	8–16	< 2	< 2
	2	256	2–4	16	2–4
	1	128	32	4	< 2
IgG anti-Fy(b)	3	256–512	< 2	< 2	16–64
	1	256	< 2	16	< 2

^{a}Number of antierythrocyte antibodies in various agglutination pattern groups.

showed a similar restriction to V$_H$I, as did IgG anti-A, and that IgM anti-B showed a restriction to the V$_H$III subgroup similar to that shown by IgG anti-B (Førre *et al.*, 1977a).

7. V$_H$ Subgroups of Membrane Immunoglobulin of Normal Human Lymphocytes

Lymphocytes from normal donors were isolated by the Isopaque–Ficoll technique (Bøyum, 1976). Lymphocytes from both normal donors and patients with chronic lymphocytic leukemias (CLLs) were tested using immunofluorescence technique as described before (Frøland and Natvig, 1973).

Lymphocytes from 20 normal blood donors were stained with FITC-conjugated anti-F(ab')$_2$, anti-V$_H$I-, anti-V$_H$II-, and anti-V$_H$III-subgroup-specific antisera. The means of the percentage of staining were 2.9, 5.0, and 5.5% for the V$_H$I, V$_H$II, and V$_H$III subgroups, respectively (Table 6) (Førre *et al.*, 1976c). In addition, the sum of the percentages of the lymphocytes stained with each of the V$_H$-subgroup-specific antisera corresponded well with the percentages of the lymphocytes stained with an anti-F(ab')$_2$ antiserum. Also, by double immunofluorescence staining as well as in various depletion experiments (Table 7) and tests with thymocytes and lymphocytes from hypogammaglobulinemic patients, it was shown that the staining with V$_H$-subgroup-specific antisera corresponded to the membrane Ig-positive cells, i.e., the B-lymphocyte population.

8. V$_H$ Subgroups of Membrane Immunoglobulin of Chronic Lymphocytic Leukemia Cells

Lymphocytes from 20 patients with CLL were studied for membrane staining by direct immunofluorescence employing anti-F(ab')$_2$-, anti-V$_H$I-, anti-V$_H$II-, and anti-V$_H$III-subgroup-specific antisera, as well as L-chain-specific antisera (Table 8).

Some lymphocyte preparations were also studied in indirect immunofluorescence using an antiserum raised against a fragment (V_H) corresponding to the V region of the H chain of a human IgG3 myeloma protein (Kup). Lymphocytes from each CLL patient demonstrated a restriction of V_H subgroups expressed on the cell membrane; 6 were restricted to the V_HI subgroup, 7 to the V_HII subgroup, and 7 to the V_HIII subgroup (Førre *et al.*, 1977c). This restriction gave further evidence for

TABLE 6. Percentages of Peripheral Blood Lymphocytes Stained with Antisera against F(ab')$_2$ as well as the V_HI, V_HII, and V_HIII Subgroups

Donor	Staining with: Anti-F(ab')$_2$	Anti-V_HI	Anti-V_HII	Anti-V_HIII
9	16	3	8	4
68	10	1	2	7
70	5	1	1	2
75	25	5	5	10
109	10	2	3	6
118	17	4	7	5
125	16	3	6	6
194	16	1	7	4
196	12	2	3	6
250	18	4	5	8
314	5	2	0	2
316	7	2	3	2
347	14	6	5	7
393	18	3	10	5
410	9	2	3	5
544	18	4	8	10
799	22	5	12	9
943	8	1	6	2
946	6	1	2	5
997	14	6	4	5
Mean	13.2	2.9	5.0	5.5
(range)	(5–25)	(1–6)	(1–12)	(2–10)

TABLE 7. Distribution of V_H Subgroups on Normal Peripheral Lymphocytes after B-Lymphocyte Depletion on Nylon Wool Columns[a]

Donor	Before fractionation F(ab')$_2$[b]	After fractionation			
		F(ab')$_2$	V_HI	V_HII	V_HIII
157	15	1	< 1	1	1
182	9	1	1	< 1	< 1
183	25	5	2	2	< 1
184	11	2	< 1	< 1	1
185	17	2	1	< 1	< 1
186	17	1	< 1	< 1	< 1
187	11	1	< 1	< 1	< 1
188	9	< 1	< 1	< 1	< 1
191	12	2	< 1	< 1	2

[a] Percentage of cells with membrane fluorescence.
[b] Anti-F(ab')$_2$ staining before fractionation on nylon wool columns.

TABLE 8. Distribution of V$_H$ Subgroups, Classes, and Light Chains on Peripheral Lymphocytes from Patients with Chronic Lymphocytic Leukemias [a]

Patient	Leukocyte count in Peripheral blood	Percentages of lymphocytes with membrane-bound Ig stained with antiserum against:								
		F(ab')$_2$	V$_H$I	V$_H$II	V$_H$III	IgG	IgM	IgD	κ	λ
		IgM or IgM and IgD								
M.F.	60,000	99	—	99	—	—	99	90	—	99
L.E.	30,000	90	—	85	—	—	85	—	88	—
Ø.A.	40,000	87	85	—	—	—	60	—	90	—
H.K.	30,000	99	—	—	98	—	98	—	99	—
H.E.	7,500	30	2	1	28	2	25	5	20	8
I.B.	150,000	96	—	90	—	6	90	50	5	95
K.D.	30,000	90	70	—	10	—	40	80	80	—
L.E.	80,000	90	—	—	90	—	70	—	—	70
O.R.	76,000	90	—	—	85	—	70	60	80	—
G.F.	20,000	90	3	80	5	—	85	40	NT	NT
K.G.	25,000	75	5	70	3	—	60	40	NT	NT
S.A.	30,000	80	2	4	80	—	70	75	NT	NT
A.K.	170,000	91	93	7	—	—	90	70	70	—
S.B.	100,000	91	78	—	—	—	80	60	80	—
		IgG								
A.S.	70,000	98	—	93	—	95	—	—	2	80
R.L.	50,000	85	—	—	80	80	—	—	60	—
		Unclassified								
K.G.	22,000	90	—	90	—	NT	NT	NT	NT	NT
B.M.	103,000	90	—	—	85	NT	NT	NT	NT	NT
R.A.	70,000	97	96	—	—	NT	NT	NT	NT	NT
A.S.	65,000	98	95	—	—	NT	NT	NT	NT	NT

[a] Not tested.

monoclonality of the membrane-bound Ig in the leukemic cell proliferation. Antiserum to a V$_H$ fragment stained closely similar percentages of CLL lymphocytes to that obtained with anti-F(ab')$_2$ antiserum. Furthermore, double staining revealed that the same cells were stained with anti-V$_H$ antiserum as were stained with anti-F(ab')$_2$ antiserum, i.e., only the B lymphocytes were stained (Førre *et al.*, 1977c).

9. Comments

V-region subgroups were first determined serologically on κ chains that corresponded with V$_κ$ subgroups revealed by amino acid sequence analysis (McLaughlin and Solomon, 1974). These studies were later extended, and serological typing was used for extensive studies on κ chains in various cross-idiotypic systems and for defining subgroups of κ chains (Capra and Kehoe, 1975a; Kunkel *et al.*, 1974). Serological methods were also used to discriminate V$_λ$ subgroups (Tischendorf *et al.*, 1970). By using carefully absorbed antisera against myeloma proteins with known V$_H$ subgroups from sequence studies and taking precautions to avoid idiotypic antibodies and antibodies to genetic determinants, L-chain antigens, and other determinants, we have been able to establish a serological typing system for the V$_H$ subgroups of H chains (Førre *et al.*, 1976a). Some other recent studies were also aimed at detecting V$_H$ subgroups serologically, particularly the V$_H$III subgroup (Rivat *et al.*, 1976; Feizi *et al.*, 1976). In our test systems, we also studied restriction to certain V_H subgroups of immune and natural human antibodies. Typing of antibodies for V_H subgroups has previously been performed only in certain rare instances of monoclonal cold agglutinins or rheumatoid factors where large amounts of protein can be obtained for sequence studies (Capra and Kehoe, 1975a; Kunkel *et al.*, 1974). The present technique had its major advantage in situations in which the chemical techniques could not be used because they require too large protein samples. V_H subgroups were determined in pooled Ig and in human immune antibodies. In the latter studies, a striking restriction was obtained in several instances. In the majority of cases of anti-Rh(D), there was a restriction to one particular V_H subgroup for a single antibody specificity in a given subject. In some cases, there was also an overall restriction in different individuals to one particular subgroup for antibodies with the same antibody specificity. This was particularly so for anti-D, which was restricted to V_HII, and for the anti-Kell, which was particularly restricted to V_HIII (Natvig *et al.*, 1976b). Similar studies on anti-A showed that this antibody activity was particularly related to V_HI, while anti-B IgG was related to V_HIII, although exceptions were found. Some preliminary studies have also been made with rheumatoid factors of the polyclonal type, which in several instances also show restriction, particularly to the V_HII or the V_HIII subgroup (Førre *et al.*, 1977b).

Anti-V_H-subgroup antisera also have an advantage in studying V_H subgroups of membrane Ig of lymphocytes. Our studies showed that V_H reagents react only with the Ig-positive B lymphocytes, and no indications were obtained for reactions with other cells than B lymphocytes (Førre *et al.*, 1976c, 1977c). Furthermore, each lymphocyte appeared to express only one V_H subgroup in the case of both normal peripheral blood lymphocytes and lymphocytes in CLL.

Recent studies on the idiotypes indicated that idiotype residues linked to the H-chain genetic markers are found on T lymphocytes (Janeway *et al.*, 1976). This might suggest that V regions of H chains are involved. It is somewhat surprising that we could not find V_H subgroup antigens by the immunofluorescence techniques utilized here on other cells than B lymphocytes. Thus, we have so far no indication for the presence of V_H-subgroup determinants described in this study on the T lymphocytes. More sensitive techniques will probably be required to see whether the framework amino acid residues that we detect by our reagents can be traced on these cells. Such studies are being performed at present.

References

Bøyum, A., 1976, Isolation of lymphocytes, granulocytes, and macrophages, *Scand. J. Immunol. Suppl.* **5**:9–15.

Capra, J. D., and Kehoe, J. M., 1975a, Hypervariable regions, idiotypy and the antibody-combining site, *Adv. Immunol.* **20**-1–40.

Capra, J. D., and Kehoe, J. M., 1975b, Distribution and association of heavy and light chain variable region subgroups among human IgA immunoglobulins, *J. Immunol.* **114**:678–681.

Engelhard, M., and Hilschmann, N., 1975, Die Aminosäuresequenz einer monoklonalen Immunglobulin-L-Kette vom λ-Typ, Subgruppe I (Bence–Jones Protein Vor), *Hoppe-Seyler's Z. Physiol. Chem.* **356**:1413–1444.

Feizi, T., Lecomte, J., Childs, R., and Solomon, A., 1976, Kappa chain (V_κIII) subgroup-related activity in an idiotypic anti-cold agglutinin serum, *Scand. J. Immunol.* **5**:629–636.

Frøland, S. S., and Natvig, J. B., 1973, Indentification of three different human lymphocyte populations by surface markers, *Transplant. Rev.* **16**:114–162.

Førre, Ø., Natvig, J. B., and Kunkel, H. B., 1976a, Serological detection of variable region (V_H) subgroups of Ig heavy chains, *J. Exp. Med.* **144**:897–905.

Førre, Ø., Michaelsen, T. E., and Natvig, J. B., 1976b, Antibody activity of heavy and light chains and recombined IgG of human IgG anti-D, *Scand. J. Immunol.* **5**:155–160.

Førre, Ø., Natvig, J. B., Frøland, S. S., and Johnson, P. M., 1976c, Distribution of heavy-chain variable-region (V_H) subgroups on human lymphocytes, *Scand. J. Immunol.* **5**:1221–1226.

Førre, Ø., Gaarder, P. I., and Natvig, J. B., 1977a, V_H subgroup restriction in human red cell antibodies: Studies on anti-A, anti-B and anti-Duffy antibodies, *Scand. J. Immunol.* **6**:149–156.

Førre, Ø., Johnson, P. M., and Natvig, J. B., 1977b, A study of the variable heavy chain (V_H) regions in human polyclonal IgM rheumatoid factors, *Scand. J. Rheumatol.* **6**:113–117.

Førre, Ø., Frøland, S. S., Natvig, J. B., Michaelsen, E., Johnson, P. M., Ly, B., and Laake, K., 1977c, A study of the variable heavy chain (V_H) region of membrane bound Ig on human chronic leukemic lymphocytes, *J. Immunol.* **118**:1513–1516.

Gergely, J., Wang, A. C., and Fudenberg, H. H., 1973, Chemical analysis of variable regions of heavy and light chains of cold agglutinins, *Vox. Sang.* **24**:432–440.

Gold, E. R., and Fudenberg, H. H., 1967, Chromic cloride: A coupling reagent for passive hemagglutination reactions, *J. Immunol.* **99**:859–866.

Janeway, C. A., Wigzell, H., and Binz, H., 1976, Two different V_H gene products make up the T-cell receptors, *Scand. J. Immunol.* **5**:993–1001.

Köhler, H., Shimizu, S., Paul, C., Moore, W., and Putman, F. W., 1970, Three variable gene pools common to IgM, IgG and IgA immunoglobulins, *Nature (London)* **227**:1318–1320.

Kunkel, H. G., Mannik, M., and Williams, R. C., 1963, Individual antigenic specificity of isolated antibodies, *Science* **140**:1218–1219.

Kunkel, H. G., Winchester, R. J., Joslin, F. G., and Capra, J. D., 1974, Similarities in the light chains of anti-γ-globulins showing cross-idiotypic specificities, *J. Exp. Med.* **139**:128–136.

McLaughlin, C. L., and Solomon, A., 1974, Immunochemical classification and nonisolated light chains of immunoglobulins, *J. Immunol.* **113**:1369–1372.

Moulin, A., Eskinazi, D., De Preval, C., and Fougereau, M., 1975, Chemical typing of human immunoglobulin V_H subgroups, *Immunochemistry* **12**-883–892.

Natvig, J. B., 1965, Quantitative determinations of incomplete anti-D antibodies in reaction with anti-Gm factors, *Acta Pathol. Microbiol. Scand.* **65**:570–580.

Natvig, J. B., and Kunkel, H. G., 1968, Genetic markers of human immunoglobulins: The Gm and Inv systems, *Ser. Haematol.* **1**:66–96.

Natvig, J. B., and Kunkel, H. G., 1973, Human immunoglobulins: Classes, subclasses, genetic variants, and idiotypes, *Adv. Immunol.* **16**:1–59.

Natvig, J. B., Kunkel, H. G., Rosenfield, R., Dalton, J. F., and Kochwa, S., 1976a, Idiotypic specificities of anti-Rh antibodies, *J. Immunol.* **116**:1536–1538.

Natvig, J. B., Førre, Ø., and Michaelsen, T., 1976b, Restriction of human immune antibodies to heavy-chain variable region subgroups, *Scand. J. Immunol.* **5**:667–675.

Nisonoff, A., Hopper, J. E., and Spring, S. B., 1975, Nature of the active site of an antibody molecule and the mechanism of antibody–hapten interactions, in: *The Antibody Molecule*, (F. J. Dixon and H. G. Kunkel, eds.), Academic Press, New York.

Rivat, L., Rivat, C., Lebreton, J.-P., and Ropartz, C., 1976, Antigenic determinants of heavy chain variable regions: Immunological typing of the human immunoglobulin V_HIII subgroup, *Eur. J. Immunol.* **6**:624–629.

Smith, G. P., Hood, L., and Fitch, W. M., 1971, Antibody diversity, *Annu. Rev. Biochem.* **40**:969–1012.

Tischendorf, F. W., Tischendorf, M. M., and Osserman, E. F., 1970, Subgroup-specific antigenic marker on immunoglobulin lambda chains: Identification of three subtypes of the variable region, *J. Immunol.* **1**-**5**:1033–1035.

14

Cryoglobulins and Pyroglobulins

HORACE H. ZINNEMAN

1. Cryoglobulins

1.1. Definition

A heterogeneous group of immunoglobulins (Ig's), each member of which exhibits a temperature-dependent solubility abnormality, are known as *cryoglobulins*. A single Ig with the property of reversible cryoprecipitation is usually monoclonal. More frequently, two Ig's combine by noncovalent bonds to form a mixed cryoglobulin, but when separated, neither is a cryoglobulin by itself. Cryoglobulins are usually found in blood serum, but occasionally may appear in body fluids and urine.

In plasma or serum or in solutions of physiological pH, these globulins precipitate or form a gel at temperatures below 37°C. The greater their concentration, the higher the maximum temperature at which cryoprecipitation takes place. Lower concentrations usually precipitate at or near 4°C. It is a characteristic and part of the definition of cryoglobulins that they promptly and completely go into solution again on being heated to 37°C. Single monoclonal cryoglobulins can be chilled and reheated for an undetermined number of times without change, whereas mixed cryoglobulins may produce progressively smaller cryoprecipitates with each cycle of chilling and heating (Volpé *et al.*, 1956; Lewis *et al.*, 1966).

1.2. Historical Notes

The first recorded observations of cryoglobulins in human serum are of relatively recent date. Wintrobe and Buell (1933) studied a patient who manifested what became to be known later as the classic syndrome of cryoglobulinemia. Since this patient's disease was multiple myeloma, the comparison of his cryoprecipitable

---

HORACE H. ZINNEMAN • Department of Medicine, Veterans Administration Hospital and University of Minnesota Medical School, Minneapolis, Minnesota.

serum protein with Bence Jones proteins, known for their abnormal thermally dependent solubility, was tempting.

Cryoglobulins and cryoglobulinemia were not recognized as an entity prior to the studies of Lerner and Watson (1947) and Lerner *et al.*, (1947). They introduced the terminology "cryoglobulin," recognizing that they were dealing with γ-globulins the solubility of which was dependent on temperature. They also recognized the effect of pH and ionization on cryoprecipitation, and their clinical studies found cryoglobulins in chronic infections, rheumatoid disease, alcoholic cirrhosis, and several neoplastic diseases.

This state of information remained essentially unchanged until advanced laboratory technology permitted detailed characterization of these abnormal Ig's. Newer laboratory techniques, such as immunoelectrophoresis, gel filtration, chromatography, analytical ultracentrifugation, and amino acid analysis revealed the heterogeneity of cryoglobulins, although all of them are Ig's, single Ig's as well as combinations of two or three. Occasionally, it was found that an intact Ig was not always necessary for the phenomenon of reversible cryoprecipitability. Light (L) chains, occurring in their free form as Bence Jones proteins in multiple myeloma, occasionally showed typical cryoglobulin properties.

The investigation and characterization of these Ig's, though fascinating in itself, also provides valuable information on the solubility of proteins in general.

1.3. Clinical Manifestations of Cryoglobulinemia

1.3.1. At the Bedside

The classic manifestations of cryoglobulinemia are observed at high serum concentrations of these abnormal proteins. Conversely, not all patients with high cryoglobulin concentrations offer typical signs or symptoms. Intolerance of cold or even cool temperatures manifested by pain of exposed parts of the body, particularly fingers, toes, nose, and ears, is found in less than 50% of afflicted patients (Brouet *et al.*, 1974). A number of these patients suffer a rather typical Raynaud's syndrome (MacKay *et al.*, 1956; Cohen *et al.*, 1967; Saha *et al.*, 1968; Hewitt *et al.*, 1970; Sargent *et al.*, 1970; Zlotnick *et al.*, 1972; Rigo *et al.*, 1973; Reza *et al.*, 1974; Rubens-Duval *et al.*, 1974), sometimes terminating in gangrene of the aforementioned areas. Bullous erythema was reported by Charmot *et al.* (1959), and urticaria, purpura, and arthralgia are common skin manifestations of the disease syndrome (Costanzi *et al.*, 1965; Flad *et al.*, 1968; Hewitt *et al.*, 1970; Charmot *et al.*, 1959; Meltzer *et al.*, 1966; Thivolet *et al.*, 1967; Lapes and Davies, 1970; Hansson and Lindström, 1973). These lesions not only appear on exposure to low temperature, but also may emerge independent of temperature, leaving residual brownish pigmentation. Their histological appearance is one of acute vasculitis with fibrinoid necrosis of vascular walls, perivascular infiltration by polymorphonuclear leukocytes, and hyaline-appearing intravascular deposits (Miescher *et al.*, 1965; Flad *et al.*, 1968; Hewitt *et al.*, 1970; Cream, 1972).

Vascular obstruction may lead to regional dermal ischemia and ulcerations at the lower extremities. The presence of chronic leg ulcers in the supramalleolar region in the absence of severe stasis dermatitis should prompt an investigation for serum cryoglobulins (Logothetis *et al.*, 1968; Hewitt *et al.*, 1970; Brody and

Samitz, 1973). Serum viscosity frequently is sufficiently increased, even in the absence of lower temperatures, to result in a hyperviscosity syndrome, including "boxcar appearance" of retinal vessels (O'Reilly and MacKenzie, 1967), amaurosis, or peripheral neuropathy (Siguier *et al.*, 1964; Logothetis *et al.*, 1968; Reza *et al.*, 1974). The central nervous system may be involved with commonly transient hemiplegia or dysarthria (Marshall and Malone, 1945; O'Reilly and MacKenzie, 1967). Muirhead *et al.* (1952) reported cryoglobulinemia with serum hyperviscosity and intracapillary pulmonary stasis, leading to severe cyanosis. Generally, it can be stated that 85% of all mixed cryoglobulins of Types II and III are associated with some type of clinical sign or symptom, whereas only 50% of single monoclonal cryoglobulineminas (Type I) are clinically symptomatic.

1.3.2. Diseases Likely to be Associated with Cryoglobulinemia

Clinically significant and symptomatic cryoglobulinemia may occur without the perceptible primary or precipitating disease (Volpé *et al.*, 1956; Domz and Feigin, 1957; Allen, 1966; Baughman and Sommer, 1966; Costanzi and Coltman, 1967; Matuhasi and Mitsuko, 1968; Wager *et al.*, 1968b; Zinneman *et al.*, 1968; Grossman *et al.*, 1972). In the majority of patients, however, the appearance of cryoglobulinemia can be attributed to primary diseases, most of which are known to be associated with abnormalities of Ig synthesis or metabolism, autoimmune or hypersensitivity phenomena, or persistent antigenic stimuli. The original observations by Wintrobe and Buell (1933) were made in a patient with multiple myeloma, and since that time, a considerable number of the monoclonal Ig's of that disease have been shown to possess the physicochemical properties of cryoglobulins (Marshall and Malone, 1954; Brauman *et al.*, 1956; Meltzer and Franklin, 1966; Cohen *et al.*, 1967; Grey *et al.*, 1968; Seligmann *et al.*, 1968; Bogaars *et al.*, 1973; Brouet *et al.*, 1974; Watanabe *et al.*, 1974). Occasionally, the free L chains of Bence Jones proteins in urine and sometimes in the serum assumed the properties of cryoglobulins (Varriale *et al.*, 1962; Alper, 1966; Liss *et al.*, 1967; Zinneman *et al.*, 1968; Cuprak *et al.*, 1970; Brouet *et al.*, 1974; Harris and Kohn, 1974). Occasionally, the monoclonal IgM of macroglobulinemia is a cryoglobulin, likely to pose the combined problems of cryoprecipitation and excessive blood viscosity (Braunsteiner *et al.*, 1954; MacKay *et al.*, 1956; Meltzer and Franklin, 1966; O'Reilly *et al.*, 1967; Bonomo *et al.*, 1970; Macris *et al.*, 1970; Caronia *et al.*, 1972; Brody and Samitz, 1973; Zinneman *et al.*, 1973; Brouet *et al.*, 1974). Diseases of hypersensitivity and autoimmunity are often associated with cryoglobulins, occasionally at concentrations sufficient to cause clinical phenomena: vasculitis (Barnett *et al.*, 1970; Cream, 1972; Klein *et al.*, 1972), scleroderma (Perrot *et al.*, 1971), polyarteritis nodosa (Logothetis *et al.*, 1968; Brouet *et al.*, 1974), and disseminated lupus erythematosus (Hanauer and Christian, 1967; Mustakallio *et al.*, 1967; Stastny and Ziff, 1969; Perrot *et al.*, 1971; Klein *et al.*, 1972). Cryoglobulinemia with monoclonal components, either singly as Type I or mixed as in Type II, has been seen in association with chronic glomerulonephritis (Porush *et al.*, 1969; McIntosh *et al.*, 1971; Kaufman and McIntosh, 1971). It must be remembered, however, that cryoglobulinemia may occur as a complicating consequence of streptococcal glomerulonephritis as well as represent the primary cause for immune-complex glomerulonephritis. Diseases associated with autoimmune phenomena may exhibit cryoglobulins in the sera of afflicted patients, although these proteins may or may not produce recognizable symptoms. In this disease group, cryoglobulins are found most often in rheumatoid arthritis (Emori *et al.*, 1973), Sjögren's syndrome (Logothetis *et al.*, 1968; Waldmann *et al.*, 1971; Klein *et al.*, 1972; Rigo *et al.*, 1973; Rubens-Duval and Kaplan, 1974), ulcerative colitis (Polčák *et al.*, 1967; Reza *et al.*, 1974), and chronic hepatitis and cirrhosis (Braunsteiner *et al.*, 1954; Biserte, 1961; Feizi and Gitlin, 1969; Jori and Buonanno, 1972; Zlotnick *et al.*, 1972; Florin-Christensen *et al.*, 1974).

Interestingly enough, persistent antigenic challenges may stimulate increased synthesis not only of "normal" Ig's, but also of cryoglobulins in rabbits (Herd, 1973a,b) and humans (Schultz and Yunis, 1975) and experimental animals (Davie *et al.*, 1968). Chronic infections are a common cause of persistent antigenic stimulation, and not surprisingly, subacute bacterial endocarditis (Caperton and Williams, 1969; Hurwitz *et al.*, 1975), chronic brucellosis (Lerner and Watson, 1947), sarcoidosis (Turkington and Buckley, 1966), lepromatous leprosy (Matthews and Trautman, 1965), rheumatic fever (Seligmann *et al.*, 1968), and others have been found to be associated with cryoglobulinemia, usually of Type III. Cryoglobulinemia may also be observed in viral infections that are considered to be acute. Thus, mixed cryoglobulins have been described by Wager *et al.* (1968), Kaplan (1968), and Capra *et al.* (1971) in infectious mononucleosis and cytomegalovirus mononucleosis (Wager *et al.*, 1968a,b; Barnett *et al.*, 1970). Antigenic challenges and stimuli may also play a role in malignant or neoplastic diseases. Cryoglobulinemia has been described in malignant lymphoma and chronic lymphatic leukemia (Lerner *et al.*, 1947; Lewis *et al.*, 1966; Logothetis *et al.*, 1968; Krauss and Sokal, 1966; Perrot *et al.*, 1971; Brouet *et al.*, 1974), carcinoma (Balázs and Fröhlich, 1966), and mycosis fungoides (Perrot *et al.*, 1971).

Cryoglobulinemia is by no means a rare laboratory finding, but in the majority of cases, serum cryoglobulins are found in small concentrations, and their significance is not always clear. In most infections, they disappear with cessation or cure of the disease, although they do not appear to be specific responses to the antigenic challenge of the primary disease (Hurwitz *et al.*, 1975).

1.3.3. Cryoglobulins in the Clinical Laboratory

Serum cryoglobulins in low concentrations may not readily be noticed unless special measures are taken to assure that none of them precipitates within the fibrin meshwork at the time of blood clot formation and retraction. Concentrations of 1.5 g/100 ml and above may be heralded by the difficulty of venipuncture caused by the precipitation of protein in the aspirating needle. If part or all of the cryoglobulin disappears within the blood clot, a determination of its serum concentration would *a priori* be erroneous, and in the case of gel-formation, the amount of serum that can be separated from the clot may be quite scanty, leading to erroneously high hematocrit and low serum globulin values. The erythrocyte sedimentation rate will be erroneously low when performed in the routine manner at room temperature; the correct value can be obtained by performing the procedure at 37°C. The properties of cold-agglutinins differ from cryoglobulins, but occasionally an IgM may possess both properties (Macris *et al.*, 1970). Some cryoglobulins, particularly the monoclonal components of mixed cryoglobulins, have antiglobulin activity, thus conferring significant latex fixation titers for "rheumatoid factor" (Costanzi *et al.*, 1965; Miescher *et al.*, 1965; Golde and Epstein, 1968; Wager *et al.*, 1968b; Zinneman *et* al., 1968; Caperton and Williams, 1969; Feizi and Gitlin, 1969; Porush *et al.*, 1969; Capra *et al.*, 1969; Bonomo *et al.*, 1970; Reza *et al.*, 1974; Takeda *et al.*, 1974). Anticomplementary activity has been ascribed to some mixed cryoglobulins by Balázs and Fröhlich (1966), Baughman and Sommer (1966), Mustakallio *et al.* (1967), and Wager *et al.* (1968b). Diminished serum complement levels have been found in all three groups of cryoglobulinemia (Brouet *et al.*, 1974), but components of complement have only occasionally been observed to be bound to circulating cryoglobulin complexes (Riethmüller *et al.*, 1966; Flad *et al.*, 1968; Wang *et al.*, 1974).

Douglas *et al.* (1970) observed reduced bactericidal activity of polymorphonuclear leukocytes in a patient with mixed cryoblobulinemia. Coating of these cells with cryoglobulin seemed to account for the defect. A similar observation involved the coating of blood platelets (Braunsteiner *et al.*, 1954) and their reduced function.

Cryoglobulinemia *per se* has not been known to be associated with leukocytosis. The advent of automatic electronic counters, however, has produced erroneously elevated leukocyte counts by registering cryoglobulin aggregates in addition to leukocytes (Emori *et al.*, 1973; Potron *et al.*, 1975).

1.3.4. Isolation and Purification of Cryoglobulins

In the majority of cases, serum cryoglobulin concentrations are small and might not be recognized unless the blood is allowed to clot at 37°C. The serum then contains cryoglobulins that will precipitate at 4°C, usually within 12 hr, but occasionally precipitation may not be complete until after 1 week. Generally, higher concentrations of cryoglobulins will precipitate more rapidly and at temperatures closer to 37°C. Repeated washings with 0.85% NaCl at 4°C will remove other serum constituents and normal Ig's, leaving cryoglobulins as a white precipitate that readily goes into solution at 37°C and reprecipitates on being chilled. Repeated warming and chilling will repeat the sequence of solution and precipitation of monoclonal cyroglobulins indefinitely. Mixed cryoglobulins are less stable and likely to yield diminishing amounts of cryoprecipitate after each reheating (Volpé *et al.*, 1956; Lewis *et al.*, 1966). Testing for purity of a cryoglobulin by immunoelectrophoresis or double-immune diffusion is best performed at 37°C.

Isolation of cryoglobulins from frozen plasma rather than from serum requires removal of fibrinogen at 37°C prior to cryoprecipitation maneuvers. Addition of $CaCl_2$ will precipitate fibrin, but may result in coprecipitation of cryoglobulin. This may be avoided by fourfold dilution of the plasma with 0.85% NaCl, followed by addition of 40 units thrombin/ml at 37°C.

1.4. Classification of Cryoglobulins

Various groupings of cryoglobulins have been arranged ever since it became evident that they did not constitute a single entity. The most meaningful system to date is the one proposed by Seligmann's group (Klein *et al.*, 1972; Brouet *et al.*, 1974). It recognizes three principal groups, the first one represented by single monoclonal Ig's; a second one of mixed cryoglobulins, consisting of one monoclonal and one polyclonal Ig; and a third group of mixed Ig's, neither of which is monoclonal.

TABLE 1. Number of Patients with Cryoglobulinemia

Classification Group & Subgroup	Specificity of H and L chains									Assoc
	Number	H chain	NG[a]	L chain κ, λ	NG[a]	Myeloma	Macro-globulinemia	Sjögren's syndrome	Chronic liver disease	SL Vasc
I. Single monoclonal	116			17 8						
IgM	42				16		42			
IgG	62	γ₁ 12		17 8	37	36		3	5	1
		γ₂ 13								
		γ₃ 8	29							
		γ₄ 0								
IgA	5	α₁ 1	4	— 2	3	5				
L chains	7			3 1	3	7				
II. Mixed with one monoclonal component	109			16 2						
IgM–IgG	89				71		1	5	9	
IgA–IgG (monoclonal IgA)	11	α₁ 1	9	1 2	8			1		
		α₂ 1								
IgG–IgG	9	γ₁ 3		5 4		9				
		γ₃ 6								
III. Mixed polyclonal	186									
IgM–IgG	168							1	13	
IgM–IgG–IgA	18								5	
TOTAL:	411					57	43	10	32	3

*(NG) Not given.

1.4.1. Monoclonal Cryoglobulins

Cryomacroglobulin IgM. This cryoglobulin has been described, analyzed, and characterized by various investigators (Saha *et al.*, 1968, 1969, 1970; Deutsch, 1969; Macris *et al.*, 1970; Andersen *et al.*, 1971; Zinneman *et al.*, 1973; Wang *et al.*, 1974). This type of cryoglobulin is likely to be associated with vascular insufficiency and ulcerations of the lower extremities (Baughman and Sommer, 1966). One IgM had the properties of a cryo- as well as of a pyroglobulin (Meltzer and Franklin, 1966).

Monoclonal IgG-Cryoglobulins. This group has been studied by Saha *et al.* (1968), Seligmann *et al.* (1968), Sargent *et al.* (1970), Virella and Hobbs (1971), Hansson and Lindström (1973), and Brouet *et al.* (1974). Brouet *et al.* (1974) and Virella (1971) found cryoprecipitability most frequently in IgG1 and IgG2. Table 1 presents a rather equal distribution between γ_1 and γ_2, a lesser incidence of γ_3, and absence of γ_4. Cryoprecipitation usually requires the intact IgG molecule. Generally, no antibody activity has been ascribed to these Ig's, but Seligmann *et al.* (1968) reported an IgG cryoglobulin with anti-streptolysin-O activity in a patient who had suffered three previous bouts of rheumatic fever. The carbohydrate components of IgG cryoglobulins have attracted little attention, but Brouet *et al.* (1974) found sialic acid to be lacking in some cryoglobulins, and an additional one under study by this author is deficient in sialic acid and fucose.

Monoclonal IgA-Cryoglobulins. These cryoglobulins have been reported infrequently (Auscher and Guinand, 1964; Porush *et al.*, 1969; Watanabe *et al.*, 1974). The ones studied by Watanabe *et al.* (1974) and Invernizzi *et al.* (1973) had the physicochemical properties of a cryoglobulin as well as of a pyroglobulin.

TABLE 1. (*continued*)   **329**

iseases			Clinical manifestations						
Chronic infection	Rheumatoid Arthritis	Ulcerative colitis	Glomerulonephritis	NG[a]	Purpura	Arthralgia	Raynaud's Syndrome	Ischemic leg ulcer	Neurological symptoms
					6	5	2	2	
			3	4	3	0	3	2	
	1		34	29	11	5		4	5
1				2	7		1	1	
61	2	4	3	79	28	22	8		
10				3					
72	3	4	40	117	55	32	14	9	5

Monoclonal Light Chains.   Whereas the majority of cryoglobulins are complete Ig molecules, and reduction and alkylation of them abolishes the property of cryoprecipitation, there are occasional myeloma patients secreting and excreting L chains, which possess all the physicochemical properties that characterize a cryoglobulin. L-chain cryoproteins have been reported by Varriale *et al.* (1962), Alper (1966), Liss *et al.* (1967), Zinneman *et al.* (1968), Cuprak *et al.* (1970), and Harris and Kohn (1974). Brouet *et al.* (1974) described a λ-chain cryoprotein that proved to be a mixture of a covalent dimer (80%) and a native monomer (20%). Neither the monomer alone nor the reduced and alkylated dimer was capable of cryoprecipitation.

1.4.2. Mixed Cryoglobulins with One Monoclonal Component

Mixed cryoglobulins are formed by two Ig's, neither of which is a cryoglobulin in the single state. Together, they form soluble aggregates at 37°C that precipitate at lower temperatures.

Combinations of a Monoclonal IgM with a Polyclonal IgG.   These are the most commonly encountered cryoglobulins in this group (Balázs and Fröhlich, 1966; Meltzer and Franklin, 1966; Grey *et al.*, 1968; Zinneman *et al.*, 1968; Capra *et al.*, 1969; Porush *et al.*, 1969; Caperton and Williams, 1969; Bonomo *et al.*, 1970; Caronia *et al.*, 1972; Zlotnick *et al.*, 1972; Cream, 1972; Herd, 1973b; Stone and Fedak, 1974). The IgM component most often is an IgMK. λ-Chain-carrying IgM is infrequent in this group. IgMK usually has antiglobulin activity (Zinneman *et al.*,

1968; Caperton and Williams, 1969; Brouet *et al.*, 1974). None of the four subclasses of IgG is preferentially represented.

Clinically, this group of cryoglobulins is associated with vasculitis, vascular insufficiency, various cutaneous manifestations, and glomerulonephritis.

Mixed IgG–IgA Cryoglobulins. These are found less commonly and have been studied by Matuhasi and Mitsuko (1968), Klein *et al.* (1972), and Takeda *et al.* (1974). IgA was the monoclonal component in three cases.

IgG–IgG Cryoglobulins. These cryoglobulins represent a mixture of a monoclonal with a polyclonal IgG (Grey *et al.*, 1968; Klein *et al.*, 1972; Brouet *et al.*, 1974). Recognition of this type is not always obvious because of the preponderance of the monoclonal component, which thus far has been found to be an IgG3. It is quite possible that some cryoglobulins that have been reported as monoclonal IgG eventually will turn out to belong in this group.

1.4.3. Mixed Polyclonal Cryoglobulins

This group is the most common of cryoglobulins, and may represent but a pathological increase of an entity that is found normally in minimal quantities in humans (Kaplan, 1968; Hijmans *et al.*, 1969; Cream, 1972) as well as in rabbits (Davie *et al.*, 1968). Even when the serum concentrations of cryoglobulins of this group are pathologically increased, they are usually from 0.1 to 1.0 mg/ml. The pathological setting of mixed polyclonal cryoglobulinemia is frequently an infectious or inflammatory disease, such as subacute bacterial endocarditis, infectious mononucleosis, disseminated lupus erythematosus, or chronic liver disease. These Ig's do not appear to be involved directly in specific antibody response. They do not possess antibody activity specifically related to the infectious process that provoked their pathological appearance (Hurwitz *et al.*, 1975). It is possible that polyclonal IgM combines with an IgG that is bound to an unknown antigen. Whereas Kaplan (1968) noted antinuclear activity in this group of cryoglobulins, Brouet *et al.* (1974) failed to find specific antibody activity.

1.4.4. Coprecipitation

Coprecipitation of other serum proteins may be integral to the process of cryoprecipitation in some cases, but it appears that in most instances, separation of these proteins leaves the property of cryoprecipitation of monoclonal or mixed cryoglobulins intact.

Coprecipitation of polyclonal IgG with a L-chain cryoglobulin was found to have no bearing on the process, and its removal left the L-chain cryoprecipitability virtually unchanged (Zinneman *et al.*, 1968). Allen (1966) as well as Lewis *et al.* (1966) found the presence of β-lipoproteins essential to cryoprecipitation, whereas others (Hanauer and Christian, 1967; Flad *et al.*, 1968) found complement and α_2-macroglobulin bound to their cryoglobulins. Recently, MacKechnie *et al.* (1975) described a cryoglobulin in a patient with systemic lupus erythematosus. The cryoglobulin complex contained DNA as well as some components of complement and had antinuclear activity. In a patient with Peetom–Meltzer syndrome (arthralgia, purpura, weakness) the mixed IgM–IgG cryoglobulin had coprecipitates of free DNA, C1g, C1s fibrinogen, α_2-macroglobulin, and β-lipoprotein (Peetom and Van

Loghem-Langereis, 1965). Coprecipitates of this type are the exception rather than the rule.

Table 1 compares the three groups of cryoglobulins in regard to associated diseases, clinical manifestations, and some of the laboratory specificities. It reflects the data of 60 studies within the past 15 years. Reports dating prior to that period could not be included, despite their merits, because they did not offer classification of Ig's. Some patients have been reported more than once, and Table 1 was corrected for these duplications whenever possible. A number of studies were concerned with immunochemical data and gave incomplete clinical information. Loss of this type is indicated in the "NG" columns. Despite these shortcomings, the table is considered meaningful, although not statistically accurate.

Compared with the finding of Brouet *et al.* (1974), the incidence of monoclonal IgG is greater in this compilation. This greater incidence may reflect regional differences, and it is also possible that some cryoglobulins were not recognized as mixed IgG–IgG with one monoclonal component and erroneously placed into the group of monoclonal IgG's.

Not surprisingly, most single monoclonal IgG, IgA, and L-chain cryoglobulins occurred in patients with multiple myeloma. The majority of mixed cryoglobulins of Group II were associated with glomerulonephritis and vasculitis, whereas the mixed polyclonal cryoglobulins of Group III were found mainly in patients with chronic infections and chronic hepatic disease.

Purpura, arthralgia, and Raynaud's syndrome were the most common clinical manifestations.

1.5. Mechanisms of Cryoprecipitation

The solubility of a protein is determined by a number of factors, especially pH, surface charges of the molecule, and ionic strength of the solution.

Hydration at the molecule's surface is an important determinant of its hydrodynamic behavior. H. F. Fisher (1965) states that the amount of water bound per gram of protein is relatively stable at 0.28 g.

Carbohydrate components of Ig's, such as hexoses, hexosamines, and fucose, are also hydration factors in the molecule solubility, whereas sialic acid contributes directly its negative electrostatic charge to the surface polarity.

Amino acid residues and their sequential as well as steric arrangements probably have the greatest effect on solubility. Most polar residues (lysine, arginine, histidine, aspartic acid, glutamic acid, threonine, serine, and tyrosine) are normally located at the surface, whereas nonpolar residues are usually buried in the anhydrous interior. Decrease in the number of tyrosine residues was thought to be responsible for the cryoprecipitability of an IgM (Zinneman *et al.*, 1973), an IgG (Cummings, 1968), and to some extent an IgM described by Uki *et al.* (1974), and a deficit of serine in the L chains was suspected to be the cause for the cryoprecipitability of an IgG (Wang *et al.*, 1974).

The concept of asphericity relating to a basically spherical molecule with a fixed layer-thickness of outer (polar) amino acid residues, is expressed by the formula (Fisher, H. F., 1964)

$$P_s = \frac{Ve}{Vi}$$

where P_s is the polarity ratio (polar/nonpolar residues, relating to a spherical shape), e is the external shell, and i is the internal mass. It follows that as the molecule's volume shrinks, P_s becomes larger, since the relative number of nonpolar groups must decrease because of the relatively greater diminution of the interior in which to bury them. Asphericity may then be defined as P/P_s. Generally, protein molecules and particularly Ig's are not spherical, and their polarity ratio (P) is greater than P_s. In this situation, the molecule equation is preserved by changes in steric conformation and shape. If P is very much greater than that of the corresponding P_s, the molecule will assume a rodlike structure. If, however, the P value of such a peptide chain becomes less than the corresponding P_s, there will be too few polar residues to cover the nonpolar core completely. This would render the molecule insoluble, unless it can satisfy the equation. This may be accomplished by increasing the weight of the molecule to a value for which P_s no longer exceeds P, in other words, by aggregation to dimers and trimers. This phenomenon is commonly observed in the soluble aggregation of abnormal monoclonal cryo- and pyroglobulins at optimal thermal conditions (Lo Spalluto et al., 1962; Balázs and Fröhlich, 1966; Kaplan, 1968; Cuprak et al., 1970; Zinneman and Seal, 1971; Hansson and Lindström, 1973; Zinneman et al., 1973; Pruzanski et al., 1973; Uki et al., 1974), indicating an abnormal deficit of polar residues. Such a deficit may be created by deletions within a peptide chain, as suggested by Zinneman et al. (1973) and Wang et al. (1974). Variations in amino acid sequence may force polar residues into the interior of the molecule, while exposing nonpolar ones, thus creating a deficit in polarity, without an actual loss of polar residues. The steric arrangement of secondary and tertiary structure is by no means rigid. It may change in response to various factors. Givol et al. (1974) observed steric changes of IgG in response to antigen-binding. Temperature changes also influence the folding and polarity of peptide chains. (Saluk and Clem, 1975). While an Ig with reduced polarity may stay in solution in optimal temperature by aggregating to dimers and trimers, cooling results in additional conformational changes and loss of polarity and solubility—in other words, cryoprecipitation. Reheating to 37°C brings the conformation of the molecule to its former soluble state. A pH of below 5 and above 8.5 usually prevents cryoprecipitation.

Complex formation of antigen–antibody type, involving noncovalent bonds, represents an alternate explanation of cryoprecipitation, with or without change of surface polarity. Saluk and Clem (1975) showed abnormalities in the Fab fraction of a monoclonal IgG3 cryoglobulin. Cooling produced conformational changes of the Fab fragment, which exposed new and unusual antibody-combining sites, which manifested themselves in temperature-dependent antibody activity against the autologous Fc fragment as well as against Fc fragments of two IgG3 and one IgG1 myeloma globulins, leading to IgG–IgG complexes at or below 24°C. Measurements of the reduced viscosity of the Fab suggested progressive opening and then closing of the Fab molecule with a peak value between 16 and 18°C. Antibodylike activity of Fab against its own Fc fragment was also observed by Saha et al. (1969).

Suppression of cryoprecipitation, which is observed in media of 2 M urea, 2 M guanidine-HCl, 1 M NaCl, and pH 4.5, is also compatible with the concept of antigen–antibody reaction.

Uki et al. (1974) could abolish cryoprecipitation of a 22 S cryoglobulin by admixing its own Fabμ-containing fragments, a reaction that appears akin to the effect of antibody excess. In this particular case, the antigen appeared to reside within L chains with intact intrachain disulfide bridges.

Enzymatic cleavage of single monoclonal cryoglobulins usually results in loss of cryoprecipitability of the separated Fab and Fc fragments (Saha *et al.*, 1970; Stone and Fedak, 1974). Pruzanski *et al.* (1973), however, reported cryoprecipitability of the (Fab')2 fragment of an IgA cryoglobulin a phenomenon that makes temperature-dependent loss of polarity more likely than antigen–antibody reaction.

As previously mentioned, the negative charge of sialic acid contributes to the solubility of an Ig, and its absence may reduce surface polarity to the extent that steric changes during cooling will render $P < P_s$, resulting in cryoprecipitation. Absence of sialic acid from the IgG component of a mixed cryoglobulin was described by Zinneman *et al.* (1968) and found to be the case by others in mixed cryoglobulins (McIntosh *et al.*, 1970; McIntosh and Grossman, 1971; Zlotnick *et al.*, 1972). Subsequent analysis of seven mixed IgM–IgG cryoglobulins in the author's laboratory found sialic acid absent in the IgG component of four. Sialic acid was also found to be missing in the monoclonal IgG cryoglobulin of a patient with Sjögren's syndrome. Sialic acid deficiency of similar cryoglobulins has also been found by others (Hansson and Lindström, 1973; Brouet *et al.*, 1974).

Carbohydrate components other than sialic acid, such as fucose, hexose, and hexosamine, carry no charge but appear to contribute to the solubility of an Ig by surface hydration. Andersen *et al.* (1971) removed some of the carbohydrate groups of an IgMK cryoglobulin by means of glycosidase. This treatment decreased solubility even at 37°C, and complete solubilization was not accomplished until the temperature was raised to 52°C. Similar observations, as yet unpublished, were made by this author during the study of an IgGK cryoglobulin, which had greatly reduced fucose and hexose components. At 37°C, this cryoglobulin was only partly soluble, whereas elevation to 52°C resulted in complete solution.

A recent contribution by Wang *et al.* (1974) evaluated nine monoclonal cryoglobulins by sequential amino acid analysis and suggests their association of L chains with PCA pyrrolidine-carboxylic acid-blocked *N*-terminus and possibly with H chains of the $V_H I$ subgroup.

There are multiple reasons and mechanisms for the cryoprecipitability of Ig's— some of them recognized, others perhaps as yet unknown—but temperature-dependent reduction of surface polarity with or without antigen–antibody-like noncovalent bonding appears to be a common property.

1.6. Possible Factors in the Emergence of Cryoglobulinemia

Review of the conditions and diseases in which cryoglobulinemia may occur suggests that synthesis of these abnormal Ig's is triggered by chronic and sometimes acute antigenic stimuli. Seligmann *et al.* (1968) found high-titered antistreptolysin activity of an IgG myeloma cryoglobulin in a 38-year-old man who previously had suffered three attacks of rheumatic fever. Schultz and Yunis (1975) reported the emergence of a mixed cryoglobulin with antibody activity to a liver antigen after prolonged administration of liver extract.

Association of cryoglobulinemia with chronic infections has been recognized from the time of the first description of cryoglobulins (Lerner and Watson, 1947), and since then by many other investigators (Meltzer and Franklin, 1966; Meltzer *et al.*, 1966; Turkington and Buckley, 1966; Barnett *et al.*, 1970; Zlotnick *et al.*, 1972; Griswold *et al.*, 1974).

Mixed polyclonal cryoglobulinemia has also been recognized in acute Epstein–Barr-virus and cytomegalovirus infections (Kaplan, 1968; Wager *et al.*, 1968b; Capra *et al.*, 1969; Barnett *et al.*, 1970). Antigenic stimuli by various forms of hepatic cirrhosis and hepatitis also have resulted in cryoglobulinemia (Zlotnick *et al.*, 1972; Florin-Christensen *et al.*, 1974).

Experimental challenges with streptococcal vaccines (Herd, 1973a,b) or live group B streptococci (Davie *et al.*, 1968) produced mixed cryoglobulinemia in rabbits. The frequent association of cryoglobulinemia with diseases of autoimmunity should not go unmentioned.

The emergence of cryoglobulinemia may represent the pathologically increased synthesis of Ig's that are normally present in minimal concentrations. Cream (1972) found mixed cryoglobulins in normal humans at an average concentration of 30 μg/ml.

Mixed cryoglobulins were also found by Hijmans *et al.* (1969) in approximately 25% of presumably normal black New Zealand mice.

1.7. Therapy

There has not been a unified or controlled approach to the treatment of cryoglobulinemia, so that reports on therapy are necessarily episodic. Therapeutic efforts have been directed at either reduction or elimination of cryoglobulin concentrations in the serum.

Plasmapheresis is beneficial in situations of emergency, ordinarily due to the hyperviscosity syndrome, although the effect is transient. Frequent plasmapheresis on a long-range treatment basis would deprive the patient of inordinate amounts of proteins, unless not only cellular elements, but also the plasma after cryoglobulins have been removed by overnight precipitation at 4°C, are returned to the patient.

Pharmaceutical approaches have failed to yield clear-cut results. A given medication would seem beneficial in one instance and useless in the hands of another investigator. This is not surprising, considering the variety of cryoglobulins and the diseases with which they are known to be associated.

Penicillamine therapy has been ineffective (Brouet *et al.*, 1974; O'Reilly and MacKenzie, 1967). Chlorambucil has also been disappointing (O'Reilly and Mac-Kenzie, 1967; Hewitt *et al.*, 1970; Rubens-Duval and Kaplan, 1974), although there is one report of limited success (Rigo *et al.*, 1973). More promising results have been achieved by combinations of adrenocorticosteroids with cytotoxic agents, such as phenylalanine mustard (Brody and Samitz, 1973), cyclophosphamide (Rubens-Duval and Kaplan, 1974), and 6-mercaptopurine (Miescher *et al.*, 1965). The author is aware of one as yet unreported case of primary cryoglobulinemia (Type II, IgM–IgG) in which complete remission was achieved by splenic irradiation. At the time of this writing, the remission has reached a duration of 4 years.

In attempting any type of therapy, one should keep in mind that it is usually directed toward the manifestations of the disease process rather than the cause, and that the effect will necessarily be limited.

2.1. Definition and Historical Notes

Pyroglobulins are Ig's with a temperature-dependent instability that transforms them into a gel at 56°C. This gel is irreversible by changes of temperature, pH, or dilution.

Pyroglobulins were so named by Martin and Mathieson (1953), but reported much earlier under the misnomer of "serum Bence Jones proteins" (Ellinger, 1898). Hammarsten et al. (1945) repeated the observation, and thanks to the availability of more sophisticated techniques, could identify their thermolabile protein as a γ-globulin that on electrophoresis presented itself as a sharp peak. These authors also believed that they were dealing with a form of Bence Jones protein. Six years later, Collier et al. (1951) reported four thermolabile serum globulins, three in patients with multiple myeloma, one in a patient with metastatic carcinoma. The abnormally thermolabile serum proteins were again mistaken for Bence Jones proteins, although they formed irreversible coagula at 56°C. Martin and Mathieson (1953) were the first to recognize pyroglobulins as an entity of γ-globulins, which differed from Bence Jones proteins, and this was corroborated by Huisman et al. (1956) on the basis of amino acid analysis. Pyroglobulinemia in association with malignant lymphoma was reported by Zinneman (1958).

In 1959, Martin et al. were able to report 20 cases of pyroglobulinemia, half of which were associated with multiple myeloma. Two of the pyroglobulins were also cryoglobulins. Subsequent studies have been devoted to further identification and characterization of pyroglobulins, and have resulted in the elucidation of some of the abnormalities responsible for the formation of pyrogel at 56°C.

2.2. Clinical Significance

2.2.1. Associated Diseases

Pyroglobulinemia has been observed most commonly in multiple myeloma. This disease was associated with roughly 50% of all reported cases (Brachfeld and Myerson, 1956; Cattaneo et al., 1970; Collier et al., 1951; Fisher, B., et al., 1963; Huisman et al., 1956; Invernizzi et al., 1973; Lipman, 1964; Martin and Mathieson, 1953; Martin et al., 1959; Patterson et al., 1965b; Solomon and Steinfeld, 1965; Sugai, 1972; Zinneman and Seal, 1971). It was also associated with macroglobulinemia (Cattaneo et al., 1970; Invernizzi et al., 1973; Martin et al., 1959; Patterson et al., 1970; Stefanini et al., 1970) and with other lymphoproliferative disorders (Patterson et al., 1968; Zinneman, 1958), systemic lupus erythematosus (Martin et al., 1959), and carcinoma (Martin et al., 1959).

Occasionally, an associated disease could not be defined, although multiple myeloma was a likely possibility (Ellinger, 1898; Hammarsten et al., 1945).

2.2.2. Clinical Signs and Symptoms

Pyroglobulins are not known to have caused clinical symptoms per se. In high concentrations, they can be responsible for a hyperviscosity syndrome (McCann et *al.*, 1976a,b), but detection always depended on heating serum to 56°C, a temperature used for complement inactivation.

2.2.3. Isolation of Pyroglobulins

IgM pyroglobulins can be isolated from serum with comparative ease if they also happen to be euglobulins. Repeated precipitation in distilled water and resolution in electrolyte solutions will suffice to purify them.

Whenever this simple procedure is not possible, the methods used for Ig's in general are applicable: gel filtration, electrophoresis, chromatography on columns of DEAE-cellulose, DEAE-Sephadex, CM-cellulose, and affinity chromatography or fractionation with ammonium sulfate, either singly or in appropriate combinations.

2.3. Classification of Pyroglobulins

IgG. Most of the reported pyroglobulins have been identified as IgG, or where identification and classification was incomplete, may be assumed to be in this class (Brachfeld and Myerson, 1956; Cattaneo *et al.*, 1970; Collier *et al.*, 1951; Fisher, B., *et al.*, 1963; Hammarsten *et al.*, 1945; Huisman *et al.*, 1956; Invernizzi *et al.*, 1973; Lipman, 1964; Martin *et al.*, 1959; Patterson *et al.*, 1965a,b; Solomon and Steinfeld, 1965; Zinneman, 1958; Zinneman and Seal, 1971). The ones that could be studied were monoclonal.

IgM. Macropyroglobulins have been studied by Cattaneo *et al.* (1970), Invernizzi *et al.* (1973), Stefanini *et al.* (1970), and Patterson *et al.* (1970) in patients with Waldenström's macroglobulinemia or lymphosarcoma, and in at least one patient without definable primary disease (McCann *et al.*, 1976a,b). All of them were monoclonal.

IgA. This monoclonal pyroglobulin is the least common. Only two have been reported thus far (Invernizzi *et al.*, 1973; Sugai, 1972), both in patients with multiple myeloma. Sugai's patient presented with the hyperviscosity syndrome.

Combined Cryopyroglobulinemia. Occasionally, an abnormal Ig shows the properties of a cryoglobulin as well as of a pyroglobulin. In the earliest recognition of two cryopyroglobulins by Martin *et al.* (1959), the Ig's involved could not be further identified. Meltzer and Franklin (1966) found one IgM globulin with these properties, Invernizzi *et al.* (1973) described three IgMs, and Watanabe *et al.* (1974) reported an IgA cryopyroglobulin.

2.4. Mechanisms

The thermodynamic principles of protein solubility, as they apply to cryoglobulins and cryoprecipitation, are also valid in the phenomenon shown by pyroglobulins. Most normal human proteins will acquire increased viscosity at 63°C and coagulate at 80°C. L chains are an exception to this rule. They do, however, form a transient precipitate at 50–60°C, a property that earlier led to the confusion of pyroglobulins with Bence Jones proteins despite obvious dissimilarities: transient and reversible precipitate of L chains and irreversible gel-formation by pyroglobu-

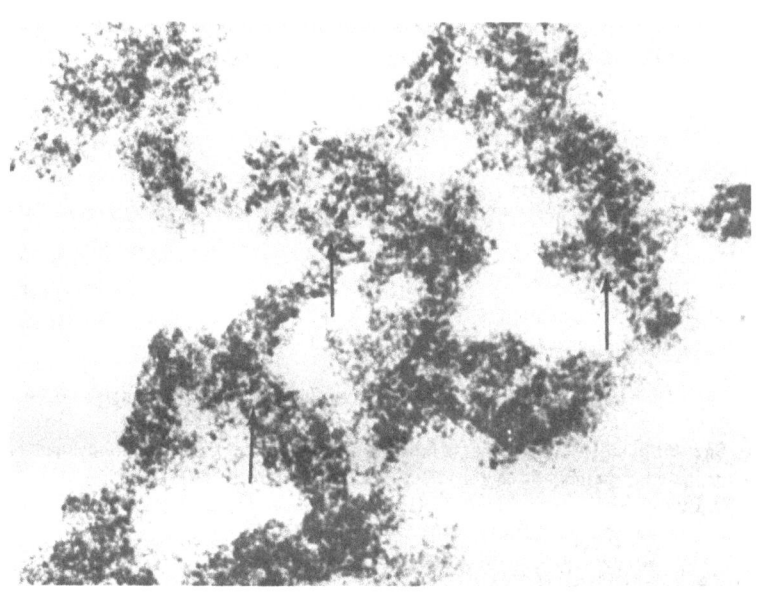

Figure 1. Gel meshwork of an IgM pyroglobulin. The preparation was stained with a combination of uranyl acetate and lead citrate. Arrows show recognizable IgM-pentamers within the meshwork. Magnification × 121,000. Electron microscopy by Akhuri A. Sinha, Ph.D.

lins. At this point, electron-microscopic evidence shows a meshwork of pyroglobu-lins, which are firmly bound together by hydrophobic bonding (Figure 1).

Amino acid analysis of several pyroglobulins has found increases of nonpolar and decreases of polar residues within the H chains. Studies of carbohydrate components have not uncovered quantitative or qualitative abnormalities. The tendency of many pyroglobulins to polymerization also suggests surface depolariza-tion. This abnormality may be due to a disproportion of hydrophilic to hydrophobic residues in favor of the latter. Where this disproportion is not found, the loss of polarity may arise from abnormalities in the primary structure of H chains, which would necessitate conformational changes, with burying of polar residues and exposing of nonpolar ones.

Reduced polarity itself is sufficient to lead to polymerization. Additional conformation changes resulting from temperature elevation to 56°C will expose additional hydrophobic residues. Whereas abnormal H chains alone do not form pyrogels, they do so together with L chains, which normally show reduced solubil-ity at 55°C. The resulting pyrogel occurs exactly at that temperature. The unfolding effect of sodium dodecyl sulfate (SDS) on the protein is caused by the interaction of the hydrophobic tail of SDS with the hydrophobic areas of the protein, leaving the sulfate group to intereact with the water shell (i.e., become a soluble Ig–SDS complex). The addition of negative charges by sulfuric acid groups is also expressed by increased anodal migration of the protein–SDS complex (Zinneman and Seal, 1971; Klein, 1973).

The formation of pyrogels at 56°C appears to differ fundamentally from heat coagulation of normal serum proteins at 80°C or above. While pyrogels are meshes of hydrophobically bonded Ig's, the gels of heat-coagulated normal Ig's have lost all appearance of ultrastructure and present the picture of amorphous protein coagula.

References

Allen, J. C., 1966, Studies on two-component cryoprecipitation, *Fed. Proc. Fed. Am. Soc. Exp. Biol.* **25**:726 (abstract).

Alper, C. A., 1966, Cryoglobulinuria: Studies of a cryo-Bence–Jones protein, *Acta Med. Scand. Suppl.* **445**:200–205.

Andersen, B. R., Tesar, J. T., Schmid, F. R., Haisty, W. K., and Hartz, W. H., Jr., 1971, Biological and physical properties of a human γM-cryoglobulin and its monomer subunit, *Clin. Exp. Immunol.* **9**:795–807.

Auscher, C., and Guinand, S., 1964, Étude d'une β_2A globuline cryo-précipitable, *Clin. Chim. Acta* **9**:40–48.

Balázs, V., and Fröhlich, M. H., 1966, Anti-heavy chain activity of the monoclonal (paraprotein) cryoglobulins with rheumatoid factor effect, *Am. J. Med. Sci.* **72**:668–674.

Barnett, E. V., Bluestone, R., Gracchiolo, A., III, Goldberg, L. S., Kantor, G. L., and McIntosh, R. M., 1970, Cryoglobulinemia and disease, *Ann. Intern. Med.* **73**:95–107.

Baughman, R. D., and Sommer, R. G., 1966, Cryoglobulinemia presenting as "factitial ulceration," *Arch. Dermatol.* **94**:725–731.

Biserte, G., 1961, Les cryoglobulinémies, *Ann. Biol. Clin.* **19**:265–287.

Bogaars, H. A., Kalderon, A. E., Cummings, F. J., Kaplan, S., Melnicoff, I., Park, C., Diamond, I., and Calabresi, P., 1973, Human IgG cryoglobulin with tubular crystal structure, *Nature (London) New Biol.* **245**:117–118.

Bonomo, L., Dammacco, F., Tursi, A., and Trizio, D., 1970, Waldenström's macroglobulinaemia with anti-IgG activity: A series of five cases, *Clin. Exp. Immunol.* **6**:531–545.

Brachfeld, J., and Myerson, R. M., 1956, Pyroglobulinemia: Diagnostic clue in multiple myeloma, *J. Am. Med. Assoc.* **161**:865–866.

Brauman, J., Duret, R., Bray, G., Potylière, P., Burtin, P., van Cutsem, J., and Lambert, P. P., 1956, Myeloma à cryoglobuline spontanément cristallisable, *Acta Clin. Belg.* **6**:518–539.

Braunsteiner, H., Falkner, R., Meumayer, A., and Pakesch, F., 1954, Makromolekuläre Kryoglobulinämie, *Klin. Wochenschr.* **32**:722–726.

Brody, J. I., and Samitz, M. H., 1973, Cutaneous signs of cryoparaproteinemia: Control with Burst Alkeran and Prednisone, *Am. J. Med.* **55**:211–214.

Brouet, J. C., Clauvel, J.-P., Danon, F., Klein, M., and Seligmann, M., 1974, Biologic and clinical significance of cryoglobulins, *Am. J. Med.* **57**:775–788.

Caperton, E. M., Jr., and Williams, R. C., Jr., 1969, *In vivo* study of IgM rheumatoid factors from mixed cryoglobulins, *J. Lab. Clin. Med.* **74**:239–249.

Capra, J. D., Winchester, R. J., and Kunkel, H. G., 1969, Cold-reactive rheumatoid factors in infectious mononucleosis and other diseases, *Arthritis Rheum.* **12**:67–73.

Capra, J. D., Kehoe, J. M., Winchester, R. J., and Kunkel, H. G., 1971, Structure–function relationships among anti-gamma globulin antibodies, *Ann. N. Y. Acad. Sci.* **190**:371–381.

Caronia, F., Patti, A., Donatuti, G., and Guarnaccia, C., 1972, Cryoglobulinemia—Report of a case with γM and γG serum gel, *Acta Haematol.* **48**:183–190.

Cattaneo, R., Bazzi, C., Simonati, V., and Balestrier, G., 1970, Studio immunochimico di tre casi di piroglobulinemia, *Prog. Immunobiol. Stand.* **4**:199–204.

Charmot, G., Laplane, G., André, L.-G., and Ferrand, J., 1959, Cryoglobulinémie essentielle avec érythème polymorphe et acroparesthésies, *Presse Med.* **67**:1939–1940.

Cohen, J. J., Goodfriend, L., and Rose, B., 1967, Studies on the solubilization of a 7S cryoglobulin, *Can. J. Biochem.* **45**:609–611.

Collier, F. C., Reich, A., and King, J. W., 1951, Multiple myeloma: A report of four cases, demonstrating Bence Jones proteinemia found during routine complement-fixation tests, *N. Engl. J. Med.* **245**:969–971.

Costanzi, J. J., and Coltman, C. A., Jr., 1967, Kappa chain cold precipitable immunoglobulin G (IgG) associated with cold urticaria, *Clin. Exp. Immunol.* **2**:167–178.

Costanzi, J. J., Clark, D. A., and Tennenbaum, J. I., 1965, Cryoglobulinemia associated with a macroglobulin, *Am. J. Med.* **39**:163–172.

Cream, J. J., 1972, Cryoglobulins in vasculitis, *Clin. Exp. Immunol.* **10**:117–126.

Cummings, N. A., 1968, Decreased tyrosine/tryptophan ratio in a 6.6S cryoglobulin, as determined by a spectrophotometric technique, *Biochem. Biophys. Res. Commun.* **33**:165–171.

Cuprak, L. J., Stollar, B. D., Kritzman, J., and Liss, M., 1970, Effects of chemical modification of a Bence–Jones cryoglobulin, *Immunochemistry* **7**:199–205.

Davie, J. M., Osterland, C. K., Miller, E. J., and Krause, R. M., 1968, Immune cryoglobulins in rabbit streptoccocal antiserum, *J. Immunol.* **100**:814–820.

Deutsch, H. F., 1969, Properties and modifications of a cryomacroglobulin possessing cold agglutinin activity, *Biopolymers* **7**:21–37.

Domz, C. A., and Feigin, E. V., 1957, Cryoglobulinemia, *AMA Arch. Intern. Med.* **100**:471–473.

Douglas, S. D., Lahav, M., and Fudenberg, H. H., 1970, A reversible neutrophil bacterial defect associated with a mixed cryoglobulin, *Am. J. Med.* **49**:274–280.

Ellinger, A., 1898–1899, Das Vorkommen des Bence–Jones'schen Körpers im Harn bei Tumoren des Knochenmarks, und seine diagnostische Bedeutung, *Dtsch. Arch. Klin. Med.* **62**:255–278.

Emori, H., Bluestone, R., and Goldberg, L. S., 1973, Pseudoleukocytosis associated with cryoglobulinemia, *Am. J. Clin. Pathol.* **60**:202–204.

Feizi, T., and Gitlin, N., 1969, Immune-complex disease of the kidney associated with chronic hepatitis and cryoglobulinemia, *Lancet* **2**:873–876.

Fisher, B., Schaer, L. R., and Messinger, S., 1963, The occurence of pyroglobulins in unsuspected myeloma, *Am. J. Clin. Pathol.* **40**:291–294.

Fisher, H. F., 1964, A limiting law relating the size and shape of protein molecules to their composition, *Proc. Natl. Acad. Sci. U.S.A.* **51**:1285–1291.

Fisher, H. F., 1965, An upper limit to the amount of hydration of a protein molecule: A corollary to the "limiting law of protein structure," *Biochim. Biophys. Acta* **109**:544–550.

Flad, H.-D., Rother, U., and Miescher, P. A., 1968, Bithermische Komplementaktivierung bei Kryoglobulinämie, *Verh. Dtsch. Ges. Inn. Med.* **74**:484–487.

Florin-Christensen, A., Roux, M. E. B., and Arana, R. M., 1974, Cryoglobulins in acute and chronic liver diseases, *Clin. Exp. Immunol.* **16**:599–605.

Givol, D., Pecht, I., Hochman, J., Schlessinger, J., and Steinberg, I. Z., 1974, Conformational changes in the Fab and Fc of the antibody as a consequence of antigen binding, in: *Progess in Immunology II* (L. Brent and J. Holborow, eds.), pp. 39–47, Nort-Holland, Amsterdam and Oxford.

Golde, D., and Epstein, W., 1968, Mixed cryoglobulins and glomerulonephritis, *Ann. Intern. Med.* **69**:1221–1227.

Grey, H. M., Kohler, P. F., Terry, W. D., and Franklin, E. C., 1968, Human monoclonal γG-cryoglobulins with anti γ-globulin activity, *J. Clin. Invest.* **47**:1875–1884.

Griswold, W. R., Koss, M., Chernack, W. J., Weil, R., III., Sutphen, J., and McIntosh, R. M., 1974, Glomerular localization of antigen and antibody in rabbits following intravenous administration of serum cryoproteins from homologous animals with acute serum sickness, *Proc. Soc. Exp. Biol. Med.* **145**:117–123.

Grossman, J., Abraham, G. M., Leddy, J. P., and Condemi, J. L., 1972, Crystalglobulinemia, *Ann. Intern. Med.* **77**:395–400.

Hammarsten, G., Lindgren, G., Olhagen, B., and Ordell, R., 1945, Hyperglobulinemia with a unique thermolabile γ-component: Report of a case, *Acta Med. Scand.* **123** (I):50–55.

Hanauer, L., and Christian, C. L., 1967, Studies of cryoproteins in systemic lupus erythematosus, *J. Clin. Invest.* **46**:400–408.

Hansson, U., and Lindström, F. D., 1973, Some factors affecting precipitation and complex formation of an IgG cryoglobulin, *Clin. Exp. Immunol.* **14**:427–435.

Harris, R. I., and Kohn, J., 1974, A urinary cryo-Bence–Jones protein gelling at room temperature, *Clin. Chim. Acta* **53**:233–237.

Herd, Z. L., 1973a, Antiglobulins and cryoglobulins in rabbits producing homogeneous streptococcal antibodies, *Immunology* **25**:923–930.

Herd, Z. L., 1973b, Experimental cryoglobulinaemia. Production and properties of streptococcus-induced rabbit cryoglobulins, *Immunology* **25**:931–939.

Hewitt, M. J., Leibowitch, M. M., Clauvel, J.-P., and Escande, J.-P., 1970, Les manifestations cutanées des cryoglobulinémies, *Soc. Fr. Dermatol. Syphilogr.* **77**:630–654.

Hijmans, W., Radema, H., Van Es, L., Feltkamp, T. E. W., Van Loghem, J. J., and Schaap, D. L., 1969, Cryoglobulins in New Zealand black mice, *Clin. Exp. Immunol.* **4**:227–239.

Huisman, T. H. J., Van der Wal, B., Groen, A., and Van der Sar, A., 1956, Investigations on a heat-coagulable globulin in the blood of a patient with multiple myeloma, *Clin. Chim. Acta* **1**:525–532.

Hurwitz, D., Quismorio, P., and Friou, G. J., 1975, Cryoglobulinemia in patients with infectious endocarditis, *Clin. Exp. Immunol.* **19**:131–141.

Invernizzi, F., Cattaneo, R., Rosso di San Secondo, V., Balestrieri, G., and Zanussi, C., 1973, Pyroglobulinemia: A report of eight patients with associated paraproteinemia, *Acta Haematol.* **50**:65–74.

Jori, G. P., and Buonanno, G., 1972, Chronic hepatitis and cirrhosis of the liver in cryoglobulinaemia, *Gut* **13**:610–613.

Kaplan, M. E., 1968, Cryoglobulinemia in infectious mononucleosis: Quantitation and characterization of the cryoproteins, *J. Lab. Clin. Med.* **71**:754–765.

Kaufman, D. B., and McIntosh, R., 1971, The pathogenesis of the renal lesion in a patient with streptococcal disease, infected ventriculoatrial shunt, cryoglobulinemia and nephritis, *Am. J. Med.* **50**:262–268.

Klein, M., 1973, Immunochemical studies of four human IgM pyroglobulins, *Immunochemistry* **10**:673–680.

Klein, M., Danon, F., Brouet, J. C., Signoret, Y., and Seligmann, M., 1972, Étude immunochimique de 130 cryoglobulines humaines, *Rev. Euro. Etud. Clin. Biol.* **17**:948–957.

Krauss, St., and Sokal, J. E., 1966, Paraproteinemia in the lymphomas, *Am. J. Med.* **40**:400–413.

Lapes, M. J., and Davis, J. S., 1970, Arthralgia—purpura—weakness—cryoglobulinemia, *Arch. Intern. Med.* **126**:287–289.

Lerner, A., and Watson, C. J., 1947, Studies of cryoglobulins. I. Unusual purpura associated with the presence of a high concentration of cryoglobulin, *Am. J. Med. Sci.* **214**:410–415.

Lerner, A., Barnum, C. P., and Watson, C. J., 1947, Studies of cryoglobulins. II. The spontaneous precipitation of protein from serum at 5°C in various disease states, *Am. J. Med. Sci.* **241**:416–421.

Lewis, L. A., Van Ommen, R. A., and Page, I. H., 1966, Association of cold-precipitability with β-lipoprotein and cryoglobulin, *Am. J. Med.* **40**:785–793.

Lipman, I. Y., 1964, Pyroglobulinemia: An unusual presenting sign in multiple myeloma, *J. Am. Med. Assoc.* **188**:1002–1004.

Liss, M., Fudenberg, H. H., and Kritzman, J., 1967, A Bence–Jones cyroglobulin: Chemical, physical and immunological properties, *Clin. Exp. Immunol.* **2**:467–475.

Logothetis, J., Kennedy, W. R., Ellington, A., and Williams, R. C., 1968, Cryoglobulinemic neuropathy: Incidence and clinical characteristics, *Arch. Neurol.* **19**:389–397.

Lo Spalluto, J., Dorward, B., Miller, W., Jr., and Ziff, M., 1962, Cryoglobulinemia based on interaction between a gamma macroglobulin and 7S gamma globulin, *Am. J. Med.* **32**:142–147.

MacKay, J. R., Eriksen, N., Motulsky, A. G., and Volwiler, W., 1956, Cryo- and macroglobulinemia: Electrophoretic, ultracentrifugal and clinical studies, *Am. J. Med.* **20**:564–587.

MacKechnie, H. L., Ogryzlo, M. A., and Pruzanski, W., 1975, Heterogeneity of IgM–IgG cryocomplexes: Immunological–clinical correlation, *J. Rheumatol.* **2**:225–240.

Macris, N. T., Capra, J. D., Frankel, G. J., Ioachim, H. L., Satz, H., and Bruno, M. S., 1970, A lambda light chain cold-agglutinin-cryomacroglobulin occurring in Waldenström's macroglobulinemia, *Am. J. Med.* **48**:524–529.

Marshall, R. J., and Malone, R. G. S., 1954, Cryoglobulinaemia with cerebral purpura, *Br. Med. J.* **2**:279–280.

Martin, W. J., and Mathieson, D. R., 1953, Pyroglobulinemia (heat-coagulable globulin in the blood), *Proc. Staff Meet. Mayo Clin.* **28**:545–554.

Martin, W. J., Mathieson, D. R., and Eigler, J. O., 1959, Pyroglobulinemia: Further observations and review of 20 cases, *Proc. Staff Meet. Mayo Clin.* **34**:95–101.

Matthews, L. J., and Trautman, J. R., 1965, Cryoproteinemia in leprosy, *Dermatol. Int.* **4**:164–168.

Matuhasi, T. U., and Mitsuko, M. N., 1968, γA–γG Mixed cryoglobulin, *Jpn. J. Exp. Med.* **38**:205–211.

McCann, S. R., Zinneman, H. H., Oken, M. M., Leary, M. M., Swaim, W. R., and Moore, M., 1976a, IgM pyroglobulinemia with erythrocytosis presenting as hyperviscosity syndrome. I. Clinical features and viscometric studies, *Am. J. Med.* **61**:316–320.

McCann, S. R., Zinneman, H. H., Oken, M. M., and Sinha, A. A., 1976b, IgM pyroglobulinemia with erythrocytosis presenting as hyperviscosity syndrome. II. Biochemical properties and mechanisms of pyrogel formation, *Am. J. Med.* **61**:321–325.

McIntosh, R. M., and Grossman, B., 1971, IgG, β_1c, fibrinogen cryoprotein in acute glomerulonephritis, *N. Engl. J. Med.* **285**:1521–1522.

McIntosh, R. M., Kaufman, D. B., Kulvinskas, C., and Grossman, B. J., 1970, Cryoglobulins. I. Studies on the nature, incidence and clinical significance of serum cryoproteins in glomerulonephritis, *J. Lab. Clin. Med.* **75**:566–577.

McIntosh, R. M., Kulvinskas, C., and Kaufman, D. B., 1971, Cryoglobulins. II. The biological and chemical properties of cryoproteins in acute post-streptococcal glomerulonephritis, *Int. Arch. Allergy* **41**:700–715.

Meltzer, M., and Franklin, E. C., 1966, Cryoglobulinemia: A study of 29 patients. I. IgG and IgM cryoglobulins and factors affecting cryoprecipitability, *Am. J. Med.* **40**:828–836.

Meltzer, M., Franklin, E. C., Elias, K., McClusky, R. T., and Cooper, N., 1966, Cryoglobulinemia: A clinical and laboratory study. II. Cryoglobulins with rheumatoid factor activity, *Am. J. Med.* **40**:837–856.

Miescher, P. A., Paronetto, F., and Koffler, D., 1965, Immune study in vasculitis associated with 19S–7S type of cryoglobulinemia, *Arthritis Rheum.* **8**:457 (abstract).

Muirhead, E. E., Montgomery, P. O. B., and Gordon, C. E., 1952, Thromboembolic pulmonary vascular sclerosis: Report of a case following pregnancy and of a case associated with cryoglobulinemia, *Arch. Intern. Med.* **89**:41–62.

Mustakallio, K. K., Lassus, A., Putkonen, T., and Wager, O., 1967, Cryoglobulins and rheumatoid factor in systemic lupus erythematosus, *Acta Dermatol. Venereol.* **47**:241–248.

O'Reilly, R. A., and MacKenzie, M. R., 1967, Primary macrocryoglobulinemia: Remission with adrenal corticosteroid therapy, *Arch. Intern. Med.* **120**:234–238.

Patterson, R., Nelson, V. L., and Pruzansky, J. J., 1965a, Pyroglobulinemia: Some characteristics of a heat labile protein, *Immunology* **9**:477–482.

Patterson, R., Roberts, M., and Pruzansky, J. J., 1965b, Localization of thermoprecipitable activity to the ''heavy'' polypeptide chain of a G-myeloma pyroglobulin, *Proc. Soc. Exp. Biol. Med.* **120**:275–278.

Patterson, R., Weiszer, I., Rambach, W., Roberts, M., and Suszko, I. M., 1968, Comparative cellular and immunochemical studies of two cases of pyroglobulinemia, *Am. J. Med.* **44**:147–153.

Patterson, R., Roberts, M., Rambach, W., and Falleroni, A., 1970, An IgM-pyroglobulin associated with lymphosarcoma, *Am. J. Med.* **48**:503–508.

Peetom, F., and Van Loghem-Langereis, E., 1965, IgM–IgG cryoglobulinemia: An autoimmune phenomenon, *Vox Sang.* **10**:281–292.

Perrot, H., Thivolet, J., Quincy, C., Fradin, G., and Later, R., 1971, Les cryoglobulinémies: À propos de 40 observations, *Lyon Med.* **226**:373–382.

Polčák, J., Wiedermann, D., Polčáková, J., and Skálová, M., 1967, Immunochemical and immunoelectrophoretic characteristics of cryoprotein and formol-gel-test in the sera of patients with ulcerative colitis, *Gastroenterologia* **107**:273–282.

Porush, J. G., Grishman, E., Alter, A. A., Mandelbaum, H., and Churg, J., 1969, Paraproteinemia and cryoglobulinemia associated with atypical glomerulonephritis and the nephrotic syndrome, *Am. J. Med.* **47**:957–964.

Potron, G., Boy, J., and Droulle, C., 1975, Fausse hyperleucocytose due à une cryoglobulinémie, *Nouv. Presse Med.* **4**:2272.

Pruzanski, W., Jancelewicz, Z., and Underdown, B., 1973, Immunological and physicochemical studies of IgA(λ) cryogelglobulinemia, *Clin. Exp. Immunol.* **15**:181–191.

Reza, M. J., Roth, B. E., Pops, M. A., and Goldberg, L. S., 1974, Intestinal vasculitis in essential, mixed cryoglobulinemia, *Ann. Intern. Med.* **81**:632–634.

Riethmüller, G., Meltzer, M., Franklin, E., and Miescher, P. A., 1966, Serum complement levels in patients with mixed (IgM–IgG) cryoglobulinaemia, *Clin. Exp. Immunol.* **1**:337–339.

Rigo, P., De Leval-Rutten, F., and Salmon, J., 1973, Cryoglobulinémie mixte I.G.M.–I.G.G.—un cas chez une malade atteinte de macroglobulinémie de Waldenström, *Nouv. Presse Med.* **2**:2603.

Rubens-Duval, A., and Kaplan, G., 1974, Manifestations articulaires des cryoglobulinémies, *Rev. Rhum.* **41**:605–613.

Rubens-Duval, A., Kaplan, G., and Nebillot, A., 1974, Cryoglobuline, macroglobuline et syndrome de Gougerot–Sjögren: Traitement par le chlorambucil et la cyclophosphamide, *Sem. Hop. Paris* **50**:1665–1671.

Saha, A., Edwards, M. A., Sargent, A. U., and Rose, B., 1968, Mechanism of cryoprecipitation. I. Characteristics of a human cryoglobulin, *Immunochemistry* **5**:341–356.

Saha, A., Sambury, S., Smart, K., Heiner, D. C., Sargent, A. U., and Rose, B., 1969, Studies on cryoprecipitation. II. Immunochemical characterization of a human cryoglobulin, *J. Immunol.* **102**:476–487.

Saha, A., Chowdhury, P., Sambury, S., Smart, K., and Rose, B., 1970, Studies on cryoprecipitation. IV. Enzymic fragments of a human cryoglobulin, *J. Biol. Chem.* **245**:2730–2736.

Saluk, P. H., and Clem, W., 1975, Studies on the cryoprecipitation of a human IgG$_3$ cryoglobulin: The effects of temperature-induced conformational changes on the primary interaction, *Immunochemistry* **12**:29–37.

Sargent, A. U., Saha, A., Klassen, G. K., and Rose, B., 1970, Studies of cryoprecipitation. III. Hemodynamic and metabolic adaptation to a circulating single component cryoglobulin, *Am. J. Med.* **48**:54–62.

Schultz, D. R., and Yunis, A. A., 1975, Immunoblastic lymphadenopathy with mixed cryoglobulinemia: A detailed case study, *N. Engl. J. Med.* **292**:8–12.

Seligmann, M., Danon, F., Basch, A., and Bernard, J., 1968, IgG myeloma cryoglobulin with antistreptolysin activity, *Nature (London)* **220**:711–712.

Siguier, F., Godeau, P., Lévy, R., Binet, J. L., and Hamida, B., 1964, À propos d'un cas de neuropathie cryglobulinémique (étude clinique et biologique), *Sem. Hop.* **40**:1928–1934.

Solomon, J., and Steinfeld, J. L., 1965, Pyroglobulinemia: Report of a case with protein turnover studies, *Am. J. Med.* **38**:937–942.

Stastny, P., and Ziff, M., 1969, Cold-insoluble complexes and complement levels in systemic lupus erythematosus, *N. Engl. J. Med.* **280**:1376–1381.

Stefanini, M., McDonnell, E. E., Andracki, E. G., Swansbro, W. J., and Durr, P., 1970, Macropyroglobulinemia: Immunochemical studies in three cases, *Am. J. Clin. Pathol.* **54**:94–101.

Stone, M. J., and Fedak, J., 1974, Studies on monoclonal antibodies. II. Immune complex (IgM–IgG) cryoglobulinemia: The mechanism of cryoprecipitation, *J. Immunol.* **113**:1377–1385.

Sugai, S., 1972, IgA pyroglobulin, hyperviscosity syndrome and coagulation abnormality in a patient with multiple myeloma, *Blood* **39**:224–237.

Takeda, K., Okumura, H., Hirose, S., and Muranaka, M., 1974, Immuno- and physiochemical studies of an IgA–IgG mixed cryoglobulin, *Int. Arch. Allergy* **46**:38–52.

Thivolet, J., Moene, Y., and Pellerat, J., 1967, Urticaire à frigore avec cryoglobulinémie, *Bull. Soc. Fr. Dermatol. Syphilogr.* **74**:392–395.

Turkington, R. W., and Buckley, C. E., 1966, Macrocryoglobulinemia and sarcoidosis, *Am. J. Med.* **40**:156–164.

Uki, J., Young, C. A., and Suzuki, T., 1974, A 22S cryomacroglobulin with antibody-like activity. I. Physico-chemical characterization and modification of its cryoproperties, *Immunochemistry* **11**:729–740.

Varriale, P., Ginsberg, D. M., and Sass, M. D., 1962, A urinary cryoprotein in multiple myeloma, *Ann. Intern. Med.* **57**:819–823.

Virella, G., 1971, IgG subclasses in relation to viscosity and cryoglobulin syndromes, *Br. Med. J.* **2**:322.

Virella, G., and Hobbs, J. R., 1971, Heavy chain typing in IgG monoclonal gammapathies with special reference to cases of serum hyperviscosity and cryoglobulinemia, *Clin. Exp. Immunol.* **9**:973–980.

Volpé, R., Bruce-Robertson, A., Fletcher, A. A., and Charles, W. B., 1956, Essential cryoglobulinaemia: Review of the literature and report of a case treated with ACTH and cortisone, *Am. J. Med.* **20**:533–553.

Wager, O., Mustakallio, K. K., and Räsänen, J. A., 1968a, Mixed IgA–IgG cryoglobulinemia: Immunologic studies and case reports of three patients, *Am. J. Med.* **44**:179–187.

Wager, O., Räsänen, J. A., Hagman, A., and Klemola, E., 1968b, Mixed cryoimmunoglobulinaemia in infectious mononucleosis and cytomegalovirus mononucleosis, *Int. Arch. Allergy* **34**:345–361.

Waldmann, T. A., Johnson, J. S., and Talal, N., 1971, Hypogammaglobulinemia associated with accelerated catabolism of IgG secondary to its interaction with an IgG-reactive monoclonal IgM, *J. Clin. Invest.* **50**:951–959.

Wang, A. C., Wells, J. V., and Fudenberg, H. H., 1974, Chemical analyses of cryoglobulins, *Immunochemistry* **11**:341–345.

Watanabe, A., Kitamura, M., and Shimizu, M., 1974, Immunoglobulin A (IgA) with properties of both cryoglobulin and pyroglobulin, *Clin. Chim. Acta* **52**:231–237.

Wintrobe, M. M., and Buell, M. V., 1933, Hyperproteinemia associated with multiple myeloma: With report of a case in which an extraordinary hyperproteinemia was associated with thrombosis of the retinal veins and symptoms suggested Raynaud's disease, *Bull. Johns Hopkins Hosp.* **52**:156–165.

Zinneman, H. H., 1958, Dysproteinemia, *Postgrad. Med.* **23**:550–560.

Zinneman, H. H., and Seal, U. S., 1971, The role of hydrophobic bonding in the thermoprecipitation of a pyroglobulin, *Eur. J. Clin. Biol. Res.* **16**:668–672.

Zinneman, H. H., Levi, D., and Seal, U. S., 1968, On the nature of cryoglobulins, *J. Immunol.* **100**:594–603.

Zinneman, H. H., Fromke, V. L., and Seal, U. S., 1973, Some biochemical properties of a cryomacroglobulin, *Clin. Chim. Acta* **43**:91–99.

Zlotnick, A., Slavin, S., and Eliakim, M., 1972, Mixed cryoglobulinemia with a monoclonal IgM component associated with chronic liver disease, *Isr. J. Med. Sci.* **8**:1968–1979.

15

Biosynthesis and Secretion of Immunoglobulins

YONG SUNG CHOI

1. Introduction

During the immune reponse, antigen induces B lymphocytes to proliferate and differentiate into plasma cells, which then actively secrete specific antibodies (Davie and Paul, 1971). Since the chemical structure of the immunoglobulin (Ig) molecule has been extensively worked out (Porter, 1973), biosynthetic studies may now have great value for the further understanding of humoral immune responses in molecular terms (Williamson, 1973), and will also provide us with an excellent experimental model for molecular studies of the differentiation of lymphocytes as well as other eukaryotic cells (Watson, 1976).

2. Methods

The methods most commonly used to study biosynthesis of Ig (Choi *et al.*, 1971a) are as follows: Solid lymphoid tissue (e.g., spleen, lymph node, myeloma tumors) is put in a tissue culture medium, cut into small pieces, and then dispersed in a glass homogenizer with a loosely fitting Teflon pestle. Cells are recovered following filtration through a sterile stainless steel screen (No. 200 mesh) and washed twice by centrifugation in the culture medium. Normal lymphocytes are further purified by Ficoll–Hypaque gradient centrifugation (Thorsby and Bratlie, 1970). All operations are performed at room temperature.

To study protein biosynthesis, the isolated lymphoid cells are incubated at a concentration of 5×10^6 to 5×10^7 cells per ml in Eagle's medium, made without leucine, containing 5% fetal calf serum and 20–40 μCi/ml [^{3}H]leucine. Incubations are usually performed in a humidified tissue-culture incubator at 37°C in 15% CO_2 and 85% air. After incubation for varying periods of time, the cultures are chilled quickly in an ice-water bath and centrifuged at 3000g for 10 min to separate the cells

YONG SUNG CHOI • Memorial Sloan-Kettering Cancer Center, New York, New York 10021.

from the incubation media that contain secreted proteins. The cells are then lysed with a nonionic detergent (i.e., 0.5–1.0% Nonidet P-40, Shell Chemical Co.), which solubilizes cytoplasm without breaking the nuclei (Borun *et al.*, 1967). Nuclei and ribosomes are removed by centrifugation at 150,000*g* for 60 min at 0°C. Both the cell lysate and the supernatant fractions are subjected to (1) trichloroacetic acid precipitation to determine the total amount of radioactive proteins synthesized and (2) serological assay to measure the radiolabeled Ig. Under ideal conditions, the amount of specific radioactivity of labeled protein per cell should be proportional to the product of the concentration and specific activity of radioactive amino acids used.

Indirect precipitation has been most commonly used for the serological assay of radiolabeled Ig (Choi *et al.*, 1971a; Melchers and Andersson, 1973), in which Ig is complexed with excess rabbit anti-Ig serum, and the complexes precipitated by goat (or sheep) antirabbit IgG. To use this assay for Ig biosynthetic experiments, the following precautions must be observed: (1) Titrations of rabbit anti-Ig and of goat antirabbit IgG must be performed using radiolabeled Ig to ensure that all radioactivity can be completely precipitated. (2) Nonspecific precipitation must be performed by similar reaction of the same amount of radiolabeled material with normal rabbit serum (or antisera against antigens other than Ig). (3) The specificity of the serological reaction must be verified by a competitive experiment that shows that the radioactivity precipitated with anti-Ig serum can be reduced to the level of the nonspecific precipitates by addition of excess purified Ig. (4) The serologically precipitated radioactivity must be examined by polyacrylamide gel electrophoresis (PAGE) (Shapiro *et al.*, 1967). PAGE of the specific serological precipitates shows that the radioactivity is recoverable in Ig peaks, whereas PAGE of the nonspecific precipitates does not show any distinctive peptide profile (Choi *et al.*, 1971a).

3. Synthesis of Light and Heavy Polypeptide Chains

Hood and Prahl (1971) provided evidence to suggest that the amino acid sequences of each Ig polypeptide chain may be encoded by two separate genes: one for the variable (V) and another for the constant (C) region. For both light (L) and heavy (H) polypeptide chains, integration of the V with the C gene information must take place at some stage to yield a single polypeptide product. Whether this integration occurs during or after transcription was tested by determining whether the whole molecule (both V and C regions) of L and H chains is synthesized from a single initiation point.

During synthesis of polypeptides, amino acids are added sequentially from the amino-terminus to the carboxyl-terminus (Dintzis, 1961). Brief pulse-labeling of polypeptides during synthesis, using a radioactive amino acid, was found to label the carboxyl-terminal portion of the molecule more heavily than the amino-terminal portion. Using this method developed to study hemoglobin synthesis, Lennox *et al.* (1967) investigated biosynthesis of the L chain in a mouse myeloma cell line secreting only the κ chain. Cell suspensions were pulse-labeled with [^{3}H]leucine, ^{3}H-labeled L chain was purified from the cell lysate and mixed with purified L chains, which were previously labeled uniformly with [^{14}C]leucine, and the mixtures were digested with trypsin. The specific activities of tryptic peptides, defined by the ratio of ^{3}H and ^{14}C, could be arranged in a sequence that was consistent with the hypothesis that the whole polypeptide chain is synthesized from a single initiation point (Knopf, 1973).

Knopf et al. (1967) also examined the synthesis of H chains in mouse myeloma cells producing IgG2a and obtained identical results. In a similar study of the H chain of rabbit IgG, Fleischman (1967) showed that the Fc and Fab portions of rabbit IgG were not synthesized separately.

If both the L and H chains are each synthesized separately from a single initiation point, this would imply the existence of separate mRNAs for L and H chains. The discovery of separate classes of polyribosomes synthesizing L and H chains clearly supports this conclusion (Shapiro et al., 1966). In normal lymphoid tissues (Norton et al., 1965; Scharff and Uhr, 1965; Becker and Rich, 1966; Voss and Bauer, 1967; Kuechler and Rich, 1969) and myeloma cells (Askonas and Williamson, 1966; Shapiro et al., 1966; Williamson and Askonas, 1967; Schubert, 1968; Schubert and Cohn, 1968), L chains are synthesized on 200 S polysomes containing 4 or 5 ribosomes, while H chains are synthesized on 300 S polysomes containing 11–18 ribosomes. The number of monosomes per polysome in each class also agrees with the length of the mRNA, estimated from the size of the L or H chains translated from them (DePetris, 1970; Swan et al., 1972; Stevens and Williamson, 1972).

4. Assembly of Immunoglobulin Molecules

The basic structure of Ig is a dimer of H and L chains (H_2L_2) stabilized by interchain disulfide bonds (see the review by Porter, 1973). The assembly of Ig from L and H chains can proceed via a number of pathways (Baumal and Scharff, 1973). This has been studied through pulse-chase experiments using labeled followed by unlabeled amino acids. Sodium dodecyl sulfate (SDS)-PAGE of pulse-labeled intracellular Ig will reveal only covalently bonded intermediates: H_2L_2, H_2L, H_2, HL, L_2. During a chase period, the relative amounts of these intermediates will change, revealing a precursor–product relationship between them. For example, in IgG2a- and IgG1-producing mouse myeloma cells (Baumal et al., 1971), relatively large amounts of L, H, H_2, and H_2L were detected shortly after pulse-labeling; immediately after the chase started, large amounts of H_2 were present. As this H_2 molecule decreased in amount during the chase period, there was first a progressive increase and then a decrease in H_2L, followed in time by an increase in H_2L_2 suggesting the assembly pathway

$$(A) \ H + H \rightarrow H_2 + L \rightarrow H_2L + L \rightarrow H_2L_2$$

In the IgG2b-producing mouse myeloma cells, however, HL was found to be the major precursor, suggesting the assembly pathway of

$$(B) \ H + L \rightarrow HL \rightarrow H_2L_2$$

Since SDS disrupts noncovalent bonds between polypeptide chains, it is more difficult to identify the various possible intermediates that are not covalently linked. For mouse IgA in which H and L chains are assembled by noncovalent bonds (Abel and Grey, 1968), monomeric L chains are bound noncovalently to H_2, and dimerization of these L chains to give H_2L_2 takes place shortly after secretion (Bevan, 1971a).

To give IgA and IgM, polymerization of H_2L_2 itself takes place during the process of secretion; monomeric IgM becomes a pentamer $(H_2L_2)_5$ and monomeric IgA a dimer $(H_2L_2)_2$. Within IgA- and IgM-producing cells, 7 S monomer (H_2L_2) was found to be a predominant form (Parkhouse, 1971; Della Corte and Parkhouse, 1973). While IgA producers utilize H_2 as a major precursor for H_2L_2 [Pathway (A)], IgM-producing myeloma cells utilize HL as the major precursor of the intracellular monomer [Pathway (B)] (Buxbaum *et al.*, 1971; Bargellesi *et al.*, 1972). Events that take place just before secretion at the time of polymerization include the incorporation of the joining (J) chain into the molecule (Parkhouse, 1972) and the addition of terminal carbohydrate residues (Parkhouse, 1972; Melchers and Andersson, 1973). Thus, a block in any biochemical event at the stage of polymerization might result in IgM monomer molecules being incorporated in the surface membrane as Ig receptors, rather than in their being secreted.

5. Secretion of Immunoglobulins

It has previously been shown that although the processes of synthesis of the L and H polypeptides and their assembly into Ig molecules takes place in less than 10 min (Shapiro *et al.*, 1966; Williamson and Askonas, 1967), secretion of newly synthesized Ig molecules does not begin until 30 min after synthesis (Helmreich *et al.*, 1961; Melchers and Knopf, 1967). The kinetics of synthesis and secretion of Ig was studied by incubating mouse myeloma cells with radioactive amino acids (Choi *et al.*, 1971b). Under continuous labeling conditions, where the rate of radioactive leucine incorporation into total protein is linear (Choi and Good, 1972a) (Figure 1a), the amount of labeled Ig inside the cells increased without a lag for about 2 hr and then remained constant (Figure 1b). Labeled Ig appeared in the medium outside the cells after a lag of 30 min. The rate of secretion of Ig increased and became constant after 1 hr. In the medium outside the cells, serologically precipitable radioactivity accounted for at least 80% of the total trichloroacetic acid precipitable radioactivity, indicating that almost all the radioactive proteins recovered outside the cells were indeed Ig. Similar kinetics of Ig secretion was observed in IgG-producing normal lymphoid cells (Choi and Good, 1972a; Melchers and Andersson, 1973).

Intracellular transport and secretion of the carbohydrate-containing L chain have been more thoroughly studied by measuring the changing distribution of [³H]leucine pulse-labeled L chains in subcellular fractions, after chase intervals long enough to allow secretion (Choi *et al.*, 1971b). Analogous to the mode of secretion of proteins by pancreatic (Jamieson and Palade, 1967) and liver cells (Campbell, 1970), L and H chains are synthesized on membrane-bound polysomes and vectorally released into the cisternae of the rough endoplasmic reticulum (Bevan, 1971b). Free ribosomes do not contain nascent L chains (Cioli and Lennox, 1973). Ig is then transported to the smooth endoplasmic reticulum containing the Golgi complex and secreted out of the cells. The mechanism of its intracellular transport and passage through plasma membrane is not known. It appears to be an energy-requiring step, however, since it can be blocked by respiration inhibitors (Jamieson and Palade, 1968) or by temperature reduction (Stevens and Williamson, 1973; Baumal and Scharff, 1973). It has been suggested that Ig may be discharged from the plasma membrane near the small vesicles of the Golgi complex by reverse pinocytosis (Zagury *et al.*, 1970; Uhr, 1970). Ig secretion is not blocked, however,

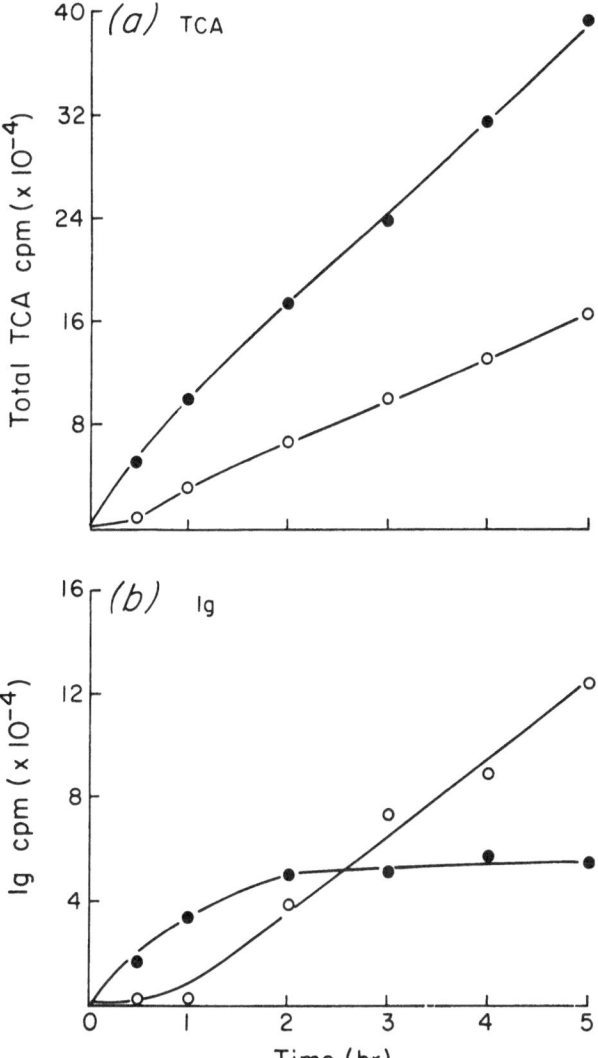

Figure 1. Kinetics of incorporation of [³H]leucine into trichloroacetic-acid-precipitable material and Ig of the spleen cells. A cell suspension (2×10^7 cells/ml) in leucine-less Eagle's medium containing 5% fetal calf serum was incubated at 37°C with [³H]leucine (16 μCi/ml). Aliquots of 1 ml each were distributed into petri dishes and the experiment was performed as described in Section 2. (●) Intracellular protein; (○) secreted protein. (a) Trichloroacetic acid-precipitable material; (b) serologically precipitable Ig. Reproduced from Choi and Good (1972a).

by cytochalasin B, which is known to inhibit pinocytosis in macrophages (Parkhouse and Allison, 1972), thus making this mechanism unlikely.

During intracellular transport, there is an orderly addition of carbohydrate residues. This conclusion is based on identification of the molecules with different carbohydrate compositions, analysis of the order in which carbohydrate residues are attached, and correlation of these data with the successive appearance in different cell fractions of L chains or Ig in transit (Choi *et al.,* 1971b; Melchers,

1971). A schematic diagram summarizing the results of these investigations, the correlation of the carbohydrate composition of the L chain with its appearance in different subcellular components during transport, is presented in Figure 2. In the rough endoplasmic reticulum, the L chain contains its full complement of glucosamine and mannose residues. In the course of transport to the smooth endoplasmic reticulum, the first, or both, galactose residues are attached; further galactose and fucose residues are attached shortly before secretion. Orderly addition of glucosamine and galactose to Ig during the secretion process has been demonstrated biochemically (Uhr and Schenkein, 1970; Melchers, 1971; Choi *et al.,* 1971b; Knopf *et al.,* 1975) as well as by electron microscopic autoradiography (Zagury *et al.,* 1970).

These studies raise the question whether or not the addition of carbohydrate is necessary for Ig secretion to occur at all (Eylar, 1965). If it is, then the requirement might be investigated using mutant myeloma cells blocked in their ability to secrete. In particular, comparison of the galactosyl transferase activity of secreting and nonsecreting cells may be revealing. In support of this hypothesis is the recent discovery that primordial IgM of chicken bursal cells is not secreted and lacks galactose in the H chains, whereas secreted IgM contains galactose (Choi and Good, 1972b). Further evidence supporting such a mechanism of secretion is the finding that 2-deoxy-D-glucose blocks intracellular transport of IgG molecules from rough to smooth membranes by inhibiting glycosylation (Melchers, 1973). In the presence of 2-deoxy-D-glucose, both glycosylation and secretion of newly synthesized IgG1 by mouse myeloma cells (MOPC 21) were completely inhibited, while the intracellular accumulation of IgG1 continued. Furthermore, most of the newly synthesized IgG1 was found in the nonsedimentable supernatant fraction, suggest-

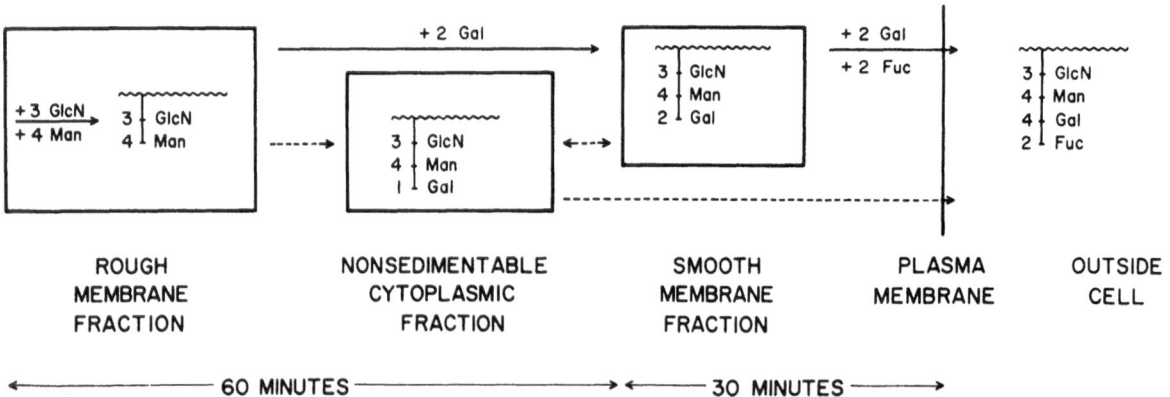

Figure 2. Subcellular distribution, carbohydrate composition, and intracellular transport of L chain. The subcellar components identified after centrifugation in the convex exponential sucrose gradient of a cell homogenate are represented by rectangles; the sucrose-gradient fractions containing these components are indicated at the top of the figure. These sucrose-gradient fractions are heterogeneous, but differ in their relative contents of rough and smooth membrane structures; the subcellular components found in highest concentrations in each fraction are given in the figure. The earliest steps of carbohydrate attachment are not specified in the figure, as they were not studied in this investigation. The average carbohydrate composition of the L chain in each fraction is given, inside the rectangles. The time scale shown in the figure represents the average transit times of L chains in the rough membrane and smooth membrane fractions; the times required for the events within each fraction remain to be determined. The horizontal lines represent the amino acid portion of L chain; vertical lines, the carbohydrate portion. (GlcN) glucosamine; (Man) mannose; (Gal) galactose; (Fuc) fucose. Reproduced from Choi *et al.* (1971b).

ing that binding to a membrane through glucosylation steps may be a signal for secretion.

It is also possible that a secretory protein may be already in the pathway to secretion before any carbohydrate has been attached. The addition of the carbohydrate moiety to the secreted Ig may be an accidental consequence of its being bound to a membrane, where the carbohydrate-attaching enzymes are distributed (Hagopian et al., 1968). In contrast to cell-associated proteins, which are made on free polysomes (Redman, 1969; Ganoza and Williams, 1969), the membrane-bound character of L and H chains synthesizing polysomes may determine that the fate of Ig is to be secreted (Cioli and Lennox, 1973). Cell-free synthesis of L chains using mRNA from mouse myeloma cells (MOPC 21 or MOPC 46) produced a slightly longer precursor polypeptide chain (Milstein et al., 1972). Peptide analysis of these precursors revealed identical tryptic peptides, except for an additional 14 or 15 amino acids at the N-terminus. Recently, a similar short-lived peptide extension was found in several precursors for dog pancreatic secretory proteins, which was synthesized in vitro by translation of its mRNA (Devillers-Thiery et al., 1975). Furthermore, amino acid sequence determination of this peptide revealed extensive homology in the 16 amino-terminal residues. It was postulated that this short amino acid sequence may provide a determinant for the postsynthetic processing. Binding to a membrane would then occur after translation of the first few condons of mRNA. There is evidence suggesting that the binding of polysomes to the membrane occurs after the initiation of protein synthesis (Rosbach, 1972; Harrison et al., 1974). These results imply that carbohydrate residues may be added to Ig as a result of their exposure to glycosyl transferase during secretion, rather than as a requirement for secretion (Williamson, 1973).

6. Differentiation of B Lymphocytes

So far, this review has focused on Ig synthesis and secretion by fully differentiated plasma cells or their malignant equivalents. Equally interesting is the synthesis of Ig by their precursors, B lymphocytes. In contrast to a homogeneous population of myeloma cells, in vitro biosynthesis of Ig by normal lymphoid cells reveals a population average of lymphoid cells used in the experiment. Using a velocity sedimentation method to separate the cells by sizes (Miller and Phillips, 1969), it has been found that plasma cells synthesize and secrete Ig in amounts 100- to 1000-fold greater than do small B lymphocytes (Melchers and Andersson, 1973; Lifter et al., 1976). Thus, a minute contamination of small B lymphocytes by plasma cells can easily lead to misinterpretation of the experimental results.

Early events in the life history of B lymphocytes are best understood in the chicken, in which a single, defined tissue, the bursa of Fabricius, supports their proliferation (Glick, 1964). It is known that hemopoietic stem cells settle in specialized epithelial microenvironments and that Ig synthesis and cell proliferation commence within a very short time (Moore and Owen, 1966). Lymphoid cells, which bear Ig on their surface, appear in the bursa of 12- to 13-day-old embryos (Kincade and Cooper, 1971). Thus, the bursa of Fabricius provides an excellent model in which to study the development of B lymphocytes, which apparently are not induced by an exogenous antigen (Cooper et al., 1972; Choi and Good, 1973).

Immunoglobulin-synthesizing cells from the spleen and bursa were fractionated by 1g centrifugation, and characterized by their ability to synthesize immunoglobulin and by staining with fluorescent antilight chain (Lifter *et al.*, 1976). Four subpopulations of immunoglobulin-synthesizing cells were identified. In the bursa, slowly sedimenting ($s = 2.3$ mm/hr) and rapidly sedimenting ($s > 3.5$ mm/hr) subpopulations with surface immunoglobulin were present; in the spleen, a slowly sedimenting ($s = 2.3$ mm/hr) subpopulation with surface immunoglobulin and plasma cells ($s > 3.5$ mm/hr) with large concentrations of intracellular immunoglobulin existed. The subpopulations differed most markedly in their ability to synthesize immunoglobulin (cpm Ig synthesized/10^6 Ig positive cells); the rates of immunoglobulin synthesis were in the ratio: 1:2/1:900. The slowly sedimenting B cells from the spleen and both subpopulations of B cells from the bursa released small amounts of immunoglobulin into the culture media, whereas the plasma cells released immunoglobulin at a rate as much as 3700 times greater. Bursal B cells could be further distinguished from splenic B cells by a greater amount of DNA synthesis.

A similar differentiation of B lymphocytes was observed after stimulation by antigen (Sterzl and Nordin, 1971). In both the mouse (Greaves *et al.*, 1970) and the guinea pig (Davie and Paul, 1971), antigen-binding cells have been detected before any significant development of antibody-secreting cells. During differentiation, B lymphocytes change morphologically into plasma cells, the latter having fully developed rough and smooth endoplasmic reticulum with cisternae-containing Ig (Shands *et al.*, 1973; Shohat *et al.*, 1973; Avrameas and Leduc, 1970). In small B lymphocytes, the synthesized Ig becomes incorporated into the plasma membrane as Ig receptors for antigen (Greaves and Hogg, 1971). Antigen, after binding to receptor Ig, induces differentiation of B lymphocytes into plasma cells that synthesize much more Ig, which is now actively secreted. Since only a very small fraction of lymphocytes (0.02% of all cells in unstimulated animals) bind a given antigen, it is very difficult, practically, to perform biochemical studies with antigen-stimulated B lymphocytes (Ada, 1970).

Melchers and Andersson (1973) used mitogens to induce a large number of B lymphocytes. Bacterial lipopolysaccharides (LPS) from *Escherichia coli* activate a larger number of B lymphocytes to proliferate and differentiate into IgM-secreting cells (Parkhouse and Allison, 1972). Small B lymphocytes of nude mice synthesize 7 S IgM that contains only glucosamine and mannose (Andersson *et al.*, 1974). Within the first hour, LPS stimulate small resting mouse B lymphocytes to an increased rate of synthesis and secretion of IgM (Melchers and Andersson, 1974a). Stimulated B lymphocytes synthesize 10–100 times more IgM than unstimulated cells and actively secrete IgM as the 19 S pentamer, whereas unstimulated cells shed only 7 S IgM. Secreted 19 S IgM contains galactose and fucose residues in addition to mannose and glucosamine; furthermore, such initial changes in the rate and type of IgM synthesis after mitogenic stimulation are not affected by actinomycin D, suggesting that such maturation of B lymphocytes is not necessarily accompanied by new mRNA synthesis (Melchers and Andersson, 1974b).

ACKNOWLEDGMENTS

I greatly appreciate both the critical reading of the manuscript and the comments of Drs. F. K. Sanders, J. Lifter, P. Kincade, and D. Kiszkiss. The secretarial skill of P. Higgins was very valuable in preparing this chapter.

The author's work is supported by grants from the National Cancer Institute and the American Cancer Society.

Abel, C. A., and Grey, H. M., 1968, Studies on the structure of mouse γA myeloma proteins, *Biochemistry* **7**:2682–2688.

Ada, G. L., 1970, Antigen binding cells in tolerance and immunity, *Transplant. Rev.* **5**:105–129.

Andersson, J., Lafleur, L., and Melchers, F., 1974, IgM in bone marrow-derived lymphocytes: Synthesis, surface deposition, turnover and carbohydrate composition in unstimulated mouse B cells, *Eur. J. Immunol.* **4**:170–180.

Askonas, B. A., and Williamson, A. R., 1966, Biosynthesis of immunoglobulins on polyribosomes and assembly of the IgG molecule, *Proc. R. Soc. London Ser. B* **166**:232–243.

Avrameas, S., and Leduc, E. H., 1970, Detection of simultaneous antibody synthesis in plasma cells and specialized lymphocytes in rabbit lymph nodes, *J. Exp. Med.* **131**:1137–1168.

Bargellesi, A., Periman, P., and Scharff, M. D., 1972, Synthesis, assembly and secretion of γ-globulin by mouse myeloma cells. IV. Assembly of IgA, *J. Immunol.* **108**:126–134.

Baumal, R., and Scharff, M. D., 1973, Synthesis, assembly and secretion of mouse immunoglobulin, *Transplant. Rev.* **14**:163–183.

Baumal, R., Potter, M., and Scharff, M. D., 1971, Synthesis, assembly and secretion of gamma globulin by mouse myeloma cells. IV. Assembly of the three subclasses of IgG, *J. Exp. Med.* **134**:1316–1334.

Becker, M. J., and Rich, A., 1966, Polyribosomes of tissues producing antibodies, *Nature (London)* **212**:142–146.

Bevan, M. J., 1971a, Interchain disulfide bond formation studied in two mouse myelomas which secrete immunoglobulin A, *Eur. J. Immunol.* **1**:133–138.

Bevan, M. J., 1971b, The vectorial release of nascent immunoglobulin peptides, *Biochem. J.* **122**:5–11.

Borun, T. W., Scharff, M. D., and Robbins, E., 1967, Preparation of mammalian polyribosomes with the detergent Nonidet P-40, *Biochim. Biophys. Acta* **149**:302–304.

Buxbaum, J., Zolla, S., Scharff, M. D., and Franklin, E. C., 1971, Synthesis and assembly of immunoglobulins by malignant human plasmacytes and lymphocytes. II. Heterogeneity of assembly in cells producing IgM proteins, *J. Exp. Med.* **133**:1118–1130.

Campbell, P. N., 1970, Functions of polyribosomes attached to membranes of animal cells, *FEBS Lett.* **7**:1–7.

Choi, Y. S., and Good, R. A., 1972a, Development of chicken lymphoid system. I. Synthesis and secretion of immunoglobulins by chicken lymphoid cells, *J. Exp. Med.* **135**:1133–1149.

Choi, Y. S., and Good, R. A., 1972b, Development of chicken lymphoid system. II. Synthesis of primordial immunoglobulin M by the bursa cells of chick embryo, *J. Exp. Med.* **136**:8–20.

Choi, Y. S., and Good, R. A., 1973, Biosynthesis and secretion of antibody by chicken lymphoid cells, *J. Immunol.* **110**:1485–1491.

Choi, Y. S., Knopf, P. M., and Lennox, E. S., 1971a, Subcellular fractionation of mouse myeloma cells, *Biochemistry* **10**:659–667.

Choi, Y. S., Knopf, P. M., and Lennox, E. S., 1971b, Intracellular transport and secretion of an immunoglobulin light chain, *Biochemistry* **10**:668–679.

Cioli, D., and Lennox, E. S., 1973, Immunoglobulin nascent chains on membrane-bound ribosomes of myeloma cells, *Biochemistry* **12**:3211–3217.

Cooper, M. D., Lawton, A. R., and Kincade, P. W., 1972, A developmental approach to the biological basis for antibody diversity, *Contemp. Top. Immunobiol.* **1**:33–47.

Davie, J. M., and Paul, W. E., 1971, Receptors on immunocompetent cells. II. Specificity and nature of receptors on dinitrophenylated guinea pig albumin—[125]I-binding lymphocytes of normal guinea pig, *J. Exp. Med.* **134**:495–516.

Della Corte, E. D., and Parkhouse, R. M. E., 1973, Biosynthesis of immunoglobulin A (IgA) and immunoglobulin M (IgM) requirement for J chain and a disulphide-exchanging enzyme for polymerization, *Biochem. J.* **136**:597–606.

DePetris, S., 1970, Electron microscopy of polyribosomes synthesizing immunoglobulin chains: Comparison with sizes determined by density-gradient-sedimentation data, *Biochem. J.* **118**:385–389.

Devillers-Thiery, A., Kindt, T., Scheele, G., and Blobel, G., 1975, Homology in amino-terminal sequence of precursors to pancreatic secretory proteins, *Proc. Natl. Acad. Sci. U.S.A.* **72**:5016–5020.

Dintzis, H. M., 1961, Assembly of the peptide chains of hemoglobin, *Proc. Natl. Acad. Sci. U.S.A.* **47**:247–261.

Eylar, E. H., 1965, On the biological role of glycoproteins, *J. Theor. Biol.* **10**:89–113.

Fleischman, J. B., 1967, Synthesis of the IgG heavy chain in rabbit lymph node cells, *Biochemistry* **6**:1311–1320.

Ganoza, M. C., and Williams, C. A., 1969, *In vitro* synthesis of different categories of specific protein by membrane-bound and free ribosomes, *Proc. Natl. Acad. Sci. U.S.A.* **63**:1370–1376.

Glick, B., 1964, The bursa of Fabricius and the development of immunologic competence, in: *The Thymus in Immunobiology* (R. A. Good and A. E. Gabrielson, eds.), pp. 343–358, Hoeber, New York.

Greaves, M. F., and Hogg, N. M., 1971, Immunoglobulin determinants on the surface of antigen binding T and B lymphocytes in mice, *Prog. Immunol.* **1**:111–126.

Greaves, M. F., Möller, E., and Möller, G., 1970, Studies on antigen-binding cells. II. Relationship to antigen-sensitive cells, *Cell. Immunol.* **1**:388–403.

Hagopian, A., Bosmann, H. B., and Eylar, E. H., 1968, Glycoprotein biosynthesis: The localization of polypeptidyl : N-acetylgalactosaminyl, collagen : glucosyl, and glycoprotein : galactosyl transferases in HeLa cell membrane fractions, *Arch. Biochem. Biophys.* **128**:387–396.

Harrison, T. M., Brownlee, G. G., and Milstein, C., 1974, Studies on polysome-membrane interactions in mouse myeloma cells, *Eur. J. Biochem.* **47**:613–620.

Helmreich, E., Kern, M., and Eisen, H. N., 1961, The secretion of antibody by isolated lymph node cells, *J. Biol. Chem.* **236**:464–473.

Hood, L., and Prahl, J., 1971, The immune system: A model for differentiation in higher organisms, *Adv. Immunol.* **14**:291–351.

Jamieson, J. D., and Palade, G. E., 1967, Intracellular transport of secretory proteins in the pancreatic exocrine cell, *J. Cell Biol.* **34**:577–596.

Jamieson, J. D., and Palade, G. E., 1968, Intracellular transport of secretory proteins in the pancreatic exocrine cell. IV. Metabolic requirements, *J. Cell Biol.* **39**:589–603.

Kincade, P. W., and Cooper, M. D., 1971, Development and distribution of immunoglobulin-containing cells in the chicken, *J. Immunol.* **106**:371–382.

Knopf, P. M., 1973, Pathways leading to expression of immunoglobulins, *Transplant. Rev.* **14**:145–162.

Knopf, P. M., Parkhouse, R. M. E., and Lennox, E. S., 1967, Biosynthetic units of an immunoglobulin heavy chain, *Proc. Natl. Acad. Sci. U.S.A.* **58**:2288–2295.

Knopf, P. M., Sasso, E., Destree, A., and Melchers, F., 1975, Polysaccharide intermediates formed during intracellular transport of a carbohydrate-containing secreted immunoglobulin light chain, *Biochemistry* **14**:4136–4143.

Kuechler, E., and Rich, A., 1969, Sequential synthesis of messenger RNA and antibodies in rabbit lymph nodes, *Nature (London)* **222**:544–547.

Lennox, E. S., Knopf, P. M., Munro, A. J., and Parkhouse, R. M. E., 1967, A search for biosynthetic subunits of light and heavy chains of immunoglobulins, *Cold Spring Harbor Symp. Quant. Biol.* **32**:249–254.

Lifter, J., Kincade, P. W., and Choi, Y. S., 1976, Subpopulations of chicken B lymphocytes, *J. Immunol.* **117**:2220–2225.

Melchers, F., 1971, Biosynthesis of the carbohydrate portion of immunoglobulins: Radiochemical and chemical analysis of the carbohydrate moieties of two myeloma proteins purified from different subcellular fractions of plasma cells, *Biochemistry* **10**:653–659.

Melchers, F., 1973, Biosynthesis, intracellular transport, and secretion of immunoglobulins: Effect of 2-deoxy-D-glucose in tumor plasma cells producing and secreting immunoglobulin G₁, *Biochemistry* **12**:1471–1476.

Melchers, F., and Andersson, J., 1973, Synthesis, surface deposition and secretion of immunoglobulin M in bone marrow-derived lymphocytes before and after mitogenic stimulation, *Transplant. Rev.* **14**:76–130.

Melchers, F., and Andersson, J., 1974a, IgM in bone marrow-derived lymphocytes: Changes in synthesis, turnover and secretion, and in numbers of molecules on the surface of B cells after mitogenic stimulation, *Eur. J. Immunol.* **4**:181–188.

Melchers, F., and Andersson, J., 1974b, Early changes in immunoglobulin M synthesis after mitogenic stimulation of bone marrow-derived lymphocytes, *Biochemistry* **13**:4645–4653.

Melchers, F., and Knopf, P. M., 1967, Biosynthesis of the carbohydrate portion of immunoglobulin chains: Possible relation to secretion, *Cold Spring Harbor Symp. Quant. Biol.* **32**:255–262.

Miller, R. G., and Phillips, R. A., 1969, Separation of cells by velocity sedimentation, *J. Cell Physiol.* **73**:191–201.

Milstein, C., Brownlee, G. G., Harrison, T. M., and Matthews, M. B., 1972, A possible precursor of immunoglobulin light chains, *Nature (London) New Biol.* **239**:117–120.

Moore, M. A. S., and Owen, J. J. T., 1966, Experimental studies on the development of the bursa of Fabricius, *Dev. Biol.* **14**:40–51.

Norton, W. L., Lewis, D., and Ziff, M., 1965, The effect of progressive immunization on polyribosomal size in lymphoid cells, *Proc. Natl. Acad. Sci. U.S.A.* **54**:851–856.

Parkhouse, R. M. E., 1971, Immunoglobulin M biosynthesis: Production of intermediates and excess of light chain in mouse myeloma MOPC 104E, *Biochem. J.* **123**:635–641.

Parkhouse, R. M. E., 1972, Biosynthesis of J-chain in mouse IgA and IgM, *Nature (London) New Biol.* **236**:9–11.

Parkhouse, R. M. E., and Allison, A. C., 1972, Failure of cytochalasin B or colchicine to inhibit secretion of immunoglobulins, *Nature (London) New Biol.* **235**:220–222.

Porter, R. R., 1973, Immunoglobulin structure, in: *Defense and Recognition* (R. R. Porter, ed.), pp. 159–197, University Park Press, Baltimore.

Redman, C. M., 1969, Biosynthesis of serum proteins and ferritin by free and attached ribosomes of rat liver, *J. Biol. Chem.* **244**:4308–4315.

Rosbach, M., 1972, Formation of membrane-bound polyribosomes, *J. Mol. Biol.* **65**:413–422.

Scharff, M. D., and Uhr, J. W., 1965, Functional ribosomal unit of gamma-globulin synthesis, *Science* **148**:646–648.

Schubert, D., 1968, Immunoglobulin assembly in a mouse myeloma, *Proc. Natl. Acad. Sci. U.S.A.* **60**:683–690.

Schubert, D., and Cohn, M., 1968, Immunoglobulin biosynthesis. III. Blocks in defective synthesis, *J. Mol. Biol.* **38**:273–288.

Shands, J. W., Peavy, D. L., and Smith, R. T., 1973, Differential morphology of mouse spleen cells stimulated *in vitro* by endotoxin, phytohemagglutinin, pokeweed mitogen, and staphylococcal enterotoxin B, *Am. J. Pathol.* **70**:1–24.

Shapiro, A. L., Scharff, M. D., Maizel, J. V., Jr., and Uhr, J. W., 1966, Polyribosomal synthesis and assembly of the H and L chains of gamma globulin, *Proc. Natl. Acad. Sci. U.S.A.* **56**:216–221.

Shapiro, A. L., Vinuela, E., and Maizel, J. V., Jr., 1967, Molecular weight estimation of polypeptide chains by electrophoresis in SDS–polyacrylamide gels, *Biochem. Biophys. Res. Commun.* **28**:815–820.

Shohat, M., Janossy, G., and Dourmashkin, R. R., 1973, Development of rough endoplasmic reticulum in mouse splenic lymphocytes stimulated by mitogen, *Eur. J. Immunol.* **3**:680–687.

Sterzl, J., and Nordin, A., 1971, The common cell precursors for cells producing different immunoglobulins, in: *Cell Interactions and Receptor Antibodies in Immune Responses* (O. Makela, A. Cross, and T. U. Kosunen, eds.), pp. 213–230, Academic Press, New York.

Stevens, R. H., and Williamson, A. R., 1972, Isolation of messenger RNA coding for mouse heavy-chain immunoglobulin, *Proc. Natl. Acad. Sci. U.S.A.* **70**:1127–1131.

Stevens, R. H., and Williamson, A. R., 1973, Translational control of immunoglobulin synthesis. I. Repression of heavy chain synthesis. *J. Mol. Biol.* **78**:505–516.

Swan, D., Aviv, H., and Leder, P., 1972, Purification and properties of biologically active messenger RNA for a myeloma light chain, *Proc. Natl. Acad. Sci. U.S.A.* **69**:1967–1971.

Thorsby, E., and Bratlie, A., 1970, A rapid method for preparation of pure lymphocyte suspension, in: *Histocompatibility Testing—1970* (P. I. Terasaki, ed.), pp. 655–656, Munksgaard, Copenhagen.

Uhr, J. W., 1970, Intracellular events underlying synthesis and secretion of immunoglobulin, *Cell. Immunol.* **1**:228–244.

Uhr, J. W., and Schenkein, I., 1970, Immunoglobulin synthesis and secretion. IV. Sites of incorporation of sugars as determined by subcellular fractionation, *Proc. Natl. Acad. Sci. U.S.A.* **66**:952–958.

Voss, E. W., and Bauer, D. C., 1967, Intracellular biosynthesis of rabbit antibody, *J. Biol. Chem.* **242**:4495–4500.

Watson, J. D., 1976, The problem of antibody synthesis, in: *Molecular Biology of the Gene,* 3rd Ed., pp. 591–640, W. A. Benjamin, New York.

Williamson, A. R., 1973, Biosynthesis of immunoglobulins, in: *Defense and Recognition* (R. R. Porter, ed.), pp. 229–255, University Park Press, Baltimore.

Williamson, A. R., and Askonas, B. A., 1967, Biosynthesis of immunoglobulins: The separate classes of polyribosomes synthesizing heavy and light chains, *J. Mol. Biol.* **23**:201–216.

Zagury, D., Uhr, J. W., Jamieson, J. D., and Palade, G. E., 1970, Immunoglobulin synthesis and secretion. II. Radioautographic studies of sites of addition of carbohydrate moieties and intracellular transport, *J. Cell Biol.* **46**:52–63.

16

Lymphocyte Membrane Immunoglobulins: An Overview

BENVENUTO PERNIS

1. Introduction

Selective concepts of antibody formation imply that preformed antibodies are present as receptors on the membrane of immunocytes and are instrumental, after interaction with the corresponding antigens, in triggering these cells to undergo a series of events that ultimately lead to antibody production. This view of the physiology of the immune response was first put forward by Ehrlich (1900), who visualized polyvalent immunocytes, each carrying on its membrane a variety of receptors for antigens; the interaction of antigen with one kind of these receptors induced a "compensatory" hyperproduction of the receptors, which then spilled into the body fluids as soluble antibodies. Almost 60 years later Burnet (1959) proposed a similar concept, but with one major difference, namely, that the combining property of the receptors present on the membrane of one cell is uniform, and that the interaction of these receptors with the corresponding antigen determines this cell to clonal expansion or deletion with the corresponding consequences of antibody production or tolerance.

On these simple concepts of antigen–receptor interaction, all modern immunology is grounded; it is therefore not surprising that since lymphocyte membrane immunoglobulins (MIg's) were first clearly demonstrated by Raff et al. (1970) and by Pernis et al. (1970), much attention and research has been concentrated on the subject, with the consequent publication of a large number of papers and the inevitable production of a number of controversies. The present rather vast field of research on lymphocyte MIg's has been the subject of good reviews (see Warner, 1974) and of several symposia (see Seligman et al., 1975). It is not the purpose of

BENVENUTO PERNIS • Departments of Microbiology and Medicine, College of Physicians and Surgeons of Columbia University, New York, New York.

this article to systematically examine the field, but simply to evidence some key points that appear important and established in our present knowledge, and to discuss some of the main problems that we have to solve to fully understand the physiology of the Ig receptors.

2. Basic Data on Membrane Immunoglobulins

Two kinds of Ig's can be found on the membranes of lymphoid cells: those produced by other cells and passively acquired through binding to Fc receptors, and those actively synthesized by the same cell that carries them. Obviously, only the latter can function as receptors for antibody formation in a selective system, and thus we are interested mainly in them. Actively synthesized Ig molecules are present on the membranes of a proportion of lymphoid cells (see below) in all vertebrate species that have been studied, their presence appearing not to be separable from the existence of a defined immune system.

These MIg's have been demonstrated by optical or electron microscopy with a variety of methods employing antibodies against the Ig's labeled with fluorochromes, electron-dense markers, radioisotopes, and enzymes; sensitized erythrocytes and appropriate antibodies have also been used in rosette tests. In addition, Ig's or their component chains have been identified, among membrane proteins labeled with radioisotopes, with physical methods such as polyacrylamide gel electrophoresis, generally with an intermediate separation from the other membrane proteins by means of anti-Ig antibodies. So we have no doubts that these molecules are present on lymphoid cell membranes; they can be removed with proteolytic enzymes (such as trypsin or pronase at appropriate concentrations) or by exposure to anti-Ig antibodies (see below). The living lymphocytes will then reconstitute their normal amount of MIg within some hours of *in vitro* culture (from 6 to 18, depending on the cells and the culture conditions), thus clearly showing active synthesis.

Each lymphocyte that carries MIg can have from 20,000 to 200,000 MIg molecules; such heterogeneity of MIg densities is clearly apparent on immunofluorescence examination of polyclonal lymphocyte populations from the blood or lymphoid organs. Monoclonal B lymphocytes, such as the human peripheral-blood lymphocytes (PBL) in cases of chronic lymphocytic leukemia (CLL), may show a more restricted range of MIg densities; this, however, is not the rule. The density of MIg on the monoclonal lymphocyte population of certain patients with non-Hodgkin's solid tissue lymphomas is often much greater than on the lymphocytes of the usual case of CLL. We do not know how the lymphocytes control the density of their MIg; definite correlations between MIg density and lymphocyte function are also not apparent.

The MIg's are oriented, as expected on the basis of their antigen-binding function, with the Fab toward the outside and the Fc in contact with the cell membrane. In fact, it was shown by Fu and Kunkel (1974) that the antigenic determinants of the heavy (H) chain domains at the carboxy-terminal end of the IgM and IgD molecules present on the membrane of human lymphocytes are not available for reaction with the corresponding antibodies. The mode of binding of the MIg H chain to the lymphocyte membrane has not yet been defined; there are two possibilities: either (1) the carboxy-terminal end of the H chain is directly embedded

359

LYMPHOCYTE
MEMBRANE
IMMUNO-
GLOBULINS:
AN OVERVIEW

in the lipid bilayer or (2) the H-chain C-terminal is specifically accepted by a non-Ig membrane protein (proreceptor). The first possibility appears more likely. Whichever the binding mechanism may be, the MIg's, like other membrane proteins, exhibit the capacity of lateral movement in the plane of the cell membrane and show the phenomena of patching and capping when interacting with multivalent ligands; it has still not been shown that these phenomena are prominent when lymphocytes interact with antigens *in vivo*, or that they play a role in lymphocyte triggering.

The biosynthesis of MIg is not known in detail. The synthesis of H and light (L) chains is required, as well as the assembly of these chains. It is therefore necessary that the synthesis of MIg take place on membrane-bound polyribosomes in some vesicle in the cytoplasm of the lymphocyte; vesicles in the Golgi area are a likely possibility.

The vesicles should be inserted in the plasma membrane, together with the membrane-bound Ig's. Taking into account the average number of MIg molecules and their half-life on the membrane (see below), a very limited synthetic activity is required to keep the steady state; it can be calculated that a few polyribosomes would be sufficient. It is clear that the biosynthesis of MIg's is under separate control from that of the molecules that accumulate in the cisternae of the endoplasmic reticulum of antibody-secreting cells. In fact, there are cells (most B lymphocytes) that have MIg but do not have easily demonstrable intracytoplasmic Ig's, and there are cells (most mature Ig G plasma cells) that have abundant Ig's in the cytoplasm (and secrete them), but are negative in all the tests for MIg's. Furthermore, there are plasma cells (Pernis *et al.,* 1971) that express different classes of Ig's on the membrane (IgM or IgM + IgG) and in the cytoplasm (IgG only). The problem of the separation in control, and presumably in intracellular topography, of the synthesis of membrane vs. secretory Ig's is a very intriguing one, since the law of the uniformity of the combining site requires that the same L chain and V_H genes control both the membrane and the secretory Ig's synthesized by a single immunocyte.

Once inserted on the membrane, the MIg molecules have a turnover that apparently is very different in different kinds of cells: in resting mouse B lymphocytes, the half-life of MIg was estimated to be as long as 40–80 hr (Melchers and Andersson, 1973). On the other hand, the half-life of radioiodinated MIg of normal human tonsil lymphoid cells was found to be approximately 6 hr, for both IgM and IgD (Ferrarini *et al.,* 1976a). A much shorter half-life of 45 min was found for the MIg of a human lymphoblastoid line continuously growing *in vitro* (Lerner *et al.,* 1972). After reaction with multivalent ligands (such as antigens or anti-Ig antibodies), the MIg molecules disappear from the membrane within 10–20 min at body temperature in most kinds of lymphoid cells. There are two ways whereby the MIg molecules can leave the lymphocyte membrane, namely, internalization in pinocytotic vesicles or shedding in the surrounding fluids. There is evidence that both occur; the shedding phemonenon is probably the normal mode of MIg turnover in the absence of cross-linkage with multivalent ligands, and was directly demonstrated to occur *in vitro* (Vitetta and Uhr, 1972). It also probably occurs *in vivo* with the liberation of very minute amounts of Ig's in the body fluid. This amount can be calculated on the basis of the number of B lymphocytes in the body, the average number of MIg molecules on their membranes, and their half-life; what one obtains from this calculation is that the concentration of Ig molecules in body fluids that can be ascribed to shedding of MIg from lymphocyte membranes is of the order of less than 100 ng/ml. It is interesting to point out that for an Ig class (IgD) that in a given species (monkeys) is only on the membranes and is not secreted, this is precisely the concentration, attributable to shedding only, that was found in the serum (Corte *et al.*, 1978). Internalization in pinocytotic vesicles is, on the other hand, the way out of the plasma membrane of those MIg molecules that have been cross-linked by anti-Ig antibodies (Taylor *et al.*, 1971); it is likely that cross-linkage by antigen has the same effect.

The fate and function of pinocytosed MIg molecules are not known; a certain proportion is probably degraded in lysosomes, but it is not excluded that some MIg molecules, endocytosed as the consequence of interreaction with polyvalent ligands, may perform an important regulatory role.

3. Cells That Carry Actively Synthesized Membrane Immunoglobulins

The methods indicated in Section 1 have identified Ig on the membranes of bone-marrow-derived (B) lymphoid cells at various stages of development, from immature lymphocytes in fetal liver to mature, Ig-secreting plasma cells in adult peripheral lymphoid tissues. On the other hand, the presence of actively synthe-sized MIg's on thymus-derived (T) lymphocytes has never been unequivocally established. Considerable debate on this subject has been going on, but the argu-ment is not settled.

The present trend of belief is that T lymphocytes have their own class of actively synthesized receptors that is different from Ig's, except perhaps for a certain portion of the variable region (V) carrying the idiotype. It is quite certain that some T lymphocytes have on their membranes Ig molecules passively acquired either through a bridge of antigen (Pernis *et al.*, 1974a; Nagy *et al.*, 1976) or through the Fc receptors that T lymphocytes have for IgG (Stout and Herzenberg, 1975) or for IgM (Moretta *et al.*, 1975). On the other hand, as stated above, the presence of actively synthesized MIg's is considered to be a marker of B lymphocytes. These cells appear in the human fetus (liver) around 9.5 weeks of gestation (Lawton *et al.*, 1972) and in the liver of the mouse at the 17–18th day of gestation (Owen *et al.*, 1977). These MIg-positive cells are preceded in the mouse liver (as well as in the spleen) by precursors that appear around the 12th day of gestation, as ascertained by organ culture *in vitro* (Owen *et al.*, 1975). It may be that some of these precursors, although devoid of MIg's, have instead intracytoplasmic Ig's (Owen *et al.*, 1977); these cytoplasmic-positive but surface-negative B lymphocytes are also present in the bone marrow of the adult mouse. B lymphocytes without surface Ig's (null cells) were also identified in adult human blood (Chess *et al.*, 1975); again, the cultivation of these cells *in vitro* supports the possibility that at least some of them may "mature" into MIg$^+$ lymphocytes. The general conclusion from this kind of studies is that MIg's are a marker of B lymphocytes that appear in these cells at a given level of development. The relationships between the developmental stage and the class of the MIg's will be considered later. Of course, MIg's are not only present on B lymphocytes, but also persist when these cells enlarge and divide and become lymphoblasts; most human lymphoblastoid lines continuously growing *in vitro* have MIg. On the other hand, the terminal stages of maturation of the B immunocytes, i.e., the Ig-secreting plasma cells, may or may not have MIg, depending on the class of Ig that is in their cytoplasm (Ferrarini *et al.*, 1976b).

361

LYMPHOCYTE
MEMBRANE
IMMUNO-
GLOBULINS:
AN OVERVIEW

4. Membrane Immunoglobulin Idiotypes, Allotypes, and Isotypes

4.1. Idiotypes

Idiotypes and antigen-binding properties of Ig's are both dependent on the V regions of H and L chains. If, as discussed at the beginning of this article, the MIg's actively synthesized by a single lymphocyte are uniform for what concerns their V regions, it follows that they should have a uniform idiotype (a set of idiotopes) and uniform antigen-binding properties.

An important experiment by Raff *et al.* (1973) supports this basic concept. In this experiment, it was established that an antigen with repeated identical determinants (polymerized flagallin) can induce the polar localization (capping) of *all* the MIg's of those lymphocytes with which it reacts; a relevant element of this experiment was that the same result was obtained with the cells of unimmunized as well as of antigen-primed mice.

Turning now to idiotypes according to their original definition, i.e., the individual antigenic properties of a monoclonal population of Ig molecules, it was likewise established (Fu *et al.*, 1974) that the MIg's of a single lymphocyte, or of a clone of lymphocytes (in human CLL), have an uniform idiotype. This work, too, made use of the capping phenomenon and showed that an antiidiotypic antiserum (prepared with serum monoclonal IgM) can cap all the MIg molecules present on the blood lymphocytes of the same CLL patient irrespective of their IgM or IgD isotype (see below).

Of course, the uniformity of the idiotype and antigen-binding properties of the MIg's of a single lymphocyte does not necessarily mean that a single lymphocyte can bind one antigen only; although in principle two different antigens will react with two different (but certainly not homogeneous) lymphocyte populations (Julius *et al.*, 1976), there will be some antigens for which double binding will be found to take place on a certain proportion of lymphocytes. This phenomenon is simply due to the existence of polyfunctional Ig molecules, i.e., molecules that can accommodate one *or* another antigenic determinant in their combining site (Richards *et al.*, 1975). Lymphocytes carrying receptors of this kind increase in number after immunization with the two antigens in sequence (Czaja *et al.*, 1977). There are, however, reports of double-binding lymphocytes that have been interpreted as indicating heterogeneity of the MIg molecules of a single cell (De Luca *et al.*, 1975).

All that we have been considering so far concerning the antigen-binding properties of lymphocyte MIg's has a functional meaning only if the antibodies secreted by the cells derived from them after stimulation react with the same antigens. This prediction was verified in experiments performed with the fluorescence-activated cell sorter (FACS) by Julius and Herzenberg (1974). The concordance of the idiotype of lymphocyte MIg's and of the molecules secreted by more mature members of the same clone was established in cases of Waldenström's macroglobulinaemia by Preud'homme and Seligmann (1972a) and in cases of CLL by Fu *et al.* (1974).

4.2. Allotypes

Only one gene, paternal or maternal, is active in the synthesis of Ig chains in plasma cells. This phenomenon, designated *allelic exclusion,* determines the syntehsis of H and L chains marked by one allotype only in plasma cells of heterozygous individuals. Without allelic exclusion, the Ig's synthesized by a single plasma cell would not be homogeneous.

Likewise, without allelic exclusion, the principle of the uniformity of the combining site of lymphocyte MIg's could not be valid. Direct study of this question by double immunofluorescence indicated complete allelic exclusion of the MIg molecules of rabbit lymphocytes, with regard to both the H and L chains (Pernis *et al.,* 1970); in fact, this observation was the first that clearly established endogenous synthesis of the lymphocyte MIg as opposed to the possibility of a passive uptake.

Different results were reported, however, by Wolf *et al.* (1971) with the use of a rosette test in a mixed antiglobulin reaction: in these experiments, a sizable porportion of lymphocytes from heterozygous rabbits expressing both allelic allotypes on their membrane was found. At present, the question is not definitely settled, but the work with the FACS (Jones *et al.,* 1974) is in favor of allelic exclusion of lymphocyte MIg; moreover, this work supports the important fact that the Ig allotypes expressed by a lymphocyte and by its progeny of Ig-secreting cells are the same. Complete concordance of allotype expression between membrane and intracytoplasmic Ig's, in those individual cells that synthesize both kinds, was also found (Pernis *et al.,* 1971).

Those who find allelic exclusion of lymphocyte MIg's also find that the relative frequency of lymphocytes with one or another allelic product is parallel to the allelic ratio in serum Ig's; it appears, therefore, that this ratio (which may be very different from 1, as, for instance, in the case of the rabbit *b4* and *b9* alleles) is the consequence of whichever process regulates the frequency of lymphocytes differentiated in either direction.

4.3. Isotypes

There are several important facts that concern the expression of L-chain types and H-chain classes (isotypes) on the membrane of single lymphocytes and the frequency of cells showing one or another MIg pattern. These facts are pertinent to the development of B immunocytes and give us a view of some unexpected features of the physiology of these cells; they will be discussed separately.

4.3.1. Light-Chain Types

L chains of MIg's have been studied mainly in human PBL. Here, there seems to be no disagreement with the view that each lymphocyte in normal blood carries either κ or λ Light chains and that the ratio of the two lymphocyte groups roughly parallels the κ/λ ratio of serum Ig's. Monoclonal lymphoid cell populations, like those of lymphoblastoid cells grown *in vitro* or of PBL in cases of CLL, show one L chain type only. The L-chain pattern is therefore simple and in agreement with the law of the uniformity of the combining site; in fact, this uniformity would not be possible if single lymphocytes synthesized both κ and λ L chains, since the two types are connected with different sets of V regions.

4.3.2. μ Heavy Chains

363

LYMPHOCYTE
MEMBRANE
IMMUNO-
GLOBULINS:
AN OVERVIEW

IgM is the major class of Ig's on the lymphocyte membrane in all species. It is the first class that appears in the development of B lymphocytes, and very few are the cells of this group that have MIg's and do not have IgM. Unlike the secreted molecules, the MIgM is exclusively in the form of 7–8 S monomer (Vitetta *et al.*, 1971). On the basis of the effects of treatment with anti-μ antibodies (discussed in later sections), it appears that MIgM plays a central role in the regulation of the Ig synthesis of B immunocytes.

4.3.3. δ Heavy Chains

Molecules of the IgD class are present in low concentration (mean 30 μg/ml) in human serum and are absent or present in nanogram amounts in the sera of other species. In contrast, MIgD molecules were found in the majority (about 80%) of peripheral blood B lymphocytes in the human newborn or adult (Rowe *et al.*, 1973), and were detected as a component quantatively comparable with IgM in the lymphocytes of peripheral lymphoid tissues of adult mice (Vitetta *et al.*, 1975). It follows from the prevalence of IgM on lymphocyte membranes noted in Section 4.3.2 that IgD must coexist with IgM on the membranes of most cells. That it does was clearly shown in the work of Rowe *et al.* (1973), in which it was also found that μ and δ chains present on the membrane of the same lymphocyte were part of separate molecules that "capped" independently under the effect of the corresponding antisera. It was also shown that in keeping with the rule that one lymphocyte carries L chains of one type only, the IgM and IgD molecules that coexisted on the same membrane had L chains of the same type. The coexistence of MIg molecules of two different classes on the same cell does not necessarily contradict the principle of the uniformity of the combining site. In fact, the different H-chain classes are under control of a closely linked cluster of genes for the constant (C) region that is in turn linked to a group of genes for the V regions; pairing between the V_H and C_H genes apparently is subject to no restrictions, so that antibodies of different classes but with the same combining properties can be synthesized by a given B immunocyte or a given clone of immunocytes either sequentially in time or even simultaneously. Proof that the IgM and IgD receptors of the same cell have either identical or closely related combining sites and idiotypes has been given (Pernis *et al.*, 1974b, Fu *et al.*, 1974, Salsano *et al.*, 1974). Since most human PBL have both IgM and IgD, it is not surprising that the majority of cases of human CLL that are due to proliferation of B lymphocytes show cells with both Ig classes on the membrane. The monoclonal CLL lymphocytes may differ from the normal ones with regard to the relative amounts of IgM and IgD on single cells: whereas normal cells show a complete range from an excess of IgM to an excess of IgD, many (but not all) CLL cases show a predominance of one or the other of the two classes.

There are two main problems that are raised by the coexistence of IgM and IgD receptors on the same cell. The first is that of the simultaneous synthesis of the two classes of H chains that, as we have seen, must have the same or closely related V_H regions. If, as appears likely, there is simultaneous synthesis of the two corresponding mRNA molecules, then the problem arises how one V_H gene can simultaneously control the corresponding part of the two different messengers. A possible model is provided by the recent studies on splicing of mRNA (Berget *et al.*, 1977).

The second problem is that of the functional roles of the two different classes of receptors that coexist on the same cell. Several hypotheses have been proposed, some of which are related to the time sequence of the expression of the two classes in the course of B-lymphocyte development. In fact, it was shown by Vitetta *et al.* (1975) that the less mature B lymphocytes in newborn mice and in the bone marrow of adult animals do not have IgD or have much less of it. On the other hand, IgD is also absent from the membrane of most memory B lymphocytes in antigen-primed mice, and in particular, it is absent from the precursors of high-affinity antibody-forming cells (see Pernis, 1977). On the basis of these data, it appears that the developmental sequence of MIg class expression by B lymphocytes is, at least for some cells, as follows:

(1) IgM only → (2) IgM + IgD → (3) IgM + IgG → (4) IgG only

The functional stages that might correspond to these four steps of MIg class expression are a matter of conjecture. Pernis (1976) hypothesized as follows: Cells of group 1 are those cells that are easily made tolerant in the absence of specific T help. Cells of group 2 are virgin B lymphocytes relatively resistant to tolerance. Cells of groups 3 and 4 are memory cells. The possibility that memory lymphocytes may be IgD-negative was also advanced by Cooper *et al.* (1976), whereas very interesting recent work by Cambier *et al.* (1977) showed that enzymatic cleavage of MIgD (IgM resists this treatment to some extent) from adult mouse spleen lymphocytes does make these cells much more susceptible to the induction of tolerance *in vitro*.

Although we are not very near to the understanding of the molecular mechanisms of the function of the simultaneously present IgM and IgD receptors, it is an easy prediction that this function will eventually show a clear requirement for *both* classes working together either in synergism or in antagonism.

4.4.4. γ Heavy Chains

The work of Winchester *et al.* (1975) showed that the percentage of lymphocytes stained with fluorescent anti-IgG antibodies may greatly exceed the number of cells really carrying receptor molecules of this class, due to a nonspecific binding of the fluorescent reagents through the Fc receptor that could be avoided with the use of conjugated F(ab')₂ anti-IgG. It appears, therefore, that IgG, i.e., the major Ig class in the serum, is present as a receptor in only a small proportion of B lymphocytes.

In view of the methodological problems mentioned above, it becomes important to consider the evidence that lymphocytes with actively synthesized IgG receptors really exist. This evidence is solid: (1) Human PBL showing allelic exclusion for membrane IgG allotypes were seen by Litwin (1972) and by Fröland and Natvig (1972). (2) Cases of human CLL in which the clone actively synthesizes MIgG were seen by Preud'homme and Seligmann (1972b); these cases are rare, in agreement with the fact that normal human lymphocytes with MIgG are also rare. (3) Mouse spleen lymphocytes with MIgG *belonging to one subclass only* were detected by Pernis *et al.* (1977). The percentage of these cells among all B lymphocytes is quite low in unstimulated populations, but may rise to 20% or more 6 hr after stimulation with lipopolysaccharide (LPS). These stimulated B lymphocytes again show only one IgG subclass per cell. This eliminates the possibility of passive uptake of these molecules; most of these stimulated cells have membrane IgG *together with* IgM. (4) Several experiments showing a specific inhibition of B-immunocyte activity after treatment *in vitro* with antibodies against IgG (see Section 5) are compatible only with the assumption that IgG receptors exist and are functional. That the IgG-bearing lymphocyte population, although small, may perform important immunological functions is indicated by work of Okumura *et al.* (1976), which shows that lymphocytes with MIgG include almost all memory cells, with the specification that memory to be expressed with production of antibodies of a given IgG subclass is borne by lymphocytes that have receptors of the same subclass. IgG molecules, however, may not be the *only* membrane receptors of memory lymphocytes; these receptors may include cells that have *both* IgM *and* IgG receptors or even primarily IgM receptors but are programmed to express IgG quickly after stimulation. An indication in this direction is given by the work of Abney *et al.* (1976).

The small percentage of lymphocytes with MIgG is, as already noted, in sharp contrast with the fact that IgG is the major Ig class in the serum. This discrepancy between membrane expression and serum concentration is also found in the case of IgD and in general for most H-chain isotypes, in contrast with what is valid for L-chain isotypes or for allotypes, where there is a good parallel between the serum concentration and the membrane representation of a given Ig kind. There is a simple explanation for this discrepancy: B-immunocytes switch the H chains of the Ig's that they synthesize so that the Ig class eventually secreted is often different from the class or classes of Ig present on the membrane of the precursors. On the other hand, there are no interallelic or inter-L-chain switches.

5. Effects of the Interaction between Membrane Immunoglobulins and Antiimmunoglobulin Antibodies

Important elements for the understanding of the function of MIg molecules can be obtained from the study of the effects of the interaction between MIg and anti-Ig antibodies. Many experiments of this kind have been performed, both *in vitro* and *in vivo:* we will limit out attention here to some *in vitro* experiments because they are simpler to analyze.

5.1. Effects on Antibody Production

The first study of this kind was that of Mitchison (1967), who showed that anti-mouse-Ig antibodies suppressed a secondary response to a hapten (4-hydroxy-3-iodo-5-nitrophenylacetyl) *in vitro*. A similar effect on the primary response to sheep erythrocytes was detected by Fuji and Jerne (1969); a significant feature of their experiments was that the addition to the cultures of an excess of mouse Ig's after 1 or 2 days reversed the inhibition, thus showing that the effect of anti-Ig antibodies was not due to killing of Ig-bearing cells.

Experiments of this nature support our belief that MIg's are essential for a specific immune response and have been performed in several laboratories (Greaves, 1970; Lesley and Dutton, 1970). Data directly implying an interaction between the antibodies and the MIg of B lymphocytes as the cause of the blocking of the *in vitro* immune reaction were provided by Mond *et al.* (1972). Pierce *et al.* (1972a,b) used class-specific antibodies and found that in the primary response, anti-μ suppressed the production of antierythrocyte antibodies of all classes, while anti-γ and anti-α eliminated only the plaques of the same class. In the secondary response, in contrast, the IgG and IgA responses were not inhibited by anti-μ, but only by the corresponding antisera.

5.2. Modulation of Membrane Immunoglobulins

The antigens of the TL system, expressed on mouse thymus lymphocytes, that are under the control of a locus (the *Tla* locus) adjacent to the region where the genes of the major histocompatability complex are located are subject to the phenomenon of antigen modulation. This phenomenon (Old *et al.*, 1968) consists in the long-lasting disappearance of the TL antigen from the lymphocyte surface after exposure to anti-TL antibodies; it can be produced *in vitro,* requires a sufficiently long contact between the cells and the antibodies, is not due to cytotoxic effects, and is blocked by actinomycin D treatment of the lymphocytes. Such an effect does not take place for a variety of other lymphocyte membrane antigens, and has been compared to the antigenic changes that occur on the membrane of *Paramecia* exposed to antisera (see Beale, 1954).

It is important to know that the MIg's show the phenomenon of antigen modulation. This phenomenon was the object of the studies of Raff *et al.* (1975). These workers showed that events very similar to antigenic modulation take place in immature mouse B lymphocytes (from fetal liver or adult bone marrow) after exposure to purified antibodies (or, less efficiently, Fab fragments thereof) directed against total mouse Ig's or mouse μ chains. On the other hand, mature lymphocytes from adult spleen quickly recover their MIg after interruption of the exposure to the antiserum, as already seen by Taylor *et al.* (1971) and Loor *et al.* (1972). Moreover, the MIg loss in immature lymphocytes requires a much lower concentration of antibodies than in mature cells and is more rapid. Sidman and Unanue (1975) independently obtained similar results. Since there is no difference in the average amount of MIg molecules present on a mature or an immature lymphocyte, we should conclude that the differences in short-term events following contact with anti-Ig antibodies (i.e., the differences in rapidity of MIg loss and in sensitivity to different antibody concentrations) must be connected with non-Ig membrane molecules that are involved in the process and that are represented differently in mature and immature lymphocytes. Possibly these molecules also play a role in the long-lasting MIg modulation by antibodies. There are several non-Ig membrane components that are expressed differently in mature and immature B lymphocytes; among them is the Fe receptor, which was shown to cocap with MIg under the effect of the F(ab')$_2$ of anti-Ig antibodies (Forni and Pernis, 1975). The conclusion is that the MIg's of immature B lymphocytes, but not those of mature cells, are subject to the phenomenon of antigen modulation. This conclusion may have important implica-

367

LYMPHOCYTE
MEMBRANE
IMMUNO-
GLOBULINS:
AN OVERVIEW

tions, as discussed by Raff *et al.* (1975), for some aspects of immunogical tolerance. Furthermore, it seems to me, antigenic modulation implies that Ig molecules play, directly or indirectly, a regulatory role on their own synthesis; the conclusion would then be that MIg's regulate themselves in immature but not in mature lymphocytes. We shall see in the next section that the MIg of *mature* cells can instead, in some conditions, regulate the synthesis of *intracytoplasmic* Ig's synthesized for secretion.

5.3. Effect of Antiimmunoglobulin Antibodies on Differentiation to Immunoglobulin-Secreting Cells Induced by Lipopolysaccharides

Several different substances, called *polyclonal B-cell activators* (PBA), induce mouse B lymphocytes to proliferation, Ig secretion, and H-chain switches; they thus activate the full range of B-immunocyte reactions. It is widely believed that the PBA (among which are the LPS endotoxins of gram-negative bacteria) operate with no meaningful interaction with the MIg's but rather through separate receptors called *mitogen receptors*. Antibodies against Ig's, however, can inhibit some or all of the effects of PBA. Andersson *et al.* (1974) found that antibodies against mouse Ig's or antibodies specific for mouse μ chains either as intact molecules or as F(ab')$_2$ fragments, blocked the maturation to Ig secretion, but not the proliferation, of adult mouse spleen lymphocytes induced by LPS. After contact with LPS, the effect is a long-lasting one, and the cells do not recover their capacity toward Ig secretion even if all anti-Ig antibodies are removed from the cells with proteolytic enzymes. It appears, therefore, that anti-Ig antibodies, obviously through an interaction with the MIg's, can, under some conditions, regulate the capacity of the B lymphocyte to develop an Ig-secreting activity.

The long-lasting nature of this effect has some analogies with the modulation of MIg induced in immature lymphocytes by anti-Ig antibodies, although clearly the case of intracytoplasmic Ig shows the inhibition of a potentiality, not the block of an existing activity; in fact, it is impossible to influence Ig secretion with anti-Ig antibodies after this process has started. Kearney *et al.* (1976) also studied the effects of anti-Ig antibodies on LPS stimulation, and they obtained similar findings, i.e., a block of maturation but not of proliferation. Moreover, they found that newborn lymphocytes are much more susceptible to the blocking effect as measured by the concentration of anti-Ig antibodies necessary to obtain it; this higher susceptibility (about 300-fold) of immature lymphocytes is parallel to that of MIg's to modulation by anti-Ig antibodies, and further implicates the MIg molecules as mediators of the anti-Ig block of maturation.

Kearney *et al.* (1975) also found that anti-μ antibodies inhibit maturation not only to IgM secretion but also to IgG secretion, so the LPS-induced H-chain switch is also blocked and the key role of MIgM in the regulation of Ig synthesis by B lymphocytes is emphasized. We obtained the same results in a similar system (Pernis, 1977; Pernis *et al.*, unpublished), finding that anti-μ antibodies inhibit the LPS-induced appearance of plasma cells with intracytoplasmic antibodies of all classes, whereas antibodies against IgG1, IgG2a, or IgG2b suppressed only the appearance of cells containing the corresponding Ig; antisera against mouse IgD did not significantly alter the plasma-cell response to LPS.

That anti-Ig antibodies inhibit LPS-induced maturation is therefore well established; not all experiments, on the other hand, show a normal (or even enhanced) proliferative response to LPS of anti-Ig-treated lymphocytes, as indicated above. Schrader (1975) found an inhibition of mitogenesis as measured by DNA synthesis of mouse lymphocytes, and this was also the result obtained by Sidman and Unanue (1976); it appears likely that these interesting differences in results are due to the use of different antisera or different experimental conditions. In the experiments of Sidman and Unanue (1976), the block of mitogenesis was much more efficient with the use of intact anti-Ig antibodies than with their $F(ab')_2$ fragments, thus suggesting a coordinate role of the Fc receptor in the inhibition of proliferation.

5.4. Stimulation of Lymphocytes by Antiimmunoglobulin Antibodies

The concept of MIg's as lymphocyte receptors immediately suggests, in a straightforward simple-minded view, that interaction of these receptors with a ligand, be it antigen or anti-Ig antibody, should determine the reactions of the lymphocyte not only in a negative direction, as discussed above, but also in a positive sense by triggering the cell to activate its different programs.

This possibility was first shown to be a real one by the work of Sell and Gell (1965), who showed that anti-allotype antisera as well as heterologous antisera directed against rabbit Ig's could consistently activate rabbit PBL to blast transformation. In fact, this work was the first that had as a direct implication the existence of MIg's. Subsequently, it was shown by Fanger et al. (1970) that cross-linkage of the MIg was necessary, since $F(ab')_2$ fragments of the anti-Ig were required to induce the transformation. Chicken lymphocytes, too, appeared to be activated to DNA synthesis by anti-Ig antibodies (Skamen and Ivanyi, 1969), but only recently was this result obtained with mouse cells (Weiner et al., 1976a); it appears that only lymphocytes of aged mice are reactive in this kind of stimulation that, as for the rabbit, requires divalent antibodies or fragments (Weiner et al., 1976b).

All these experiments showed that anti-Ig antibodies can stimulate lymphocytes to proliferation, but not to maturation and Ig secretion. Even the latter effect, however, has now been obtained: Kishimoto and Ishizaka (1975) showed that polyclonal production of Ig's of different classes can be obtained by treating rabbit lymphocytes with the corresponding antibodies, provided that an enhancing factor produced by T lymphocytes was added to the cultures. Finally, Platts-Mills and Ishizaka (1975) induced primed human tonsil lymphocytes to secrete antibody (antidiphtheria toxin) by treating them with anti-IgG in the absence of any added enhancing factor.

At first sight, we may be confused by the apparently contradictory results of much experimental work discussed in this final section:

Anti-Ig antibodies may block antibody production induced by antigen, but they may also, in the absence of the antigen, stimulate by themselves the same event in primed cells.

Again, anti-Ig antibodies can block the polyclonal cell proliferation induced by LPS, but they can, on the other hand, act as mitogens by themselves. Different aspects of B-lymphocyte triggering, namely, proliferation, maturation to Ig secretion, and H-chain switches, may be very differently affected by anti-Ig antibodies, often with opposing effects.

369

LYMPHOCYTE
MEMBRANE
IMMUNO-
GLOBULINS:
AN OVERVIEW

A closer view shows, however, that this heterogeneity of results is not the consequence of inadequate experiments, but truly reflects the complexity of the problem. It appears that, on one side, the specificity and the concentration of anti-Ig antibodies may be responsible for different results, and, on the other, the lymphocytes can react very differently according to their maturity, age of donors, species, and other parameters. On the whole, this complexity is probably connected with the crucial and sophisticated function of the MIg's in determining *one or the other* of the two basic reactions of lymphocytes to antigens, namely, stimulation or paralysis. This function of the MIg's is certainly correlated with that of a variety of other non-Ig receptors of B-lymphocyte membranes such as the Fc receptor, the postulated receptors for T antibodies and for mitogens, Ia antigens, and so on. The unraveling of the cellular and molecular events in this system of lymphocyte regulation will be an essential stage in our progress toward the understanding of the physiology of these cells, and ultimately of the entire immune system.

References

Abney, E. R., Keeler, K. D., Parkhouse, R. M. E., and Willcox, H. N. A., 1976, Immunoglobulin M receptors on memory cells of IgG antibody-forming cell clones, *Eur. J. Immunol.* 6:443–450.

Andersson, J., Bullock, W. W., and Melchers, F., 1974, Inhibition of mitogenic stimulation of mouse lymphocytes by anti-mouse immunoglobulin antibodies, *Eur. J. Immunol.* 4:715–722.

Beale, G. H., 1954, *The Genetics of Paramecium aurelia,* Cambridge University Press, Cambridge, England.

Burnet, F. M., 1959, *The Clonal Selection Theory of Acquired Immunity,* Cambridge University Press, Cambridge, England.

Cambier, J. C., Vitetta, E. S., Kettmann, J. R., Wetzel, G. M., and Uhr, J. W., 1977, B cell tolerance. III. Effect of papain-mediated cleavage of cell surface IgD on tolerance susceptibility of murine B cells, *J. Exp. Med.* 146:107–117.

Chess, L., Levine, H., McDermott, R. P., and Schlossman, S. F., 1975, Immunologic function of isolated human lymphocyte subpopulations. VI. Further characterization of the surface-Ig-negative, E-rosette-negative (null cell) subset, *J. Immunol.* 115:1483–1487.

Cooper, M. D., Kearney, J. F., Lawton, A. R., Abney, E. R., Parkhouse, R. M. E., Preud'homme, J. L., and Seligman, M., 1976, Generation of immunoglobulin class diversity in B cells: A discussion with emphasis on IgD development, *Ann. Immunol. (Inst. Pasteur)* 127C:573–581.

Corte, G., Ferrarini, M., Tonda, P., Bargellesi, A., and Pernis, B., 1978, Membrane IgD on monkey lymphocytes, *Eur. J. Immunol.* (in press).

Czaja, M. J., Richards, F. F., and Varga, J. M., 1977, Multispecific lymphoid Cell Surface Receptors. *Proc. Natl. Acad. Sci. U.S.A.* 74:1224–1228.

De Luca, D., Miller, A., and Sercarz, E., 1975, Antigen binding to lymphoid cells from unimmunized mice. II. High frequency of antigen binding cells for several protein antigens by a morphologically distinct Ig-bearing population of T and B lymphocytes, *Cell. Immunol.* 18:255–273.

Ehrlich, P., 1900, Croonian lecture: On immunity with special reference to cell life, *Proc. R. Soc. London Ser. B* 66:424–448.

Fanger, M. W., Hart, D. A., Wells, J. V., and Nisinoff, A., 1970, Requirement for cross-linkage in the stimulation of transformation of rabbit peripheral lymphocytes by antiglobulin reagents, *J. Immunol.* 105:1484–1492.

Forni, L., and Pernis, B., 1975, Interactions between Fc receptors and membrane immunoglobulins on B lymphocytes, in: *Membrane Receptors of Lymphocytes* (M. Seligmann, J. L. Preud'homme, and F. M. Kourilsky, eds.), pp. 193–202, North-Holland, Amsterdam and Oxford.

Fröland, S. S., and Natvig, J. B., 1972, Class, subclass, and allelic exclusion of membrane-bound Ig of human B lymphocytes, *J. Exp. Med.* 136:409–414.

Fu, S. M., and Kunkel, H. G., 1974, Membrane immunoglobulins of B lymphocytes: Inability to detect certain characteristic IgM and IgD antigens, *J. Exp. Med.* 140:895–903.

Fu, S. M., Winchester, R. J., Feizi, T., Walzer, P. D., and Kunkel, H. G., 1974, Idiotype specificity of surface immunoglobulin and the maturation of leukemic bone-marrow derived lymphocytes, *Proc. Natl. Acad. Sci. U.S.A.* **71**:4487–4490.

Fuji, H., and Jerne, N. K., 1969, Primary immune response *in vitro:* Reversible suppression by anti-globulin antibodies, *Ann. Inst. Pasteur* **117**:801–805.

Ferrarini, M., Corte, G., Viale, G., Durante, M. L., and Bargellesi, A., 1976a, Membrane Ig on human lymphocytes: Rate of turnover of IgD and IgM on the surface of human tonsil cells, *Eur. J. Immunol.* **6**:372–378.

Ferrarini, M., Viale, G., Risso, A., and Pernis, B., 1976b, A study of the immunoglobulin classes present on the membrane and in the cytoplasm of human tonsil plasma cells, *Eur. J. Immunol.* **6**:562–565.

Greaves, M. F., 1970, Biological effects of anti-immunoglobulins: Evidence for immunoglobulin receptors on T and B lymphocytes, *Transplant. Rev.* **5**:45.

Jones, P. P., Cebra, J. J., and Herzenberg, L. A., 1974, Restriction of gene expression in B lymphocytes and their progeny. II. Commitment to immunoglobulin allotype, *J. Exp. Med.* **139**:581–599.

Julius, M. H., and Herzenberg, L. A., 1974, Isolation of antigen binding cells from unprimed mice: Demonstration of antibody-forming cell precursor, activity and correlation between precursor and secreted antibody avidities, *J. Exp. Med.* **140**:904–920.

Julius, M. H., Janeway, C. A., and Herzenberg, L. A., 1976, Isolation of antigen binding cells from unprimed mice. II. Evidence for monospecificity of antigen binding cells, *Eur. J. Immunol.* **6**:288–292.

Kearney, J. F., Cooper, M. D., and Lawton, A. R., 1976, B lymphocyte differentiation induced by lipopolysaccharide. III. Suppression of B cell maturation by anti-mouse immunoglobulin antibodies, *J. Immunol.* **116**:1664–1668.

Kishimoto, T., and Ishizaka, K. J., 1975, Regulation of antibody response *in vitro*. IX. Induction of secondary anti-hapten IgG antibody response by anti-immunoglobulin and enhancing soluble factor, *J. Immunol.* **114**:585–591.

Lawton, A. R., Selg, K. S., Royal, S. A., and Cooper, M. D., 1972, Ontogeny of B lymphocytes in the human fetus, *Clin. Immunol. Immunopathol.* **1**:84–93.

Lerner, R. A., McConhaey, P. J., Jansen, I., and Dixon, F. J., 1972, Synthesis of plasma-membrane associated and secretory immunoglobulins in diploid lymphocytes, *J. Exp. Med.* **135**:136–149.

Lesley, J., and Dutton, R. W., 1970, Antigen receptor molecules: Inhibition by antiserum against kappa light chains, *Science* **169**:487–488.

Litwin, S. D., 1972, Allelic and class exclusion of membrane-associated immunoglobulins of human lymphocytes, *J. Immunol.* **108**:1129–1131.

Loor, F., Forni, L., and Pernis, B., 1972, The dynamic state of the lymphocyte membrane: Factors affecting the distribution and turnover of surface immunoglobulins, *Eur. J. Immunol.* **2**:203–212.

Melchers, F., and Andersson, J., 1973, Synthesis, surface deposition and secretion of immunoglobulin M in bone-marrow derived lymphocytes, before and after mitogenic stimulation, *Transplant, Rev.* **14**:76–130.

Mitchison, N. A., 1967, Antigen recognition responsible for the induction *in vitro* of the secondary response, *Cold Spring Harbor Symp. Quant. Biol.* **32**:431–440.

Mond, J. J., Takahashi, R., and Thorbecke, G. J., 1972, Surface antigens of immunocompetent cells. III. *In vitro* studies of the role of B and T cells in immunological memory, *J. Exp. Med.* **136**:663–675.

Moretta, L., Ferrarini, M., Durante, M. L., and Mingari, M. C., 1975, Expression of a receptor for IgM by human T cells *in vitro*, *Eur. J. Immunol.* **5**:565–569.

Nagy, Z., Elliot, B. E., Nabholz, M., Krammer, P. H., and Pernis, B., 1976, Surface binding of alloantigens to T cells activated in the mixed lymphocyte reaction, *J. Exp. Med.* **143**:648–659.

Okumura, K., Julius, M. H., Tsu, T., Herzenberg, L. A., and Herzenberg, L. A., 1976, Demonstration that IgG memory is carried by IgG-bearing cells, *Eur. J. Immunol.* **6**:467–472.

Old, L. J., Stockert, E., Boyse, E. A., and Kim, J. H., 1968, Loss of TL antigens from cells exposed to TL antibody: Study of the phenomenon *in vitro*, *J. Exp. Med.* **127**:523–539.

Owen, J. J. T., Raff, M. C., and Cooper, M. D., 1975, Studies on the generation of B lymphocytes in the mouse embryo, *Eur. J. Immunol.* **5**:468–473.

Owen, J. J. T., Wright, D. E., Habu, S., Raff, M. C., and Cooper, M. D., 1977, Studies on the generation of B lymphocytes in fetal liver and bone-marrow, *J. Immunol.* **118**:2067–2072.

Pernis, B., 1976, IgD Receptors, in: *Immunopathology VII: International Symposium, Bad Schachen, Germany* (P. Miescher, ed.), pp. 74–81, Schwabe and Co., Basel and Stuttgart.

Pernis, B., 1977, Lymphocyte membrane IgD, *Immunological Reviews* **37**:210–218.

371

LYMPHOCYTE
MEMBRANE
IMMUNO-
GLOBULINS:
AN OVERVIEW

Pernis, B., Forni, L., and Amante, L., 1970, Immunoglobulin spots on the surface of rabbit lymphocytes, *J. Exp. Med.* **132**:1001–1018.

Pernis, B., Forni, L., and Amante, L., 1971, Immunoglobulins as cell receptors, *Ann. N. Y. Acad. Sci.* **190**:420–429.

Pernis, B., Miller, J. F. A. P., Forni, L., and Sprent, J., 1974a, Immunoglobulin on activated T cells detected by indirect immunofluorescence, *Cell. Immunol.* **10**:476–482.

Pernis, B., Brouet, J. C., and Seligmann, M., 1974b, IgD and IgM on the membrane of lymphoid cells in macroglobulinemia: Evidence for identity of membrane IgD and IgM antibody activity in a case with anti-IgG receptors, *Eur. J. Immunol.* **4**:776–778.

Pernis, B., Forni, L., and Luzzati, A. L., 1977, Synthesis of multiple immunoglobulin classes by single lymphocytes, *Cold Spring Harbor Symp. Quant. Biol.* **41**:175–183.

Pierce, C. W., Solliday, S. M., and Asofsky, R., 1972a, Immune responses *in vitro*. IV. Suppression of primary γM, γG and γA plaque-forming cell responses in mouse cell cultures by class-specific antibody to mouse immunoglobulins, *J. Exp. Med.* **135**:675–697.

Pierce, C. W., Solliday, S. M., and Asofsky, R., 1972b, Immune responses *in vitro*. V. Supression of γ-M, γ-G and γA plaque-forming cell responses in cultures of primed mouse spleen cells by class-specific antibody to mouse immunoglobulins, *J. Exp. Med.* **135**:698–710.

Platts-Mills, T. A. E., and Ishizaka, K., 1975, IgG diphtheria antitoxin responses from human tonsil lymphocytes induced by anti-γ-chain antibodies, *J. Immunol.* **114**:1605–1610.

Preud'homme, J. L., and Seligmann, M., 1972a, Immunoglobulins on the surface of lymphoid cells in Waldenström's macroglobulinemia, *J. Clin. Invest.* **51**:701–705.

Preud'homme, J. L., and Seligmann, M., 1972b, Surface bound immunoglobulins as a cell marker in human lymphoproliferative diseases *Blood.* **40**:777–794.

Raff, M. C., Sternberg, M., and Taylor, R. B., 1970, Immunoglobulin determinant on the surface of mouse lymphoid cells, *Nature (London)* **225**:553–554.

Raff, M. C., Feldman, M., and de Petris, S., 1973, Monospecificity of bone-marrow derived lympho-cytes, *J. Exp. Med.* **137**:1024–1030.

Raff, M. C., Owen, J. J. T., Cooper, M. D., Lawton, A. R., Megson, M., and Gathings, W., 1975, Differences in susceptibility of mature and immature mouse B lymphocytes to anti-immunoglobulin induced immunoglobulin suppression *in vitro*: Possible implications for B cell tolerance to self, *J. Exp. Med.* **142**:1052–1064.

Richards, F. F., Konigsberg, W. H., Rosenstein, R. W., and Varga, J. M., 1975, On the specificity of antibodies: Biochemical and biophysical evidence indicates the existence of polyfunction antibody combining regions, *Science* **187**:130–137.

Rowe, D. S., Hug, K., Forni, L., and Pernis, B., 1973, Immunoglobulin D as a lymphocyte receptor, *J. Exp. Med.* **138**:965–972.

Salsano, F., Froland, S. S., Natvig, J. B., and Michaelsen, T. E., 1974, Same idiotype of B lymphocyte membrane IgD and IgM: Evidence for monoclonality of chronic lymphocytic leukemia cells, *Scand. J. Immunol.* **3**:841–846.

Schrader, J. W., 1975, Antagonism of B lymphocyte: Mitogenesis by anti-immunoglobulin antibody, *J. Immunol.* **115**:323–326.

Seligmann, M., Preud'homme, J. L., and Kourisky, F. M. (eds.), 1975, *Membrane Receptors of Lymphocytes*, North-Holland, Amsterdam and Oxford.

Sell, S., and Gell, P. G. H., 1965, Studies on rabbit lymphocytes *in vitro*. I. Stimulation of blast transformation with an antiallotype serum, *J. Exp. Med.* **122**:423–439.

Sidman, C. L., and Unanue, E. R., 1975, Receptor-mediated inactivation of early B lymphocytes, *Nature (London)* **257**:149–151.

Sidman, C. L., and Unanue, E. R., 1976, Control of B-lymphocyte function. I. Inactivation of mitogene-sis by interactions with surface immunoglobulin and Fc-receptor molecules, *J. Exp. Med.* **144**:882–896.

Skamen, E., and Ivanyi, J., 1969, Lymphocyte transformation by H-chain specific anti-immunoglobulin sera, *Nature (London)* **221**:681–682.

Stout, R. D., and Herzenberg, L. A., 1975, The Fc receptor of thymus-derived lymphocytes. I. Detection of a subpopulation of murine T lymphocytes bearing the Fc receptor, *J. Exp. Med.* **142**:611–621.

Taylor, R. B., Duffus, P. H., Raff, M. C., and de Petris, S., 1971, Redistribution and pinocytosis of lymphocyte surface immunoglobulin molecules induced by anti-immunoglobulin antibody, *Nature (London) New Biol.* **233**:225–229.

Vitetta, E., and Uhr, J., 1972, Cell surface immunoglobulin. V. Release from murine splenic lymphocytes, *J. Exp. Med.* **135**:675–695.

Vitetta, E., Baur, S., and Uhr, J., 1971, Cell surface immunoglobulin. II. Isolation and characterization of immunoglobulin from mouse splenic lymphocytes, *J. Exp. Med.* **134**:242–264.

Vitetta, E. S., Melcher, U., McWilliams, M., Phillips-Quagliata, J., Lamm, M., and Uhr, J., 1975, Cell surface Ig. IX. The appearance of an IgD-like molecule on murine lymphoid cells during ontogeny, *J. Exp. Med.* **141**:206–215.

Warner, N. L., 1974, Membrane immunoglobulins and antigen receptors on B and T lymphocytes, *Adv. Immunol.* **19**:67–216.

Weiner, H. L., Moorhead, J. W., and Claman, H. N., 1976a, Anti-immunoglobulin stimulation of murine lymphocytes. I. Age dependency of the proliferative response, *J. Immunol.* **116**:1656–1661.

Weiner, H. L., Moorhead, J. W., Yamaga, K., and Kubo, R. T., 1976b, Anti-immunoglobulin stimulation of murine lymphocytes. II. Identification of cell surface target molecules and requirements for cross-linkage, *J. Immunol.* **117**:1527–1531.

Winchester, R., Fu, S. M., and Kunkel, H. G., 1975, IgG on lymphocyte surfaces: Technical problems and the significance of a third cell population, *J. Immunol.* **114**:1210–1212.

Wolf, B., Janeway, C. A., Jr., Coombs, R. R. A., Carry D., Gell, P. G. H., and Kelus, A. S., 1971, Immunologlobulin determinants on the lymphocytes of normal rabbits. III. As4 and As6 determinants on individual lymphocytes and the concept of allelic exclusion, *Immunology* **20**:931–944.

Index

Activator, polyclonal, of B cell, 367
Adrenocorticosteroid, 334
Affinity of antibody, 85–116, 125, 126
Agglutinin, 206–208
    see Cold agglutinin
Allelic exclusion, 244, 362
Allergen, variable region specificity, 180
Allotype
    of gamma-chain constant region, 231
    of heavy-chain variable region, 230–231
    marker, 230
    of membrane immunoglobulin, 361–365
    and regulatory gene, hypothetical, 231
Amia calva, immunoglobulin of, 210
Amino acid sequence analysis, 3, 16–18, 21–22,
        27, 30, 135, 137, 157–159, 163–165, 199,
        220–221, 275, 276, 280, 288, 311, 313,
        351
Anaphylaxis, passive cutaneous, 184, 190–191
    as assay for antibody quantity, 184
    method described, 184
Anguilla rostrata hemagglutinin, 209
Antibody, 10, 106–108, 119
    affinity, 85–116, 125, 126
        cellular studies, 102–103
        combining site, 112–113
        intrinsic, 86–95
        for ligand, 88–104
        multivalence, role of, 104–112
        selectivity, 86–87
        specificity, 86–87
        variation, temporal, 95–104
    anti-DNP, 91, 93
    anti-DNA, 46–47
    as antigen, 123, 179–186
    antigen-binding, 135–142
        biological significance, 142–147
    antihapten, 176
    antiidiotypic, 123
    antiimmunoglobulin, 367–369
    antilactose, 93–98, 107
    antiovalbumin, 90

Antibody (*cont.*)
    antiphosphorylcholine, 104
    antiprotein, 90
    bivalent, 105–107, 110, 122
    combining regions, 117–154, 284
        location, 122
        probes, 123–130
        structural determination by X-ray
            crystallography, 130–135
        structure, 122–135
    crystalline, 130
    crystallography by X ray, 130–135
    effector function, 173
    Fab, *see* Immunoglobulin
    Fc, *see* Immunoglobulin
    function, 37
    hapten, 54, 93
    heavy chain, *see* Chain, heavy
    heteroclitic, 117
    hypervariable region, 284
    increase, 146
    induction, model of, 176
        allosteric, 176
        associative, 176
        distortive, 176
        ligand complex, 86–87, 91–92, 110–111
    maturation pattern, 146, 147
    number of, 118–119
    and plasma cell, 37
    probes for combining sites, 123–129
    reaginic, 300–301
    secretion, 99–100
    selectivity, 86–87
    specificity, 28, 86–87, 119, 145–146
    structure, 42–43
        of combining site, 122–135
        domain hypothesis, 132, 187
    see also Immunoglobulin
Antigalactosidase antibody, 96, 197
Antigen, 147, 357
    amino acid sequence and specificity, 135
    and antibody, 174–186

Antigen (*cont.*)
-binding, 5, 53, 118, 134, 138–147, 352
dissimilar antigens to a single combining region, 120
functional correlates of, 135–142
specificity, 135
structural correlates of, 135–142
combining, 120–121
heterogeneity, 139–140
modulation, 366
number of, 118
original antigenic sin, 146
specificity, 135, 281–282
variable region, 136
Antiserum
hyperimmune, 312
to variable group, 312
Asphericity, 331
Autoimmune disease and virus, 302
Autoimmunity, 325, 334
Avidity, *see* Antibody affinity
Azulene reagent, 126

B lymphocyte, *see* Lymphocyte
Bacillus amyloliquefaciens strain H restriction enzyme, 234
Bacteriophage
f-2, 208
hapten-conjugated, 193
ϕX174, 106–107
Basophil, 189
and immunoglobulin E, 179–180
Bence Jones protein, 2, 11, 25, 324, 325, 334–336
Binding, 122, 128, 135–142, 181–182, 189–190
antigen, *see* Antigen
constant, intrinsic, 121
energy, physiological significance, 121
kinetics, 176
Bivalent interaction, 106
monogamous, 106
Blast transformation, 368
Bragg's law, 8
Bromine, 186
Brucella abortus, 208–209
Brucellosis, chronic, 326
Bufo marinus antibody, 212
Burkitt's lymphoma, 266
Bursectomy in chick embryo, 246

C region, 274, 346
gene, 197, 276
transition, 276
Carassius auratus immunoglobulin, 211
Carbene, activated, 126
Carbohydrate in immunoglobulin, 157, 199
Cell membrane, *see* Membrane

Chain in immunoglobulin
alpha, bond, 160, 164
heavy, 3, 19, 20, 27, 28, 38, 121, 122, 128, 363–365
amino acid sequence, 3
binding, 128
disease, *see* Heavy-chain disease
domain, 38
homology, 3
hypervariable region, 3
immunoglobulin fold, 14
isotope, 20
and L chain, association with, 27–28
region, 135
synthesis, 346–347
variable subgroups, 311–321
J, 58, 155–172
alpha chain, 164
amino acid, composition of, 163
antigenicity, 164
attachment of, 164
carbohydrate composition, 163–164
detection of, 166
mu chain, 164
physicochemical data, 162–164
molecular weight, 162–163
secretory component, 155–169
properties, chemical, 156–159
species cross-reactions, 164
light, 3, 16, 21, 30, 38, 121, 122–128
amino acid sequence analysis, 3, 16
association with heavy chain, 27–28
binding, 122, 128
carbohydrate composition, 348, 350
dimer, 134
domain, 38
heavy chain, association with, 27–28
homology region analysis, 3
hypervariable region analysis, 3, 21, 286
immunoglobulin fold, 14
isotype, 20
origin, 280
pattern, phylogenetic, 280
region, 135
sequence analysis, 311
amino acid, 3, 16
homology region, 3
hypervariable region, 3, 21, 286
structure, three-dimensional, 10, 12, 30
synthesis, 346–347
transport, intracellular, 348–349
types, 362
variable region, 288
Chelonia mydas immunoglobulin, 212
Chelydra serpentina immunoglobulin, 212, 216
Chordapa aves, 213
antibody against 2,4-dinitrophenol, 216
immunized with bacteria, 213

Chromic chloride method, 312
Clone
  antibody-producing cells, number of, 119, 142
  dominance of, 120, 136
  selection
    concept, 285
    hypothesis, 273
Cluster analysis, 136
Codon, universality of, 199
Cold agglutinin, 326
Combining sites, 112–113, 120, 122, 144, 146
  structure, 122–135
Complement
  activation, 37, 175
  cascade, 175
    activation, 175
    C3, 177
  fixation,
    alternate pathway, 177, 189
    classical pathway, 174–177, 187–189
Complementarity
  combining region of antibody and interacting
    ligand, 87
  determining region, 274, 276
  residue, 30
Coprecipitation, 330–331
Counterbalance, renal, 15
Crassostrea virginica agglutinin, 207
Cryoglobulin, 323–343
  classification, 327–331
  in clinical laboratory, 326–327
  definition, 323
  first observed (1933), 323
  history, 323–324
  isolation, 327
  mixed, 328–330
  monoclonal, 328
  polyclonal, 330
  purification, 327
Cryoglobulinemia, 324, 336
  and chronic infection, 333
  clinical manifestation, 324–327
  patients, number of, 329
  therapy, 334
Cryoprecipitability, reversible, 324
Cryoprecipitation
  asphericity, 331–332
  mechanism of, 331–333
Crystallography, 8
  see also X-ray crystallography
Cyanosis, 325
Cyclophosphamide, 334
Cyprinus carpio immunoglobulin, 211
Cytomegalovirus, 334

Determinant, idiotypic, 281–283
Dextran, 124

Diazonium fluoroborate, 125
Diffraction techniques, 6–7
  see also X-ray diffraction
Dimethylnaphthalenesulfonyl (DNS), 142
  anti-antibody, 4, 46, 47, 91–94, 101, 106, 108
  hapten, 103
Dinitrophenol (DNP)
  antibody to, 216
  anti-antibody, 91, 93
  as hapten, 103, 274
Disulfide bridge in immunoglobulin chains, 160,
    161, 164, 347
Domain, 38–39
  hypothesis of antibody structure, 132, 187,
    274
Duck immunized with bacteria, 213
Duffy antibody, 317

Effector
  of antibody, 173
    function listed, 174
  of Edelman, 174
Ehrlich's (1900) physiology of the immune
    response, 357
Elasmobranch lymphocyte with antibody, 219
Electron microscopy, 4
Elongation of L chain, 266
Emission anisotropy, 63
Enhancement factor
  evaluation, 106
    quantitative, 105
  formulation, mathematical, 110
  system, simplest to consider, 109
Epimetheus and evolution, 199
Epinephelus itaira immunoglobulin, 211
Episome theory, 286
Epstein–Barr virus, 334
Eptatretus stoutii immunoglobulin, 208
Escherichia coli, 185, 200, 235, 252
  antiphagocytic, 185
  β-galactosidase, 235
Evolution
  Epimethean, 199
  humoral, 205
  Promethean, 200
Exclusion, allelic, 244, 362
Exocrine gland cells, mucosal epithelial, 161

Fab segment of immunoglobulin, 12, 29, 39, 40,
    44, 51, 112, 177, 186, 217
  crystal, 130
  dimension of molecule, 14
  Fc interaction, 177
  flexibility of arms, 51–52
  fragments, 12, 112
  hapten complex, 23–26, 30
  model of, 13, 14, 19, 21

Fab segment of immunoglobulin (*cont.*)
New, 12–14, 16, 21–28, 130
combining site, 25
model, 13, 14, 21
structure, 12
protein, basic, 134
X-ray crystallographic model, 14
region, 40
structure in myeloma protein immunoglobulin, 44–45, 112
Fc segment of immunoglobulin, 9–10, 173, 177
Fab interaction, 177
G, 186
localization, submolecular, by complement fixation, 187
region, 39, 40
structure, three-dimensional, of human fragment, 30
Flagellin, 305, 361
Flexibility, segmental, 51–53
of Fab, 51–52
of immunoglobulin, 215
Fluorescence
depolarization technique, 46
energy, transfer technique, 143
system, 90
Fourier map, 8–9, 11
Fourier transform, 7
Framework region, invariant, 276

Gadolinium, 129
Gallus domesticus immunoglobulin, 213
Gammopathy
double, 245, 246
triple, 245
Gangrene, 324
Gene
activation, 243–244
cluster, 197
constant region, 197
duplication in evolution of Ig, 197
evolution of immunoglobulin, duplication in, 197
expression, 243–244
fundamental tenet of, 287
HLA complex, 198
interaction model, 287
region
constant, 197
variable, 197
regulatory, 244
Germ-line theory, 285–286
objection to, 286
validity of, 285
Ginglymostoma cirratum immunoglobulin, 209, 216, 278
Globulin, *see* Lepore-type hybrid gamma-globulin

H-2, *see* Histocompatibility
H chain, *see* Chain, heavy
Haemulon album, immunoglobulin, 211
Hapten, 23–26, 55, 102, 119, 136, 142
aromatic, 121
in bacteria, 24
-binding kinetics, 176
-Fab complex, 23–26, 30
see also DNP
Heavy-chain disease (HCD), 243
deletion of the C1 domain, 243
failure to synthesize L chain, 269
hypervariable region, 243
properties, listed, 258
protein, alpha, 258–263
alpha, 261–262, 268
gamma, 258–261, 269
mu, 262–263
Helix pomatia, agglutinin, 207
Hemagglutination inhibition test, 312, 316
Hemocyanin, keyhole limpet, 208
Hemoglobin, 9, 12
X-ray analysis of, 9
Heterodontus francisci immunoglobulin, 210, 218–219, 222–223, 278
Heterogeneity
degree of, 140
index, 141
"Hinge" region of immunoglobulin, 3, 39, 48, 49, 51–53, 56
connecting Fab and Fc segments, 3
peptides of IgA, 161
see also Flexibility
Histocompatibility complex, major (MHC), 298
locus, 198, 301–303
nomenclature, 300
HLA, *see* Histocompatibility locus
Homarus americanus agglutinin, 207
Homology subunits, structure of, 16
Horse antibody against pneumococcal polysaccharide, 56
Hydrogen bonds between main chain atoms, 17
Hypergammaglobulinemia purpura, 136
Hypersensitivity
delayed, 302
immediate, 37, 179, 302
Hypervariable region, 135–137, 274, 284
sequence of, 21
Hyperviscosity syndrome, 335

Ictalurus punctatus immunoglobulin, 214
Idiotypy, nature of, 281–284
determinant, 282, 283
localization, molecular, 281–282
of membrane Ig, 361–365
shared, 282
specificity, 282

Immune response, 37, 88, 95, 146, 297
gene (*Ir*), 298–299
control, 297, 299
identification by antigen, 298
maturation, 95
physiology, 357
Ehrlich's view, 357
Immune serum
as a population phenomenon, 145
specificity, 143
Immune system in vertebrate, 198
evolution
Epimethean, 199
humoral, 205
Promethean, 200
mutation, somatic, 202
Immunity
cell-mediated, 37
humoral, in invertebrate, 206–208
Immunochemistry, 1
central problems in, 1
Immunodeficiency disease, 306–307
Immunoglobulin (Ig)
amino acid sequence, 231, 233
antibody combining site, 21–23
antigen dissimilar, bound to a single combining
region, 120
-dependent, 187–189
complement fixation, 189
opsonic activity, 189
-independent, 189–191
anaphylaxis, passive cutaneous, 190–191
binding lymphocyte, 190
binding macrophage, 189
catabolism of Ig, regulation of, 190
interaction with protein 'A' of
Staphylococcus aureus, 191
regulation of intestinal passage, 190
regulation of placental passage, 190
in antihapten antiserum, 144
assembly, 168–169, 347–348
atypical, 257–272
structure of, 257–272
and B lymphocyte differentiation, 351–352
biosynthesis of, 345–355
C region, *see* constant region
catabolism, regulation of, 183–184, 190
on cell surface, 219–223
chain
heavy, in association with light chain, 27–28
light chain in association with heavy chain,
27–28
polypeptide, diagram of, 15
structure of four chains conceptualized, 118
cleavage, proteolytic, 217
combining region, 117, 215
multispecificity, 28–29
polyfunctional, 144

Immunoglobulin (*cont.*)
combining region (*cont.*)
structure, 122–135
subgroups, 28
conformation, 214–217
constant region (C region), 217–221, 231–234,
273–295
fusion of C and V region, 235–241
copy–splice mechanism, 235
crossing over mechanism, 235
looping out mechanism, 235
sharing of a single constant region, 231–232
constant sequences, 26–27
control, genetic, of variable regions, 26–29
deletion, 27, 262, 263, 268
of carboxy terminal sequence, 264–265
of heavy chain, 264–264
of hinge region, 263–264
internal, 265
of last domain of heavy chain, 264
degradation, rate of, 183
2,4-dinitrophenol combining site, 216
diversity of, 268
domain hypothesis, 187, 229
and evolution, 197–204
Fab fragment, structure of, 12–21, 23–26
high-resolution studies, 14–21
low-resolution studies, 12–14
Fc fragment, 9–10, 184
flexibility, segmental, 37–83, 215
"fold," 14, 15
fusion of C and V regions, 235–241
mechanism, *see* constant region, fusion of
gene duplication, 197–204
gene translocation model for C and V region. 236
genetic control, of synthesis, *see* synthesis
heavy chain, 276
disease, *see* Heavy-chain disease
synthesis, 346–347
variant, 258–263
heterogeneous populations of, 117
insertion of sequences observed, 27
insertional theory, 286–290
hypervariable model, 288
instructive template hypothesis, 285
junction of C and V regions, 236–241, 276
amino acid sequence, 236–241
light chain, 19
elongation, 266
synthesis, 346–347
linkage groups, 241–242
localization, submolecular, 186–191
lymphocyte with membrane Ig, 357–372
lymphoid cell, bone marrow-derived, with
membrane Ig, 360
on membrane of lymphocyte, 357–372
anti-antibody interaction, 365–366
allotype, 361–365

Immunoglobulin (*cont.*)
    on membrane of lymphocyte (*cont.*)
        cells carrying, 360–361
        data, basic, 358–360
        idiotype, 361–365
        isotype, 361–365
        leaving the membrane via pinocytic vesicle, 359
        leaving the membrane via shedding, 359
    on membrane of lymphoid cell, 360
    origin, phylogenetic, 205–228
    passage
        intestinal, 182–183
        placental, 182
        regulation of, 182–183
    peptide mapping analysis, 231
    polyfunctional property, 173
    polypeptide chain, 276
        heavy, 229
        light, 229
        synthesis, 346–347
        two gene hypothesis, 229
    population, heterogeneous, 117
        subpopulations, 118
    primary structure, 217–219
    property, biological, 173–196
        antigen-dependent, 174
        antigen-independent, 174
        and structure, 173–196
    region sequence
        constant, 219, *see* constant region
        variable, 218, *see* variable region
    secretion, 345–355, 367–368
        kinetics, 348–350
        methods, 345–346
    segmental flexibility, 37–83
    sequences, 27, 218–219
    serum concentration, 183
    site, active, 214–217
    solution conformation, 37–83
    structure, 219–223
        of active site, 214–217
        and biological properties, 173–196
        of Fab fragments, 12–21
        of Fc fragments, 9–10
        primary, 217–219
        three-dimensional, 1–36
    synthesis
        genetic control, 229–230, 297–310
        kinetics, 348–350
        rate, 183
    unit, basic model, 230
    variable region, 17, 217–221, 273–295
        fusion with constant region, 235–241
            mechanism, *see* constant region
        genetic control, 26–29
        idiotypy, 281–284
        localization, molecular, 281–282

Immunoglobulin (*cont.*)
    variable region (*cont.*)
        origin, genetic, 284–291
        sharing of a single constant region, 231–232
    of vertebrate
        ostracoderm-derived, 208–209
        placoderm-derived, 209–213
            amphibia, 212
            aves, 213
            chondrichthyes, 209–210
            osteichthyes, 210–212
            reptilia, 212–213
    X-ray crystallography, 5–9
Immunoglobulin type
    A, 44, 67–70, 112, 133, 159–162, 167, 168, 603
    D, 70–72, 305, 316, 320, 363
        anti-, 316, 320
    E, 72–76, 300–301
        anti-, 186
        and basophil affinity, 179
        -cell receptor interaction, 180
        and mast cell, 179
        models
            associative, 180
            bridging, 180
    G, 1–5, 9, 29, 31, 39–56, 75, 89, 100, 103, 104, 364–366
        absence, 307
        affinity, temporal variation of, 95–101
        anti-A, 317
        anti-B, 317
        anti-D, 316
        anti-Fy, 317
        antigen modulation, 366
        Fab segment, 29, 44, 112, 186, 217
            New, 16, 22, 24, 27, 28, 130
        Fc segment, 181, 186, 217
        flexibility, 50
        Gm
            allotype, 303–305
            factor, 303
            gene complex, 303
            phenotype, 304
        isotypic variation, 303
        model of G2, 232
        papain treatment, 122, 217
        structure, primary, 38–40, 45, 187
        subclass, 183, 303, 304
        viscosity, 129
    M, 56–67, 93, 94, 103–104, 107–109, 305
        absence, 307
        affinity, 93, 101–104, 108
        anti-, 108, 288
        antihapten, 176
        antilactose, 101–102
        conformation, 56–61
        control, genetic, 103
        equine, 65, 101

Immunoglobulin type (*cont.*)
M (*cont.*)
in fish, 198
flexibility, 61–67
model, 232
nurse shark, 65–66
polymerization, 168
receptor, 363
secreting cell, maturation of, 102
in vertebrates, 223
and X chromosome, 306
Infection, chronic, 326
Intestine
regulation of passage, 190
Isotype, 2
membrane Ig, 361–365

Keyhole limpet hemocyanin, 208
Kol protein, 44, 45, 53
electron-density map, 45
X-ray crystallography, 53

Lanthanide, 129
Leg ulcer, chronic, 324
Lepisosteus osseus immunoglobulin, 210
Lepisosteus platyrhincus immunoglobulin, 210–
Lepomis macrochirus immunoglobulin, 272
Lepore-type hybrid gamma-globulin, 266
Leprosy, 326
Leukemia, chronic lymphocytic, 326, 363
cell with membrane Ig, 317–319
V_H subgroup, 317–319
and mu-heavy-chain disease, 262
Ligand
and antibody, 110–111
affinity of monovalent, 88–104
-binding, 107
bivalent, 110
complex, 86–87, 91–92, 110–111
distribution, calculated, 111
monovalent and affinity for antibody, 88–104
probe, polymeric, 124, 125
specificity, 135
Limulus polyphemus agglutinin, 207
Lipopolysaccharide-induced maturation, 368
Lupus erythematosus, disseminated, 325
Lymphocyte, 365
B, 345
activation, polyclonal (PBA), 367
differentiation, 351–352
immunoglobulin synthesis, 351
life history, 351
receptor of antibody, 181
synthesis of Ig, 351
-binding, 181–182, 190
membrane Ig, 311–321
V_H subgroups, 317–319
stimulation, 368

Lymphoid cell, 273, 360
Lymphoma, Mediterranean, 261
Lysozyme, 135

Macroglobulinemia, 61, 335, 361
Macromolecule pattern, internal, 127
Macrophage, 177
-binding, 181, 189
Mammal, 278
species, 278
Mast cell, 189
and IgE, 179
Maturation
phenomenon, 98–101
process, 101
Measles virus, 302
Mediterranean lymphoma, 261
Membrane
of cell, destruction of, 175
immunoglobulin on, 361–365
of lymphocyte, 311–321
V subgroup of H chain, 311–321
Menadione, 142
6-Mercaptopurine, 334
Mitogen, 352
receptor, 367
see also individual mitogens
Monocyte, 177–179
membrane receptor on, 178
Mononucleosis
cytomegalovirus, 326
infectious, 326
Mouse myeloma protein, 68–69
Fab fragment of IgA, 112
Mucosa of epithelial cell of exocrine gland, 161
Multigene theory, 285
Mutation, somatic, of immune system, 202
Multivalent interaction analysis based on viral neutralization, 106
Mycosis fungoides, 326
Myeloma protein, 1, 10, 12, 23, 24, 31, 125, 127, 130, 133, 142, 245, 325
and antigen, 23–24
and Bence Jones protein, 324
combining region, 125
crystallized, 12
GOE, 261
and hapten, 23
heavy chain
altered, 263–265
V subgroup, 311–321
LA, 261
and light chain, altered, 265–266
mouse protein, 263
relationship, 315
V_H subgroup, 314–316
peptide analysis, 314

Myoglobulin, 9
  of sperm whale, 91
  X-ray analysis, 9

Natural selection has only hindsight, 199, 203
Necturus maculosus immunoglobulin, 212
Neoceratodus forsteri immunoglobulin, 211
Neuropathy, peripheral, 325
Neutralization reaction, 107
Neutrophil, 177–179
  IgG, 177
  membrane receptor, on, 178
Nitrogen receptor, 367
Nitroxide spin label, 129
Null cell, 360
Nurse shark, 94
  anti-DNP antibody in, 94

Opsonin, 189
Opsonization, 177–179
  defined, 178
Oryctalagus cuniculus immunoglobulin, 216

Papain, 73
Parasite, evolution of, 200
Patterson function, 7
Penicillamine therapy, 334
Peptide map, 157
Petromyzon marinus immunoglobulin, 208
  immunized with bacteria, 209
    with bacteriophage, 208
    with group O human red blood cells, 209
Phenylalanine mustard, 334
ϕX174 bacteriophage, 106–107
Phosphorylcholine, 123, 128
Placenta, regulation of passage across, 190
Plaque-forming cell, 100
Plasma cell, 359
  failure of immunoglobulin synthesis, 261
  tumor, 261
Plasmapheresis, 334
Pleuronectes platessa immunoglobulin, 209
Polyasparagine, 125
Polyclonal B-cell activator (PBA), 367
Polyodon spathula immunoglobulin, 210
Polymorphism, genetic, 199
Polypeptide
  chain, 2
    one chain–two genes, 179, 229–255
      evidence, 229–255
      history, 229–230
    fold, 134
    synthesis, 346
Polyribosome
  and chain synthesis on, 347
  membrane-bound, 359
Precipitation, indirect, 346

Probes of antibody combining regions
  affinity probe, 125–127
  electron microscope probe, 129–130
  photoaffinity probe, 125–127
  physiochemical probe, 127–129
  polymeric ligand probe, 124–125
  serological probe, 123–124
Promethean evolution, 199–201
  of the immune system, 200
  strategy of, 201–203
Protopterus aethiopicus immunoglobulin, 211
Pseudemys scripta immunoglobulin, 212
Protein biosynthesis, 345
Protein crystallization, 6
Pyrogel formation, 337
Pyroglobulin, 335–338
  amino acid analysis, 337
  -associated disease, 335–338
  classification, 336
  clinical picture, 335–338
  definition, 335
  history, 335
  immunoglobulin M, 337
  isolation, 336
  mechanism, 336–338
  symptom, 335–336

Ragweed hay fever, 300
  antigen E, 301
Rana catesbiana immunoglobulin, 212
Raynaud's syndrome, 324, 331
Reagin, 300–301
Renal counterbalance, 15
Residue, phylogenetically associated, 280
Restriction enzyme, bacterial, 234
Rh
  anti-antibody, 316
  erythrocyte, 302–303
Rheumatic
  arthritis, 326
  factor, 174, 185–186
    is an anti-antibody, 185
    antigenic determinant, 191
    anti-IgE antibody, 186
    and IgG1 subclass, 186
    reactivity, specific, 186
RNA–DNA hybridization, 234–235
Rubella virus, 302

Salmo gairdneri immunoglobulin, 216
Salmonella anti-antibody, 245
  S. adelaide flagellin, 305
  S. typhi antigen, 299
  and shark, 217
Scatchard plot, 139, 140
  of ligand-binding to antibody, 140
Scleroderma, 325

Secretory component, 155–161
  amino acid composition, 158
  bound, 155
  free, 155
  molecular weight, 156
  role, physiological, 161
Sequence analysis, comparative, 123
Serum viscosity, 325
Shark immunoglobulin, 209–210
Sialic acid, 333
Sjögren's syndrome, 326
Somatic recombination theory, 290
  main objections to, 291
  major difficulty of, 290
  mutation theory, 290–291
Specificity of shared idiotype, 123
Staphylococcus aureus, 178
  antiphagocytic, 185
  polysaccharide, 136
  protein A, 185, 191
    and IgG, 185
Stopped flow technique, 141
Subgroup
  defined, 277
  distribution in phylogeny, 277
  origin, phylogenetic, 279
Sugar (D-), 157, 163–164
  six carbon, dominates the biological world,
    199
Suppressor function, 37
Switch, genetic, 245–246

T-cell helper, 37
Terminal NH$_2$ sequences, 157, 159
Thymic-type lymphoma within thymus,
    93
Thymus containing lymphoma, 93
Transformation, allosteric, 177
Trypsin digestion, 73
Tryptophan, 128

V region, *see* Variable region of antibody
Variable region of antibody, 26, 39, 136, 197,
    201, 203, 274, 346, 360
  amino acid sequence, primary, 137, 288
  anti-antiserum, 312
  conservation, 137
  defined, 274
  determinant, idiotypic, 282
  evolution, 203
  genes for, 276
  of heavy chain, 279
  in myeloma protein, 275
  origin, genetic, 284–291
    theories of, 285–291
  structure, 131
    genetic control of, 26, 284–285
  subgroup, 278, 279
    of H chain, 311–321
    of L chain, 311–321
  transition, 276
Vasculitis, 325
Vertebrate
  immune system of
    gene duplication, 198
    gene evolution, 198
    immunoglobulin M in, 223
    species, phylogenetic emergence, 206
Vesicle, 359
Virus neutralization, 106
  see also individual viruses
Viscosity of serum, 325
Vitamin K, 128

Waldenström's macroglobulinemia, *see*
    Macroglobulinemia

X chromosome, 306
X-ray crystallography, 1, 128, 130–135
  conclusions from, 134–135
X-ray diffraction, 5–7, 39
Xenopus laevis immunoglobulin, 212